SANFORD GUIDE

熱病

Antimicrobial Stewardship Since 1969

THE SANFORD GUIDE
To Antimicrobial Therapy 2020

50th Edition

David N. Gilbert, M.D.
Henry F. Chambers, M.D.
Michael S. Saag, M.D.
Andrew T. Pavia, M.D.

Douglas Black, Pharm.D.
Helen W. Boucher, M.D.
David O. Freedman, M.D.
Kami Kim, M.D.
Brian S. Schwartz, M.D.

THE SANFORD GUIDE
To Antimicrobial Therapy
2020

50th Edition

Editors

David N. Gilbert, M.D.
Chief of Infectious Diseases,
Providence Portland Medical Center, Oregon
Professor of Medicine,
Oregon Health Sciences University

Henry F. Chambers, M.D.
San Francisco General Hospital
Professor of Medicine Emeritus
University of California, San Francisco

Michael S. Saag, M.D.
Associate Dean for Global Medicine
Director, UAB Center for AIDS Research
Professor of Medicine and Director,
Division of Infectious Diseases,
University of Alabama, Birmingham

Andrew T. Pavia, M.D.
George & Esther Gross Presidential Professor
Chief, Division of Pediatric Infectious Diseases,
University of Utah, Salt Lake City

Contributing Editors

Douglas Black, Pharm.D.
Professor of Pharmacy,
University of Washington, Seattle

Brian S. Schwartz, M.D.
Associate Professor of Medicine,
University of California, San Francisco

Helen W. Boucher, M.D.
Chief, Division of Geographic Medicine
and Infectious Diseases
Professor of Medicine
Tufts Medical Center, Boston, Massachusetts

David O. Freedman, M.D.
Emeritus Professor of Medicine,
University of Alabama, Birmingham

Kami Kim, M.D.
Professor of Internal Medicine,
Division of Infectious Diseases
and International Medicine,
Morsani College of Medicine,
University of South Florida, Tampa

Publisher

Antimicrobial Therapy, Inc.

Managing Editor

Jeb C. Sanford

The GUIDE TO ANTIMICROBIAL THERAPY is updated annually and published by:

ANTIMICROBIAL THERAPY, INC.
11771 Lee Highway, P.O. Box 276
Sperryville, VA 22740-0276 USA
Tel 540-987-9480 Fax 540-987-9486
Email: info@sanfordguide.com
www.sanfordguide.com

Acknowledgements
Thanks to Silvina Trapé, Jonatan Bohman and their team for manuscript design and layout of this edition of the SANFORD GUIDE.

Note to Readers
Since 1969, the SANFORD GUIDE has been independently prepared and published. Decisions regarding the content of the SANFORD GUIDE are solely those of the editors and the publisher. We welcome questions, comments and feedback concerning the SANFORD GUIDE. All of your feedback is reviewed and taken into account in updating the content of the SANFORD GUIDE.

Every effort is made to ensure accuracy of the content of this guide. However, current full prescribing information available in the package insert for each drug should be consulted before prescribing any product. The editors and publisher are not responsible for errors or omissions or for any consequences from application of the information in this book and make no warranty, express or implied, with respect to the currency, accuracy, or completeness of the contents of this publication. Application of this information in a particular situation remains the professional responsibility of the practitioner.

For the most current information, subscribe to webedition.sanfordguide.com or Sanford Guide mobile device applications

Printed in the United States of America
ISBN 978-1-944272-14-2
Spiral Edition (English)

—TABLE OF CONTENTS—

ABBREVIATIONS

3TC = lamivudine
AB,% = percent absorbed
ABC = abacavir
ABCD = amphotericin B colloidal dispersion
ABLC = ampho B lipid complex
ABSSSI = acute bacterial skin & skin structure infection
AD = after dialysis
ADF = adefovir
AG = aminoglycoside
AIDS = Acquired Immune Deficiency Syndrome
Amox-clav = amoxicillin-clavulanate
AM-CL-ER = amoxicillin-clavulanate extended release
AMK = amikacin
Amox = amoxicillin
AMP = ampicillin
Ampho B = amphotericin B
Amp-sulb = ampicillin-sulbactam
AP = atovaquone proguanil
APAG = antipseudomonal aminoglycoside
ARDS = acute respiratory distress syndrome
ARF = acute rheumatic fever
ASA = aspirin
ATS = American Thoracic Society
ATV = atazanavir
AUC = area under the curve
Azithro = azithromycin
bid = 2x per day
BL/BLI = beta-lactam/beta-lactamase inhibitor
BSA = body surface area
BW = body weight
C&S = culture & sensitivity
C/S = culture & sensitivity
CABP = community-acquired bacterial pneumonia
CAPD = continuous ambulatory peritoneal dialysis
CARB = carbapenems
CDC = U.S. Centers for Disease Control
Cefpodox = cefpodoxime proxetil
Ceftaz = ceftazidime
Ceph= cephalosporin
CFB = ceftobiprole
CFP = cefepime
Chloro = chloramphenicol
CIP = ciprofloxacin; **CIP-ER** = CIP extended release
Clarithro = clarithromycin; **ER** = extended release
Clav = clavulanate
Clinda = clindamycin
CLO = clofazimine
Clot = clotrimazole
CMV = cytomegalovirus
Cobi = cobicistat
CQ = chloroquine phosphate
CrCl = creatinine clearance
CrCln = CrCl normalized for BSA
CRBSI = catheter-related bloodstream infection
CRE = carbapenem resistant enteric
CRRT = continuous renal replacement therapy
CSD = cat-scratch disease
CSF = cerebrospinal fluid
CXR = chest x-ray
d4T = stavudine
Dapto = daptomycin
DBPCT = double-blind placebo-controlled trial
dc = discontinue
ddC = zalcitabine
ddI = didanosine
DIC = disseminated intravascular coagulation
Diclox = Dicloxacillin
div = divided
DLV = delavirdine
DORI = doripenem
DOT = directly observed therapy
Doxy = doxycycline
DR = delayed release
DRSP = drug-resistant S. pneumoniae
DBRPCT = Double blind, randomized, placebo-controlled trial
DS = double strength
EBV = Epstein-Barr virus
EES = erythromycin ethyl succinate
EFZ = efavirenz
ELV = elvitegravir
EMB = ethambutol
ENT = entecavir
ER = extended release
ERTA = ertapenem
Erythro = erythromycin
ESBLs = extended spectrum β-lactamases
ESR = erythrocyte sedimentation rate
ESRD = endstage renal disease
Flu = fluconazole
Flucyt = flucytosine
FOS-APV = fosamprenavir
FQ = fluoroquinolone
FTC = emtricitabine
G = generic
GAS = Group A Strep
Gati = gatifloxacin
GC = gonorrhea
Gemi = gemifloxacin
Gent = gentamicin
gm = gram
GNB = gram-negative bacilli
Grazo = grazoprevir
Griseo = griseofulvin
Gtts = drops
H/O = history of
HEMO = hemodialysis
HHV = human herpesvirus
HIV = human immunodeficiency virus

ABBREVIATIONS (2)

HLR = high-level resistance
HSCT = hematopoietic stem cell transplant
HSV = herpes simplex virus
IA = injectable agent/anti-inflammatory drugs
IDV = indinavir
IFN = interferon
IM= intramuscular
IMP = imipenem-cilastatin
INH = isoniazid
Inv = investigational
IP = intraperitoneal
IT = intrathecal
Itra = itraconazole
IV = intravenous
IVDU = intravenous drug user
IVIG = intravenous immune globulin
Keto = ketoconazole
kg = kilogram
KPC = serine carbapenemase
LAB = liposomal ampho B
LCM = lymphocytic choriomeningitis virus
LCR = ligase chain reaction
Levo = levofloxacin
LP/R = lopinavir/ ritonavir
MBL = metallo beta lactamase
mcg (or µg) = microgram
MDR = multi-drug resistant
MER = meropenem
Metro = metronidazole
Mino = minocycline
mL = milliliter
Moxi = moxifloxacin
MQ = mefloquine
MSM = men who have sex with men
MSSA/MRSA = methicillin-sensitive/resistant S. aureus
MTB = Mycobacterium tuberculosis
NAF = Nafcillin

NAI = not FDA-approved (indication or dose)
NB = name brand
NF = nitrofurantoin
NFR = nelfinavir
NNRTI = non-nucleoside reverse transcriptase inhibitor
NOS = not otherwise specified mechanism of resistance
NRTI = nucleoside reverse transcriptase inhibitor
NSAIDs = non-steroidal
NUS = not available in the U.S.
NVP = nevirapine
O Ceph = oral cephalosporins
Oflox = ofloxacin
P Ceph = parenteral cephalosporins
PCR = polymerase chain reaction
PEP = post-exposure prophylaxis
PI = protease inhibitor
Pip-tazo = piperacillin-tazobactam
po = oral dosing
PQ = primaquine
PRCT = Prospective randomized controlled trials
PTLD = post-transplant lymphoproliferative disease
Pts = patients
Pyri = pyrimethamine
PZA = pyrazinamide
q wk = dose weekly
q[x]h = every [x] hours, e.g., q8h = every 8 hrs
qid = 4x per day
QS = quinine sulfate
Quinu-dalfo = **Q-D** = quinupristin-dalfopristin
R = resistant
RDBPCT = randomized double blind placebo controlled trial
RFB = rifabutin
RFP = rifapentine
Rick = Rickettsia
RIF = rifampin
RSV = respiratory syncytial virus
RTI = respiratory tract infection

RTV = ritonavir
rx = treatment
SA = Staph. aureus
sc = subcutaneous
SSPE = Subacute sclerosing panencephalitis
SD = serum drug level after single dose
Sens = sensitive (susceptible)
SM = streptomycin
Sofos = sofosbuvir
SQV = saquinavir
SS = steady state serum level
STD = sexually transmitted disease
subcut = subcutaneous
Sulb = sulbactam
Sx = symptoms
TAF = tenofovir alafenamide
Tazo = tazobactam
TBc = tuberculosis
TDF = tenofovir
TEE = transesophageal echocardiography
Teico = teicoplanin
Telithro = telithromycin
Tetra = tetracycline
tid = 3x per day
TMP-SMX = trimethoprim-sulfamethoxazole
TNF = tumor necrosis factor
Tobra = tobramycin
TPV = tipranavir
TST = tuberculin skin test
UTI = urinary tract infection
Vanco = vancomycin
Velpat = velpatasvir
VISA = vancomycin intermediately resistant S. aureus
VL = viral load
Vori = voriconazole
VZV = varicella-zoster virus
ZDV = zidovudine

ABBREVIATIONS OF JOURNAL TITLES

AAC: Antimicrobial Agents & Chemotherapy
Adv PID: Advances in Pediatric Infectious Diseases
AHJ: American Heart Journal
AIDS Res Hum Retrovir: AIDS Research & Human Retroviruses
AAP: American Academy of Pediatrics
AJG: American Journal of Gastroenterology
AJM: American Journal of Medicine
AJRCCM: American Journal of Respiratory Critical Care Medicine
AJTMH: American Journal of Tropical Medicine & Hygiene
Aliment Pharmacol Ther: Alimentary Pharmacology & Therapeutics
Am J Hlth Pharm: American Journal of Health-System Pharmacy
Amer J Transpl: American Journal of Transplantation
AnEM: Annals of Emergency Medicine
AnIM: Annals of Internal Medicine
Ann Pharmacother: Annals of Pharmacotherapy
AnSurg: Annals of Surgery
Antivir Ther: Antiviral Therapy
ArDerm: Archives of Dermatology
ArIM: Archives of Internal Medicine
ARRD: American Review of Respiratory Disease
BMJ: British Medical Journal
BMT: Bone Marrow Transplantation
Brit J Derm: British Journal of Dermatology
Can JID: Canadian Journal of Infectious Diseases
Canad Med J: Canadian Medical Journal
CCM: Critical Care Medicine
CCTID: Current Clinical Topics in Infectious Disease
CDSR: Cochrane Database of Systematic Reviews
CID: Clinical Infectious Diseases
Clin Micro Inf: Clinical Microbiology and Infection
CMN: Clinical Microbiology Newsletter
Clin Micro Rev: Clinical Microbiology Reviews
CMAJ: Canadian Medical Association Journal
COID: Current Opinion in Infectious Disease
Curr Med Res Opin: Current Medical Research and Opinion
Derm Ther: Dermatologic Therapy
Dermatol Clin: Dermatologic Clinics
Dig Dis Sci: Digestive Diseases and Sciences
DMID: Diagnostic Microbiology and Infectious Disease
EID: Emerging Infectious Diseases
EJCMID: European Journal of Clin. Micro. & Infectious Diseases
Eur J Neurol: European Journal of Neurology
Exp Mol Path: Experimental & Molecular Pathology
Exp Rev Anti Infect Ther: Expert Review of Anti-Infective Therapy
Gastro: Gastroenterology
Hpt: Hepatology
ICHE: Infection Control and Hospital Epidemiology
IDC No. Amer: Infectious Disease Clinics of North America
IDCP: Infectious Diseases in Clinical Practice
IJAA: International Journal of Antimicrobial Agents
Inf Med: Infections in Medicine
J AIDS & HR: Journal of AIDS and Human Retrovirology
J All Clin Immun: Journal of Allergy and Clinical Immunology
J Am Ger Soc: Journal of the American Geriatrics Society
J Chemother: Journal of Chemotherapy
J Clin Micro: Journal of Clinical Microbiology
J Clin Virol: Journal of Clinical Virology
J Derm Treat: Journal of Dermatological Treatment
J Hpt: Journal of Hepatology
J Inf: Journal of Infection
J Med Micro: Journal of Medical Microbiology
J Micro Immunol Inf: Journal of Microbiology, Immunology, & Infection
J Ped: Journal of Pediatrics
J Viral Hep: Journal of Viral Hepatitis
JAC: Journal of Antimicrobial Chemotherapy
JACC: Journal of American College of Cardiology
JAIDS: JAIDS Journal of Acquired Immune Deficiency Syndromes
JAMA: Journal of the American Medical Association
JAVMA: Journal of the Veterinary Medicine Association
JCI: Journal of Clinical Investigation
JCM: Journal of Clinical Microbiology
JIC: Journal of Infection and Chemotherapy
JID: Journal of Infectious Diseases
JNS: Journal of Neurosurgery
JPIDS: Journal of Pediatric Infectious Diseases Society
JTMH: Journal of Tropical Medicine and Hygiene
Ln: Lancet
LnID: Lancet Infectious Disease
Mayo Clin Proc: Mayo Clinic Proceedings
Med Lett: Medical Letter
Med Mycol: Medical Mycology
MMWR: Morbidity & Mortality Weekly Report
NEJM: New England Journal of Medicine
Neph Dial Transpl: Nephrology Dialysis Transplantation
OFID: Open Forum Infectious Diseases
Ped Ann: Pediatric Annals
Peds: Pediatrics
Pharmacother: Pharmacotherapy
PIDJ: Pediatric Infectious Disease Journal
QJM: Quarterly Journal of Medicine
Scand J Inf Dis: Scandinavian Journal of Infectious Diseases
Sem Resp Inf: Seminars in Respiratory Infections
SGO: Surgery Gynecology and Obstetrics
SMJ: Southern Medical Journal
Surg Neurol: Surgical Neurology
Transpl Inf Dis: Transplant Infectious Diseases
Transpl: Transplantation
TRSM: Transactions of the Royal Society of Medicine

TABLE 1 – CLINICAL APPROACH TO INITIAL CHOICE OF ANTIMICROBIAL THERAPY*

Treatment based on presumed site or type of infection. In selected instances, treatment and prophylaxis based on identification of pathogens. Regimens should be reevaluated based on pathogen isolated, antimicrobial susceptibility determination, and individual host characteristics. *(Abbreviations on 2)*

ANATOMIC SITE/DIAGNOSIS/ MODIFYING CIRCUMSTANCES	ETIOLOGIES (usual)	SUGGESTED REGIMENS*		ADJUNCT DIAGNOSTIC OR THERAPEUTIC MEASURES AND COMMENTS
		PRIMARY	ALTERNATIVE§	
ABDOMEN: *See Peritoneum, page 49; Gallbladder, page 18; and Pelvic Inflammatory Disease, page 28*				
BONE: Osteomyelitis. Microbiologic diagnosis is essential. If blood culture negative, need culture of bone *(Eur J Clin Microbiol Infect Dis 33:371, 2014)*. Culture of sinus tract drainage not predictive of bone culture. For comprehensive review of antimicrobial penetration into bone, *see Clinical Pharmacokinetics 48:89, 2009.*				
Hematogenous Osteomyelitis *(see IDSA guidelines for vertebral osteo: CID July 29, 2015)*				
Empiric therapy—Collect bone and blood cultures before empiric therapy				
Newborn (<4 mos.)	S. aureus, Gm-neg. bacilli, Group B strep, Kingella kingae in children	**MRSA possible: Vanco** + (**Ceftaz or CFP**)	**MRSA unlikely:** (**Nafcillin** or **Oxacillin**) + (**Ceftaz or CFP**)	Severe allergy or toxicity: (**Linezolid**[NAI] 10 mg/kg IV/po q8h + **Aztreonam**).
Children (>4 mos.) — Adult: Osteo of extremity *(NEJM 370:352, 2014)*	S. aureus, Group A strep, Gm-neg. bacilli rare, Kingella kingae in children	**MRSA possible: Vanco** 40 mg/kg/day div q6h	**MRSA unlikely:** (**Nafcillin** or **Oxacillin**) 150 mg/kg/day div q6h (max 12 gm)	Severe allergy or toxicity: **Clinda** or **TMP-SMX** or **Linezolid**[NAI]. Adults: **Ceftaz** 2 gm IV q8h, **CFP** 2 gm IV q12h. For children **Vanco** dosed at 60 mg/kg/d div q6 or q8h.
		Add **Ceftaz or CFP** if Gm-neg. bacilli on Gram stain **Adult doses below.**		
Adult (>21 yrs) **Vertebral osteo ± epidural abscess** *(see IDSA guidelines for vertebral osteo: CID 61:859, 2015)* **Blood & bone cultures essential.**	S. aureus most common but variety other organisms. Brucella, M. tuberculosis, Coccidioides important in regions of high endemicity for the organisms	**Vanco** 15-20 mg/kg IV q 8-12h for trough of 15-20 µg/mL + (**Ceftriaxone** 2 gm q24h OR **CFP** 2 gm q8h OR **Levo** 750 mg q24h)	**Dapto** 8-10 mg/kg IV q24h OR **Linezolid** 600 mg q12h + (**Ceftriaxone** 2 gm q24h OR **CFP** 2 gm q8h OR **Levo** 750 mg q24h)	**Ceftriaxone** should not be used if pseudomonas suspected. **Piperacillin/Tazobactam** another option for pseudomonas or other Gram-negative coverage. **Dx: MRI diagnostic test of choice, indicated to rule out epidural abscess. Risk factors for recurrence:** end-stage renal disease, MRSA infection, undrained paravertebral or psoas abscess; pathogen-specific therapy for >8 wks recommended if any of these are present *(CID 62:1262, 2016)*; 6 wks of pathogen-specific therapy comparable to 12 wks for less complicated infection *(CID 62:1261, 2016 and Lancet 385:875, 2015)*. Whenever possible empirical therapy should be administered after cultures are obtained.

* **PRIMARY REGIMENS SUGGESTED** are for adults (unless otherwise indicated) with clinically severe (often life-threatening) infections. Dosages also assume normal renal function, and not severe hepatic dysfunction.

§ **ALTERNATIVE REGIMENS INCLUDE** these considerations: allergy, pregnancy, pharmacology/pharmacokinetics, compliance, costs, local resistance profiles.

TABLE 1 (2)

ANATOMIC SITE/DIAGNOSIS/ MODIFYING CIRCUMSTANCES	ETIOLOGIES (usual)	SUGGESTED REGIMENS*		ADJUNCT DIAGNOSTIC OR THERAPEUTIC MEASURES AND COMMENTS
		PRIMARY	ALTERNATIVE§	
BONE/Hematogenous Osteomyelitis *(continued)*				
Specific therapy—Culture and in vitro susceptibility results known. *See CID Jul 29, 2015 for IDSA Guidelines*				
	MSSA	**Nafcillin** or **Oxacillin** 2 gm IV q4h or **Cefazolin** 2 gm IV q8h	**Vanco** 15-30 mg/kg IV q 8-12h for trough of 15-20 µg/mL OR **Dapto** 8-10 mg/kg IV q24h OR **Linezolid** 600 mg IV/po q12h	**Other options if susceptible in vitro and allergy/toxicity issues *(see NEJM 362:11, 2010):*** 1) **TMP-SMX** 8-10 mg/kg/d po/IV div q8h + **RIF** 300-450 mg bid: limited data, particularly for MRSA *(see AAC 53:2672, 2009)*; 2) **Levo** 750 mg po q24h) + **RIF** 600 mg po q24h; 3) **Fusidic acid**[NUS] 500 mg IV q8h + **RIF** 300 mg po bid. *(CID 42:394, 2006)*; 4) **Ceftriaxone** 2 gm IV q24h *(CID 54:585, 2012) (MSSA only)*: Duration of therapy: 6 weeks, provided that epidural or paravertebral abscesses can be drained; consider longer course in those with extensive infection or abscess particularly if not amenable to drainage because of increased risk of treatment failure *(OFID Dec 5:1, 2014)* (although data are lacking that this approach improves efficacy versus a 6 wks course) and >8 weeks in patients undergoing device implantation *(CID 60:1330, 2015)*.
	MRSA—*See Table 6, page 90; IDSA Guidelines CID 52:e18-55, 2011; CID 52:285-92, 2011*	**Vanco** 15-20 mg/kg IV q 8-12h for trough of 15-20 µg/mL ± **RIF** 300-450 mg bid.	**Linezolid** 600 mg q12h IV/po ± **RIF** 300 mg po/IV bid OR **Dapto** 8-10 mg/kg q24h IV ± **RIF** 300-450 mg po/IV bid	
Hemoglobinopathy: Sickle cell/thalassemia	Salmonella; other Gm-neg. bacilli	**CIP** 400 mg IV q12h OR **CIP** 750 mg po bid	**Levo** 750 mg IV/po q24h	Thalassemia: transfusion and iron chelation risk factors. Because of decreasing levels of susceptibility to fluoroquinolones among Salmonella spp. and growing resistance among other gram-negative bacilli, would add a second agent (e.g., third-generation cephalosporin) until susceptibility test results available. Alternative for salmonella is Ceftriaxone 2 gm IV q24h if nalidixic acid resistant which is predictive of fluoroquinolone resistance.
Contiguous Osteomyelitis Without Vascular Insufficiency				
Empiric therapy: Get cultures!				
Foot bone osteo due to nail through tennis shoe	P. aeruginosa	**CIP** 750 mg po bid or **Levo** 750 mg po q24h	**Ceftaz** 2 gm IV q8h or **CFP** 2 gm IV q8h	*See Skin—Nail puncture, page 60*. Need debridement to remove foreign body.
Long bone, post-internal fixation of fracture	S. aureus, Gm-neg. bacilli, P. aeruginosa	**Vanco** 15-20 mg/kg q8-12h IV q 8-12h for trough of 15-20 µg/mL + [**Ceftaz** or **CFP**]. *See Comment*	**Linezolid** 600 mg IV/po bid[NAI] + (**Ceftaz** or **CFP**). *See Comment*	Often necessary to remove hardware after union to achieve eradication. May need revascularization. **Regimens listed are empiric.** Adjust after culture data available. If susceptible Gm-neg. bacillus, **CIP** 750 mg po bid or **Levo** 750 mg po q24h. For other *S. aureus* options: *See Hem. Osteo. Specific Therapy, page 6.*
Osteonecrosis of the jaw	Probably rare adverse reaction to bisphosphonates	Infection may be secondary to bone necrosis and loss of overlying mucosa. Treatment: minimal surgical debridement, chlorhexidine rinses, antibiotics (e.g. Pip-tazo). Evaluate for concomitant actinomycosis, for which specific long-term antibiotic treatment would be warranted.		
Prosthetic joint	*See prosthetic joint, page 35*			
Spinal implant infection	S. aureus, coag-neg staphylococci, gram-neg bacilli	Onset within 30 days: culture, treat for 3 mos.	Onset after 30 days remove implant, culture & treat	*See CID 55:1481, 2012*
Sternum, post-op	S. aureus, S. epidermidis, occasionally, gram-negative bacilli	**Vanco** 15-20 mg/kg q8-12h IV for trough of 15-20 µg/mL recommended for serious infections.	**Linezolid** 600 mg po/IV[NAI] bid	Sternal debridement for cultures & removal of necrotic bone. For *S. aureus* options: *Hem. Osteo. Specific Therapy, page 6*. If setting or gram stain suggests possibility of gram-negative bacilli, add appropriate coverage based on local antimicrobial susceptibility profiles (e.g., cefepime, Pip-tazo).

 **NOTE: All dosage recommendations are for adults (unless otherwise indicated) and assume normal renal function. § Alternatives consider allergy, PK, compliance, local resistance, cost.*

TABLE 1 (3)

ANATOMIC SITE/DIAGNOSIS/ MODIFYING CIRCUMSTANCES	ETIOLOGIES (usual)	SUGGESTED REGIMENS* PRIMARY	SUGGESTED REGIMENS* ALTERNATIVE§	ADJUNCT DIAGNOSTIC OR THERAPEUTIC MEASURES AND COMMENTS
BONE *(continued)*				
Contiguous Osteomyelitis With Vascular Insufficiency.				
Most pts are **diabetics** with peripheral neuropathy & infected skin ulcers *(see Diabetic foot, page 18)*	Polymicrobic [Gm+ cocci (to include MRSA) (aerobic & anaerobic) and Gm-neg. bacilli (aerobic & anaerobic)]	Debride overlying ulcer & submit bone for histology & culture. Select antibiotic based on culture results & treat for 6 weeks. **No empiric therapy unless acutely ill.** If acutely ill, *see suggestions, Diabetic foot, page 18.* Revascularize if possible.		**Diagnosis of osteo:** Culture bone biopsy (gold standard). Poor concordance of culture results between swab of ulcer and bone – need bone. Sampling by needle puncture inferior to biopsy *(CID 48:888, 2009).* Osteo likely if ulcer >2 cm², positive probe to bone, ESR >70 & abnormal plain x-ray *(JAMA 299:806, 2008).* **Treatment:** (1) **Revascularize if possible;** (2) Culture bone; (3) Specific antimicrobial(s).
Chronic Osteomyelitis: Specific therapy By definition, implies presence of dead bone. **Need valid cultures**	S. aureus, Enterobacteriaceae, P. aeruginosa	**Empiric rx not indicated.** Base systemic rx on results of culture, sensitivity testing. If acute exacerbation of chronic osteo, rx as acute hematogenous osteo. Surgical debridement important.		**Important adjuncts:** removal of orthopedic hardware, surgical debridement; vascularized muscle flaps, distraction osteogenesis (Ilizarov) techniques. Antibiotic-impregnated cement & hyperbaric oxygen adjunctive. **NOTE: RIF + (Vanco or β-lactam)** effective in animal model and in a clinical trial of S. aureus chronic osteo.
BREAST: Mastitis—*Obtain culture; need to know if MRSA present. Review of breast infections: BMJ 342:d396, 2011.*				
Postpartum mastitis *(Cochrane Review: Cochrane Database Syst Rev 2013 Feb 28;2:CD005458; see also CID 54:71, 2012)*				
Mastitis without abscess	S. aureus; less often S. pyogenes (Gp A or B), E. coli, bacteroides species, maybe Corynebacterium sp., & selected coagulase-neg. staphylococci (e.g., S. lugdunensis)	**NO MRSA:** **Outpatient: Diclox** 500 mg po qid or **Cephalexin** 500 mg po qid. **Inpatient: Nafcillin/ Oxacillin** 2 gm IV q4-6h	**MRSA Possible:** **Outpatient: TMP-SMX-DS** tabs 1-2 po bid or, if susceptible, **Clinda** 300 mg po tid **Inpatient: Vanco** 1 gm IV q12h; if over 100 kg, 1.5 gm IV q12h.	If no abscess & controllable pain, ↑ freq of nursing may hasten response.
Mastitis with abscess				For painful abscess I&D is standard; needle aspiration reported successful. Resume breast feeding from affected breast as soon as pain allows. *(Breastfeed Med 9:239, 2014)*
Non-puerperal mastitis with abscess	S. aureus; less often Bacteroides sp., peptostreptococcus (Peptoniphilus sp.), & selected coagulase-neg. staphylococci	*See regimens for Postpartum mastitis, page 7.*		Smoking and diabetes may be risk factors *(BMJ 342:d396, 2011).* **If subareolar & odoriferous**, most likely anaerobes; need to **add Metro** 500 mg IV/po tid. If not subareolar, staph. Need pretreatment aerobic/anaerobic cultures. Surgical drainage for abscess. **I&D standard.** Corynebacterium sp. assoc. with chronic granulomatous mastitis *(JCM 53:2895, 2015).* **Consider TB in chronic infections.**
Breast implant infection	Acute: S. aureus, S. pyogenes. TSS reported. Chronic: Look for rapidly growing Mycobacteria	Acute: **Vanco** 15-20 mg/kg IV q8-12h.	Chronic: Await culture results. *See Table 12A* for mycobacteria treatment.	Risk of complications higher with late-onset infection (>30 days post implantation). Antibiotics alone may be sufficient for minor infections; explantation often required for more serious infections. *Plast. Reconstr. Surg 139:20, 2017.*

Abbreviations on page 2. **NOTE: All dosage recommendations are for adults (unless otherwise indicated) and assume normal renal function. § Alternatives consider allergy, PK, compliance, local resistance, cost.*

TABLE 1 (4)

ANATOMIC SITE/DIAGNOSIS/ MODIFYING CIRCUMSTANCES	ETIOLOGIES (usual)	SUGGESTED REGIMENS* PRIMARY	SUGGESTED REGIMENS* ALTERNATIVE§	ADJUNCT DIAGNOSTIC OR THERAPEUTIC MEASURES AND COMMENTS
CENTRAL NERVOUS SYSTEM				
Brain abscess				
Primary or contiguous source Review: *NEJM 371:447, 2014.*	Streptococci (60–70%), bacteroides (20–40%), Enterobacteriaceae (25-33%), S. aureus (10-15%), S. anginosus grp. Rare: Nocardia *(below)*, Listeria. *See S. aureus Comment*	(**Cefotaxime** 2 gm IV q4h or **Ceftriaxone** 2 gm IV q12h) + (**Metro** 7.5 mg/kg q6h or 15 mg/kg IV q12h) Add **Vanco** 15-20 mg/kg IV q8-12h or **Linezolid** 600 mg IV/po q12h to the regimen if S. aureus is a possibility Duration of rx unclear; usually 4-6 wks or until resolution by neuro-imaging (CT/MRI)	**Pen G** 3-4 million units IV q4h + **Metro** 7.5 mg/kg q6h or 15 mg/kg IV q12h	If CT scan suggests cerebritis or abscesses <2.5 cm and pt neurologically stable and conscious, start antibiotics and observe. Otherwise, surgical drainage necessary. If blood cultures or other clinical data do not yield a likely etiologic agent, aspirate even small abscesses for diagnosis if this can be done safely. S. anginosus grp esp. prone to produce abscess. Ceph/metro does not cover listeria.
Post-surgical, post-traumatic. Review: *NEJM 371:447, 2014.*	S. aureus, Enterobacteriaceae	**For MSSA:** (**Nafcillin** or **Oxacillin**) 2 gm IV q4h + (**Ceftriaxone** or **Cefotaxime**)	**For MRSA: Vanco** 15-20 mg/kg IV q 8-12h for trough of 15-20 mcg/mL + (**Ceftriaxone** or **Cefotaxime**)	Empiric coverage, de-escalated based on culture results. **Aspiration of abscess usually necessary for dx & rx. If P. aeruginosa suspected, substitute (Cefepime or Ceftazidime) for (Ceftriaxone or Cefotaxime).**
HIV-1 infected (AIDS)	Toxoplasma gondii	*See Table 13A, page 166*		
Nocardia: Haematogenous abscess	N. farcinica, N. asteroides & N. brasiliensis *See AAC 58:795, 2014* for other species.	**TMP-SMX:** 15 mg/kg/day of TMP & 75 mg/kg/day of SMX, IV/po div in 2-4 doses + **IMP** 500 mg q6h IV. If multiorgan involvement some add **Amikacin** 7.5 mg/kg q12h. After 3-6 wks of IV therapy, switch to po therapy. Immunocompetent pts: **TMP-SMX**, **minocycline** or **Amox-clav** x 3+ months. Immunocompromised pts: Treat with 2 drugs x 1 yr.	**Linezolid** 600 mg IV or po q12h + meropenem 2 gm q8h	**Linezolid** 600 mg po bid reported effective. For in vitro susceptibility testing: Wallace (+1) 903-877-7680 or U.S. CDC (+1) 404-639-3158. **TMP-SMX** remains a drug of choice for CNS nocardia infection: in vitro resistance to TMP-SMX may be increasing *(CID 51:1445, 2010)*, but whether this is associated with worse outcomes is not known and a recent study casts doubt on this with only 2.5% of 552 isolates resistant; difficulties with end-point determinations might account for discrepancies in reported rates of resistance *(JCM 50:670, 2012)*. **If sulfonamide resistant or sulfa-allergic**, **Amikacin** plus one of: **IMP**, **MER**, **Ceftriaxone** or **Cefotaxime**. *N. farcinica* is resistant to third-generation cephalosporins, which should not be used for treatment of infection caused by this organism. If TMP-SMX resistance reported, *see JCM 50:670, 2012* (before stopping TMP-SMX).
Subdural empyema: In adult 60–90% is extension of sinusitis or otitis media. Rx same as primary brain abscess. Surgical emergency: must drain. Review in *LnID 7:62*, 2007.				
Encephalitis/encephalopathy *IDSA Guideline: CID 47:303, 2008; Intl diagnosis consensus: CID 57:1114, 2013. (For Herpes see Table 14A, page 181 and for rabies, Table 20B, page 257)*	H. simplex (42%), VZV (15%), M. TB (15%), Listeria (10%) *(CID 49:1838, 2009)*. Other: arbovirus, West Nile, rabies, Lyme, Parvo B19, Cat-scratch, Mycoplasma, EBV and others.	Start IV **Acyclovir** while awaiting results of CSF PCR for H. simplex. For amebic encephalitis *see Table 13A*. Start **Doxy** 100 mg q12h if setting suggests R. rickettsii, Anaplasma, Ehrlichia or Mycoplasma. **Ceftriaxone** 2 gm IV q24h or **Doxy** 100 mg q12h x 14 days for Lyme encephalitis.		Increasing recognition of autoimmune antibody-mediated encephalitis, e.g., anti-N-methyl aspartate receptors & others. Dx: CSF antibody panel. Ref: *NEJM 2018,378:840*. Review of acute viral encephalitis *(NEJM 2018;379:557)*
Meningitis, "Aseptic": Pleocytosis of up to 100s of cells, CSF glucose normal, neg. culture for bacteria *(See Table 14A, page 178)* Ref: *CID 47:783, 2008*	Enteroviruses, HSV-2, LCM, HIV, VZV, other viruses, syphilis, drugs [NSAIDs, metronidazole, carbamazepine, lamotrigine TMP-SMX, IVIG, (e.g., detuximab, infliximab)], rarely leptospirosis, Lyme.	For all but leptospirosis, IV fluids and analgesics. D/C drugs that may be etiologic. For lepto (**Doxy** 100 mg IV/po q12h) or (**Pen G** 5 million units IV q6h) or (**AMP** 0.5–1 gm IV q6h). Repeat LP if suspect partially-treated bacterial meningitis. **Acyclovir** 5-10 mg/kg IV q8h sometimes given for HSV-2 meningitis (**NOTE:** distinct from HSV encephalitis where early rx is mandatory).		If available, PCR of CSF for enterovirus. VZV, HSV-2: concurrent or history of prior genital lesions often absent *(see J Neurovirol 19:166, 2013)*. For lepto, positive epidemiologic history and concomitant hepatitis, conjunctivitis, dermatitis, nephritis. For list of implicated drugs: *Inf Med 25:331, 2008.* CNS Lyme: Varies – palsy, encephalitis, aseptic meningitis: *see page 62.* Etiologies: *Med 95:e2372, 2016.*

 **NOTE: All dosage recommendations are for adults (unless otherwise indicated) and assume normal renal function. § Alternatives consider allergy, PK, compliance, local resistance, cost.*

TABLE 1 (5)

ANATOMIC SITE/DIAGNOSIS/ MODIFYING CIRCUMSTANCES	ETIOLOGIES (usual)	SUGGESTED REGIMENS*		ADJUNCT DIAGNOSTIC OR THERAPEUTIC MEASURES AND COMMENTS
		PRIMARY	ALTERNATIVE§	
CENTRAL NERVOUS SYSTEM *(continued)*				
Meningitis, Bacterial, Acute: Goal is empiric therapy, then CSF exam within 30 min. If focal neurologic deficit, give empiric therapy, then head CT, then LP. If no focal deficit, empiric therapy, LP & then head CT *(CID 2018,66:321)*. For distribution of pathogens by age group, *see NEJM 364:2016, 2011.*				
Empiric Therapy—CSF Gram stain is negative—immunocompetent				
Age: Preterm to <1 mo *LnID 10:32, 2010*	Group B strep 49%, E. coli 18%, listeria 7%, misc. Gm-neg. 10%, misc. Gm-pos. 10%	**AMP** 75-100 mg/kg IV q6h + **Cefotaxime** 75 mg/kg IV q6h + **Genta** 2.5 mg/kg IV q8h or 5-7 mg/kg IV q24h. Intraventricular treatment not recommended.	**AMP** 75-100 mg/kg IV q6h + **Cefotaxime** 75 mg/kg IV q6h OR **AMP** 75-100 mg/kg IV q6h + **Gent** 2.5 mg/kg IV q8h	Regimens active vs. Group B strep, most coliforms, & listeria. If premature infant with long nursery stay, S. aureus, enterococci, and resistant coliforms potential pathogens. **If high risk of MRSA,** use vanco + cefotaxime. Alter regimen after culture/ sensitivity data available.
Age: 1 mo– 50 yrs Recent review: *Lancet Infect Dis 16:339, 2016.*	S. pneumo, meningococci, H. influenzae now uncommon, **listeria unlikely if young adult & immunocompetent** (add **Ampicillin** if suspect listeria: 2 gm IV q4h)	Adult: [(**Cefotaxime** 2 gm IV q4–6h OR **Ceftriaxone** 2 gm IV q12h)] + **Dexamethasone** + **Vanco** **Dexamethasone:** 0.15 mg/kg IV q6h x 2–4 days. **Give with, or just before, 1st dose of antibiotic** *(see Comment).* *See footnote[1] for Vanco Adult dosage and[2] for ped. dosage*	[(**MER** 2 gm IV q8h) (Peds: 40 mg/kg IV q8h)] + IV **Dexamethasone** + **Vanco**[1]	For patients with severe **β-lactam allergy,** *see below (Empiric Therapy—positive gram stain and Specific Therapy)* for alternative therapies.
Age: >50 yrs or alcoholism or other **debilitating assoc diseases** or **impaired cellular immunity**	S. pneumo, listeria, meningococci, Gm-neg. bacilli	(**AMP** 2 gm IV q4h) + (**Ceftriaxone** 2 gm IV q12h or **Cefotaxime** 2 gm IV q4-6h) + **Vanco** + IV **Dexamethasone** **For Vanco dose,** *see footnote[1]*. **Dexamethasone dose:** 0.15 mg/kg IV q6h x 2–4 days; 1st dose before, or concomitant with, 1st dose of antibiotic.	**MER** 2 gm IV q8h + **Vanco** + IV **Dexamethasone**. *For severe Pen allergy, see Comment*	For patients with severe **β-lactam allergy,** *see below (Empiric Therapy—positive gram stain and Specific Therapy)* for alternative agents that can be substituted to cover likely pathogens. LP without CT for patients with altered level of consciousness and non-focal neurological exam associated with earlier treatment and improved outcome *(CID 60:1162, 2015)*
Post-neurosurgery Ventriculostomy/lumbar catheter; ventriculoperitoneal (atrial) shunt or penetrating trauma w/o basilar skull fracture Shunt-related meningitis IDSA Guidelines: *CID 64:e34, 2017.*	S. epidermidis, S. aureus, Cutibacterium acnes. Facultative and aerobic gram-neg bacilli, including: P. aeruginosa & A. baumannii (may be multi-drug resistant)	**Vanco** (to achieve trough level of 15-20 mg/mL) + (**Cefepime** or **Ceftaz** 2 gm IV q8h) • **If severe Pen/Ceph allergy,** for possible gram-neg, substitute either: **Aztreonam** 2 gm IV q6-8h or **CIP** 400 mg IV q12h. **Intraventricular antibiotic dosing** (lower dose for slit ventricles, intermediate dose for normal size ventricles, higher dose for enlarged ventricles): **Amikacin** 30 mg, **Gent** 4-8 mg in adults, 1-2 mg in infants, children, **Polymyxin E** (Colistin) 10 mg, **Tobra** 5-20 mg, **Vanco** 5-20 mg, **Dapto** 5 mg. **Frequency of administration** depends on drainage output: < 50 ml/24h: every 3rd day, 50-100 ml/24h: every second day, 100-150 ml/day: once daily, 150-200 ml/24h: increase dose of vancomycin by 5 mg, gentamicin by 1 mg, 200-250 ml/24h: increase dose of vancomycin by 5 mg, gentamicin by 1 mg	**Vanco** (to achieve trough level of 15-20 mg/mL) + (**MER** 2 gm IV q8h)	• Remove infected shunt and place external ventricular catheter for drainage or pressure control. • Intraventricular therapy used if the shunt cannot be removed or cultures fail to clear with systemic therapy. • **Shunt reimplantation:** If coagulase-negative staphylococci, diphtheroids, or C. acnes: no CSF abnormalities, day 3 after externalization if CSF cultures are negative at 48h; CSF abnormalities present: 7-10 days after the last positive CSF culture. If S. aureus or Gram-negative organism: 10 days after last positive CSF culture.

[1] **Vanco adult dose:** 15-20 mg/kg IV q8 -12h to achieve trough level of 15-20 µg/mL

[2] **Dosage of drugs used to treat children age ≥1 mo: Cefotaxime** 50 mg/kg per day IV q6h; **Ceftriaxone** 50 mg/kg IV q12h; **Vanco** 15 mg/kg IV q6h to achieve trough level of 15-20 µg/mL.

Abbreviations on page 2. **NOTE: All dosage recommendations are for adults (unless otherwise indicated) and assume normal renal function. § Alternatives consider allergy, PK, compliance, local resistance, cost.*

TABLE 1 (6)

ANATOMIC SITE/DIAGNOSIS/ MODIFYING CIRCUMSTANCES	ETIOLOGIES (usual)	SUGGESTED REGIMENS*		ADJUNCT DIAGNOSTIC OR THERAPEUTIC MEASURES AND COMMENTS
		PRIMARY	ALTERNATIVE§	
CENTRAL NERVOUS SYSTEM/Meningitis, Bacterial, Acute/Empiric Therapy—CSF Gram stain is negative—immunocompetent *(continued)*				
Trauma with basilar skull fracture	S. pneumoniae, H. influenzae, S. pyogenes	**Vanco** (to achieve trough level of 15-20 mg/mL) + (**Ceftriaxone** 2 gm IV q12h or **Cefotaxime** 2 gm IV q6h) + [**Dexamethasone** 0.15 mg/kg IV q6h x 2-4 d (1st dose with or before 1st antibiotic dose)]. *See Clin Micro Rev 21:519, 2008.*		
Empiric Therapy—Positive CSF Gram stain				
Gram-positive diplococci	S. pneumoniae	(**Ceftriaxone** 2 gm IV q12h or **Cefotaxime** 2 gm IV q4–6h) + **Vanco** 15-20 mg/kg IV q8-12h (to achieve 15-20 µg/mL trough) + **Dexamethasone** 0.15 mg/kg IV q6h; first dose is given 15-20 minutes prior to first antibiotic dose, and then continued for 4 days for confirmed pneumococcal infection.		**Alternatives: MER** 2 gm IV q8h or **Moxi** 400 mg IV q24h.
Gram-negative diplococci	N. meningitidis	(**Cefotaxime** 2 gm IV q4–6h or **Ceftriaxone** 2 gm IV q12h)		**Alternatives: Pen G** 4 mill. units IV q4h or **AMP** 2 gm q4h or **Moxi** 400 mg IV q24h or **Chloro** 1 gm IV q6h (Chloro less effective than other alternatives: *see JAC 70:979, 2015*)
Gram-positive bacilli or coccobacilli	Listeria monocytogenes	**AMP** 2 gm IV q4h ± **Genta** 2 mg/kg IV loading dose then 1.7 mg/kg IV q8h		If pen allergic use **TMP/SMX** 5 mg/kg (TMP component) q6-8h. Use of meropenem associated with increased 30-day mortality *(Clin Microbiol Infect 22: 725, 2016)*. Data showing beneficial effect of gentamicin combination therapy are inconclusive.
Gram-negative bacilli	H. influenzae, enterics, P. aeruginosa	(**Ceftazidime** or **Cefepime** 2 gm IV q8h) + **Genta** 2 mg/kg IV 1st dose then 1.7 mg/kg IV q8h		**Alternatives: MER** 2 gm IV infused over 4h q8h (covers ESBLs); **Aztreonam** 2 gm IV q6-8h (safe in beta-lactam allergic patient). **Dexamethasone not recommended for Gram-negatives other than suspected H. influenza infection** administered as 0.15 mg/kg IV q6h; first dose is given 15-20 minutes prior to first antibiotic dose, and then continued for 4 days if H. influenza infection is confirmed.
Specific Therapy—Positive culture of CSF with in vitro susceptibility results available				
H. influenzae	β-lactamase positive	**Ceftriaxone** 2 gm IV q12h (adult), 50 mg/kg IV q12h (peds) + **Dexamethasone** 0.15 mg/kg IV q6h; first dose is given 15-20 minutes prior to first antibiotic dose, and then continued for 4 days in microbiologically confirmed cases.		**Pen. allergic: Chloro** 12.5 mg/kg IV q6h (max. 4 gm/day.) (Chloro less effective than other alternatives: *see JAC 70:979, 2015*); **CIP** 400 mg IV q8-12h; **Aztreonam** 2 gm q6-8h.
Listeria monocytogenes *(CID 43:1233, 2006)*		**AMP** 2 gm IV q4h ± **Genta** 2 mg/kg IV loading dose, then 1.7 mg/kg IV q8h		If pen allergic use **TMP/SMX** 5 mg/kg (TMP component) q6-8h. Use of meropenem associated with increased 30-day mortality *(Clin Microbiol Infect 22: 725, 2016)*. Data showing beneficial effect of gentamicin combination therapy are inconclusive.
N. meningitidis		**Pen G** (adult dose 4 million units q4h) x 7 days or **Ceftriaxone** 2 gm IV q12h x 7 days (preferred if MIC is 0.1 to 1.0 µg/ml); if β-lactam allergic, **Chloro** 12.5 µg/kg (up to 1 gm) IV q6h (but less effective than other alternatives: *see JAC 70:979, 2015*).		Other alternatives: **MER** 2 gm IV q8h or **Moxi** 400 mg q24h. Rare isolates resistant to Chloro; FQ-resistant isolates encountered rarely. Increased risk of invasive meningococcal infection in recipients of eculizumab *(MMWR 66:734, 2017)*.

 **NOTE: All dosage recommendations are for adults (unless otherwise indicated) and assume normal renal function. § Alternatives consider allergy, PK, compliance, local resistance, cost.*

TABLE 1 (7)

ANATOMIC SITE/DIAGNOSIS/ MODIFYING CIRCUMSTANCES	ETIOLOGIES (usual)	SUGGESTED REGIMENS*		ADJUNCT DIAGNOSTIC OR THERAPEUTIC MEASURES AND COMMENTS
		PRIMARY	ALTERNATIVE§	
CENTRAL NERVOUS SYSTEM/Meningitis, Bacterial, Acute/Specific Therapy—Positive culture of CSF with in vitro susceptibility results available *(continued)*				
S. pneumoniae **Notes:** 1. Dexamethasone 0.15 mg/kg IV q6h; first dose 15-20 minutes prior to first antibiotic dose, and then continued for 4 days. 2. If MIC ≥1, repeat CSF exam after 24–48h. 3. Treat for 10–14 days	Pen G MIC <0.1 mcg/mL	**Pen G** 4 million units IV q4h or **AMP** 2 gm IV q4h		**Alternatives: Ceftriaxone** 2 gm IV q12h, **Chloro** 1 gm IV q6h (Chloro less effective than other alternatives: *see JAC 70:979, 2015*)
	0.1–1 mcg/mL	**Ceftriaxone** 2 gm IV q12h or **Cefotaxime** 2 gm IV q4–6h		**Alternatives: Cefepime** 2 gm IV q8h or **MER** 2 gm IV q8h
	≥2 mcg/mL	**Vanco** 15-20 mg/kg IV q8-12h (15-20 µg/mL trough target) + (**Ceftriaxone** or **Cefotaxime** as above)		**Alternatives: Moxi** 400 mg IV q24h
	Ceftriaxone MIC >0.5 mcg/mL	**Vanco** 15-20 mg/kg IV q8-12h (15-20 µg/mL trough target) + (**Ceftriaxone** or **Cefotaxime** as above)		**Alternatives: Moxi** 400 mg IV q24h If MIC to Ceftriaxone ≥2 mcg/mL, add **RIF** 600 mg po/IV 1x/day to **Vanco** + (**Ceftriaxone** or **Cefotaxime**).
E. coli, other coliforms, or P. aeruginosa	**Consultation advised**— need susceptibility results	(**Ceftazidime** or **Cefepime** 2 gm IV q8h) + **Genta** 2 mg/kg IV x 1 dose, then 1.7 mg/kg IV q8h x 21 days.		**Alternatives: MER** 2 gm IV infused over 4h q8h; **CIP** 400 mg IV q8h (need to confirm susceptibility) **Reculture CSF after 4-5 days of therapy;** If culture is still positive, may need adjunctive intrathecal or intraventricular antibiotic therapy.
Prophylaxis for H. influenzae and N. meningitidis				
Haemophilus influenzae type B Household or close contact group defined as persons who reside with the patient or a nonresident who has spent 4 hours or more with the index patient for at least 5 of the 7 days preceding the day of hospitalization of the patient.		**RIF** 20 mg/kg (not to exceed 600 mg) once daily x 4 days for individuals ≥1 mo; 10 mg/mg once daily x 4 days for age <1 mo.		**Household or Close Contacts:** RIF chemoprophylaxis recommended for index patients (unless treated with Cefotaxime or Ceftriaxone) and all household contacts in households with members aged <4 years who are not fully vaccinated or members aged <18 years who are immunocompromised, regardless of their vaccination status. **Childcare Contacts:** RIF chemoprophylaxis recommended in childcare settings when two or more cases of invasive Hib disease have occurred within 60 days and unimmunized or underimmunized children attend the facility; when prophylaxis is indicated, it should be prescribed for all attendees, regardless of age or vaccine status, and for childcare providers.
Prophylaxis for Neisseria meningitidis exposure (close contact)		**RIF** 10 mg/kg (max dose 600 mg) q12h x 2 days (adult or child ≥1 mo); 5 mg/kg q12h x 2 dose child <1 mo OR **Ceftriaxone** single IM dose of 250 mg (adult) or 125 mg (child age <15 years) OR **CIP** single po 500 mg dose (age ≥18; not recommended in pregnant or lactating women, or if CIP resistant isolates circulating in the local community).		**Spread by respiratory droplets**, not aerosols, hence close contact req. ↑ risk if close contact for at least 4 hrs during wk before illness onset (e.g., housemates, day care contacts, cellmates) or exposure to pt's nasopharyngeal secretions (e.g., kissing, mouth-to-mouth resuscitation, intubation, nasotracheal suctioning).
Meningitis, chronic Defined as symptoms + CSF pleocytosis for ≥4 wks	MTB cryptococcosis, other fungal, neoplastic, Lyme, syphilis, Whipple's disease	Treatment depends on etiology. No urgent need for empiric therapy, but when TB suspected treatment should be expeditious.		Long list of possibilities: bacteria, parasites, fungi, viruses, neoplasms, vasculitis, and other miscellaneous etiologies—*see Neurol Clin 28:1061, 2010. See NEJM 370:2408, 2014* for diagnosis of neuroleptospirosis by next generation sequencing technologies.
Meningitis, eosinophilic *Hawaii J Med Public Health, 72(6 Suppl 2):35, 2013*	Angiostrongyliasis, gnathostomiasis, baylisascaris	Corticosteroids	Anti-helminthic therapy probably not beneficial	1/3 lack peripheral eosinophilia. Need serology to confirm diagnosis. Steroid ref.: *Cochrane Database Syst Rev. 2015 Feb 17;(2):CD009088*
Meningitis, HIV-1 infected (AIDS) *See Table 11, Sanford Guide to HIV/AIDS Therapy*	As in adults, >50 yrs: also consider cryptococci, M. tuberculosis, syphilis, HIV aseptic meningitis, Listeria monocytogenes	If etiology not identified: treat as adult >50 yrs + obtain CSF/serum cryptococcal antigen *(see Comments)*	For crypto rx, *see Table 11A, page 136*	C. neoformans most common etiology in AIDS patients. H. influenzae, pneumococci, listeria, TBc, syphilis, viral, histoplasma & coccidioides also need to be considered. Obtain blood cultures.

Abbreviations on page 2. *NOTE: All dosage recommendations are for adults (unless otherwise indicated) and assume normal renal function. § Alternatives consider allergy, PK, compliance, local resistance, cost.*

TABLE 1 (8)

ANATOMIC SITE/DIAGNOSIS/ MODIFYING CIRCUMSTANCES	ETIOLOGIES (usual)	SUGGESTED REGIMENS*		ADJUNCT DIAGNOSTIC OR THERAPEUTIC MEASURES AND COMMENTS
		PRIMARY	ALTERNATIVE§	
EAR				
External otitis				
Acute external otitis: "Swimmer's ear", ear buds, headsets Ref: *JAMA 2018;320:1375*	*S. aureus, P. aeruginosa*	Ear drops: 1) **CIP** + (dexamethasone or hydrocortisone) bid x 7 days; 2) **Oflox** qd x 7 days; 3) **CIP** single dose		In Cochrane meta-analysis, antiseptics, acidifying agents, glucocorticoids & topical antibiotics have similar outcomes *(Cochr Sys Rev 2010;1:CD004740)*. Topical antibiotic therapy favored with cure rates of 65-90%; all are expensive ($70-300).
Chronic	Usually 2° to seborrhea	Eardrops: [(**Polymyxin B** + **Neomycin** + **hydrocortisone** qid) + **selenium sulfide shampoo**]		Control seborrhea with dandruff shampoo containing selenium sulfide (Selsun) or [(ketoconazole shampoo) + (medium potency steroid solution, triamcinolone 0.1%)].
Fungal	Candida species	**Fluconazole** 200 mg po x 1 dose & then 100 mg po x 3-5 days.		
"Necrotizing (malignant) otitis externa" Risk groups: Diabetes mellitus, AIDS, chemotherapy. *See Am J Otolaryngol 37:425, 2016.*	Pseudomonas aeruginosa in >95% *(Otol & Neurotology 34:620, 2013)*	**CIP** 400 mg IV q8h; 750 mg po q8-12h only for early disease	**Pip-tazo** 3.375 gm q4h or extended infusion (3.375 gm over 4 hrs q8h) + **Tobra**	Very high ESRs are typical. Debridement usually required. R/O osteomyelitis: CT or MRI scans. If bone involved, treat for 6–8 wks. Other alternatives if P. aeruginosa is susceptible: **IMP** 0.5 gm q6h or **MER** 1 gm IV q8h or **CFP** 2 gm IV q12h or **Ceftaz** 2 gm IV q8h.
Otitis media—infants, children, adults *(Cochrane review: Cochrane Database Syst Rev. Jan 31;1:CD000219, 2013); American Academy of Pediatrics Guidelines: Pediatrics 131:e964, 2013)*				
Acute Two RCTs indicate efficacy of antibiotic rx if age <36 mos & definite AOM *(NEJM 364:105, 116 & 168, 2011)*				
Initial empiric therapy of acute otitis media (AOM) **NOTE: Treat children <2 yrs old**. If >2 yrs old, fever <39C, mild or no ear pain, neg./questionable exam— consider analgesic treatment without antimicrobials. Favorable results in mostly afebrile pts with waiting 48hrs before deciding on antibiotic use *(JAMA 296:1235, 1290, 2006)*	Overall detection in middle ear fluid: No pathogen 4% Virus 70% Bact. + virus 66% Bacteria 92% Bacterial pathogens from middle ear: S. pneumo 49%, H. influenzae 29%, M. catarrhalis 28%. Ref.: *CID 43:1417 & 1423, 2006.* Children 6 mos-3 yrs, 2 episodes AOM/yrs & 63% are virus positive *(CID 46:815 & 824, 2008).*	**If NO antibiotics in prior month:** **Amox** 80-90 mg/kg/d divided q8h or q12h (**preferred regimen**) OR **Amox-clav** 90/6.4 mg/kg/d divided bid Options for nonIgE PCN allergy: **Cefdinir** 14 mg/kg/d divided q12h or once q24h **Cefpodoxime proxetil** 10 mg/kg/d divided q12h or once q24h **Cefprozil** 15 mg/kg/d divided q12h **Cefuroxime axetil** 30 mg/kg/d divided q12h **All doses are pediatric** **Duration of rx:** <2 yrs old x 10 days; ≥2 yrs x 5–7 days. Appropriate duration unclear. 5 days may be inadequate for severe disease *(NEJM 347:1169, 2002)* **For adult doses, *see Sinusitis, page 53, and Table 10A***	**Received antibiotics in prior month: Amox-clav** 90/6.4 mg/kg/d divided bid OR **Ceftriaxone** 50 mg/kg IV or IM once daily for 3 days Other options include oral **Cefdinir, Cefpodoxime proxetil, Cefprozil,** or **Cefuroxime axetil** but these may be less effective for pen-non-susceptible S. pneumoniae. For adults also: **Levo** or **Moxi**	**β-lactam allergy:** If history unclear or rash, oral ceph OK; avoid ceph if IgE-mediated allergy, e.g., anaphylaxis. **TMP-SMX:** high failure rate if etiology is DRSP or H. influenza. **Macrolides:** limited efficacy against S. pneumo and H. influenza, use only if β-lactam not an option. **Drug-resistant S. pneumo:** Risk ↑ if age <2 yrs, antibiotics last 3 mos, &/or daycare attendance. Selection of drug based on (1) effectiveness against β-lactamase producing H. influenzae & M. catarrhalis & (2) effectiveness against S. pneumo, inc. DRSP. Cefaclor, Loracarbef, & Ceftibuten less active vs. S. pneumo (Pen resistant) than other β-lactams. **Otitis media with effusion:** no benefit of antibiotics *(Cochrane Database Syst Rev. Sep 12:9:CD009163, 2012).* **Persistent otorrhea with PE tubes:** Hydrocortisone/Bacitracin/Colistin eardrops[NUS] 5 drops tid x 7 d more effective than po Amox-clav *(NEJM:370:723, 2014).* **Refractory or recurrent AOM, age 6 months to 5 years:** Levofloxacin 20 mg/kg/d in divided doses q12h if other options have failed. Tympanostomy tubes may prevent recurrent AOM.

 **NOTE: All dosage recommendations are for adults (unless otherwise indicated) and assume normal renal function. § Alternatives consider allergy, PK, compliance, local resistance, cost.*

TABLE 1 (9)

ANATOMIC SITE/DIAGNOSIS/ MODIFYING CIRCUMSTANCES	ETIOLOGIES (usual)	SUGGESTED REGIMENS* PRIMARY	SUGGESTED REGIMENS* ALTERNATIVE§	ADJUNCT DIAGNOSTIC OR THERAPEUTIC MEASURES AND COMMENTS
EAR/Otitis media—infants, children, adults *(continued)*				
Treatment for clinical failure after 3 days	Drug-resistant S. pneumoniae main concern	**NO antibiotics in month prior to last 3 days:** **Amox-clav HD** or **Cefdinir** or **Cefpodoxime** or **Cefprozil** or **Cefuroxime Axetil** or IM **Ceftriaxone** x 3 days *For dosage, see footnote*[3] **All doses are pediatric** Duration of rx as above	**Antibiotics in month prior to last 3 days:** [(IM **Ceftriaxone**) or (**Clinda**) and/or tympanocentesis] *See Comments*	**Clindamycin** not active vs. H. influenzae or M. catarrhalis. S. pneumo resistant to macrolides is usually also resistant to clindamycin. Definition of failure: no change in ear pain, fever, bulging TM or otorrhea after 3 days of therapy. Tympanocentesis will allow culture. **Levo** 20 mg/kg/d in divided doses q12h if other options have failed (not FDA approved).
After >48 hrs of nasotracheal intubation	Pseudomonas sp., klebsiella, enterobacter	**Ceftazidime** or **CFP** or **IMP** or **MER** or (**Pip-tazo**) or **CIP**. *(For dosages, see Ear, Necrotizing (malignant) otitis externa, page 12)*		With nasotracheal intubation >48 hrs, about ½ pts will have otitis media with effusion.
Prophylaxis: acute otitis media **Antimicrobial Stewardship: Use of antibiotics to prevent otitis media is a major contributor to emergence of antibiotic-resistant S. pneumo.**	Pneumococci, H. influenzae, M. catarrhalis, Staph. aureus, Group A strep *(see Comments)*	**Antimicrobial prophylaxis is not recommended.**	Pneumococcal protein conjugate vaccine decreases frequency of acute otitis media infections. Tympanostomy tube may prevent recurrent AOM *(Otolaryn Head Neck Surg 156(4S):S88, 2017)*. Evidence supporting benefits of adenoidectomy are inconclusive *(Cochrane Database Syst Rev 2010:CD008282)* Avoid FQ ear drops post-T-tubes; increased risk of chronic perforation *(NEJM 2017;64:1052)*	
Mastoiditis: Complication of acute or chronic otitis media. If chronic, look for cholesteatoma (Keratoma)				
Acute				
Generally too ill for outpatient therapy.	*1st episode:* S. pneumoniae H. influenzae M. catarrhalis *If secondary to chronic otitis media:* S. aureus P. aeruginosa S. pneumoniae	Obtain cultures, then empiric therapy. 1st episode: **Ceftriaxone** 2 gm IV once daily OR **Levo** 750 mg IV once daily	Acute exacerbation of chronic otitis media: Surgical debridement of auditory canal, then [**Vanco** (dose to achieve tough of 15-20 mcg/mL) + **Pip-tazo** 3.375 gm IV q6h] OR [**Vanco** (dose as above) + **CIP** 400 mg IV q8h]	• Diagnosis: CT or MRI • Look for complication: osteomyelitis, suppurative lateral sinus thrombophlebitis, purulent meningitis, brain abscess • ENT consultation for possible mastoidectomy
Chronic				
Generally not ill enough for parenteral antibiotics	As per 1st episode and: S. aureus P. aeruginosa Anaerobes Fungi	Culture ear drainage. May need surgical debridement. Topical Fluoroquinolone ear drops. ENT consult.		• Diagnosis: CT or MRI

[3] **Drugs & peds dosage (all po unless specified) for acute otitis media: Amoxicillin UD (usual dose)** = 40 mg/kg per day div q12h or q8h. **Amoxicillin HD (high dose)** = 90 mg/kg per day div q12h or q8h. **AM-CL HD** = 90 mg/kg per day of amox component. **Extra-strength Amox-clav oral suspension** (Augmentin ES-600) available with 600 mg AM & 42.9 mg CL / 5 mL—dose: 90/6.4 mg/kg per day div bid. **Cefuroxime axetil** 30 mg/kg per day div q12h. **Ceftriaxone** 50 mg/kg IM x 3 days. **Clindamycin** 20–30 mg/kg per day div qid (may be effective vs. DRSP but no activity vs. H. influenzae). **Other drugs suitable for drug (e.g., Penicillin) - sensitive S. pneumo: TMP-SMX** 4 mg/kg of TMP q12h. **Erythro-sulfisoxazole** 50 mg/kg per day of erythro div q6–8h. **Clarithro** 15 mg/kg per day div q12h; **Azithro** 10 mg/kg per day x 1 & then 5 mg/kg q24h on days 2–5. Other FDA-approved regimens: 10 mg/kg q24h x 3 days & 30 mg/kg x 1. **Cefprozil** 15 mg/kg q12h; **Cefpodoxime proxetil** 10 mg/kg per day as single dose; **Cefaclor** 40 mg/kg per day div q8h. **Cefdinir** 7 mg/kg q12h or 14 mg/kg q24h.

Abbreviations on page 2. **NOTE: All dosage recommendations are for adults (unless otherwise indicated) and assume normal renal function. § Alternatives consider allergy, PK, compliance, local resistance, cost.*

TABLE 1 (10)

ANATOMIC SITE/DIAGNOSIS/ MODIFYING CIRCUMSTANCES	ETIOLOGIES (usual)	SUGGESTED REGIMENS*		ADJUNCT DIAGNOSTIC OR THERAPEUTIC MEASURES AND COMMENTS
		PRIMARY	ALTERNATIVE§	
EYE				
Eyelid: *(See Cochrane Database Syst Rev 5:CD005556, 2012)*				
Blepharitis	Etiol. unclear. Factors include Staph. aureus & Staph. epidermidis, seborrhea, rosacea, & dry eye	Lid margin care with baby shampoo & warm compresses q24h. Artificial tears if assoc. dry eye *(see Comment)*.		Topical ointments of uncertain benefit *(Cochrane Database Syst Rev. 2017 Feb 7;2:CD011965)*. If associated rosacea, add doxy 100 mg po bid for 2 wks and then q24h.
Hordeolum (Stye) Cochrane review of effectiveness of non-surgical interventions found no evidence for or against non-surgical interventions for treatment of acute internal hordeola *(Cochrane Database Syst Rev. 2017 Jan 9;1:CD00774)*.				
External (eyelash follicle)	Staph. aureus	Hot packs only. Will drain spontaneously		Infection of superficial sebaceous gland.
Internal (Meibomian glands): Can be acute, subacute or chronic.	Staph. aureus, MSSA	Oral **Diclox** + hot packs		Also called acute meibomianitis. Rarely drain spontaneously; may need I&D and culture. Role of fluoroquinolone eye drops is unclear. MRSA often resistant to lower conc.; may be susceptible to higher concentration of FQ in ophthalmologic solutions of gati, levo or moxi.
	Staph. aureus, MRSA	**TMP-SMX-DS**, tabs ii po bid		
	Staph. aureus, MRSA (MDR)	**Linezolid** 600 mg po bid		
Conjunctiva: Review: *JAMA 310:1721, 2013.*				
Conjunctivitis of the newborn (ophthalmia neonatorum): by day of onset post-delivery—all dose pediatric				
Onset 1st day	Chemical due to silver nitrate prophylaxis	None		Usual prophylaxis is erythro ointment; hence, silver nitrate irritation rare.
Onset 2–4 days	N. gonorrhoeae	**Ceftriaxone** 25–50 mg/kg IV x 1 dose *(see Comment)*, not to exceed 125 mg		Treat mother and her sexual partners. Hyperpurulent. Topical rx inadequate. **Treat neonate for concomitant Chlamydia trachomatis.**
Onset 3–10 days	Chlamydia trachomatis	**Erythro base or ethylsuccinate syrup** 12.5 mg/kg q6h x 14 days. No topical rx needed.		Diagnosis by NAAT. Alternative: **Azithro suspension** 20 mg/kg po q24h x 3 days. Treat mother & sexual partner.
Onset 2–16 days	Herpes simplex types 1, 2	Topical anti-viral rx under direction of ophthalmologist.		Also give Acyclovir 60 mg/kg/day IV div 3 doses *(Red Book online, accessed Jan 2011)*.
Ophthalmia neonatorum prophylaxis: **Erythro** 0.5% ointment x 1 or **Tetra** 1% ointment[NUS] x 1 application; effective vs. gonococcus but not C. trachomatis				
Pink eye (viral conjunctivitis) Usually unilateral	Adenovirus (types 3 & 7 in children, 8, 11 & 19 in adults)	No treatment. If symptomatic, artificial tears may help. (some studies show 2 day reduction of symptoms with steroids; not recommended)		Highly contagious. Onset of ocular pain and photophobia in an adult suggests associated keratitis—rare.
Inclusion conjunctivitis (adult) Usually unilateral & concomitant genital infection	Chlamydia trachomatis	**Azithro** 1 gm once	**Doxy** 100 mg po bid x 7 days	Oculogenital disease. Diagnosis NAAT. Urine NAAT for both GC & chlamydia. Treat sexual partner. May need to repeat dose of azithro.
Trachoma —a chronic bacterial keratoconjunctivitis linked to poverty	Chlamydia trachomatis	**Azithro** 20 mg/kg po single dose—78% effective in children; Adults: 1 gm po.	**Doxy** 100 mg po bid x minimum of 21 days or **Tetracycline** 250 mg po qid x 14 days.	Starts in childhood and can persist for years with subsequent damage to cornea. Topical therapy of marginal benefit. Avoid doxy/tetracycline in young children. Mass treatment works.
Suppurative conjunctivitis, bacterial: Children and Adults (Eyedrops speed resolution of symptoms: *Cochrane Database Syst Rev. Sep 12;9:CD001211, 2012)*				
JAMA 310:1721, 2013	Staph. aureus, S. pneumoniae, H. influenzae, Viridans Strep., Moraxella sp.	FQ ophthalmic solns: **CIP** (generic); others expensive (**Besi, Levo, Moxi**) All 1-2 gtts q2h while awake 1st 2 days, then q4–8h up to 7 days.	**Polymyxin B + TMP** solution 1–2 gtts q3–6h x 7–10 days.	**FQs** best spectrum for empiric therapy. High concentrations ↑ likelihood of activity vs. S. aureus—even MRSA. **TMP** spectrum may include MRSA. Polymyxin B spectrum only Gm-neg. bacilli but no ophthal. prep of only **TMP**. Most S. pneumo resistant to Gent & Tobra.
Gonococcal (peds/adults)	N. gonorrhoeae	**Ceftriaxone** 25-50 mg/kg IV/IM (not to exceed 125 mg) as one dose in children; 1 gm IM/IV as one dose in adults		

Abbreviations on page 2. **NOTE: All dosage recommendations are for adults (unless otherwise indicated) and assume normal renal function. § Alternatives consider allergy, PK, compliance, local resistance, cost.*

TABLE 1 (11)

ANATOMIC SITE/DIAGNOSIS/ MODIFYING CIRCUMSTANCES	ETIOLOGIES (usual)	SUGGESTED REGIMENS*		ADJUNCT DIAGNOSTIC OR THERAPEUTIC MEASURES AND COMMENTS
		PRIMARY	ALTERNATIVE§	
EYE *(continued)*				
Cornea (keratitis): Usually serious and often sight-threatening. Prompt ophthalmologic consultation essential for diagnosis, antimicrobial and adjunctive therapy! Herpes simplex most common etiology in developed countries; bacterial and fungal infections more common in underdeveloped countries.				
Viral				
H. simplex *(See Clin Exp Ophthalmol 44:824, 2016)* Adenovirus uncommon etiology *(Cur Opin Ophthalmology 29: 365-72, 2018)*	H. simplex, types 1 & 2	**Trifluridine** ophthalmic sol'n, one drop q2h up to 9 drops/ day until re-epithelialized, then one drop q4h up to 5x/ day, for total not to exceed 21 days. *See Comment*	**Ganciclovir** 0.15% ophthalmic gel: Indicated for acute herpetic keratitis. One drop 5 times per day while awake until corneal ulcer heals; then, one drop three times per day for 7 days.	**For severe infection or immunocompromised host**, consider adding **acyclovir** 400 mg po 5x daily or **valacyclovir** 1000 mg bid. Topical acyclovir 3% ointment 5x daily is a first-line treatment for HSV epithelial keratitis outside the United States. Approx 30% recurrence rate within one year; consider prophylaxis with acyclovir 400 mg bid for 12 months or valacyclovir 500 mg once daily to prevent recurrences.
Varicella-zoster ophthalmicus	Varicella-zoster virus	**Famciclovir** 500 mg po tid or **Valacyclovir** 1 gm po tid x 10 days	**Acyclovir** 800 mg po 5x/day x 10 days	Clinical diagnosis most common: dendritic figures with fluorescein staining in patient with varicella-zoster of ophthalmic branch of trigeminal nerve.
Bacterial		**All treatment listed for bacterial, fungal, protozoan is topical unless otherwise indicated**		
Acute: No comorbidity	*S. aureus, S. pneumo., S. pyogenes, Haemophilus sp.*	**Moxi:** ophthalmic 0.5%: 1 drop q1h for the first 48h then taper according to response	**CIP** 0.3% ophthal or **Levo** 0.5% ophthal. 1-2 gtts/hr x 24-72 hrs, then taper OR **Gati** eye drops: 1-2 gtts q2h while awake x 2 days, then q4h x 3-7 days	Regimens vary: some start rx by applying drops q5 min for 5 doses; some apply drops q15-30 min for several hours; some extend interval to q2h during sleep. In a clinical trial, drops were applied q1h for 48-72h, then q2h through day 6; then q2h during waking hours on days 7-9; then q6h until healing *(Cornea 29:751, 2010)*. **NOTE:** despite high concentrations, may fail vs. MRSA. Prior use of fluoroquinolones associated with increased MICs *(JAMA Ophthalmol. 131:310, 2013)*; high MICs associated with poorer outcome *(Clin Infect Dis 54:1381, 2012)*.
Contact lens users	P. aeruginosa	**CIP** 0.3% ophthalmic solution or **Levo** 0.5% ophthalmic solution 1-2 gtts hourly x24-72h, taper based on response.	**Gent** or **Tobra** 0.3% ophthalmic solution 1-2 gtts hourly x24h then taper based on clinical response.	Recommend alginate swab culture and susceptibility testing; refer to ophthalmologist. **Cornea abrasions:** treated with Tobra, Gent, or CIP gtts qid for 3-5 days; referral to ophthalmologist recommended cornea infiltrate or ulcer, visual loss, lack of improvement or worsening symptoms *(Am Fam Physician. 87:114, 2013)*.
Dry cornea, diabetes, immunosuppression	Staph. aureus, S. epidermidis, S. pneumoniae, S. pyogenes, Enterobacteriaceae, listeria	**CIP** 0.3% ophthalmic solution 1-2 gtts hourly x24-72 hrs, then taper based on clinical response.	**Vanco** (50 mg/mL) + **Ceftaz** (50 mg/mL) hourly for 24-72h, taper depending upon response. *See Comment.*	Specific therapy guided by results of alginate swab culture.
Fungal	Aspergillus, fusarium, candida and others.	**Natamycin** (5%): 1 drop q1-2h for several days; then q3-4h for several days; can reduce frequency depending upon response.	**Amphotericin B** (0.15%): 1 drop q1-2h for several days; can reduce frequency depending upon response.	Obtain specimens for fungal wet mount and cultures. Numerous other treatment options (**Itra** 1% topical x 6 wks, **Itra** 100 mg po bid x 3 wks, Vori 1% topical x 2 wks, **Miconazole** 1% topical 5x daily, **silver sulphadiazine** 0.5-1% topical 5x daily) appear to have similar efficacy *(Cochrane Database Syst Rev 2:004241, 2012)*

 **NOTE: All dosage recommendations are for adults (unless otherwise indicated) and assume normal renal function. § Alternatives consider allergy, PK, compliance, local resistance, cost.*

TABLE 1 (12)

ANATOMIC SITE/DIAGNOSIS/ MODIFYING CIRCUMSTANCES	ETIOLOGIES (usual)	SUGGESTED REGIMENS*		ADJUNCT DIAGNOSTIC OR THERAPEUTIC MEASURES AND COMMENTS
		PRIMARY	ALTERNATIVE§	
EYE/Cornea (keratitis) *(continued)*				
Mycobacteria: Post-refractive eye surgery	*M. chelonae; M. abscessus*	**Gati** or **Moxi** eye drops: 1 gtt qid in conjunction with other active antimicrobial eyedrops (**Amikacin** 50 mg/L and **Clarithro** 10 mg/L).		**Alternative:** systemic rx: **Doxy** 100 mg po bid + **Clarithro** 500 mg po bid *(PLoS One 10:doi16236, 2015).*
Protozoan Soft contact lens users. Ref: *CID 35:434, 2002.* Uncommon. Trauma and soft contact lenses are risk factors.	Acanthamoeba, sp.	Topical 0.02%-0.2% biguanide chlorhexidine or 0.02%-0.06% Polyhexamethylene biguanide (PHMB) in combination with propamidine (0.1 %) or hexamidine (0.1 %). Start with lower dose of PHMB and titrate to clinical response.		Initially, drops should be applied up to hourly day and night for the first 48 hours then hourly during the daytime for the first week, then with subsequent taper over 3 - 4 weeks. Debridement may also be warranted *(https://www.cdc.gov/parasites/acanthamoeba/health_professionals/acanthamoeba_keratitis_hcp.html).*
Lacrimal apparatus				
Canaliculitis	Actinomyces Staph., Strept. Rarely, Arachnia, fusobacterium, nocardia, candida	Apply hot packs to punctal area 4x/day. Refer to ophthalmologist for removal of granules and local irrigation with an antibiotic solution.		Digital pressure produces exudate at punctum; Gram stain confirms diagnosis.
Dacryocystitis (lacrimal sac)	S. pneumo, S. aureus, H. influenzae, S. pyogenes, P. aeruginosa	Often consequence of obstruction of lacrimal duct. Empiric systemic antimicrobial therapy based on Gram stain of aspirate—*see Comment.*		Need ophthalmologic consultation. Surgery may be required. Can be acute or chronic. Culture to detect MRSA.
Endophthalmitis: Endogenous (secondary to bacteremia or fungemia) and exogenous (post-injection, post-operative) types. **Ophthalmologic consult imperative.**				
Bacterial: Haziness of vitreous key to diagnosis. Needle aspirate of both vitreous and aqueous humor for culture prior to therapy. Intravitreal administration of antimicrobials essential.				
Postocular surgery (cataracts)				
Early, acute onset (incidence 0.05%)	S. epidermidis 60%, Staph. aureus, streptococci, & enterococci each 5–10%, Gm-neg. bacilli 6%	**Immediate ophthal. consult.** If only light perception or worse, immediate vitrectomy + intravitreal vanco 1 mg & intravitreal ceftazidime 2.25 mg.		
Low grade, chronic	Cutibacterium acnes, S. epidermidis, S. aureus (rare)	Intraocular **Vanco**. Usually requires vitrectomy, lens removal.		
Post filtering blebs for glaucoma	Strep. species (viridans & others), H. influenzae	Referral to ophthalmologist for intravitreal **Vanco** 1 mg + **Ceftaz** 2.25 mg and a topical ophthalmic antimicrobial.		
Post-penetrating trauma	Bacillus sp., S. epiderm.	Referral to ophthalmologist for intravitreal **Vanco** 1 mg + (**Ceftaz** 2.25 mg or **Amikacin** 0.4 mg) + systemic **Vanco** 15-20 mg/kg IV q8-12h + [**Ceftaz** 1 g IV q8h or **CIP** 400 mg IV/po q12h]. Vitrectomy may be required.		
Hematogenous	S. pneumoniae, N. meningitidis, Staph. aureus, Grp B Strep, K. pneumo	(**Cefotaxime** 2 gm IV q4h or **Ceftriaxone** 2 gm IV q24h) + **Vanco** 30-60 mg/kg/day IV in 2-3 div doses to achieve target trough serum concentration of 15-20 mcg/mL pending cultures. Intravitreal antibiotics as with early postocular surgery. Urgent ophthalmological consultation.		
IV heroin abuse	S. aureus, Bacillus cereus, Candida sp.	Empirically, as above for hematogenous with definitive therapy based on etiology and antimicrobial susceptibility. Urgent ophthalmological consultation.		

 **NOTE: All dosage recommendations are for adults (unless otherwise indicated) and assume normal renal function. § Alternatives consider allergy, PK, compliance, local resistance, cost.*

TABLE 1 (13)

ANATOMIC SITE/DIAGNOSIS/ MODIFYING CIRCUMSTANCES	ETIOLOGIES (usual)	SUGGESTED REGIMENS*		ADJUNCT DIAGNOSTIC OR THERAPEUTIC MEASURES AND COMMENTS
		PRIMARY	ALTERNATIVE§	
EYE/Endophthalmitis *(continued)*				
Mycotic (fungal): Broad-spectrum antibiotics, often corticosteroids, indwelling venous catheters	Candida sp., Aspergillus sp.	Intravitreal **Ampho B** 0.005–0.01 mg in 0.1 mL. *Also see Table 11A, page 135 for concomitant systemic therapy. See Comment.*		Patients with *Candida* spp. chorioretinitis usually respond to systemically administered antifungals *(Clin Infect Dis 53:262, 2011)*. Intravitreal ampho and/or vitrectomy may be necessary for those with vitritis or endophthalmitis. *(IDSA guidelines CID 62:409, 2016).*
Retinitis				
Acute retinal necrosis	Varicella zoster virus (VZV), Herpes simplex	IV **Acyclovir** 10–12 mg/kg IV q8h x 5–7 days, then **Acyclovir** 800 mg po 5 x/day OR **Valacyclovir** 1000 mg po tid OR **Famciclovir** 500 mg po tid		Strong association of VZ virus with atypical necrotizing herpetic retinopathy. Ophthalmology consultation.
HIV+ (AIDS) CD4 usually <100/mm³	Cytomegalovirus	*See Table 14A, page 180*		Occurs in 5–10% of AIDS patients
Progressive outer retinal necrosis	VZV, H. simplex, CMV (rare)	**Acyclovir** 10-12 mg/kg IV q8h for 1-2 weeks, then (**Valacyclovir** 1000 mg po tid, or **Famciclovir** 500 mg po tid, or **Acyclovir** 800 mg po tid). Ophthalmology consultation imperative: approaches have also included intra-vitreal injection of anti-virals (foscarnet, ganciclovir implant). In rare cases due to CMV use **Ganciclovir/Valganciclovir** *(see CMV retinitis, Table 14A).*		Most patients are highly immunocompromised (HIV with low CD4 or transplantation). In contrast to Acute Retinal Necrosis, lack of intraocular inflammation or arteritis. May be able to stop oral antivirals when CD4 recovers with ART *(Ocul Immunol Inflammation 15:425, 2007).*
Orbital cellulitis *(see page 57 for erysipelas, facial)*	S. pneumoniae, H. influenzae, M. catarrhalis, S. aureus, anaerobes, group A strep, occ. Gm-neg. bacilli post-trauma	**Vanco** 15-20 mg/kg IV q8-12h (target trough serum concentrations of 15-20 μg/mL) + ([**Ceftriaxone** 2 gm IV q24h + **Metro** 1 gm IV q12h] OR **Pip-tazo** 3.375 gm IV q6h		**If Penicillin/Ceph allergy: Vanco** + **Moxi** 400 mg IV q24h. Problem is frequent inability to make microbiologic diagnosis. Image orbit (CT or MRI). Risk of cavernous sinus thrombosis. If vanco intolerant, another option for S. aureus is dapto 8-10 mg/kg IV q24h.

 **NOTE: All dosage recommendations are for adults (unless otherwise indicated) and assume normal renal function. § Alternatives consider allergy, PK, compliance, local resistance, cost.*

TABLE 1 (14)

ANATOMIC SITE/DIAGNOSIS/ MODIFYING CIRCUMSTANCES	ETIOLOGIES (usual)	SUGGESTED REGIMENS*		ADJUNCT DIAGNOSTIC OR THERAPEUTIC MEASURES AND COMMENTS
		PRIMARY	ALTERNATIVE§	
FOOT				
"Diabetic foot"—Two thirds of patients have triad of neuropathy, deformity and pressure-induced trauma. IDSA Guidelines *CID 54:e132, 2012.*				
Ulcer without inflammation	Colonizing skin flora	No antibacterial therapy.		**General:** 1. Glucose control, eliminate pressure on ulcer 2. **Assess for peripheral vascular disease** 3. Caution in use of TMP-SMX in patients with diabetes, as many have risk factors for hyperkalemia (e.g., advanced age, reduced renal function, concomitant medications) *(Arch Intern Med 170:1045, 2010).* 4. Improved outcomes in healing of diabetic foot ulcer with negative-pressure wound therapy (See *Curr Opin Infect Dis 29:145, 2016* for review). **Principles of empiric antibacterial therapy:** 1. Obtain culture; cover for MRSA in moderate, more severe infections pending culture data, local epidemiology. 2. Severe limb and/or life-threatening infections require initial parenteral therapy with predictable activity vs. Gm-positive cocci including MRSA, coliforms & other aerobic Gm-neg. rods, & anaerobic Gm-neg. bacilli. 3. **NOTE:** The regimens listed are suggestions consistent with above principles. Other alternatives exist & may be appropriate for individual patients. 4. Risk of associated osteomyelitis is increased if ulcer area >2 cm², positive probe to bone *(CID 2016,63:944),* ESR >70 and abnormal plain x-ray. Negative MRI reduces likelihood of osteomyelitis *(JAMA 299:806, 2008).* MRI is best imaging modality *(CID 47:519 & 528, 2008).*
Mild infection	*S. aureus (assume MRSA), S. agalactiae (Gp B), S. pyogenes predominate*	**Oral therapy: Diclox** or **Cephalexin** or **Amox-clav** (not MRSA) **Doxy** or **TMP-SMX-DS** (MRSA) **Clinda** (covers MSSA, MRSA, strep) *Dosages in footnote*[4]		
Moderate infection. **Osteomyelitis** *See Comment.*	As above, plus coliforms possible	**Oral:** As above **Parenteral therapy:** [based on prevailing susceptibilities: (**Amp-sulb** or **Pip-tazo** or **ERTA** or other carbapenem)] plus [**Vanco** (or alternative anti-MRSA drug as below) until MRSA excluded]. *Dosages in footnotes*[5,6]		
Extensive local inflammation plus systemic toxicity.	As above, plus anaerobic bacteria. Role of enterococci unclear.	**Parenteral therapy:** (**Vanco** plus **β-lactam/β-lactamase inhibitor**) or (**vanco** plus [**DORI** or **IMP** or **MER**]). Other alternatives: 1. **Dapto** or **Linezolid** for vanco 2. (**CIP** or **Levo** or **Aztreonam**) plus **Metronidazole** for β-lactam/β-lactamase inhibitor *Dosages in footnote*[6] **Assess for arterial insufficiency!**		
Onychomycosis: *See Table 11, page 138, fungal infections*				
Puncture wound: Nail/Toothpick	P. aeruginosa (Nail), S. aureus, Strept (Toothpick)	Cleanse. Tetanus booster. Observe.		*See Osteomyelitis, page 5.* 1–2% evolves to osteo.
GALLBLADDER				
Cholecystitis, cholangitis, biliary sepsis, or common duct obstruction (partial: 2nd to tumor, stones, stricture).	Enterobacteriaceae 68%, enterococci 14%, bacteroides 10%, Clostridium sp. 7%, rarely candida	(**Pip-tazo** or **Amp-sulb**) If life-threatening: **IMP** or **MER** or **DORI** *Dosages in footnote*[6] *on page 18.* * Add **Vanco** for empiric activity vs. enterococci	(**P Ceph 3*** + **Metro**) or (**Aztreonam*** + **Metro**) or (**CIP*** + **Metro**) or **Moxi**	In severely ill pts, antibiotic therapy complements adequate biliary drainage. 15-30% pts will require decompression: surgical, percutaneous or ERCP-placed stent. Gallbladder bile is culture pos. in 40-60% *(J Infect 51:128, 2005).* No benefit to continuation of antibiotics after surgery in pts with acute calculous cholecystitis *(JAMA 3312:145, 2014).*

[4] **TMP-SMX-DS** 1-2 tabs po bid, **Minocycline** 100 mg po bid, **Pen VK** 500 mg po qid, (O Ceph 2, 3: **Cefprozil** 500 mg po q12h, **Cefuroxime axetil** 500 mg po q12h, **Cefdinir** 300 mg po q12h or 600 mg po q24h, **Cefpodoxime** 200 mg po q12h), **CIP** 750 mg po bid. **Levo** 750 mg po q24h. **Diclox** 500 mg qid. **Cephalexin** 500 mg qid. **Amox-clav** 875/125 bid. **Doxy** 100 mg bid (now considered safe, regardless of age, for rx ≤21 days). **Clinda** 300-450 mg tid.

[5] **AM-CL-ER** 2000/125 mg po bid, **TMP-SMX-DS** 1-2 tabs po bid, **CIP** 750 mg po bid, **Levo** 750 mg po q24h, **Moxi** 400 mg po q24h, **Linezolid** 600 mg po bid.

[6] **Vanco** 1 gm IV q12h, (**parenteral β-lactam/β-lactamase inhibitors**; **Amp-sulb** 3 gm IV q6h, **Pip-tazo** 3.375 gm IV q6h or 4.5 gm IV q8h or 4 hr infusion of 3.375 gm q8h; **carbapenems: Doripenem** 500 mg (1-hr infusion) q8h, **ERTA** 1 gm IV q24h, **IMP** 0.5 gm IV q6h, **MER** 1 gm IV q8h, **Dapto** 6 mg per kg IV q24h, **Linezolid** 600 mg IV q12h, **Aztreonam** 2 gm IV q8h. **CIP** 400 mg IV q12h, **Levo** 750 mg IV q24h, **Moxi** 400 mg IV q24h, **Metro** 1 gm IV loading dose & then 0.5 gm IV q6h or 1 gm IV q12h.

Abbreviations on page 2. **NOTE: All dosage recommendations are for adults (unless otherwise indicated) and assume normal renal function. § Alternatives consider allergy, PK, compliance, local resistance, cost.*

TABLE 1 (15)

ANATOMIC SITE/DIAGNOSIS/ MODIFYING CIRCUMSTANCES	ETIOLOGIES (usual)	SUGGESTED REGIMENS*		ADJUNCT DIAGNOSTIC OR THERAPEUTIC MEASURES AND COMMENTS
		PRIMARY	ALTERNATIVE§	
GASTROINTESTINAL				
Gastroenteritis—Empiric Therapy (laboratory studies not performed or culture, microscopy, toxin results NOT AVAILABLE) *NEJM 370:16, 2014*; **IDSA Guideline (Diarrhea):** ***CID 2017,65:1963 & e45.***				
Premature infant with necrotizing enterocolitis	Associated with intestinal flora	Treatment should cover broad range of intestinal bacteria using drugs appropriate to age and local susceptibility patterns, rationale as in diverticulitis/peritonitis, *page 24*.		Pneumatosis intestinalis, if present on x-ray confirms diagnosis. Bacteremia-peritonitis in 30-50%. If Staph. epidermidis isolated, add vanco (IV). For review and general management, *see NEJM 364:255, 2011.*
Mild diarrhea (≤3 unformed stools/day, minimal associated symptomatology)	Bacterial *(see Severe, below)*, viral (norovirus), parasitic. Viral usually causes mild to moderate disease. For traveler's diarrhea, *see page 22*	Fluids only + lactose-free diet, avoid caffeine		**Rehydration: For po fluid replacement,** *see Cholera, page 21.* **Antimotility** (Do not use if fever, bloody stools, or suspicion of HUS): Loperamide (Imodium) 4 mg po, then 2 mg after each loose stool to max. of 16 mg per day. Bismuth subsalicylate (Pepto-Bismol) 2 tablets (262 mg) po qid. **Hemolytic uremic syndrome (HUS):** Risk in **children** infected with E. coli 0157:H7 is 8-10%. Early treatment with TMP-SMX or FQs ↑ risk of HUS. **Norovirus:** Etiology of over 90% of non-bacterial diarrhea (± nausea/ vomiting). Lasts 12-60 hrs. Hydrate. No effective antiviral. **Other potential etiologies (parasitic):** Cryptosporidia—no treatment in immunocompetent host. Cyclospora—usually chronic diarrhea, responds to TMP-SMX *(see Table 13A)*. Klebsiella oxytoca identified as cause of antibiotic-associated hemorrhagic colitis (cytotoxin positive): *NEJM 355:2418, 2006.*
Moderate diarrhea (≥4 unformed stools/day &/or systemic symptoms)		Antimotility agents *(see Comments)* + fluids		
Severe diarrhea (≥6 unformed stools/day, &/or temp ≥101°F, tenesmus, blood, or fecal leukocytes). **NOTE: Severe afebrile bloody diarrhea should ↑ suspicion of Shiga-toxin E. coli 0157:H7 & others** *(MMWR 58 (RR-12):1, 2009).*	Shigella, salmonella, C. jejuni, Shiga toxin + E. coli, toxin-positive C. difficile, Klebsiella oxytoca, E. histolytica. *For typhoid fever, see page 65*	**Azithro** 1000 mg po x 1 dose or 500 mg po q12h x 3 days	**CIP** 750 mg po x 1 dose, continue for 3 days if not resolved OR 500 mg po q12 x 3 days	
		If recent antibiotic therapy (C. difficile toxin colitis possible) *promptly test stool for C. diff. toxin*		
Gastroenteritis—Specific Therapy (results of culture, microscopy, toxin assay AVAILABLE) Ref.: *NEJM 370:1532, 2014*; IDSA infectious diarrhea guideline *(CID 2017,65:1963).*				
If culture negative, probably **Norovirus (Norwalk)** other virus *(EID 17:1381, 2011) — see Norovirus, page 187*	**Aeromonas/Plesiomonas**	**CIP** 750 mg po bid x 3 days.	**TMP-SMX DS** tab 1 po bid x 3 days	Aeromonas ref: *Eur J Clin Microbiol ID. 36:1393, 2017.*
	Amebiasis (Entamoeba histolytica, Cyclospora, Cryptosporidia and **Giardia)**, *see Table 13A*			
NOTE: WBC >15,000 suggestive of C. difficile in hospitalized patient.	**Campylobacter jejuni** History of fever in 53-83%. Self-limited diarrhea in normal host.	**Azithro** 500 mg po q24h x 3 days OR 1000 mg po one dose	**Erythro stearate** 500 mg po qid x 5 days or **CIP** 500 mg po bid (CIP resistance increasing) *(CID 2017;65:1624).*	**Post-Campylobacter Guillain-Barré;** assoc. 15% of cases *(Ln 366:1653, 2005).* Assoc. with small bowel lymphoproliferative disease; may respond to antimicrobials *(NEJM 350:239, 2004).* **Reactive arthritis** another potential sequelae. *See Traveler's diarrhea, page 22.*
	Campylobacter fetus Diarrhea uncommon. More systemic disease in debilitated hosts	**Genta** *(see Table 10C)*	**AMP** 100 mg/kg/day IV div q6h or **IMP** 500 mg IV q6h	Draw blood cultures. In bacteremic pts, FQ resistance common in *C. fetus*. Meropenem inhibits C. fetus at low concentrations in vitro. Clinical review: *CID 58:1579, 2014.*

 **NOTE: All dosage recommendations are for adults (unless otherwise indicated) and assume normal renal function. § Alternatives consider allergy, PK, compliance, local resistance, cost.*

TABLE 1 (16)

ANATOMIC SITE/DIAGNOSIS/ MODIFYING CIRCUMSTANCES	ETIOLOGIES (usual)	SUGGESTED REGIMENS* PRIMARY	SUGGESTED REGIMENS* ALTERNATIVE§	ADJUNCT DIAGNOSTIC OR THERAPEUTIC MEASURES AND COMMENTS
GASTROINTESTINAL/Gastroenteritis—Specific Therapy (results of culture, microscopy, toxin assay AVAILABLE) *(continued)*				
Differential diagnosis of toxin-producing diarrhea: • *C. difficile* • *Klebsiella oxytoca* • *S. aureus* • Shiga toxin producing *E. coli* (STEC) • Enterotoxigenic *B. fragilis*	**C. difficile toxin positive antibiotic-associated colitis. Probiotics:** Cochrane review found moderate quality evidence the probiotics prevents C. diff. associated diarrhea *(Cochrane Database Syst Rev. 2017 Dec 19;12:CD006095).*			
	po meds okay; WBC <15,000; no increase in serum creatinine.	**Vanco** 125 mg po qid x 10 days	*See Comment*	**D/C antibiotic if possible; avoid antimotility agents, hydration, enteric isolation.** Recent review suggests antimotility agents can be used cautiously in certain pts with mild disease who are receiving rx *(CID 48:598, 2009).* **Relapse in 10-20%.** Note: **Metro 500 mg tid no longer recommended as first-line therapy and should be used only if resources prelude access to Vanco or Fidaxomicin.**
IDSA Guidelines *(C. diff)*: *CID 2018,66:987* Rarely, *C. diff.* infection can involve small intestine in post-colectomy pts *(OFID doi:10.1093/ofid/ofy409)*	po meds okay; Sicker; WBC >15,000; ≥50% increase in baseline creatinine	**Vanco** 125 mg po qid x 10 days. For oral use of IV Vanco, *see Table 10A, page 119.*	**Fidaxomicin** 200 mg po bid x 10 days	**Vanco superior to metro in sicker pts.** Relapse in 10-20%. Fidaxomicin had lower rate of recurrence than Vanco for diarrhea with non-NAP1 strains *(N Engl J Med 364:422, 2011).* Bezlotoxumab 1 dose IV + standard rx reduced relapse rate 11-14% *(NEJM 2017, 376:305).*
	Post-treatment relapse	**Vanco** 125 mg po qid x 10-14 days, then immediately start taper *(See Comments)*	**Fidaxomicin** 200 mg po bid x 10 days	**Vanco taper** (all doses 125 mg po): week 1 – tid, week 2 – bid week 3 – q24h week 4 – q48h, week 5 – q72h. Ref: *CID 2017;65:1624.* **Fecal transplant** more efficacious than Vanco (15/16 [93%] versus 7/26 [27%]) in curing recurrent C. difficile infection *(New Engl J Med 368:407, 2013).* Pre-transplant Vanco taper increases success of fecal transplants *(CID 2017;65:1214).* **Bezlotoxumab**, anti C. diff toxin B approved, decreases recurrence 10% but very expensive *CID 68:699, 2019.* If **Metro** used for initial therapy can use standard 10-day course of **Vanco**.
	Post-op ileus; severe disease with toxic megacolon *(NEJM 359:1932, 2008; CID 61:934, 2015).*	**Metro** 500 mg IV q8h + **Vanco** 500 mg q6h via nasogastric tube (or naso-small bowel tube) ± vanco 500 mg q6h retention enema. *See comment* for dosage. No data on efficacy of **Fidaxomicin** in severe life-threatening disease.		For vanco instillation into bowel, add 500 mg vanco to 500 mL of saline. **NOTE: IV vanco not effective.** Indications for colectomy, *see ICHE 31:431, 2010.*
	Enterohemorrhagic E. coli (EHEC): 0157:H7 & 0104:H4 & others. Hemolytic uremic syndrome complicates 6-9% *(see Comment)*	Treatment: 1. If afebrile, bloody diarrhea: a. Hydration b. Avoid antiperistaltic drugs c. No antibiotics 2. If febrile, bloody diarrhea, risk of bacteremia: **Azithro** 500 mg IV/po once daily x 3 d		**Risk of antibiotic therapy is HUS due to Shiga toxin production.** HUS = renal failure, hemolytic anemia, thrombocytopenia. Risk of HUS with antibiotic use for EHEC: OR 2.24 (CI 1.45-3.46). Hence, restrict antibiotics to patients with increased risk of, or documentation of, bacteremia due to EHEC. Refs: *CID 2016,62:1251 & 1259; CID 2012,55:33; Infection 1992,20:25; JID 2000,181:664.*
	Klebsiella oxytoca— antibiotic-associated diarrhea	Responds to stopping antibiotic		Suggested that stopping NSAIDs helps. Ref.: *NEJM 355:2418, 2006.*
(Continued on next page)	**Listeria monocytogenes**	Usually self-limited. Value of oral antibiotics (e.g., AMP or TMP-SMX) unknown, but their use might be reasonable in populations at risk for serious listeria infections. Those with bacteremia/meningitis require parenteral therapy: *see pages 10 & 65.*		Recognized as a cause of food-associated febrile gastroenteritis. Not detected in standard stool cultures. Populations at ↑ risk of severe systemic disease: pregnant women, neonates, the elderly, and immunocompromised hosts *(MMWR 57:1097, 2008).*

 **NOTE: All dosage recommendations are for adults (unless otherwise indicated) and assume normal renal function. § Alternatives consider allergy, PK, compliance, local resistance, cost.*

TABLE 1 (17)

ANATOMIC SITE/DIAGNOSIS/ MODIFYING CIRCUMSTANCES	ETIOLOGIES (usual)	SUGGESTED REGIMENS* PRIMARY	SUGGESTED REGIMENS* ALTERNATIVE§	ADJUNCT DIAGNOSTIC OR THERAPEUTIC MEASURES AND COMMENTS
GASTROINTESTINAL/Gastroenteritis—Specific Therapy (results of culture, microscopy, toxin assay AVAILABLE) *(continued)*				
(Continued from previous page)	**Salmonella, non-typhi—** For typhoid (enteric) fever, *see page 65* Fever in 71–91%, history of bloody stools in 34%	**If asymptomatic or illness mild, antimicrobial therapy not indicated. Treat if:** age <1 yr or >50 yrs, immunocompromised, vascular grafts or prosthetic joints, bacteremic, hemoglobinopathy, or hospitalized with fever and severe diarrhea *(see typhoid fever, page 65)*.		
		(**CIP** 500 mg bid) or (**Levo** 500 mg q24h) x 7-10 days (14 days if immunocompromised).	**Azithro** 500 mg po once daily x 7 days (14 days if immunocompromised).	↑ resistance to TMP-SMX and chloro. Ceftriaxone, cefotaxime usually active if IV therapy required *(see footnote⁹ on page 27, for dosage)*. CLSI has established new interpretive breakpoints for susceptibility to CIP: susceptible strains, MIC ≤0.06 µg/mL *(Clin Infect Dis 55:1107, 2012)*. **Primary treatment of enteritis is fluid and electrolyte replacement.**
	Shigella Fever in 58%, history of bloody stools 51%	**CIP** 750 mg qd or po bid x 3 days	**Azithro** 500 mg po once daily x 3 days	**Immunocompromised children & adults: Treat for 7–10 days.** Pockets of resistance: *S. flexneri* resist to CIP & Ceftriaxone *(MMWR 59:1619, 2010)*; *S. sonnei* resist to CIP in travelers *(MMWR 64:318, 2015)*; *S. sonnei* suscept to CIP but resist to azithro in MSM *(MMWR 64:597, 2015)*. CDC recommends avoiding CIP if MIC ≥0.12 µg/mL *(CDC Health Alert Network, Apr 18, 2017)*. For most individuals, treatment not necessary. May be associated with traveler's diarrhea, where one dose of treatment may be sufficient.
		Pockets of resistance *(see Comment)* **Peds doses: Azithro** 10 mg/kg/day once daily x 3 days. For severe disease, **Ceftriaxone** 50–75 mg/kg per day x 2–5 days. **CIP** suspension 10 mg/kg bid x 5 days.		
	Spirochetosis (Brachyspira pilosicoli)	Benefit of treatment unclear. Susceptible to **Metro**, **Ceftriaxone**, and **Moxi**.		Anaerobic intestinal spirochete that colonizes colon of domestic & wild animals plus humans. Called enigmatic disease due to uncertain status *(Digest Dis & Sci 58:202, 2013)*.
	Vibrio cholerae (toxigenic - 01 & 039) Treatment decreases duration of disease, volume losses, & duration of excretion	**Primary therapy is rehydration.** Select antibiotics based on susceptibility of locally prevailing isolates. Options include: **Doxy** 300 mg po single dose, **Azithro** 1 gm po single dose, **Tetra** 500 mg po qid x 3 days, **Erythro** 500 mg po qid x 3 days.	**Pregnancy: Azithro** 1 gm po single dose **OR Erythro** 500 mg po qid x 3 days **Peds: Azithro** 20 mg/kg po as single dose; for other age-specific alternatives, *see CDC website http://www.cdc.gov/haiticholera/hcp_goingtohaiti.htm*	**Antimicrobial therapy shortens duration of illness, but rehydration is paramount.** When IV hydration is needed, use Ringer's lactate. Switch to po repletion with Oral Rehydration Salts (ORS) as soon as able to take oral fluids. ORS are commercially available for reconstitution in potable water. If not available, WHO suggests a substitute can be made by dissolving ½ teaspoon salt and 6 level teaspoons of sugar per liter of potable water *(http://www.who.int/cholera/technical/en/)*. CDC recommendations for other aspects of management developed for Haiti outbreak can be found at *http://www.cdc.gov/haiticholera/hcp_goingtohaiti.htm* Isolates from this outbreak demonstrate reduced susceptibility to ciprofloxacin and resistance to sulfisoxazole, nalidixic acid and furazolidone. Vaccine for cholera available *(Med Lett Drugs Ther. 58:113, 2016)*.
	Vibrio parahaemolyticus, V. mimicus, V. fluvialis	**Antimicrobial rx does not shorten course. Hydration.**		Shellfish exposure common. Treat severe disease: **FQ, Doxy, P Ceph 3**
	Vibrio vulnificus Usual presentation is skin lesions & bacteremia; life-threatening	Adult: (**Doxy** or **Minocycline** 100 mg IV/po bid) + (**Ceftriaxone** 2 gm IV once daily or **Ceftaz** 1 gm IV q8h). Peds: **Doxy** 4.4 mg/kg/day div bid (max 200 mg/day). Alternatives: **Levo** or **CIP**. Ref: *Epidemiol Infect. 142:878, 2014.*		
	Yersinia enterocolitica Fever in 68%, bloody stools in 26%	**No treatment unless severe.** If severe, **Doxy** 100 mg IV bid + (**Tobra** or **Gent** 5 mg/kg per day once q24h). **TMP-SMX** or **FQs** are alternatives.		Mesenteric adenitis pain can mimic acute appendicitis. Lab diagnosis difficult: requires "cold enrichment" and/or yersinia selective agar. Desferrioxamine therapy increases severity, discontinue if pt on it. Iron overload states predispose to yersinia.

 *NOTE: All dosage recommendations are for adults (unless otherwise indicated) and assume normal renal function. § Alternatives consider allergy, PK, compliance, local resistance, cost.

TABLE 1 (18)

ANATOMIC SITE/DIAGNOSIS/ MODIFYING CIRCUMSTANCES	ETIOLOGIES (usual)	SUGGESTED REGIMENS*		ADJUNCT DIAGNOSTIC OR THERAPEUTIC MEASURES AND COMMENTS
		PRIMARY	ALTERNATIVE§	
GASTROINTESTINAL *(continued)*				
Gastroenteritis—Specific Risk Groups–Empiric Therapy				
Anoreceptive intercourse				
Proctitis (distal 15 cm only)	Herpes viruses, gonococci, chlamydia, syphilis. *See Genital Tract, page 24*			
Colitis	Shigella, salmonella, campylobacter, E. histolytica *(see Table 13A)*			*See specific GI pathogens, Gastroenteritis, above.*
HIV-1 infected (AIDS): >10 days diarrhea	G. lamblia Acid fast: Cryptosporidium parvum or hominis, Cyclospora cayetanensis Other: Isospora belli, microsporidia (Enterocytozoon bieneusi, Septata intestinalis)			*See Table 13A*
Neutropenic enterocolitis or "typhlitis" *(CID 56:711, 2013) (World J Gastroenterol 23: 42, 2017)*	Mucosal invasion by **Clostridium septicum** and others. Occasionally caused by C. sordellii or P. aeruginosa	Bowel rest and **Pip-tazo** 4.5 gm IV q6h or **IMP** 500 mg IV q6h or **MER** 2 gm IV q8h	**Cefepime** 2 gm IV q8h + **Metro** 500 mg IV q8h	Tender right lower quadrant may be clue, but may be diffuse or absent in immunocompromised. Need surgical consult. Surgical resection controversial but may be necessary. **NOTE:** Resistance of clostridia to clindamycin reported. Pip-tazo, IMP, MER, DORI should cover most pathogens.
Traveler's diarrhea, self-medication. Patient often afebrile **Single dose therapy** is the recommended guideline *(Am J Gastro 111:602, 2016; J Trav Med 24:S63, 2017; JAMA 2017;318:957)* Advise patient: 1 dose usually sufficient, continue for 3d if not resolved after 1 dose	**Acute**: 60% due to diarrheagenic E. coli; shigella, salmonella, or campylobacter. C. difficile, amebiasis *(see Table 13A)*. **If chronic**: cyclospora, cryptosporidia, giardia, isospora	**Adult: Azithro** 1000 mg po once or 500 mg po q24h for 3 days **CIP** 750 mg po x 1 dose or 500 mg po x 3 days **OR** **Levo** 500 mg po q24h for 1-3 days **OR** **Oflox** 300 mg po bid for 3 days **OR** **Rifaximin** 200 mg po tid for 3 days **OR** **Rifamycin SB** 2 tabs bid x 3 days **Peds: Azithro** 10 mg/kg/day as a single dose for 3 days or **Ceftriaxone** 50 mg/kg/day as single dose for 3 days. Avoid FQs. **Pregnancy:** Use Azithro. Avoid FQs. **For loperamide**, *see Comment*.		**Antimotility agent:** For non-pregnant adults with no fever or blood in stool, add **loperamide** 4 mg po x 1, then 2 mg po after each loose stool to a maximum of 16 mg per day. **Rifaximin** approved only for ages 12 and older. Works only for diarrhea due to non-invasive E. coli; do not use if fever or bloody stool. **Rifamycin SB**: adult only; for E. coli. Do not use if fever or bloody diarrhea. **Ref:** *NEJM 361:1560, 2009; Clin Micro Inf 21:744, 2015.* **NOTE:** Self treatment with FQs associated with acquisition of resistant Gm-neg bacilli *(CID 60:837, 847, 872, 2015)*. Increasing resistance of Campylobacter to FQ, particularly in Asia. Azithro now first line choice.
Prevention of Traveler's diarrhea	**Not routinely indicated.** Current recommendation is to take **Imodium** with 1st loose stool.			

 NOTE: All dosage recommendations are for adults (unless otherwise indicated) and assume normal renal function. § Alternatives consider allergy, PK, compliance, local resistance, cost.

TABLE 1 (19)

ANATOMIC SITE/DIAGNOSIS/ MODIFYING CIRCUMSTANCES	ETIOLOGIES (usual)	SUGGESTED REGIMENS* PRIMARY	SUGGESTED REGIMENS* ALTERNATIVE§	ADJUNCT DIAGNOSTIC OR THERAPEUTIC MEASURES AND COMMENTS
GASTROINTESTINAL *(continued)*				
Gastrointestinal Infections by Anatomic Site: Esophagus to Rectum				
Esophagitis	Candida albicans, HSV, CMV	*See Table 11A and Table 14A.*		
Duodenal/Gastric ulcer; gastric cancer, MALT lymphomas (not 2°NSAIDs) Comparative effectiveness & tolerance of treatment Review: *NEJM 380:1158, 2018*	**Helicobacter pylori** *See Comment* Prevalence of pre-treatment resistance increasing, especially clarithro *(AAC 2017,61:e02530-16).* Ask about previous antibiotics and try to avoid prior antibiotic given. Consensus recs slightly different but rec all H. pylori + should be treated. Test & treat without EGD if age <45 yrs.	**Quadruple therapy:** (**Bismuth subsalicylate** 2 tabs qid + **Tetra** 500 mg qid + **Metro** 500 mg tid + **PPI**) x 14 days. For doses, *see footnote*[7] *& Comments*	(**PPI** + **Amox** 1000 mg bid + metro 500 mg bid + **Clarithro** 500 mg bid) x 14 days.	**Comment:** Any one of these **proton pump inhibitors (PPI)** may be used: omeprazole 20 mg bid, Lansoprazole 30 mg bid, esomeprazole 20 mg bid, pantoprazole 40 mg bid, rabeprazole 20 mg bid. In many locations, 20% failure rates with previously recommended *triple* regimens **(PPI + Amox + Clarithro)**. Exercise caution regarding potential interactions with other drugs, contraindications in pregnancy and warnings for other special populations. **Dx: Stool antigen**—Monoclonal EIA >90% sens. & 92% specific. Other tests: if endoscoped, rapid urease &/or histology &/or culture; serology less sens & spec; urea breath test, but some office-based tests underperform. Testing ref: *BMJ 344:44, 2012.* **Test of cure:** Repeat stool antigen and/or urea breath test >8 wks post-treatment. **Treatment outcome:** Failure rate of triple therapy 20% due to clarithro resistance.
Small intestine: Whipple's disease *(NEJM 356:55, 2007; LnID 8:179, 2008)* Treatment: *JAC 69:219, 2014. See Infective endocarditis, culture-negative, page 32.*	Tropheryma whipplei	(**Doxy** 100 mg po bid + **Hydroxychloroquine** 200 mg pot id) x 1 year, then **Doxy** 100 mg po bid for life (Peds dose, *see Comment*) Immune reconstitution inflammatory response (IRIS) reactions occur: Thalidomide therapy may be better than steroids for IRIS reaction *(J Infect 60:79, 2010)*		In vitro susceptibility testing and collected clinical experience *(JAC 69:219, 2014).* In vitro resistance to TMP-SMX plus frequent clinical failures & relapses. Frequent in vitro resistance to carbapenems. Ceftriaxone demonstrates high MICs against intracellular organisms in vitro *(AAC 48: 747, 2004).* **Peds: Doxy** considered safe regardless of age for duration of 21 days or less: 4.4 mg/kg div bid *(AAP Redbook 2018).*
Appendicitis, acute	Aerobic & anaerobic gram-negative bacilli	**Uncomplicated, no apparent perforation**		
		No surgery: **Ceftriaxone** 2 gm IV x 1 + **Metro** (max 1500 mg x 1) then (**Cefdinir** 600 mg po q24h + **Metro** 500 mg po q8h) x 7-10 days or **Erta** 1 gm IV q24h	*Surgery:* Peds: **Ceftriaxone** 50 mg/kg IV q24h + **Metro** 30 mg/kg (max 1500 mg) IV q24h. Adult: **Pip-tazo** 3.375 gm IV load then 3.375 gm IV over 4 hrs q8h or **Levo** 750 mg IV q24h + **Metro** 500 mg IV q8h	Goal: Activity vs. both aerobic & anaerobic bacteria. Usually no need to cover Staph., enterococci or candida. Active vs; anaerobes: Metro. Active vs. aerobic gram neg bacilli: AG, P Ceph 2/3/4, Aztreonam, Cip, Levo, Ceftaz-avi. Active vs. both: Pip-tazo, Amox-clav, carbapenems, eravacycline, Moxi, Delaflox. Refs: Non-operative rx of uncomplicated appendicitis *(J Trauma Acute Care Surg 86:722, 2019; JAMA 32:1245 & 1259, 2018).* Note: No firm guidance on dose for Metro: range 500 mg q6-8h to 30 mg/kg IV once daily (max 1500 mg).
		Perforation, peritonitis, shock *Emergency surgery:* **MER** 1 gm IV q8h or CIP 400 mg IV q8h + Metro 500 mg IV q8h *(See Comments for other options)*		

[7] **Bismuth preparations:** (1) In U.S., **bismuth subsalicylate (Pepto-Bismol)** 262 mg tabs; adult dose for helicobacter is 2 tabs (524 mg) qid. (2) Outside U.S., **colloidal bismuth subcitrate** (De-Nol) 120 mg chewable tablets; dose is 1 tablet qid. In the U.S., bismuth subcitrate is available in combination cap only (Pylera: each cap contains bismuth subcitrate 140 mg + Metro 125 mg + Tetracycline 125 mg), given as 3 caps po 4x daily for 10 days **together with** a twice daily PPI.

TABLE 1 (20)

ANATOMIC SITE/DIAGNOSIS/ MODIFYING CIRCUMSTANCES	ETIOLOGIES (usual)	SUGGESTED REGIMENS* PRIMARY	ALTERNATIVE§	ADJUNCT DIAGNOSTIC OR THERAPEUTIC MEASURES AND COMMENTS
GASTROINTESTINAL/Gastrointestinal Infections by Anatomic Site: Esophagus to Rectum *(continued)*				
Diverticulitis, perirectal abscess, peritonitis *Also see Peritonitis, page 49* *NEJM 2018;379:1635*	Enterobacteriaceae, occasionally P. aeruginosa, Bacteroides sp., enterococci	**Outpatient rx—mild diverticulitis, drained perirectal abscess:** [(**TMP-SMX-DS** bid) or (**CIP** 750 mg bid or **Levo** 750 mg q24h)] + **Metro** 500 mg q6h. All po x 7–10 days.	**Amox-clav-ER** 1000/62.5 mg 2 tabs po bid x 7–10 days **OR Moxi** 400 mg po q24h x 7-10 days	Must "cover" both Gm-neg. aerobic & Gm-neg. anaerobic bacteria. **Drugs active only vs. anaerobic Gm-neg. bacilli:** clinda, metro. **Drugs active only vs. aerobic Gm-neg. bacilli:** APAG[8], P Ceph 2/3/4 *(see Table 10A, page 114)*, aztreonam, CIP, Levo. **Drugs active vs. both aerobic/anaerobic Gm-neg. bacteria:** cefoxitin, cefotetan, TC-CL, Pip-tazo, Amp-sulb, ERTA, DORI, IMP, MER, Moxi, & tigecycline. **Increasing resistance of B. fragilis group** **Clinda / Moxi / Cefoxitin / Cefotetan** % Resistant: 42-80 / 34-45 / 48-60 / 19-35 *Ref: Anaerobe 17:147, 2011; AAC 56:1247, 2012; Surg Infect 10:111, 2009.*
		Mild-moderate disease—Inpatient—Parenteral Rx: (e.g., focal periappendiceal peritonitis, peridiverticular abscess, endomyometritis) **Pip-tazo** 3.375 gm IV q6h or 4.5 gm IV q8h or **Erta** 1 gm IV q24h or **Moxi** 400 mg IV q24h	[(**CIP** 400 mg IV q12h) or (**Levo** 750 mg IV q24h)] + (**Metro** 500 mg IV q6h or 1 gm IV q12h) **OR Moxi** 400 mg IV q24h	
		Severe life-threatening disease, ICU patient: **IMP** 500 mg IV q6h **or MER** 1 gm IV q8h **or Dori** 500 mg q8h (1-hr infusion). For **Ceftolo-tazo** & **Ceftaz-avi** dosing, *see Peritonitis, page 49.*	**AMP** + **Metro** + (**CIP** 400 mg IV q12h or **Levo** 750 mg IV q24h) **OR** [**AMP** 2 gm IV q6h + **Metro** 500 mg IV q6h + **Aminoglycoside**[8] *(see Table 10C, page 128)*]	**Resistance (B. fragilis):** Metro, Pip-tazo rare. Resistance to FQ increased in enteric bacteria, particularly if any FQ used recently. **Ertapenem** poorly active vs. P. aeruginosa/Acinetobacter sp. **Concomitant surgical management important**, esp. with moderate-severe disease. **Role of enterococci remains debatable**. Probably pathogenic in infections of biliary tract. Probably need drugs active vs. enterococci in pts with valvular heart disease.
		Severe penicillin/cephalosporin allergy: (**Aztreonam** 2 gm IV q6h to q8h) + [**Metro** (500 mg IV q6h) or (1 gm IV q12h)] **OR** [(**CIP** 400 mg IV q12h) or (**Levo** 750 mg IV q24h) + **Metro**].		**Tigecycline: Black Box Warning:** All cause mortality higher in pts treated with tigecycline (2.5%) than comparators (1.8%) in meta-analysis of clinical trials. Cause of mortality risk difference of 0.6% (95% CI 0.1, 1.2) not established. Tigecycline should be reserved for use in situations when alternative treatments are not suitable *(FDA MedWatch Sep 27, 2013)*. AGA guidelines recommend antibiotics be used selectively in acute, uncomplicated diverticulitis *(Gastro 149: 1944, 2015)*.
GENITAL TRACT: Mixture of empiric & specific treatment. Divided by sex of the patient. For sexual assault (rape), *see Table 15A, page 219.* ***See CDC Guidelines for Sexually Transmitted Diseases:*** *MMWR 64(RR-3):1, 2015; Med Lett 2017;59:105.*				
Both Women & Men:				
Chancroid *(Curr Op Inf Dis 29:52, 2016)* Ulcer is painful.	H. ducreyi	**Ceftriaxone** 250 mg IM single dose OR **Azithro** 1 gm po single dose	**CIP** 500 mg bid po x 3 days OR **Erythro base** 500 mg po tid x 7 days.	In HIV+ pts, failures reported with single dose azithro *(CID 21:409, 1995)*. Evaluate after 7 days, ulcer should objectively improve. All patients treated for chancroid should be tested for HIV and syphilis. All sex partners of pts with chancroid should be examined and treated if they have evidence of disease or have had sex with index pt within the last 10 days.
Non-gonococcal or post-gonococcal urethritis, cervicitis **NOTE: Assume concomitant N. gonorrhoeae** (Chlamydia conjunctivitis, *see page 14)*	Chlamydia 50%, Mycoplasma genitalium (30%). Other known etiologies (10–15%): trichomonas, herpes simplex virus, *see JID 206:357, 2012.* Ref: *CID 61:S774, 2015*	(**Doxy** 100 mg bid po x 7 days) or (**Azithro** 1 gm po as single dose). Evaluate & treat sex partner **Pregnancy: Azithro** 1 gm po single dose OR **Amox** 500 mg po tid x 7 days.	(**Erythro base** 500 mg qid po x 7 days) or (**Oflox** 300 mg q12h po x 7 days) or (**Levo** 500 mg q24h x 7 days) **In pregnancy: Erythro** base 500 mg po qid for 7 days **Doxy & FQs contraindicated**	**Diagnosis:** NAAT for C. trachomatis & N. gonorrhoeae on urine or cervix or urethra specimens *(AnIM 142:914, 2005)*. Test all urethritis/cervicitis pts for HIV & syphilis. **Evaluate & treat sex partners.** Re-test for cure in pregnancy. Azithromycin 1 gm was superior to doxycycline for M. genitalium male urethritis *(CID 48:1649, 2009)*, but may select resistance leading to ↑ failure of multi-dose azithromycin retreatment regimens *(CID 48:1655, 2009)*.

[8] **Aminoglycoside = antipseudomonal aminoglycosidic aminoglycoside, e.g., Amikacin, Gentamicin, Tobramycin, Plazomicin**

Abbreviations on page 2. **NOTE: All dosage recommendations are for adults (unless otherwise indicated) and assume normal renal function. § Alternatives consider allergy, PK, compliance, local resistance, cost.*

TABLE 1 (21)

ANATOMIC SITE/DIAGNOSIS/ MODIFYING CIRCUMSTANCES	ETIOLOGIES (usual)	SUGGESTED REGIMENS*		ADJUNCT DIAGNOSTIC OR THERAPEUTIC MEASURES AND COMMENTS
		PRIMARY	ALTERNATIVE§	
GENITAL TRACT/Both Women & Men *(continued) - CDC Guidelines: MMWR 64(RR-3):1, 2015*				
Non-gonococcal urethritis: **Mycoplasma genitalium**	Mycoplasma genitalium. Ref: *CID 61:S802, 2015.*	**Azithro** 500 mg po x1 then 250 mg po once daily x 4 days or **Azithro** 1 gm po x 1 dose	**Moxi** 400 mg once daily x 10-14 days	Diagnosis by NAAT, but usually not available. **Doxy ineffective.** No cell wall so beta-lactams ineffective. Cure with single dose Azithro only 67% *(CID 61:1389, 2015)*. Emerging resistance with no good alternatives *(Em Inf Dis 23:809, 2017)*. Pristinamycin may work *(CID 2015;60:1228)*.
Recurrent/persistent urethritis	**C. trachomatis** (43%), **M. genitalium** (30%), **T. vaginalis** (13%) *(CID 52:163, 2011)*.	**Metro** 2 gm po x 1 dose + **Azithro** 1 gm po x 1 dose	**Tinidazole** 2 gm po x 1 + **Azithro** 1 gm po x 1	High failure rate of Azithro if M. genitalium *(CID 56:934, 2013)*. Can try Moxi 400 mg po once daily x 10 days if Azithro failure *(PLoS One 3:e3618, 2008)*. New FQ resistance in Japan *(JAC 69:2376, 2014)*.
Rectal, proctitis MSM and increasingly in women	C. trachomatis, M. genitalium, N. gonorrhoeae, syphilis, HSV	Treat for GC and chlamydia; **Doxy** 100 bid x 7 days preferred over Azithro	If LGV suspected treat **Doxy** 100 bid x 21 days	**Proctitis:** prefer Doxy x 7 days *(Sex Trans Dis 41:79, 2014)*. Higher failures with azithro *(JAC 70:961, 2015)*.
Gonorrhea. **FQs no longer recommended for treatment of gonococcal infections** *(See CDC Guidelines MMWR 64(RR-3):1, 2015; CID 61:S785, 2015)*. **Cephalosporin resistance:** *JAMA 309:163 & 185, 2013.* Case report of Azithro/Ceph resist strain treated with ERTA in UK *(Eurosurv 23:5 2018)*.				
Conjunctivitis (adult)	N. gonorrhoeae	**Ceftriaxone** 1 gm IM or IV single dose + **Azithro**		Consider one-time saline lavage of eye.
Disseminated gonococcal infection (DGI, dermatitis-arthritis syndrome)	N. gonorrhoeae	**Ceftriaxone** 1 gm IV q24h + **Azithro** 1 gm po x 1	(**Cefotaxime** 1 gm q8h IV or **Ceftizoxime** 1 gm q8h IV) + **Azithro** 1 gm po x 1	**Treat for a minimum of 7 days.** Owing to high-level resistance to oral cephalosporins and fluoroquinolones in the community, "Step-down" therapy should be avoided unless susceptibilities are known and demonstrate full activity of cephalosporin or fluoroquinolone R/O meningitis/endocarditis. **Treat presumptively for concomitant C. trachomatis.** Azithro now recommended to cover resistant GC (usually tetra resistant, too) and C. trachomatis
Endocarditis	N. gonorrhoeae	**Ceftriaxone** 1-2 gm IV q12-24 hours x 4 weeks + **Azithro** 1 gm po x 1		GC endocarditis may occur in the absence of concomitant urogenital symptoms *(Infection 42: 425, 2014)*. Severe valve destruction may occur. Ceftriaxone resistance in *N. gonorrhoeae* has been reported *(AAC 55: 3538, 2011)*; determine susceptibility of any isolate recovered.
Pharyngitis Dx: NAAT	N. gonorrhoeae	**Ceftriaxone** 250 mg IM x 1 + (**Azithro** 1 gm po x 1).	Due to resistance concerns, **do not use FQs**.	Pharyngeal GC more difficult to eradicate. **Repeat NAAT 14 days post-rx. Spectinomycin[NUS], cefixime, cefpodoxime & cefuroxime not effective**
Urethritis, cervicitis, proctitis (uncomplicated) For prostatitis, *see page 29.* **Diagnosis:** Nucleic acid amplification test (NAAT) on vaginal swab, urine or urethral swab *MMWR 64(RR-3):1, 2015*	N. gonorrhoeae (50% of pts with urethritis, cervicitis have concomitant C. trachomatis — **treat for both even if NAAT indicates single pathogen**).	**Ceftriaxone** 250 mg IM x 1 + **Azithro** 1 gm po x 1 **Rx failure: Ceftriaxone** 500 mg IM x 1 + **Azithro** 2 gm po x 1; treat partner; NAAT for test of cure 1 wk post-treatment **Severe Pen/Ceph allergy**: (**Gent** 240 mg IM + **Azithro** 2 gm po x 1 dose) OR (**Gemi** 320 mg + **Azithro** 2 gm po x 1 dose) *(CID 59:1083, 2014)* (nausea in >20%)		Screen for syphilis. **Other alternatives for GC (Test of Cure recommended one week after Rx for ALL of these approaches listed below):** • **Oral cephalosporin use is no longer recommended** as primary therapy owing to emergence of resistance, *MMWR 61:590, 2012.* • Other single-dose cephalosporins: ceftizoxime 500 mg IM, cefotaxime 500 mg IM, cefoxitin 2 gm IM + probenecid 1 gm po.
Pregnancy		**Ceftriaxone** 250 mg IM x 1 + **Azithro** 1 gm po x 1		
Granuloma inguinale (Donovanosis)	Klebsiella (formerly Calymmatobacterium) granulomatis	**Azithro** 1 gm po q wk x 3 wks	**TMP-SMX** one DS tablet bid x 3 wks **OR Erythro** 500 mg po qid x 3 wks OR **CIP** 750 mg po bid x 3 wks OR **Doxy** 100 mg po bid x 3 wks	Clinical response usually seen in 1 wk. **Rx until all lesions healed,** may take 4 wks. Treatment failures & recurrence seen with Doxy & TMP-SMX. Relapse can occur 6-18 months after apparently effective Rx. If improvement not evidence in first few days, some experts add Gent 1 mg/kg IV q8h.
Herpes simplex virus	*See Table 14A, page 181*			
Human papilloma virus (HPV)	*See Table 14A, page 187*			

Abbreviations on page 2. **NOTE: All dosage recommendations are for adults (unless otherwise indicated) and assume normal renal function. § Alternatives consider allergy, PK, compliance, local resistance, cost.*

TABLE 1 (22)

ANATOMIC SITE/DIAGNOSIS/ MODIFYING CIRCUMSTANCES	ETIOLOGIES (usual)	SUGGESTED REGIMENS* PRIMARY	SUGGESTED REGIMENS* ALTERNATIVE§	ADJUNCT DIAGNOSTIC OR THERAPEUTIC MEASURES AND COMMENTS
GENITAL TRACT/Both Women & Men *(continued)*				
Lymphogranuloma venereum Ref: *CID 61:S865, 2015*	Chlamydia trachomatis, serovars. L1, L2, L3	**Doxy** 100 mg po bid x 21 days	**Erythro** 500 mg po qid x 21 days or **Azithro** 1000 mg po q wk x 3 wks (clinical data lacking)	Dx based on serology; biopsy contraindicated because sinus tracts develop. Nucleic acid ampli tests for *C. trachomatis* will be positive. In MSM, presents as fever, rectal ulcer, anal discharge *(CID 39:996, 2004; Dis Colon Rectum 52:507, 2009)*.
Phthirus pubis **(pubic lice, "crabs")** & scabies	Phthirus pubis & Sarcoptes scabiei	*See Table 13A, page 172*		
Syphilis Diagnosis: *JAMA 312:1922, 2014*; treatment: *JAMA 312:1905, 2014;* management: *CID 61:S818, 2015.* Overview: *Lancet 389: 1550, 2017.*				
Early: primary, secondary, or latent <1 yr. Screen with treponema-specific antibody or RPR/VDRL, *see JCM 50:2 & 148, 2012; CID 58:1116, 2014.* **Chancre is painless.**	T. pallidum **NOTE:** Test all pts with syphilis for HIV; test all HIV patients for latent syphilis. Screen MSM and/or HIV pts every 3-12 mos *(JAMA 315:2321 & 2328, 2016).* Pregnancy: screen all *(JAMA 2018;320:911)*	**Benzathine pen G (Bicillin L-A)** 2.4 million units IM x 1 *(See Comment)*	(**Doxy** 100 mg po bid x 14 days) or (**Tetra** 500 mg po qid x 14 days) or (**Ceftriaxone** 1 gm IM/IV q24h x 10–14 days). Follow-up mandatory. Ceftriaxone efficacy *(CID 2017;65:1683)* Doxy considered safe regardless of age for rx ≤21 days *(AAP Redbook 2018)*	If early or congenital syphilis, **quantitative VDRL at 0**, 3, 6, 12 & 24 mos after rx. If 1° or 2° syphilis, VDRL should ↓ 2 tubes at 6 mos, 3 tubes 12 mos, & 4 tubes 24 mos. Update on congenital syphilis *(MMWR 64(RR-3):1, 2015).* Early latent: 2 tubes ↓ at 12 mos. With 1°, 50% will be RPR seronegative at 12 mos, 24% neg. FTA/ABS at 2–3 yrs *(AnIM 114:1005, 1991).* If titers fail to fall, examine CSF; if CSF (+), treat as neurosyphilis; if CSF is negative, retreat with benzathine Pen G 2.4 mu IM weekly x 3 wks. **If no other options: Azithro** 2 gm po x 1 dose (equivalent to **Benzathine pen** 2.4 M x 1 dose in early syphilis *(J Infect Dis 201:1729, 2010).* **Azithro-resistant syphilis** documented in California, Ireland, & elsewhere. **NOTE:** Use of **benzathine procaine penicillin** is inappropriate!!
More than 1 yr's duration (latent of indeterminate duration, cardiovascular, late benign gumma)	For penicillin desensitization method, *see Table 7, page 91* and *MMWR 64(RR-3):1, 2015*	**Benzathine pen G (Bicillin L-A)** 2.4 million units IM q week x 3 = 7.2 million units total	**Doxy** 100 mg po bid x 28 days or **Tetra** 500 mg po qid x 28 days; **Ceftriaxone** 1 gm IV or IM daily for 10-14 days MAY be an alternative (No clinical data; consult an ID specialist)	No published data on efficacy of alternatives. **Indications for LP (CDC): neurologic symptoms, treatment failure, any eye or ear involvement, other evidence of active syphilis (aortitis, gumma, iritis).** Neurosyphilis *(NEJM 381:1358, 2019).*
Neurosyphilis—Very difficult to treat. Includes ocular (retro-bulbar neuritis) syphilis **All need CSF exam.**		**Pen G** 18-24 million units per day either as continuous infusion or as 3–4 million units IV q4h x 10–14 days.	(**Procaine pen G** 2.4 million units IM q24h + **probenecid** 0.5 gm po qid) both x 10–14 days—*See Comment*	**Ceftriaxone** 2 gm (IV or IM) q24h x 14 days. For penicillin allergy: either desensitize to penicillin or obtain infectious diseases consultation. **Serologic criteria for response to rx: 4-fold or greater ↓ in VDRL titer over 6–12 mos.**
HIV infection (AIDS) CDC STD guidelines: *MMWR 64 (3), June 5, 2015*		Treatment same as HIV uninfected with closer follow-up. Treat early neurosyphilis for 10-14 days regardless of CD4 count: *MMWR 56:625, 2007.*		*See Syphilis discussion in CDC Guidelines MMWR 64(RR-3):1, 2015.* Treat for neurosyphilis if CSF VDRL negative but >20 CSF WBCs *(STD 39:291, 2012).*
Pregnancy and syphilis		Same as for non-pregnant, some recommend 2nd dose (2.4 million units) **Benzathine Pen G** 1 wk after initial dose esp. in 3rd trimester or with 2° syphilis	Skin test for penicillin allergy. Desensitize if necessary, as parenteral pen G is only therapy with documented efficacy!	Monthly quantitative VDRL or equivalent. If 4-fold ↑, re-treat. Doxy, tetracycline contraindicated. Erythro not recommended because of high risk of failure to cure fetus.

 **NOTE: All dosage recommendations are for adults (unless otherwise indicated) and assume normal renal function. § Alternatives consider allergy, PK, compliance, local resistance, cost.*

TABLE 1 (23)

ANATOMIC SITE/DIAGNOSIS/ MODIFYING CIRCUMSTANCES	ETIOLOGIES (usual)	SUGGESTED REGIMENS*		ADJUNCT DIAGNOSTIC OR THERAPEUTIC MEASURES AND COMMENTS
		PRIMARY	ALTERNATIVE§	
GENITAL TRACT/Both Women & Men/Syphilis *(continued)*				
Congenital syphilis *(Update on Congenital Syphilis: MMWR 64(RR-3):1, 2015)*	T. pallidum	**Aqueous crystalline Pen G** 50,000 units/kg per dose IV q12h x 7 days, then q8h for 10 day total.	**Procaine Pen G** 50,000 units/kg IM q24h for 10 days	Another alternative: **Ceftriaxone** ≤30 days old, 75 mg/kg IV/IM q24h (use with caution in infants with jaundice) or >30 days old 100 mg/kg IV/IM q24h. Treat 10–14 days. If symptomatic, ophthalmologic exam indicated. If more than 1 day of rx missed, restart entire course. **Need serologic follow-up!**
Warts, anogenital	*See Table 14A, page 187*			
Women:				
Amnionitis, septic abortion Data on antibiotic rx poor *(Cochrane Database (12) CD0010976, 2014)*	Bacteroides, esp. Prevotella bivia; Group B, A streptococci; Enterobacteriaceae; C. trachomatis. Rarely U. urealyticum, Mycoplasma sp.	**Pip-tazo** or **Mer/IMP/Erta** *Dosage: see footnote[9]* **NOTE:** in US and Europe, 1/3 of Grp B Strep resistant to clindamycin.	**Ceftriaxone** + **Metro**. Do not favor Amp + Gent	D&C of uterus. **In septic abortion,** Clostridium perfringens may cause fulminant intravascular hemolysis. **In postpartum patients** with enigmatic fever and/or pulmonary emboli, **consider septic pelvic vein thrombophlebitis** *(see Vascular septic pelvic vein thrombophlebitis, page 72)*. Add doxy for C. trachomatis, Ureaplasma or Mycoplasma. Review: *Frontiers Pharm 8:97, 2017.*
Cervicitis, mucopurulent Treatment based on results of nucleic acid amplification test	N. gonorrhoeae	Treat for Gonorrhea, *page 25*		Criteria for diagnosis: 1) (muco) purulent endocervical exudate and/or 2) sustained endocervical bleeding after passage of cotton swab. >10 WBC/hpf of vaginal fluid is suggestive. Intracellular gram-neg diplococci are specific but insensitive. If in doubt, send swab or urine for culture, EIA or nucleic acid amplification test and treat for both.
	Chlamydia trachomatis	Treat for non-gonococcal urethritis, *page 25*. If due to *Mycoplasma genitalium*, less likely to respond to doxy than azithro and emerging resistance to both azithro and FQ.		
Endomyometritis/septic pelvic phlebitis				
Early postpartum (1st 48 hrs) (usually after C-section)	Bacteroides, esp. Prevotella bivia; Group B, A streptococci; Enterobacteriaceae; C. trachomatis	[(**Cefoxitin** or **Erta** or **IMP** or **MER** or **Amp-sulb** or **Pip-tazo**) + **Doxy**] or [**Clinda** + (**Aminoglycoside** or **Ceftriaxone**)] *Dosage: see footnote[9]*		*See Comments under Amnionitis, septic abortion, above*
Late postpartum (48 hrs to 6 wks) (usually after vaginal delivery)	Chlamydia trachomatis, M. hominis	**Doxy** 100 mg IV or po q12h times 14 days		Tetracyclines not recommended in nursing mothers; discontinue nursing. M. hominis sensitive to tetra, clinda, not erythro.
Fitzhugh-Curtis syndrome	C. trachomatis, N. gonorrhoeae	Treat as for pelvic inflammatory disease immediately below.		Perihepatitis (violin-string adhesions). Sudden onset of RUQ pain. Associated with salpingitis. Transaminases elevated in <30% of cases.
Pelvic actinomycosis; usually tubo-ovarian abscess	A. Israelii most common	**AMP** 200 mg/kg/day in 3-4 divided doses x 4-6 wks then Pen VK 2-4 gm/day in 4 divided doses x 6-12 mo	**Doxy** or **Ceftriaxone** or **Clinda**	Complication of intrauterine device (IUD). Remove IUD. Can use **Pen G** 10-20 million units/day IV instead of **AMP** x 4-6 wks.

[9] **P Ceph 2** (**Cefoxitin** 2 gm IV q6–8h, **Cefotetan** 2 gm IV q12h, Cefuroxime 750 mg IV q8h); **Amp-sulb** 3 gm IV q6h; **Pip-tazo** 3.375 gm q6h or for nosocomial pneumonia: 4.5 gm IV q6h or 4-hr infusion of 3.375 gm q8h; **Doxy** 100 mg IV/po q12h; **Clinda** 450–900 mg IV q8h; **Aminoglycoside** (**Gent**, *see Table 10C, page 128*); **P Ceph 3** (**Cefotaxime** 2 gm IV q8h, **Ceftriaxone** 2 gm IV q24h); **Dori** 500 mg IV q8h (1-hr infusion); **Erta** 1 gm IV q24h; **IMP** 0.5 gm IV q6h; **MER** 1 gm IV q8h; **Azithro** 500 mg IV q24h; **Linezolid** 600 mg IV/po q12h; **Vanco** 1 gm IV q12h

Abbreviations on page 2. **NOTE: All dosage recommendations are for adults (unless otherwise indicated) and assume normal renal function. § Alternatives consider allergy, PK, compliance, local resistance, cost.*

TABLE 1 (24)

ANATOMIC SITE/DIAGNOSIS/ MODIFYING CIRCUMSTANCES	ETIOLOGIES (usual)	SUGGESTED REGIMENS*		ADJUNCT DIAGNOSTIC OR THERAPEUTIC MEASURES AND COMMENTS
		PRIMARY	ALTERNATIVE§	
GENITAL TRACT/Women *(continued)*				
Pelvic Inflammatory Disease (PID), salpingitis, tubo-ovarian abscess				
Outpatient rx: limit to pts with temp <38°C, WBC <11,000 per mm³, minimal evidence of peritonitis, active bowel sounds & able to tolerate oral nourishment *NEJM 372:2039, 2015; CDC Guidelines MMWR 64(RR-3):1, 2015*	N. gonorrhoeae, chlamydia, bacteroides, Enterobacteriaceae, streptococci, especially S. agalactiae Less commonly: G. vaginalis, Haemophilus influenzae, cytomegalovirus (CMV), M. genitalium, U. urealyticum	**Outpatient rx:** [(**Ceftriaxone** 250 mg IM or IV x 1) (± **Metro** 500 mg po bid x 14 days) + (**Doxy** 100 mg po bid x 14 days)]. **OR** (**Cefoxitin** 2 gm IM with **Probenecid** 1 gm po both as single dose) plus (**Doxy** 100 mg po bid with **Metro** 500 mg bid—both times 14 days)	**Inpatient regimens:** [(**Cefotetan** 2 gm IV q12h or **Cefoxitin** 2 gm IV q6h) + (**Doxy** 100 mg IV/po q12h)] (**Clinda** 900 mg IV q8h) + (**Gent** 2 mg/kg loading dose, then 1.5 mg/kg q8h or 4.5 mg/kg once per day), then **Doxy** 100 mg po bid x 14 days	**Another alternative parenteral regimen:** **Amp-sulb** 3 gm IV q6h + **Doxy** 100 mg IV/po q12h. Recommended treatments don't cover M. genitalium so if no response after 7-10 days consider M. genitalium NAAT and treat with **Moxi** 400 mg/day 14 days. Remember: Evaluate and treat sex partner. FQs not recommended due to increasing resistance *MMWR 64(RR-3):1, 2015 & www.cdc.gov/std/treatment)*. Suggest initial inpatient evaluation/therapy for pts with tubo-ovarian abscess. For inpatient regimens, continue treatment until satisfactory response for ≥ 24-hr before switching to outpatient regimen. Improved routine testing for chlamydia and N. gonorrhoeae among outpatients resulted in reduced hospitalization and ectopic pregnancy rates *(J Adolescent Health 51:80, 2012)*
Vaginitis— *MMWR 64(RR-3):1, 2015*				
Candidiasis Pruritus, thick cheesy discharge, pH <4.5 *See Table 11A, page 134*	Candida albicans 80–90%. C. glabrata, C. tropicalis may be increasing—they are less susceptible to azoles	**Oral azoles: Fluconazole** 150 mg po x 1; **Itraconazole** 200 mg po bid x 1 day. For milder cases, Topical Therapy with one of the over the counter preparations usually is successful (e.g., clotrimazole, butoconazole, miconazole, or tioconazole) as creams or vaginal suppositories.	**Butoconazole, Clotrimazole, Miconazole, Tioconazole** or **Terconazole** (all intravaginal): variety of strengths - from 1 dose to 7–14 days *(See Table 11A, page 134)*	Nystatin vag. tabs times 14 days less effective. Other rx for azole-resistant strains: gentian violet, boric acid. If recurrent candidiasis (4 or more episodes per yr): 6 mos. suppression with: fluconazole 150 mg po q week or itraconazole 100 mg po q24h or clotrimazole vag. suppositories 500 mg q week.
Trichomoniasis *(CID 61:S837, 2015)* Copious foamy discharge, pH >4.5 Treat sexual partners—*see Comment*	Trichomonas vaginalis **Dx:** NAAT & PCR available & most sensitive; wet mount not sensitive. Ref: *JCM 54:7, 2016.*	**Metro** 500 mg po bid x 7 days OR 2 gm single dose. 7 days more effective in RCT, If HIV+ always give 7 day course OR **Tinidazole** 2 gm po single dose **Pregnancy:** *See Comment*	**For rx failure:** Re-treat with metro 500 mg po bid x 7 days; if 2nd failure: metro 2 gm po q24h x 3–5 days. If still failure, **Tinidazole** 2 gm po q24h x 5 days	**Treat male sexual partners: Metro** 2 gm x 1 dose Nearly 20% men with NGU are infected with trichomonas *(JID 188:465, 2003)*. For alternative option in refractory cases, *see CID 33:1341, 2001.* **Pregnancy:** No data indicating metro teratogenic or mutagenic. For discussion of treating trichomonas, including issues in pregnancy, *see MMWR 64(RR-3):1, 2015; Curr Drug Safety 2015,10:170.*
Bacterial vaginosis (BV) Malodorous vaginal discharge, pH >4.5	Etiology unclear: associated with Gardnerella vaginalis, mobiluncus, Mycoplasma hominis, Prevotella sp., & Atopobium vaginae et al.	**Metro** 0.5 gm po bid x 7 days or **Metro vaginal gel**[10] (1 applicator intravaginally) 1x/day x 5 days OR 2% **Clinda vaginal cream** 5 gm intravaginally at bedtime x 7 days	**Clinda** 0.3 gm bid po x 7 days or **Clinda ovules** 100 mg intravaginally at bedtime x 3 days. **Secnidazole** 2 gm packet (granules on applesauce, yogurt, pudding) x 1 dose over 30 min.	Reported 50% ↑ in cure rate if abstain from sex or use condoms: *CID 44:213 & 220, 2007.* **Treatment of male sex partner not indicated unless balanitis present. Pregnancy:** Oral **Metro** or oral **Clinda** 7-day regimens *(see CDC STD Guidelines: MMWR 64(RR-3):1, 2015)*. If recurrent BV, can try adding **boric acid** to suppressive regimen: Metro 0.5 gm po bid x 7 days, then vaginal boric acid gelatin capsule 600 mg hs x 21 days, followed by Metro vaginal gel 2x/week x 16 weeks *(Sex Trans Dis 36:732, 2009)*.

[10] 1 applicator contains 5 gm of gel with 37.5 mg metronidazole

Abbreviations on page 2. **NOTE: All dosage recommendations are for adults (unless otherwise indicated) and assume normal renal function. § Alternatives consider allergy, PK, compliance, local resistance, cost.*

TABLE 1 (25)

ANATOMIC SITE/DIAGNOSIS/ MODIFYING CIRCUMSTANCES	ETIOLOGIES (usual)	SUGGESTED REGIMENS* PRIMARY	ALTERNATIVE§	ADJUNCT DIAGNOSTIC OR THERAPEUTIC MEASURES AND COMMENTS
GENITAL TRACT *(continued)*				
Men:				
Balanitis	Candida 40%, Group B strep, gardnerella	**Metro** 2 gm po x 1 dose OR **Fluconazole** 150 mg po x 1 dose OR **Itra** 200 mg po bid x 1 day.		Occurs in 1/4 of male sex partners of women infected with candida. Exclude circinate balanitis (Reiter's syndrome); (non-infectious) responds to hydrocortisone cream.
Epididymo-orchitis *(CID 61:S770, 2015)*				
Age <35 years	N. gonorrhoeae, Chlamydia trachomatis	(**Ceftriaxone** 250 mg IM x 1 + **Doxy** 100 mg po bid x 10 days) + bed rest, scrotal elevation, analgesics.		Enterobacteriaceae occasionally encountered. Test all pts age <35 yrs for HIV and syphilis.
Age >35 years or MSM (insertive partners in anal intercourse)	Enterobacteriaceae (coliforms)	[**Levo** 500-750 mg IV/po once daily] OR [(**Oflox** 300 mg po bid) or (400 mg IV twice daily)] for 10-14 days. If STI unlikely, low local resistance, **TMP-SMX** 1 DS bid x 10-14 days. **Amp-sulb**, **P Ceph 3**, **Pip-tazo** *(Dosage: see footnote[9] on page 27)* for MSM can be mixed GC/chlamydia with enterics so treat with FQ AND Ceftriaxone 250 mg IM x1) Also: bed rest, scrotal elevation, analgesics		Midstream pyuria and scrotal pain and edema. **NOTE:** Do urine NAAT (nucleic acid amplification test) to ensure absence of N. gonorrhoeae with concomitant risk of FQ-resistant gonorrhoeae or of chlamydia if using agents without reliable activity. Other causes include: mumps, brucella, TB, intravesicular BCG, B. pseudomallei, coccidioides, Behcet's.
Non-gonococcal urethritis	*See page 25 (CID 61:S763, 2015)*			
Prostatitis—Review: *CID 50:1641, 2010. See Guidelines 2015 http://onlinelibrary.wiley.com/doi/10.1111/bju.13101/epdf*				
Acute Uncomplicated (with risk of STD; age <35 yrs)	N. gonorrhoeae, C. trachomatis	**Ceftriaxone** 250 mg IM x 1 then **Doxy** 100 mg bid x 10 days.		FQs no longer recommended for gonococcal infections. Test for HIV. In AIDS pts, prostate may be focus of Cryptococcus neoformans.
Uncomplicated with low risk of STD	Enterobacteriaceae (coliforms)	**FQ** *(dosage: see Epididymo-orchitis, >35 yrs, above)* or **TMP-SMX** 1 DS tablet (160 mg TMP) po bid x 10–14 days (minimum). Some authorities recommend 4 weeks of therapy.		Treat as acute urinary infection, 14 days (not single dose regimen). Some recommend 3–4 wks therapy. If uncertain, do NAAT for C. trachomatis and N. gonorrhoeae. If resistant enterobacteriaceae, use ERTA 1 gm IV qd. If resistant pseudomonas, use IMP or MER (500 mg IV q6 or q8 respectively)
Chronic bacterial	Enterobacteriaceae 80%, enterococci 15%, P. aeruginosa	**CIP** 500 mg po bid x 4-6 wks OR **Levo** 750 mg po q24h x 4 wks.	**TMP-SMX-DS** 1 tab po bid x 1–3 mos (Fosfomycin: *see Comment*)	**With treatment failures** consider infected prostatic calculi. FDA approved dose of levo is 500 mg; editors prefer higher dose. Fosfomycin penetrates prostate; case report of success with 3 gm po q24h x 12-16 wks *(CID 61:1141, 2015)* or 3 gm q3d x 6 wks *(AAC 60:1854, 2016)*.
Chronic prostatitis/chronic pain syndrome	The most common prostatitis syndrome. Etiology is unknown.	α-adrenergic blocking agents are controversial *(AnIM 133:367, 2000)*.		Pt has sx of prostatitis but negative cultures and no cells in prostatic secretions. Rev.: *JAC 46:157, 2000*. In randomized double-blind study, CIP and an alpha-blocker of no benefit *(AnIM 141:581 & 639, 2004)*.
HAND *(Bites: See Skin)*				
Paronychia				
Nail biting, manicuring	Staph. aureus (maybe MRSA)	Incision & drainage; culture	**TMP-SMX-DS** 1-2 tabs po bid while waiting for culture result.	*See Table 6 for alternatives*. Occasionally--candida, gram-negative rods.
Contact with saliva— dentists, anesthesiologists, wrestlers	Herpes simplex (Whitlow)	**Acyclovir** 400 mg tid po x 10 days	**Famciclovir** or **Valacyclovir**, *see Comment*	Gram stain and routine culture negative. Famciclovir/valacyclovir for primary genital herpes; *see Table 14A, page 181*
Dishwasher (prolonged water immersion)	Candida sp.	**Clotrimazole** (topical)		Avoid immersion of hands in water as much as possible.

Abbreviations on page 2. **NOTE: All dosage recommendations are for adults (unless otherwise indicated) and assume normal renal function. § Alternatives consider allergy, PK, compliance, local resistance, cost.*

TABLE 1 (26)

ANATOMIC SITE/DIAGNOSIS/ MODIFYING CIRCUMSTANCES	ETIOLOGIES (usual)	SUGGESTED REGIMENS*		ADJUNCT DIAGNOSTIC OR THERAPEUTIC MEASURES AND COMMENTS
		PRIMARY	ALTERNATIVE§	
HEART				
Infective endocarditis—Native valve—empirical rx awaiting cultures—No IV illicit drugs	**Diagnostic criteria** include evidence of continuous bacteremia (multiple positive blood cultures), new murmur (worsening of old murmur) of valvular insufficiency, definite emboli, and echocardiographic (transthoracic or transesophageal) evidence of valvular vegetations. Refs.: *Circulation 132:1435, 2015.* For antimicrobial prophylaxis, *see Table 15C, page 223.*			
Valvular or congenital heart disease but no modifying circumstances *See Table 15C, page 223 for prophylaxis*	Viridans strep 30–40%, "other" strep 15–25%, enterococci 5–18%, staphylococci 20-35% (including coag-neg staphylococci- *CID 46:232, 2008).*	**Vanco** 15-20 mg/kg q8-12h (target trough conc of 15-20 µg/mL) + **Ceftriaxone** 2g 24h OR **Vanco** 15-20 mg/kg q8-12h (target trough conc of 15-20 µg/mL) + **Gent** 1 mg/kg q8h IV/IM	Substitute **Dapto** 6 mg/kg IV q24h (or q48h for CrCl <30 mL/min) for **Vanco**	If patient not acutely ill and not in heart failure, wait for blood culture results. If initial 3 blood cultures neg. after 24–48 hrs, obtain 2–3 more blood cultures before empiric therapy started. Gent dose is for CrCl of 80 mL/min or greater; even low-dose Gentamicin for only a few days carries risk of nephrotoxicity *(CID 48:713, 2009)*. Gent is used for synergy; peak levels need not exceed 4 µg/mL and troughs should be <1 µg/mL. Coagulase-negative staphylococci can occasionally cause native valve endocarditis *(CID 46:232, 2008)*. Modify therapy based on identification of specific pathogen as soon as possible to obtain best coverage and to avoid toxicities. **Surgery indications:** *See NEJM 368:1425, 2013.* Role of surgery in pts with left-sided endocarditis & large vegetation *(NEJM 366:2466, 2012)*. No difference in 15 yr survival between bioprosthetic and mechanical valve *(JAMA 312:1323, 2014)*.
Infective endocarditis—Native valve—culture positive Ref: *Circulation 132:1435, 2015.*				
Viridans strep, S. bovis *(S. gallolyticus)* with **pen G MIC ≤0.12 mcg/mL**	**Viridans strep, S. bovis (S. gallolyticus subsp. gallolyticus)**	(**Pen G** 12–18 million units/ day IV, divided - q4h x 4 wks) **OR** (**Ceftriaxone** 2 gm IV q24h x 4 wks)	[(**Pen G or Ceftriaxone** 2 gm IV q24h) + **Gent** 3 mg per kg IV q24h] x 2 wks.	4-wks regimen preferred for most patients. Avoid 2-wks regimen for patients age >65 years, those with cardiac or extracardiac abscess, creatinine clearance of <50 mL/min, impaired eighth cranial nerve function, or Abiotrophia, Granulicatella, or Gemella spp infection. Vancomycin 15 mg/kg q12h x 4 weeks, dose adjusted to achieve trough concentrations of 10-15 µg/mL for patients allergic to or intolerant of Pen or Ceftriaxone.
Viridans strep, S. bovis (S. gallolyticus) with **pen G MIC >0.12 to <0.5 mcg/mL**	**Viridans strep, S. bovis (S. gallolyticus subsp. gallolyticus)**	**Pen G** 24 million units/day IV (divided q4h) x 4 wks + **Gent** 3 mg/kg IV q24h x 2 wks	**Vanco** 15 mg/kg q12h x 4 wks, dose adjusted to achieve trough concentrations of 10-15 µg/mL	If the isolate is Ceftriaxone susceptible (MIC <0.5 µg/mL), then Ceftriaxone x 4 wks alone is an option.
For viridans strep or S. bovis with **pen G MIC ≥0.5 mcg/mL** **NOTE:** Inf. Dis. consultation suggested	**Viridans strep, S. bovis, nutritionally variant streptococci** (new names are: Abiotrophia sp. & Granulicatella sp.)	[(**Pen G** 24 million units per 24h IV, divided q4h x 4 wks) + (**Gent** 3 mg/kg/d in 2-3 divided doses x 4 wks)] OR (**AMP** 12 gm/day IV, divided q4h + **Gent** as above x 4 wks)	**Vanco** 15 mg/kg q12h x 4 wks, dose adjusted to achieve trough concentrations of 10-15 µg/mL	For streptococci with Ceftriaxone MIC <0.5 µg/mL, Ceftriaxone 2 gm q24h can be substituted for ampicillin or penicillin. For gentamicin given 1 mg/kg q8h target peak serum concentration of 3-4 µg/mL and trough serum concentration of <1 µg/mL.

 **NOTE: All dosage recommendations are for adults (unless otherwise indicated) and assume normal renal function. § Alternatives consider allergy, PK, compliance, local resistance, cost.*

TABLE 1 (27)

ANATOMIC SITE/DIAGNOSIS/ MODIFYING CIRCUMSTANCES	ETIOLOGIES (usual)	SUGGESTED REGIMENS*		ADJUNCT DIAGNOSTIC OR THERAPEUTIC MEASURES AND COMMENTS
		PRIMARY	ALTERNATIVE§	
HEART/Infective endocarditis—Native valve—culture positive *(continued)* Ref: *Circulation 132:1435, 2015.*				
Enterococci, penicillin and aminoglycoside susceptible	E. faecalis E. faecium	[(**AMP** 2 gm IV q4h or **Pen G** 24 million units) + **Gent** 3 mg/kg/d IV in 2-3 divided doses] x 4-6 wks	(**AMP** 2 gm IV q4h + **Ceftriaxone** 2 gm IV q12h) x 6 wks Penicillin-intolerant patient only: (**Vanco** 30 mg/kg/d IV in 2 divided doses + **Gent** 1 mg/kg IV q8h) x 6 wks	**Native valve:** 4 wks Pen or AMP + Gent if symptoms <3 mo; 6 wks if symptoms >3 mo; **prosthetic valve:** 6 wks. Target **Vanco** trough of 15-20 µg/mL. Adjust dose of **Gent** to achieve peak serum conc. of 3-4 µg/mL and trough of <1 µg/mL. **AMP+Ceftriaxone** preferred for patients with creatinine clearance <50 mL/min or who develop such on gent regimen. Vanco + Gent toxic: consider pen desensitization.
Enterococci, Penicillin susceptible, Gentamicin resistant (MIC >500 µg/mL), streptomycin susceptible (MIC <1500 µg/mL)	E. faecalis E. faecium	(**AMP** 2 gm IV q4h + **Ceftriaxone** 2 gm IV q12h) x 6 wks	[(**AMP** 2 gm IV q4h or **Pen G** 24 million units) + **streptomycin** 15 mg/kg IV q24h] x 4-6 wks	May have to consider surgical removal of infected valve. Must confirm streptomycin MIC for synergy if strep combo used. **AMP + Ceftriaxone** regimen preferred, if creatinine clearance <50 mL/min, concern for impaired eighth nerve function.
Enterococci, Penicillin, aminoglycoside, Vancomycin resistant	E. faecalis E. faecium	**Dapto** 8-12 mg/kg IV q24h + **AMP** 2 gm IV q4h	**Linezolid** 600 mg IV/po q12h	**Quinupristin-Dalfopristin** 7.5 mg/kg IV q8h (via central line for E. faecium, not active vs E. faecalis). Duration of therapy ≥8 weeks, expert consultation strongly advised. Valve replacement often required for cure.
Infective endocarditis, Gram-negative bacilli	Enterobacteriaceae or P. aeruginosa	Optimal therapy unknown, infectious diseases consult recommended: an aminoglycoside (**Tobra** if P. aeruginosa) + (**Cefepime** or **MER**) is a reasonable option.		Choice of agents based on in vitro susceptibilities, fluoroquinolone an option instead of aminoglycoside, but few data.
Infective endocarditis, fungal	Candida sp. Aspergillus	Optimal therapy unknown, infectious diseases consultation recommended; an azole or echinocandin is a reasonable empirical choice. High failure rate with medical therapy alone, consider early surgery		
Staphylococcal endocarditis **Aortic &/or mitral valve infection—MSSA** Surgery indications: *see Comment page 30.*	**Staph. aureus, methicillin-sensitive**	**Nafcillin/Oxacillin** 2 gm IV q4h x 4–6 wks	[(**Cefazolin** 2 gm IV q8h x 4–6 wks) OR **Vanco** 30-60 mg/kg/d in 2-3 divided doses to achieve trough of 15-20 mcg/mL x 4–6 wks	If IgE-mediated penicillin allergy, 10% cross-reactivity to cephalosporins *(AnIM 141:16, 2004)*. **Cefazolin** and **Nafcillin** probably similar in efficacy and Cefazolin better to erated *(CID 65:100, 2017; Clin Micro Infect 24:152, 2018)*. Presence of cefazolin inoculum effect may limit efficacy *(Open Forum Infect Dis. 2018 May 23;5(6):ofy123)*.
Aortic and/or mitral valve—MRSA	**Staph. aureus, methicillin-resistant**	**Vanco** 30-60 mg/kg per day in 2-3 divided doses to achieve target trough concentrations of 15-20 mcg/mL recom-mended for serious infections.	**Dapto** 8-12 mg/kg q24h IV (Not FDA approved for this indication or dose)	For other alternatives, *see Table 6, page 90.* Daptomycin references: *JAC 68:936 & 2921, 2013.* Case reports of success with Telavancin *(JAC 65:1315, 2010; AAC 54 5376, 2010; JAC 66: 2186, 2011)* and ceftaroline *(JAC 67:1267, 2012; J Infect Chemother 19: 42, 2013).*
Tricuspid valve infection (usually IVDUs): MSSA, uncomplicated	**Staph. aureus, methicillin-sensitive**	**Nafcillin/Oxacillin** 2 gm IV q4h x 2 wks (uncomplicated)	**If penicillin allergy:** **Vanco** 30-60 mg/kg/d in 2-3 divided doses to achieve trough of 15-20 mcg/mL x 4 wks OR **Dapto** 8-12 mg/kg IV q24h x 4 wks OR **Cefazolin** 2 gm IV q8h x 4 wks	**2-week regimen not long** enough if metastatic infection (e.g., osteo) or left-sided endocarditis. **Dapto** resistance can occur de novo, after or during vanco, or after/during dapto therapy. *See Comments on MSSA above.*

 **NOTE: All dosage recommendations are for adults (unless otherwise indicated) and assume normal renal function. § Alternatives consider allergy, PK, compliance, local resistance, cost.*

TABLE 1 (28)

ANATOMIC SITE/DIAGNOSIS/ MODIFYING CIRCUMSTANCES	ETIOLOGIES (usual)	SUGGESTED REGIMENS*		ADJUNCT DIAGNOSTIC OR THERAPEUTIC MEASURES AND COMMENTS
		PRIMARY	ALTERNATIVE§	
HEART/Infective endocarditis—Native valve—culture positive *(continued)*				
Tricuspid valve--MRSA	**Staph. aureus, methicillin-resistant**	**Vanco** 15-20 mg/kg q8-12h to achieve target trough concentrations of 15-20 mcg/mL recommended for serious infections x 4–6 wks	**Dapto** 8-12 mg/kg IV q24h x 4-6 wks *(NEJM 355: 653, 2006). (See Comments & table 6, page 90)*	**Dapto** 8-12 mg/kg not FDA-approved dose.
Slow-growing fastidious Gm-neg. bacilli--any valve	**HACEK group** *(see Comments).*	**Ceftriaxone** 2 gm IV q24h x 4 wks OR **CIP** 400 mg IV q12h x 4 wks	**Amp-sulb** 3 gm IV q6h x 4 wks OR **Levo** 750 mg po/IV q24h x 4 wks OR **Moxi** 400 mg po/ IV q24h x 4 wks	**HACEK** (acronym for Haemophilus parainfluenza, Aggregatibacter, Actinobacillus, Cardiobacterium, Eikenella, Kingella). **AMP** 2 gm IV q4h an option if growth of isolate in vitro is sufficient for reliable determination of ampicillin susceptibility.
Bartonella species--any valve	B. henselae, B. quintana	**Doxy** 100 mg IV/po bid x 6 weeks + **Gent** 3 mg/kg/day IV divided in 3 equal doses x 2 wks	If can't use gentamicin: **Doxy** 100 mg IV/po bid x 6 wks + **RIF** 300 mg IV/po bid x 2 wks	**Dx:** Immunofluorescent antibody titer ≥1:800; blood cultures only occ. positive, or PCR of tissue from surgery *(J Clin Micro 57:e00114, 2019).* B. quintana transmitted by body lice among homeless. **Doxy** considered safe regardless of age for rx ≤21 days *(AAP Redbook 2018).*
Infective endocarditis— "culture negative"				
Fever, valvular disease, and ECHO vegetations ± emboli and neg. cultures.		Etiology in 348 cases studied by serology, culture, histopath, & molecular detection: C. burnetii 48%, Bartonella sp. 28%, and rarely (Abiotrophia elegans (nutritionally variant strep), Mycoplasma hominis, Legionella pneumophila, Tropheryma whipplei—together 1%), & rest without etiology identified (most on antibiotic). *See CID 51:131, 2010 for approach to work-up.* Chronic Q fever: *CID 2017,65:1872. AHA treatment guidelines Circulation 132:1435, 2015.* Study from Germany suggests T. whipplei is 4th most common cause *(J Clin Micro 50:216, 2012).*		
Infective endocarditis—Prosthetic valve—empiric therapy (cultures pending) S. aureus now most common etiology *(JAMA 297:1354, 2007).*				
Early (<2 mos post-op)	S. epidermidis, S. aureus. Rarely, Enterobacteriaceae, diphtheroids, fungi	**Vanco** 15-20 mg/kg q8-12h + **Gent** 1 mg/kg IV q8h + **RIF** 600 mg po q24h		Early surgical consultation advised especially if etiology is S. aureus, evidence of heart failure, presence of diabetes and/or renal failure, or concern for valve ring abscess. Early valve surgery not associated with improved 1 year survival in patients with S. aureus prosthetic valve infection *(CID 60:741, 2015).*
Late (>2 mos post-op)	S. epidermidis, viridans strep, enterococci, S. aureus			
Infective endocarditis— Prosthetic valve—positive blood cultures **Surgical consultation advised:** Indications for surgery: severe heart failure, S. aureus infection, prosthetic dehiscence, resistant organism, emboli due to large vegetation *(See AHA guidelines; Circulation 132:1435, 2015).*	Staph. epidermidis	(**Vanco** 15-20 mg/kg IV q8-12h + **RIF** 300 mg po q8h) x 6 wks + **Gent** 1 mg/kg IV q8h x 14 days.		If S. epidermidis is susceptible to nafcillin/oxacillin in vitro (not common), then substitute nafcillin (or oxacillin) for vanco. Target vanco trough concentrations 15-20 μg/mL. Some clinicians prefer to wait 2-3 days after starting vanco/ gent before starting RIF, to decrease bacterial density and thus minimize risk of selecting rifampin-resistant subpopulations.
	Staph. aureus	Methicillin sensitive: (**Nafcillin/Oxacillin** 2 gm IV q4h + **RIF** 300 mg po q8h) x 6 wks + **Gent** 1 mg per kg IV q8h x 2 wks. Methicillin resistant: (**Vanco** 15-20 mg/kg IV q8-12h (to achieve a target trough of 15-20 mcg/mL) + **RIF** 300 mg po q8h) x 6 wks + **Gent** 1 mg per kg IV q8h x 2 wks.		
	Viridans strep, enterococci	*See infective endocarditis, native valve, culture positive, page 30.* Treat for 6 weeks.		
	Enterobacteriaceae or P. aeruginosa	[(**Cefepime** 2 gm IV q8h or **MER** 1 gm IV q8h) or (**Pip-tazo** 4.5 gm IV q6h) + **Tobra** 1.5-2 mg/kg IV q8h]		In theory, could substitute CIP for aminoglycoside, but no clinical data and resistance is common. Select definitive regimen based on susceptibility results. Can occur with native valves also.
	Candida, aspergillus	*Table 11, page 132*		High mortality. Valve replacement plus antifungal therapy standard therapy but some success with antifungal therapy alone.

 **NOTE: All dosage recommendations are for adults (unless otherwise indicated) and assume normal renal function. § Alternatives consider allergy, PK, compliance, local resistance, cost.*

TABLE 1 (29)

ANATOMIC SITE/DIAGNOSIS/ MODIFYING CIRCUMSTANCES	ETIOLOGIES (usual)	SUGGESTED REGIMENS*		ADJUNCT DIAGNOSTIC OR THERAPEUTIC MEASURES AND COMMENTS
		PRIMARY	ALTERNATIVE§	
HEART *(continued)*				
Infective endocarditis—Q fever *Emerg Infect Dis 21:1183, 2015* *JCM 52:1637, 2014*	Coxiella burnetii	**Doxy** 100 mg po bid + **hydroxychloroquine** 600 mg/day for at least 18 mos *(Mayo Clin Proc 83:574, 2008)*. *Pregnancy: Need long term* **TMP-SMX** *(see CID 45:548, 2007)*.		**Dx:** IFA > 800 phase I IgG plus evidence of endocarditis or vasculopathy or signs of chronic Q fever **OR** positive Coxiella burnetii PCR of blood or tissue. Possible chronic Q fever = IFA > 800 phase I IgG. Treatment duration: 18 mos for native valve, 24 mos for prosthetic valve. Monitor serologically for 5 yrs.
Pacemaker/defibrillator infections	S. aureus (40%), S. epidermidis (40%), Gram-negative bacilli (5%), fungi (5%).	**Device removal + Vanco** 15-20 mg/kg IV q8-12h (methicillin-resistant strain). If methicillin-susceptible staphylococci: **Nafcillin/Oxacillin** 2 gm IV q4h OR **Cefazolin** 2 gm IV q8h	**Device removal + Dapto** 8-10 mg per kg IV q24h[NAI]	**Duration of rx after device removal:** For "pocket" or subcutaneous infection, 10–14 days; if lead-assoc. endocarditis, 4–6 wks depending on organism. Device removal and absence of valvular vegetation assoc. with significantly higher survival at 1 yr *(JAMA 307:1727, 2012)*. British guidelines: *JAC 70:325, 2015*. Prophylaxis: Antibiotic eluting envelope (Tyrx) reduced infection of implantable devices *(NEJM 380:1895, 2019)*.
Pericarditis, bacterial	Staph. aureus, Strep. pneumoniae, Group A strep, Enterobacteriaceae	[**Vanco** 15-20 mg/kg q8-12h + (**Ceftriaxone** 2 gm q24h OR **Cefepime** 2 gm IV q8h)] *(Dosage, see footnote[11])*	**Vanco + CIP** 400 mg q12h *(see footnote[11])*	Drainage required if signs of tamponade. Adjust regimen based on results of organism ID and susceptibility. Use Nafcillin, Oxacillin, or Cefazolin for confirmed MSSA infection.
Rheumatic fever with carditis Ref.: *Ln 366:155, 2005*	Post-infectious sequelae of Group A strep infection (usually pharyngitis)	ASA, and usually prednisone 2 mg/kg po q24h for symptomatic treatment of fever, arthritis, arthralgia. May not influence carditis.		Clinical features: Carditis, polyarthritis, chorea, subcutaneous nodules, erythema marginatum. Prophylaxis: *see page 65.* ASA dose: 80-100 mg/kg/day (pediatric), 4-8 gm/day (adult). Eradication of group A streptococcus also recommended: Child, Penicillin V, 250 mg po tid x 10 days; adult, Penicillin V 500 mg po tid x 10 days.
Ventricular assist device-related infection Manifest & mgmt: *CID 57:1438, 2013* Prevent & mgmt: *CID 64: 222, 2017*	S. aureus, S. epidermidis, aerobic gm-neg bacilli, Candida sp	After culture of blood, wounds, drive line, device pocket and maybe pump: **Vanco** 15-20 mg/kg IV q8-12h + (**Cefepime** 2 gm IV q12h) + **Fluconazole** 800 mg IV q24h.		Can substitute **Daptomycin** 10 mg/kg/d[NAI] for **Vanco,** (**CIP** 400 mg IV q12h or **Levo** 750 mg IV q24h) for cefepime, and (**Vori, Caspo, Micafungin or Anidulafungin**) for **Fluconazole**. Modify regimen based on results of culture and susceptibility tests. Higher than FDA-approved Dapto dose because of potential emergence of resistance.
JOINT—*Also see Lyme Disease, page 62*				
Reactive arthritis				
Reiter's syndrome *(See Comment for definition)*	Occurs wks after infection with C. trachomatis, Campylobacter jejuni, Yersinia enterocolitica, Shigella/Salmonella sp.	Only treatment is non-steroidal anti-inflammatory drugs		**Definition:** Urethritis, conjunctivitis, arthritis, and sometimes uveitis and rash. **Arthritis:** asymmetrical oligoarthritis of ankles, knees, feet, sacroiliitis. **Rash:** palms and soles—keratoderma blennorrhagica; circinate balanitis of glans penis. HLA-B27 positive predisposes to Reiter's.
Poststreptococcal reactive arthritis *(See Rheumatic fever, above)*	Immune reaction after strep pharyngitis: (1) arthritis onset in <10 days, (2) lasts months, (3) unresponsive to ASA	Treat strep pharyngitis and then NSAIDs (prednisone needed in some pts)		A reactive arthritis after a β-hemolytic strep infection in absence of sufficient Jones criteria for acute rheumatic fever. Ref.: *Pediatr Emerg Care 28:1185, 2012.*

[11] **Aminoglycosides** *(see Table 10C, page 128)*, **IMP** 0.5 gm IV q6h, **MER** 1 gm IV q8h, **Nafcillin** or **Oxacillin** 2 gm IV q4h, **Pip-Tazo** 3.375 gm IV q6h or 4.5 gm q8h, **Amp-sulb** 3 gm IV q6h, **P Ceph** 1 (**cephalothin** 2 gm IV q4h or **cefazolin** 2 gm IV q8h), **CIP** 750 mg po bid or 400 mg IV bid, **Vanco** 1 gm IV q12h, **RIF** 600 mg po q24h, **Aztreonam** 2 gm IV q8h, **Cefepime** 2 gm IV q12h

TABLE 1 (30)

ANATOMIC SITE/DIAGNOSIS/ MODIFYING CIRCUMSTANCES	ETIOLOGIES (usual)	SUGGESTED REGIMENS*		ADJUNCT DIAGNOSTIC OR THERAPEUTIC MEASURES AND COMMENTS
		PRIMARY	ALTERNATIVE§	
JOINT *(continued)*				
Septic arthritis: Treatment requires both adequate drainage of purulent joint fluid and appropriate antimicrobial therapy. **There is no need to inject antimicrobials into joints.** Empiric therapy after collection of blood and joint fluid for culture; review Gram stain of joint fluid. 2 wk of oral step-down after surgical drainage and 1-2 days of IV therapy non-inferior to 4 wk for septic arthritis, principally hand or wrist, in adults *(Ann Rheum Dis 2019; 78:1114)*.				
Infants <3 mos (neonate)	Staph. aureus, Enterobacteriaceae, Group B strep	**If MRSA not a concern:** (**Nafcillin** OR **Cefazolin**) + **Cefotaxime**	**If MRSA a concern:** **Vanco + Cefotaxime**	Blood cultures frequently positive. Adjacent bone involved in 2/3 pts. Group B strep and gonococci most common community-acquired etiologies. Kingella kingae suscept. to ceftriaxone *(Ped Infect Dis J 2016, 35:340)*.
Children (3 mos–14 yrs) *K. kingella* most common for age 6-48 mos.	S. aureus 27%, S. pyogenes & S. pneumo 14%, H. influ 3%, Gm-neg. bacilli 6%, other (GC, N. mening) 14%, unk 36%	MRSA prevalence high: **Vanco** + **Cefotaxime** MRSA prevalence low: **Cefazolin**		Marked ↓ in H. influenzae since use of conjugate vaccine. **NOTE:** Septic arthritis due to salmonella has no association with sickle cell disease, unlike salmonella osteomyelitis. Usual duration is 3 weeks for S. aureus, 2-3 weeks others. 10 days of therapy as effective as a 30-day treatment course if there is a good clinical response and CRP levels normalize quickly *(CID 48:1201, 2009)*.
Adults *(review Gram stain): See page 62 for Lyme Disease and page 62 for gonococcal arthritis*				
Acute monoarticular				
At risk for sexually-transmitted disease	**N. gonorrhoeae** *(see page 25)*, S. aureus, streptococci, rarely aerobic Gm-neg. bacilli	**Gram stain negative:** **Ceftriaxone** 1 gm IV q24h or **Cefotaxime** 1 gm IV q8h or **Ceftizoxime** 1 gm IV q8h	If Gram stain shows Gm+ cocci in clusters: **Vanco** 15-20 mg/kg IV q8-12h.	Suspected gonococcal infections (GC): culture urethra, cervix, anal canal, throat, blood, joint fluid. For treatment comments, *see Disseminated GC, page 25.* **Add Azithromycin 1 gm po or Doxycycline 100 mg po twice daily for 7 days if GC proven or suspected**.
Not at risk for sexually-transmitted disease	S. aureus, streptococci, Gm-neg. bacilli	Gram stain shows Gram-pos. cocci: **Vanco** 15-20 mg/kg IV q8-12h Gram stain shows Gram-neg bacilli: **Cefepime** 2 gm q8h IV OR **Meropenem** 1 gm q8h IV Gram stain neg: **Vanco** 15-20 mg/kg IV q8-12h + [**Ceftriaxone** 1 gm IV q24h OR **Cefepime** 2 gm q8h IV q8h (preferred for possible healthcare-associated infection)] *For treatment duration, see Table 3, page 77*		Differential includes gout and chondrocalcinosis (pseudogout). **Look for crystals in joint fluid.** Adjust regimen based on culture and susceptibility. **NOTE:** *See Table 6* for MRSA treatment.
Chronic monoarticular	Brucella, nocardia, mycobacteria, fungi	*See specific bacterial organism (Table 2) and/or mycobacteria (Table 12)*		
Polyarticular, usually acute	**Gonococci,** B. burgdorferi (Lyme), acute rheumatic fever; viruses, e.g., hepatitis B, rubella vaccine, parvo B19, staph and strep may also cause polyarticular infections	Gram stain usually negative for GC. If sexually active, culture urethra, cervix, anal canal, throat, blood, joint fluid, and then: **Ceftriaxone** 1 gm IV q24h. No STD risk, Gram stain negative: **Vanco** + **Ceftriaxone** OR **Cefepime**.		GC may be associated with pustular/hemorrhagic skin lesions and tenosynovitis; treat with **Ceftriaxone** for 7 days and with **Azithromycin** 1 gm po x1 OR **Doxycycline** 100 mg po twice daily for 7 days if GC proven or suspected. Consider Lyme disease if exposure areas known to harbor infected ticks *(see page 62)*; usually large joint. Vanco+ CIP or Levo also an option if low STD risk. Expanded differential includes gout, pseudogout, reactive arthritis (HLA-B27 pos.).
Septic arthritis, post intra-articular injection	MSSE/MRSE 40%, MSSA/ MRSA 20%, P. aeruginosa, Propionibacteria, AFB	**NO empiric therapy.** Arthroscopy for culture/sensitivity, crystals, washout		Treat based on culture results x 14 days (assumes no foreign body present).

Abbreviations on page 2. **NOTE: All dosage recommendations are for adults (unless otherwise indicated) and assume normal renal function. § Alternatives consider allergy, PK, compliance, local resistance, cost.*

TABLE 1 (31)

ANATOMIC SITE/DIAGNOSIS/ MODIFYING CIRCUMSTANCES	ETIOLOGIES (usual)	SUGGESTED REGIMENS*		ADJUNCT DIAGNOSTIC OR THERAPEUTIC MEASURES AND COMMENTS
		PRIMARY	ALTERNATIVE§	
JOINT *(continued)*				
Infected prosthetic joint (PJI) • Suspect infection if sinus tract or wound drainage; acutely painful prosthesis; chronically painful prosthesis; or high ESR/CRP assoc. w/painful prosthesis. • **Empiric therapy is NOT recommended.** Treat based on culture and sensitivity results. • **3 surgical options:** 1) debridement and prosthesis retention (if sx <3 wks or implantation <30 days); 2) 1 stage, direct exchange; 3) 2 stage: debridement, removal, reimplantation • **IDSA Guidelines:** *CID 56:e1, 2013.* • Data do not allow assessment of value of adding antibacterial cement to temporary joint spacers *(CID 55:474, 2012).* • Evidence of systemic absorption of Tobra from antibiotic-impregnated cement spacers *(CID 58:1783, 2014).* *(Continued on next page)*	MSSA/MSSE	**Debridement/Retention**: (**Nafcillin/Oxacillin** 2 gm IV q4h + **RIF** 300 mg po bid) OR (**Cefazolin** 2 gm IV q8h + **RIF** 300 mg po bid) x 2-6 wks followed by [(**CIP** 750 mg po bid OR **Levo** 750 mg po q24h) + **RIF** 300 mg po bid] for 3-6 months (shorter duration for total hip arthroplasty) **1-stage exchange:** IV/po regimen as above for 3 mos **2-stage exchange:** regimen as above for 4-6 wks	(**Dapto** 8-10 mg/kg IV q24h OR **Linezolid** 600 mg po/IV bid) ± **RIF** 300 mg po bid	• **Confirm isolate susceptibility to fluoroquinolone and rifampin:** for fluoroquinolone-resistant isolate consider using other active highly bioavailable agent, e.g., TMP-SMX, Doxy, Minocycline, Amoxicillin-Clavulanate, Clindamycin, or Linezolid. • Enterococcal infection: addition of aminoglycoside optional. • *P. aeruginosa* infection: consider adding aminoglycoside if isolate is susceptible, (but if this improves outcome unclear). • Prosthesis retention most important risk factor for treatment failure *(Clin Microbiol Infect 16:1789, 2010).* (Linezolid 600 mg + Rifampin 300 mg) may be effective as salvage therapy if device removal not possible *(Antimicrob Agents Chemother 55:4308, 2011)* • If prosthesis is retained, consider long-term, suppressive therapy, particularly for staphylococcal infections: depending on in vitro susceptibility options include TMP-SMX, Doxycycline, Minocycline, Amoxicillin, Ciprofloxacin, Cephalexin. • Culture yield may be increased by sonication of prosthesis *(N Engl J Med 357:654, 2007).* • Other treatment consideration: Rifampin is bactericidal vs. biofilm-producing bacteria. Never use Rifampin alone due to rapid development of resistance. Rifampin 300 mg po/IV bid + Fusidic acid[NUS] 500 mg po/IV tid is another option *(Clin Micro Inf 12(S3):93, 2006).* • Watch for toxicity if Linezolid is used for more than 2 weeks of therapy. • Role of longer durations of therapy or chronic suppressive therapy in Gram-negative or Pseudomonas PJI not established. • Alpha-defensin immunoassay (Synovasure) with a sensitivity ~0.8-0.9 and specificity ~0.9-0.95 may be a useful biomarker for diagnosis of PJI. *(Continued on next page)*
	MRSA/MRSE	**Debridement/Retention:** (**Vanco** 15-20 mg/kg IV q8-12h + **RIF** 300 mg po bid) x 2-6 weeks *followed by* [(**CIP** 750 mg po bid OR **Levo** 750 mg po q24h) + **RIF** 300 mg po bid] for 3-6 months (shorter duration for total hip arthroplasty) **1-stage exchange:** IV/po regimen as above for 3 mos **2-stage exchange:** regimen as above for 4-6 wks	(**Dapto** 8-10 mg/kg IV q24h OR **Linezolid** 600 mg po/IV bid) ± **RIF** 300 mg po bid	
	Streptococci (Grps A, B, C, D, viridans, other)	**Debridement/Retention** (Poorer outcomes with retention compared with removal and exchange, *CID 64:1742, 2017*): **Pen G** 20 million units IV continuous infusion q24h or in 6 divided doses OR **Ceftriaxone** 2 gm IV q24h x 4-6 wks **1 or 2 stage exchange:** regimen as above for 4-6 wks	**Vanco** 15 mg/kg IV q12h	

 **NOTE: All dosage recommendations are for adults (unless otherwise indicated) and assume normal renal function. § Alternatives consider allergy, PK, compliance, local resistance, cost.*

TABLE 1 (32)

ANATOMIC SITE/DIAGNOSIS/ MODIFYING CIRCUMSTANCES	ETIOLOGIES (usual)	SUGGESTED REGIMENS*		ADJUNCT DIAGNOSTIC OR THERAPEUTIC MEASURES AND COMMENTS
		PRIMARY	ALTERNATIVE§	
JOINT/Infected prosthetic joint (PJI) *(continued)*				
(Continued from previous page)	Enterococci	**Debridement/Retention:** **Pen-susceptible:** (**AMP** 200 mg/kg/day IV in divided doses q6h or **Pen G** 20 million units/day IV by continuous infusion or in 6 divided doses) x 4-6 wks **Pen-resistant: Vanco** 15 mg/kg IV q12h x 4-6 wks **1 or 2 stage exchange:** regimen as above for 4-6 wks	**Dapto** 8-10 mg/kg IV q24h OR **Linezolid** 600 mg po/IV bid	*(Continued from previous page)*
	Cutibacterium acnes (Hold broth cultures, especially in infections of the shoulder, for 10 days with blind subculture to maximize recovery of C. acnes *(J Clin Microbiol 54:3043, 2016)*).	**Debridement/Retention:** **Pen G** 20 million units IV continuous infusion or in 6 divided doses OR **Ceftriaxone** 2 gm IV q24h x 4-6 wks **1 or 2 stage exchange:** regimen as above for 4-6 wks	**Vanco** 15 mg/kg IV q12h OR **Clinda** 300-450 mg po qid	
	Gm-neg enteric bacilli	**Debridement/Retention:** **Erta** 1 gm q24h IV OR other beta-lactam (e.g., **Ceftriaxone** 2 gm IV q24h OR **Cefepime** 2 gm IV q12h, based on susceptibility) x 4-6 wks **1 or 2 stage exchange:** regimen as above for 4-6 wks	**CIP** 750 mg po bid	
	P. aeruginosa	**Debridement/Retention:** **Cefepime** 2 gm IV q12h OR **MER** 1 gm IV q8h + **Tobra** 5.1 mg/kg once daily IV x 4-6 wks **1 or 2 stage exchange:** regimen as above for 4-6 wks	**CIP** 750 mg po bid or 400 mg IV q8h	
Rheumatoid arthritis	**TNF inhibitors** (adalimumab, certolizumab, etanercept, golimumab, infliximab) and other anti-inflammatory biologics (tofacitinib, rituximab, tocilizumab, abatacept) ↑ risk of TBc, fungal infection, legionella, listeria, and malignancy. Hep B flare may be fatal. *See Med Lett 55:1, 2013 for full listing.*			
Septic bursitis: Olecranon bursitis; prepatellar bursitis	Staph. aureus >80%, M. tuberculosis (rare), M. marinum (rare)	(**Nafcillin/Oxacillin** 2 gm IV q4h or **Cefazolin** 2 gm IV q8h if **MSSA**. Oral step-down: **Diclox** 500 mg po qid	(**Vanco** 15-20 mg/kg IV q8-12h or **Linezolid** 600 mg po bid) if **MRSA**. Another option: **Dapto** 6 mg/kg IV q24h	Empiric MRSA coverage recommended if risk factors are present and in high prevalence areas. Immunosuppression, not duration of therapy, is a risk factor for recurrence; 7 days of therapy may be sufficient for immunocompetent patients undergoing one-stage bursectomy *(JAC 65:1008, 2010)*.

 **NOTE: All dosage recommendations are for adults (unless otherwise indicated) and assume normal renal function. § Alternatives consider allergy, PK, compliance, local resistance, cost.*

TABLE 1 (33)

ANATOMIC SITE/DIAGNOSIS/ MODIFYING CIRCUMSTANCES	ETIOLOGIES (usual)	SUGGESTED REGIMENS*		ADJUNCT DIAGNOSTIC OR THERAPEUTIC MEASURES AND COMMENTS
		PRIMARY	ALTERNATIVE§	
KIDNEY & BLADDER *(Reviewed in Nature Rev 13:269, 2015; IDSA Guidelines CID 52: e103, 2011)*				
Acute Uncomplicated Cystitis & Pyelonephritis in Women				
Cystitis Diagnosis: dysuria, frequency, urgency, suprapubic pain & no vaginal symptoms *See AAC 60:2860, 7535 & 7536, 2016*	E. coli (75-95%) P. mirabilis K. pneumoniae S. saprophyticus Presence of enterococci, Grp B streptococcus, other S. epidermidis suggests contamination Often no need for culture if uncomplicated	**Nitrofurantoin (Macrobid)** 100 mg po bid x 5 d OR **TMP-SMX DS** 1 tab po bid x 3 days (Avoid TMP-SMX if 20% or more local E. coli are resistant) OR **Fosfomycin** 3 gm po x 1 dose (less effective than nitrofurantoin in RCT, *JAMA 2018,319:1771 & 1781)*	• **CIP** 250 mg bid or extended release 500 mg q24h x 3 days • **Levo** 250 mg q24h x 3 days • **Amox-clav** 875/125 mg bid x 5-7 days • **Cephalexin** 500 mg bid x 5-7 days • **Cefdinir** 300 mg bid x 3-7 days • **Pivmecillinam** (NUS) 400 mg bid for 3-7 days	• **Pyridium** (phenazopyridine) may hasten resolution of dysuria. • Beta lactams are less effective. • Nitrofurantoin & Fosfomycin active vs. ESBLs; however, if early pyelonephritis avoid these drugs due to low renal concentrations. • Vaginitis can mimic symptoms of cystitis. • Outpatient therapy of UTIs due to MDR bacteria: - Fosfomycin & nitrofurantoin usually active. - Increasing TMP-SMX & FQ resistance *(AAC 2016,60:2680).* - Beta-lactams least efficacious. - Ref: *CID 2016,63:960.* • In prospective comparative study, no benefit to replacement of needed chronic Foley catheter *(J Am Geriatric Soc 2018;66:1779).*
Pyelonephritis Diagnosis: fever, CVA, pain, nausea/vomiting	Same as for Cystitis, above. Need urine culture & sensitivity testing	*LOW RISK for resistant bacteria:* (**CIP** 500 mg po bid OR **CIP-ER** 1000 mg po once daily OR **Levo** 750 mg po once daily) x 5-7 days OR **Ceftriaxone** 1 gm IV qd x 10 days (can transition to po FQ or TMP-SMX 1 DS bid if suscept) *HIGH RISK for MDR bacteria* consider **Erta** 1 gm IV qd or, if critically ill and/or had recent Pseudomonas infection, **MER** 1 gm IV q8h	*Low risk for resistant bacteria:* **Erta** 1 gm IV q24 or **Gent** 5mg/kg IV qd. When transitioning to po, if FQ or TMP-SMX not an option, consider oral B-lactams to complete 14 days (may be less effective): **Cefixime** 400 mg po qd *(Emerg Med J 2002; 19:19)* **Amox-clav** 875 mg/125 mg po bid	• When tolerating po fluids, can transition to oral therapy; drug choice based on culture/sens results. • Consider imaging (US / CT) if critical illness, new renal failure, history of nephrolithiasis, ureteral colic, obstructive uropathy, urine pH ≥ 7.0, or failure to respond to appropriate therapy. • **HIGH-RISK for resistant bacteria include prior highly-resistant bacteria in urine, recent inpatient health-care facility stay, obstructive uropathy, recent fluoroquinolone or B-lactam exposure, recent travel to Asia, Middle East or Africa in past 3 months)**
Pregnancy: Asymptomatic bacteriuria & cystitis Drug choice based on culture / sensitivity results; do follow-up culture one week after last dose of antibiotic	E. coli (70%) Klebsiella sp. Enterobacter sp. Proteus sp. Grp B Streptococcus	**Nitrofurantoin (Macrobid)** (but not in 3rd trimester) 100 mg po q12h x 5-7 days OR **Amox-clav** 500 mg po q8h x 3-7 days OR **Cephalexin** 500 mg po bid x 3-7 days	**TMP-SMX DS** (but not in 1st trimester or at term) 1 tab po q12h x 3 days OR **Cefpodoxime** 100 mg po q12h x 3-7 days	• Treatment recommended to avoid progression to cystitis or pyelonephritis. • Untreated bacteriuria associated with increased risk of low birth wt, preterm birth & increased perinatal mortality. • If post-treatment culture positive, re-treat with different drug of longer course of same drug. • Avoid nitrofurantoin in 3rd trimester due to risk of hemolytic anemia in newborn.
Pregnancy: Acute pyelonephritis Diagnosis: CVA pain, fever, nausea/vomiting in 2nd/3rd trimester. *See Comment*	Same as for Cystitis, above Regimens are empiric therapy *(see Comment)*	**Moderately ill**: **Ceftriaxone** 1 gm IV q24h OR **Cefepime** 1 gm IV q12h. If Pen-allergic, **Aztreonam** 1 gm IV q8h (no activity vs. Gram-pos cocci)	**Severely ill**: **Pip-Tazo** 3.375 gm IV q6h OR **MER** 500 mg IV q8h OR **Erta** 1 gm IV q24h	• Differential dx includes: placental abruption & infection of amniotic fluid. • Try to avoid FQs and AGs during pregnancy. • Switch to po therapy after afebrile x 48 hrs. • **Treat for 10-14 days.** • If pyelo recurs, re-treat. Once asymptomatic continue suppressive therapy for duration of pregnancy: Nitrofurantoin 50-100 mg po qhs OR Cephalexin 250-500 mg po qhs.

 **NOTE: All dosage recommendations are for adults (unless otherwise indicated) and assume normal renal function. § Alternatives consider allergy, PK, compliance, local resistance, cost.*

TABLE 1 (34)

ANATOMIC SITE/DIAGNOSIS/ MODIFYING CIRCUMSTANCES	ETIOLOGIES (usual)	SUGGESTED REGIMENS* PRIMARY	ALTERNATIVE§	ADJUNCT DIAGNOSTIC OR THERAPEUTIC MEASURES AND COMMENTS
KIDNEY & BLADDER/Acute Uncomplicated Cystitis & Pyelonephritis in Women *(continued)*				
Recurrent UTIs in Women (2 or more infections in 6 mos/ 3 or more infections in 1 yr) Risk factors: family history, spermicide use, presence of cystocele, elevated post-void residual urine volume	Same as for Cystitis, above Regimens are options for antimicrobial prophylaxis	Preventive strategies include avoid spermicide, increase fluid intake (additional 1.5L/ day) *(JAMA Intern Med 2018; 178:1509)*, Methenamine hippurate 1gm PO BID *(Cochrane Database Syst Rev 2012)*, post-coital antibiotics (**Nitrofurantoin** 100 mg OR TMP-SMX 80 mg/400 mg OR TMP 100 mg OR **Cephalexin** 250 mg immediately after intercourse *(JAMA 1993; 264: 703)*. In post-menopausal women use Intravaginal estrogen: 0.5 mg Estriol cream intravaginal daily x 2 weeks and then twice weekly as maintenance *(N Engl J Med 1993; 329: 753)*	When primary options fail, consider daily abx prophylaxis based on susceptibilities of pathogen. Can include **TMP-SMX SS**, **cephalexin** 250 mg, or **nitrofurantoin** 50-100 mg daily)	• No strong evidence to support use of cranberry juice. • Probiotics need more study. • In DBRPCT of women age >65 yrs in nursing home, cranberry capsules resulted in no difference in bacteriuria/pyuria *(JAMA 2016,316:1873 & 1879)*.
Asymptomatic Bacteriuria in Women Defined: 2 consecutive clean catch urine cultures with ≥105 CFU/mL of same organism	Same as for Cystitis, above	**Treatment indicated:** pregnancy, urologic procedure causing bleeding from mucosa	**No treatment indicated:** non-pregnant premenopausal women, spinal cord injury pts, elderly women in/out of nursing home, prosthetic joint surgery	• Asymptomatic bacteriuria & pyuria are discordant. 60% of pts with pyuria have no bacteriuria and pyuria commonly accompanies asymptomatic bacteriuria. • In DBRPCT of women in nursing homes, compared cranberry capsules vs. placebo; no difference in bacteriuria/pyuria *(JAMA 2016;316:1873 (ed) & 1879)*.
Acute Uncomplicated Cystitis & Pyelonephritis in Men. Risk of uncomplicated UTI increased with history of insertive anal sex & lack of circumcision. *See also, Complicated UTIs in Men & Women, below*				
Cystitis	E. coli (75-95%) Rarely other enterobacteriaceae	**TMP-SMX DS** 1 tab po bid x 7 days OR (**CIP** 500 mg po bid OR **CIP-ER** 1000 mg po once daily OR **Levo** 750 mg po once daily) x 5 days		• If recurrent, evaluate for prostatitis. • Cystitis plus symptoms of bladder outlet obstruction suggests concomitant acute bacterial prostatitis. • Consider presence of STDs. Recommend NAAT for C. trachomatis & N. gonorrhoeae. • Avoid Nitrofurantoin due to low renal concentration in prostate. • If any hint of obstructive uropathy, image collecting system asap. • Case report: Fosfomycin 3 gm daily used for MDR gm-neg bacilli *(CID 61:1141, 2015)*.
Pyelonephritis	Pockets of FQ-resistant ESBL producing E. coli *(EID 2016,22:1594)*	*Low risk of MDR-GNB:* (**CIP** 400 mg IV q12h OR **Levo** 750 mg IV once daily) x 7-14 days	*High risk of MDR GNB:* **MER** 0.5-1 gm IV q8h x 7-14 days OR **Erta** 1gm IV q12. If critically illness or recent Pseudomonas infection use **MER** 1 gm IV q8h.	

 **NOTE: All dosage recommendations are for adults (unless otherwise indicated) and assume normal renal function. § Alternatives consider allergy, PK, compliance, local resistance, cost.*

TABLE 1 (35)

ANATOMIC SITE/DIAGNOSIS/ MODIFYING CIRCUMSTANCES	ETIOLOGIES (usual)	SUGGESTED REGIMENS*		ADJUNCT DIAGNOSTIC OR THERAPEUTIC MEASURES AND COMMENTS
		PRIMARY	ALTERNATIVE§	
KIDNEY & BLADDER *(continued)*				
Acute Complicated UTIs in Men & Women				
Defined: UTI plus co-morbid condition that increases infection severity & risk of failure, e.g., diabetes, pregnancy, late diagnosis, chronic foley catheter, suprapubic tube, obstruction secondary to stone, anatomic abnormalities, immunosuppression	E. coli or Other enterobacteriaceae plus: P. aeruginosa Enterococci S. aureus Candida sp.	Prior to empiric therapy: urine culture & sensitivity. If hypotensive: blood cultures. If obstructive uropathy suspected, need imaging of urinary tract asap. *See Comments*		• Uncontrolled infection, esp. if obstruction, can result in emphysematous pyelonephritis, renal abscess, carbuncle, papillary necrosis or perinephric abscess. • Due to co-morbidities & frequent infections, increased risk of drug-resistance pathogens. • Due to high incidence of resistance and infection severity, Nitrofurantoin, Fosfomycin & TMP-SMX should not be used for empiric therapy. • If enterococci cultured, need to adjust therapy based on in vitro susceptibility. • Duration of treatment varies with status of co-morbid conditions, need for urologic procedures & individualized pt clinical response. • Pip-Tazo inferior to MER vs. ceftriaxone-resistant E. coli/K. pneumo *(JAMA 2018;320:979 & 984)*.
		Low risk of MDR GNB: **Levo** 750 mg IV once daily OR **Ceftriaxone** 1 gm IV once daily OR **Cefepime** 1 gm IV q12h OR **Pip-Tazo** 3.375 gm IV q6h OR **Gent** 5 mg/kg IV Once daily. If **Pen-allergic: Aztreonam** 2 gm IV q8h	*Risk of MDR GNB ≥20%:* **MER** 0.5-1 gm IV q8h OR **Ceftolo-tazo** 1.5 gm IV q8h OR **Ceftaz-avi** 2.5 gm IV q8h **MER-vabor** 4 gm IV q8h, *see Comment*	
LIVER *(for Primary (Spontaneous) Bacterial Peritonitis (SBP), see page 49)*				
Cholangitis		*See Gallbladder, page 18*		
Cirrhosis & variceal bleeding	Esophageal flora	**CIP** 400 mg IV q12h x max. of 7 days	**Ceftriaxone** 1 gm IV once daily for max. of 7 days	Short term prophylactic antibiotics in cirrhotics with G-I hemorr, with or without ascites, decreases rate of bacterial infection & ↑ survival *(J Hepatol 60:1310, 2014)*.
Hepatic abscess Klebsiella liver abscess ref.: *Ln ID 12:881, 2012*	Enterobacteriaceae (esp. Klebsiella sp.), bacteroides, enterococci, Entamoeba histolytica, Yersinia enterocolitica (rare), Fusobacterium necrophorum *(Lemierre's)*. *For echinococcus, see Table 13, page 171. For cat-scratch disease (CSD), see pages 48 & 61*	**Metro** + (**Ceftriaxone** OR **Cefoxitin** OR **Pip-Tazo** OR **Amp-sulb** OR **CIP** or **Levo**.	**Metro** (for amoeba) + either **IMP**, **MER** OR **Dori**	**Serological tests for amebiasis should be done on all patients;** if neg., surgical drainage or percutaneous aspiration. In pyogenic abscess, ½ have identifiable GI source or underlying biliary tract disease. If amoeba serology positive, treat with **Metro** alone without surgery. Empiric **Metro** included for both E. histolytica & bacteroides. **Hemochromatosis** associated with Yersinia enterocolitica liver abscess; regimens listed are effective for yersinia. Klebsiella pneumonia genotype K1 associated ocular & CNS Klebsiella infections.
Hepatic encephalopathy	Urease-producing gut bacteria	**Rifaximin** 550 mg po bid (take with lactulose)		Ref: *NEJM 375:1660, 2016*.
Leptospirosis	Leptospirosis, *see page 64*			
Peliosis hepatis in AIDS pts	Bartonella henselae and B. quintana	*See page 61*		
Post-transplant infected "biloma"	Enterococci (incl. VRE), candida, Gm-neg. bacilli (P. aeruginosa 8%), anaerobes 5%	**Linezolid** 600 mg IV bid + **Pip-Tazo** 4.5 gm IV q6h + **Fluconazole** 400 mg IV q24h	**Dapto** 6 mg/kg per day + **Levo** 750 mg IV q24h + **Fluconazole** 400 mg IV q24h	Suspect if fever & abdominal pain post-transplant. Exclude hepatic artery thrombosis. Presence of candida and/or VRE bad prognosticators.
Viral hepatitis	Hepatitis A, B, C, D, E, G	*See Table 14E and Table 14F*		

 **NOTE: All dosage recommendations are for adults (unless otherwise indicated) and assume normal renal function. § Alternatives consider allergy, PK, compliance, local resistance, cost.*

TABLE 1 (36)

ANATOMIC SITE/DIAGNOSIS/ MODIFYING CIRCUMSTANCES	ETIOLOGIES (usual)	SUGGESTED REGIMENS*		ADJUNCT DIAGNOSTIC OR THERAPEUTIC MEASURES AND COMMENTS
		PRIMARY	ALTERNATIVE§	
LUNG/Bronchi				
Bronchiolitis/wheezy bronchitis (expiratory wheezing)				
Infants/children (≤ age 5) *See RSV, Table 14A page 188* Ref: *Ln 368:312, 2006*	**Respiratory syncytial virus** (RSV) 50%, parainfluenza 25%, human metapneumovirus	Antibiotics not useful, mainstay of therapy is oxygen and hydration. Ribavirin not recommended for bronchiolitis except HSCT and perhaps other transplant pts		RSV most important. Rapid diagnosis with antigen detection methods. For prevention a humanized mouse monoclonal antibody, **palivizumab**. *See Table 14A, page 188*. RSV immune globulin is no longer available. Guidance from the American Academy of Pediatrics recommends use of Palivizumab only in newborn infants born at 29 weeks gestation (or earlier) and in special populations (e.g., those infants with significant heart disease). *(Pediatrics 2014;134:415–420)*
Bronchitis				
Infants/children (≤ age 5)	<Age 2: Adenovirus; age 2–5: Respiratory syncytial virus, parainfluenza 3 virus, human metapneumovirus		Antibiotics indicated only with associated sinusitis or heavy growth on throat culture for S. pneumo., Group A strep, H. influenzae or no improvement in 1 week. Otherwise rx is symptomatic.	
Adolescents and adults with acute tracheobronchitis (Acute bronchitis) Ref.: *JAMA 312:2678, 2014*	Usually viral. M. pneumoniae 5%; C. pneumoniae 5%. *See Persistent cough (Pertussis)*	**Antibiotics not indicated.** Antitussive ± inhaled bronchodilators. Throat swab PCR available for Dx of mycoplasma or chlamydia.		Purulent sputum alone not an indication for antibiotic therapy. Expect cough to last 2 weeks. If fever/rigors, get chest x-ray. **If mycoplasma documented, prefer doxy over macrolides due to increasing macrolide resistance** *(AAC 57:e00968-19, 2019)*.
Persistent cough (>14 days), afebrile during community outbreak: Pertussis (whooping cough) 10–20% adults with cough >14 days have pertussis (Review: *Chest 146:205, 2014*)	Bordetella pertussis & occ. Bordetella parapertussis. Also consider asthma, gastro-esophageal reflux, post-nasal drip, mycoplasma and also chlamydia.	**Peds doses: Azithro/ Clarithro** OR **Erythro estolate**[12] OR **Erythro base**[12] OR **TMP-SMX** *(doses in footnote[12])*	**Adult doses: Azithro** po 500 mg day 1, 250 mg q24h days 2–5 OR **Erythro Estolate** 500 mg po qid x 14 days OR **TMP-SMX-DS** 1 tab po bid times 14 days OR (**Clarithro** 500 mg po bid or 1 gm **extended release** q24h x 7 days)	**3 stages of illness:** catarrhal (1–2 wks), paroxysmal coughing (2–4 wks), and convalescence (1–2 wks). Treatment may abort or eliminate pertussis in catarrhal stage, but does not shorten paroxysmal stage. **Diagnosis:** PCR on nasopharyngeal secretions or ↑ pertussis-toxin antibody. **Rx aimed at eradication of NP carriage.** In non-outbreak setting, likelihood of pertussis increased if post-tussive emesis or inspiratory whoop present.
Pertussis: Prophylaxis of household contacts	Drugs and doses as per treatment immediately above. Vaccination of newborn contacts: *CID 58:830, 2014*.			Recommended by Am. Acad. Ped. Red Book 2006 for all household or close contacts; community-wide prophylaxis not recommended.
Acute bacterial exacerbation of chronic bronchitis (ABECB), adults (almost always smokers with COPD) Ref: *NEJM 359:2355, 2008.*	Viruses 20–50%, C. pneumoniae 5%, M. pneumoniae <1%; role of S. pneumo, H. influenzae & M. catarrhalis controversial. Tobacco use, air pollution contribute.	**Severe ABECB** = ↑ dyspnea, ↑ sputum viscosity/purulence, ↑ sputum volume. For severe ABECB: (1) consider chest x-ray, esp. if febrile &/or low O_2 sat.; (2) inhaled anticholinergic bronchodilator; (3) oral corticosteroid for just 5 days (*JAMA 309:2223, 2013*); (4) D/C tobacco use; (5) non-invasive positive pressure ventilation. **Role of antimicrobial therapy is debated even for severe disease,** but study of >80,000 patients shows value of antimicrobial therapy in patients hospitalized with severe disease *(JAMA 303(20):2035, 2010)*. **For mild or moderate disease, no antimicrobial treatment** or maybe **Amox**, **Doxy**, **TMP-SMX**, or **O Ceph. For severe disease, Amox-clav**, **Azithro/Clarithro**, or **O Ceph** or FQs with enhanced activity vs. drug-resistant S. pneumo (**Gemi**, **Levo**, **Moxi** or **Pruliflox**). *Drugs & doses in footnote.* **Duration** varies with drug: range 3–10 days. Limit **Gemi** to 5 days to decrease risk of rash. **Azithro** 250 mg daily x 1 yr modestly reduced frequency of acute exacerbations in pts with milder disease *(NEJM 365:689, 2011)*.		

[12] **ADULT DOSAGE: Amox-clav** 875/125 mg po bid or 500/125 mg po q8h or 2000/125 mg po bid; **Azithro** 500 mg po x 1 dose, then 250 mg q24h x 4 days or 500 mg po q24h x 3 days; *Oral cephalosporins:* **Cefaclor** 500 mg po q8h or 500 mg extended release q12h; **Cefdinir** 300 mg po q12h or 600 mg po q24h; **Cefditoren** 200 mg tabs—2 tabs bid; **Cefixime** 400 mg po q24h; **Cefpodoxime proxetil** 200 mg po q12h; **Cefprozil** 500 mg po q12h; **Ceftibuten** 400 mg po q24h; **Cefuroxime axetil** 250 or 500 mg q12h; **Loracarbef** 400 mg po q12h; **Clarithro** extended release 1000 mg po q24h; **Doxy** 100 mg po bid; **Erythro base** 40 mg/kg/day po div q6h; **Erythro estolate** 40 mg/kg/day po div qid; FQs: **CIP** 750 mg po q12h; **Gemi** 320 mg po q24h; **Levo** 500 mg po q24h; **Moxi** 400 mg po q24h; **Prulifloxacin** 600 mg po q24h (where available); **TMP-SMX** 1 DS tab po bid.

PEDS DOSAGE: Azithro 10 mg/kg/day po on day 1, then 5 mg/kg po q24h x 4 days; **Clarithro** 7.5 mg/kg po q12h; **Erythro base** 40 mg/kg/day div q6h; **Erythro estolate** 40 mg/kg/day div q8-12h; **TMP-SMX** (>6 mos. of age) 8 mg/kg/day (TMP component) div bid.

 **NOTE: All dosage recommendations are for adults (unless otherwise indicated) and assume normal renal function. § Alternatives consider allergy, PK, compliance, local resistance, cost.*

TABLE 1 (37)

ANATOMIC SITE/DIAGNOSIS/ MODIFYING CIRCUMSTANCES	ETIOLOGIES (usual)	SUGGESTED REGIMENS*		ADJUNCT DIAGNOSTIC OR THERAPEUTIC MEASURES AND COMMENTS
		PRIMARY	ALTERNATIVE§	
LUNG/Bronchi *(continued)*				
Bronchiectasis *Thorax 65 (Suppl 1): i1, 2010; Am J Respir Crit Care Med 188:647, 2013.* Acute exacerbation	H. influ., P. aeruginosa, and rarely S. pneumo.	**Gemi**, **Levo**, or **Moxi** x 7-10 days. *Dosage in footnote*[12].		Many potential etiologies: obstruction, ↓ immune globulins, cystic fibrosis, dyskinetic cilia, tobacco, prior severe or recurrent necrotizing bronchitis: e.g. pertussis.
Prevention of exacerbation	Not applicable	Two randomized trials of **Erythro** 250 mg bid *(JAMA 309:1260, 2013)* or **Azithro** 250 mg qd *(JAMA 309:1251, 2013)* x 1 year showed significant reduction in the rate of acute exacerbations, better preservation of lung function, and better quality of life versus placebo in adults with non-cystic fibrosis bronchiectasis.		**Caveats:** higher rates of macrolide resistance in oropharyngeal flora; potential for increased risk of a) cardiovascular deaths from macrolide-induced QTc prolongation, b) liver toxicity, or c) hearing loss *(see JAMA 309:1295, 2013)*. **Pre-treatment screening:** baseline liver function tests, electrocardiogram; assess hearing; sputum culture to exclude mycobacterial disease.
Specific organisms	Aspergillus *(see Table 11)* MAI *(Table 12)* and P. aeruginosa *(Table 5B)*.			
Pneumonia: CONSIDER TUBERCULOSIS IN ALL PATIENTS; ISOLATE ALL SUSPECT PATIENTS				
Neonatal: Birth to 1 month	**Viruses:** CMV, rubella, H. simplex **Bacteria:** Group B strep, listeria, coliforms, S. aureus, P. aeruginosa **Other:** Chlamydia trachomatis, syphilis	**AMP** + **Gent** ± **Cefotaxime**. Add **Vanco** if MRSA a concern. For chlamydia therapy, **Erythro** 12.5 mg per kg po or IV qid times 14 days.		Blood cultures indicated. Consider C. trachomatis if afebrile pneumonia, staccato cough, IgM >1:8; therapy with erythro or sulfisoxazole. If MRSA documented, **Vanco**, **Clinda**, & **Linezolid** alternatives. **Linezolid** dosage from birth to age 11 yrs is 10 mg per kg q8h.
Age 1–3 months				
Pneumonitis syndrome. Usually afebrile	C. trachomatis, RSV, parainfluenza virus 3, human metapneumovirus, Bordetella, S. pneumoniae, S. aureus (rare)	**Outpatient: po** **Amox** 90-100 mg/kg/d x 10-14 days OR **Azithro** 10 mg/kg x 1 dose then 5 mg/kg once daily x 4 days	**Inpatient:** • **If afebrile: Erythro** 10 mg/kg IV q6h or **Azithro** 2.5 mg/kg IV q12h *(see Comment)*. • **If febrile: Cefotaxime** 200 mg/kg per day div q8h OR **Ceftriaxone** 75-100 mg/kg q24h	Pneumonitis syndrome: Cough, tachypnea, dyspnea, diffuse infiltrates, afebrile. Usually requires hospital care. Reports of hypertrophic pyloric stenosis after erythro under age 6 wks; not sure about azithro; bid azithro dosing theoretically might ↓ risk of hypertrophic pyloric stenosis. If lobar pneumonia, give AMP 200–300 mg per kg per day for S. pneumoniae. No empiric coverage for S. aureus, as it is rare etiology.
		For **RSV**, *see Bronchiolitis, page 40*		
Infants and Children, age >3 months to 18 yrs (IDSA Treatment Guidelines: *CID 53:617, 2011*).				
Outpatient	RSV, human metapneumovirus, rhinovirus, influenza virus, adenovirus, parainfluenza virus, Mycoplasma, H. influenzae, S. pneumoniae, S. aureus (rare)	**Amox** 90 mg/kg in 2 divided doses x 5 days	**Azithro** 10 mg/kg x 1 dose (max 500 mg), then 5 mg/kg (max 250 mg) x 4 days OR **Amox-clav** 90 mg/kg (Amox comp) in 2 divided doses x 5 days	Antimicrobial therapy may not be necessary for preschool-aged children with CAP as most infections are viral etiologies. 2011 Guidelines recommend 10-14 days but shorter duration (5-7 days) equally effective in adults.

 **NOTE: All dosage recommendations are for adults (unless otherwise indicated) and assume normal renal function. § Alternatives consider allergy, PK, compliance, local resistance, cost.*

TABLE 1 (38)

ANATOMIC SITE/DIAGNOSIS/ MODIFYING CIRCUMSTANCES	ETIOLOGIES (usual)	SUGGESTED REGIMENS*		ADJUNCT DIAGNOSTIC OR THERAPEUTIC MEASURES AND COMMENTS
		PRIMARY	ALTERNATIVE§	
LUNG/Bronchi/Pneumonia *(continued)*				
Inpatient (3 mos - 18 yrs)	As above	Fully immunized: **AMP** 50 mg/kg IV q6h Not fully immunized: **Cefotaxime** 150 mg/kg IV divided q8h or **Ceftriaxone** 75-100 mg/kg/day	Fully immunized: **Cefotaxime** 150 mg/kg IV divided q8h	If atypical infection suspected, add **Azithro** 10 mg/kg x 1 dose (max 500 mg), then 5 mg/kg (max 250 mg) x 4 days. If community MRSA suspected, add **Vanco** 15-20 mg/kg q8-12h OR **Clinda** 40 mg/kg/day divided q6-8h. Duration of therapy: 10-14 days. Depending on clinical response, may switch to oral agents as early as 2-3 days.
Adults (over age 18) — IDSA/ATS Guideline for CAP in adults: *Am J Crit Care Med 2019, 200:e45.*				
Community-acquired, empiric therapy for outpatient CAP patients with Pneumonia Severity Index (PSI) ≤90 (level I, II, or III) are candidates for out-patient therapy	S. pneumo, atypicals and mycoplasma in particular, Hemophilus, Moraxella, viral pathogens: up to 30% of cases	**No co-morbidity**: **Amox** 1 gm po tid OR **Doxy** 100 mg po bid **Co-morbidity present**: [(**Amox-clav** 875 mg/125 mg po bid x 5-7d + (**Azithro** 500 mg po x1, then 250 mg daily x 4d OR **Levo** 750 mg po q24h x 5d	**No co-morbidity**: if local rates of macrolide resistant S. pneumo < 25%: **Azithro** 500 mg po x 1 dose then 250 mg po q24h x 4 days OR **Clarithro** 500 mg po bid x 7 days **Co-morbidity present**: **Amox-clav + Doxy**	Levo substitutes: **Moxi** 400 mg po q24h or **Gemi** 320 mg po q24h Amox-clav substitutes: **Cefpodoxime** 200 mg po bid or **Cefuroxime** 500 mg po bid. **Treat for 5-7 days**
Community-acquired, empiric therapy for patient admitted to hospital	As above plus *S. aureus* in IVDU or influenza-associated CAP; legionella. No pathogen detected in majority of patients, virus > bacteria *(NEJM 373:415, 2015)*	(**Ceftriaxone** 1-2 gm IV q24h or **Ceftaroline** 600 mg IV q12h) + **Azithro** 500 mg IV q24h OR **Levo** 750 mg IV/po q24h **(not recommended as monotherapy for severe CAP)** For severe CAP use beta-lactam + macrolide	(**Ceftriaxone** 1-2 gm IV q24h or **Ceftaroline** 600 mg IV q12h) + **Doxy** 100 mg IV/po q12h OR **Moxi** 400 mg IV/po q24h For severe CAP beta-lactam + respiratory fluoroquinolone	Sputum and blood cultures recommended for in-patients, especially for severe CAP. Coverage for MRSA or *P. aeruginosa* not routinely recommended in absence of risk factors (e.g., prior isolation of the pathogen or hospitalization AND treatment with parenteral antibiotics within prior 90 days; additional risk factors for MRSA include IVDU and influenza-associated CAP. if empirical coverage is used obtain cultures/nasal PCR to allow de-escalation (cultures negative) or confirmation for need of continued therapy (cultures positive). **Treat for 5-7 days** *(NEJM 370:543, 2014 and Am J Respir Crit Care Med 200:e45-e67, 2019)*. Safe to discontinue antibiotics with normalization of procalcitonin to 0.1-0.2 mcg/mL.

Abbreviations on page 2. **NOTE: All dosage recommendations are for adults (unless otherwise indicated) and assume normal renal function. § Alternatives consider allergy, PK, compliance, local resistance, cost.*

TABLE 1 (39)

ANATOMIC SITE/DIAGNOSIS/ MODIFYING CIRCUMSTANCES	ETIOLOGIES (usual)	SUGGESTED REGIMENS* PRIMARY	SUGGESTED REGIMENS* ALTERNATIVE§	ADJUNCT DIAGNOSTIC OR THERAPEUTIC MEASURES AND COMMENTS
LUNG/Bronchi/Pneumonia *(continued)*				
Hospital-acquired or Ventilator-associated pneumonia IDSA guidelines: *CID 63:e61, 2016*	As above + MDR Gram-negatives. In 39 of 174 pts with non-ventilator HAP, respiratory virus detected *(Resp Med 2017,122:76)*	**Cefepime** 2 gm IV q12h OR **Pip-tazo** 4.5 gm q6h Note: no supportive evidence for use of nebulized/inhaled antibiotics *(CCM 47: 890 & e470, 2019)*. Suscept. testing may identify other active agents, e.g., **Ceftaz-avi**, **MER-vabor**.	**MER** 1 gm IV q8h OR **Levo** 750 mg IV/po q24h	Add **Vanco** or **Linezolid** if unit or hospital MRSA prevalence >10-20%, prior IV antibiotic use within 90 days, acute renal replacement therapy prior to VAP onset, septic shock or high risk of mortality, ARDS preceding VAP, unknown MRSA prevalence or presence of MRSA risk factors (e.g., IVDU, prior MRSA infection or colonization). For suspected pseudomonas or high risk of mortality add **CIP** 400 mg IV q8h or **Levo** 750 mg IV q24h or **Tobra** 5 mg/kg IV q24h or **AMK** 15 mg/kg IV q24h. **Aztreonam** 2 gm IV q8h can substitute for other beta-lactams if there is beta-lactam hypersensitivity, but lacks coverage for S. aureus. Consider addition of Colistin if carbapenem-resistant Gram-negative is suspected.
Pneumonia —Selected specific therapy after culture results (sputum, blood, pleural fluid, etc.) available. *Also see Table 2, page 73*				
Acinetobacter baumannii *(See also Table 5B); CID 2018;67:1455; AAC 2017;61:e01268-16*	Patients with VAP; long ICU stay with repeated antibiotic exposure	**Empiric rx:** positive culture, no in vitro suscept results, prevalence of resistance < 20%: **Cefepime**, **Ceftazidime**, **Amp-sulb** *(Doses in footnote[13]). If prevalence of resistance > 20%:* (**Amp-sulb** + **MER** + **Polymyxin B**) *(See Comments for dosing)*	**Specific rx:** culture & suscept results known, susceptible organism: **Cefepime**, **Ceftazidime**, **Amp-sulb** or **FQ**. If MDR organism & critically ill: **MER** + **Amp-sulb** + **Polymyxin B**	Combination rx for XDR strains in critically ill pts. Based on in vitro hollow-fiber data *(AAC 2017;61:e01268-16)* High dose Amp-sulb safe & effective in prospective observational clin studies *(J Infect 2008;56:432; Scand J Inf Dis 2007;39:38)*. Regimen details: **Amp-sulb** 8/4 gm IV over 4 hr q8h + **MER** 2 gm IV q8h – **Polymyxin B** 2.5 mg/kg IV over 2 hr (loading dose), then 12 hr later start 1.43 mg/kg IV q12h (maint dose).
Actinomycosis	A. Israelii and rarely others	**AMP** 200 mg/kg/day in 3-4 divided doses x 4-6 wks then **Pen** VK 2-4 gm/day in 4 divided doses x 6-12 mo	**Doxy** or **Ceftriaxone** OR **Clinda** IV x 4-6 wks, then po x 6-12 mo	Can use **Pen G** instead of AMP: 10-20 million units/day IV x 4-6 wks, then Pen VK po 6-12 mo.

[13] Doses of antibiotics used to treat pneumonia due to Acinetobacter sp., Klebsiella sp. and Pseudomonas sp. Penicillins: **Pip-Tazo** loading dose 4.5 gm over 30 min, then, 4 hrs later, start 3.375 gm IV over 4 hrs & repeat q8h; **Amp-sulb** 3 gm IV q6h. *Cephalosporins:* **Ceftazidime** 2 gm IV q8h; **Ceftaz-avi** 2.5 gm IV q8h; **Ceftolo-tazo** 3 gm IV q8h. **Aztreonam** 2 gm IV q8h. *FQs:* **CIP** 400 mg IV q8h (septic shock: may need 600 mg q8h); **Levo** 750 mg IV q24h. Carbapenems: **MER** 1-2 gm IV q8h; **MER-vabor** 4 gm IV over 3 hrs q8h; **IMP** 0.5-1 gm q8h. Aminoglycosides: **Gent/Tobra** 7 mg/kg IV x 1, then 5 mg/kg IV q8h. **Polymyxin B** 2.5 mg/kg IV over 2 hrs, then 12 hrs later, 1.5 mg/kg over 1 hr & repeat q12h. **Minocycline** 200 mg IV x 1, then 100 mg IV q12h

Abbreviations on page 2. **NOTE: All dosage recommendations are for adults (unless otherwise indicated) and assume normal renal function. § Alternatives consider allergy, PK, compliance, local resistance, cost.*

TABLE 1 (40)

ANATOMIC SITE/DIAGNOSIS/ MODIFYING CIRCUMSTANCES	ETIOLOGIES (usual)	SUGGESTED REGIMENS*		ADJUNCT DIAGNOSTIC OR THERAPEUTIC MEASURES AND COMMENTS
		PRIMARY	ALTERNATIVE§	
LUNG/Bronchi/Pneumonia/Selected specific therapy after culture results (sputum, blood, pleural fluid, etc.) available. *(continued)*				
Anthrax **Inhalation** (applies to oropharyngeal & gastrointestinal forms): **Treatment** (Cutaneous: *See page 54)* Ref: *www.bt.cdc.gov;* *CDC panel recommendations for adults: Emerg Infect Dis 20(2). Doi: 10.3201/ eid2002.130687.* *AAP recommendations for children: Pediatrics 133:e1411, 2014.*	Bacillus anthracis **To report possible bioterrorism event: 770-488-7100** Plague, tularemia: *See page 46.* Chest x-ray: mediastinal widening & pleural effusion	**Adults (including pregnancy): CIP** 400 mg IV q8h + (**Linezolid** 600 mg IV q12h or **Clinda** 900 mg IV q8h) + **Meropenem** 2 gm IV q8h *(see comments)* + **raxibacumab** 40 mg/kg IV over 2 hrs). Switch to po after 2 wks if stable: **CIP** 500 mg q12h or **Doxy** 100 mg q12h to complete 60-day regimen.	**Children: CIP** 10 mg/kg IV q8h (max 400 mg per dose) + [**Linezolid** 10 mg/kg IV q8h (age <12 yr) or **Linezolid** 15 mg/kg q12h (age >12 yr) (max 600 mg per dose)] + **MER** 40 mg/kg IV q8h (max 2 gm per dose) *(see comments)* + **raxibacumab** 40-80 mg/kg IV over 2 hrs. Switch to po after 2 wks if stable: **CIP** 15 mg/kg q12h or **Doxy** 2.2 mg/kg q12h (<45 kg) or 100 mg q12h (>45 kg) q12h to complete 60-day regimen for oral dosage.	1. Meropenem if meningitis cannot be excluded; Linezolid preferred over Clinda for meningitis. 2. Pen G 4 million units IV (adults) or 67,000 units/kg (children, max 4 million units per dose) IV q4h can be substituted for Meropenem for pen-susceptible strain. 3. For children <8 years of age tooth staining likely with Doxy for 60 days. Alternatives for oral switch include Clinda 10 mg/kg q8h (max dose 600 mg) or Levo 8 mg/kg (max dose 250 mg) q12h for <50 kg, 500 mg q24h >50 kg or for pen-susceptible strains Amox 25 mg/kg (max dose 1 gm) q8h or Pen VK 25 mg/kg (max dose 1 gm) q8h. 4. Levo and Moxi are alternatives to CIP 5. Anthrax immune globulin (**Anthrasil**) FDA approved for emergency use (U.S. strategic national stockpile). 6. Obiltoxaximab 16 mg/kg an alternative to Raxibacumab.
Anthrax, prophylaxis: *See: Emerg Infect Dis 20(2). doi: 10.3201/eid2002.130687.* 60 days of **antimicrobial prophylaxis** + 3-dose series of **Biothrax Anthrax Vaccine Adsorbed**.	Info: *www.bt.cdc.gov*	**Adults (including pregnancy): CIP** 500 mg po q12h or **Doxy** 100 mg po q12h x 60 days + 3-dose series of Biothrax Anthrax Vaccine Adsorbed	**Children: CIP** or **Doxy** *(see above for dosing)* x 60 days +3-dose series of Biothrax (not FDA approved, to be made available on investigational basis)	1. Consider alternatives to Doxy for use in pregnancy. 2. Alternatives include Clinda, Levo, Moxi, and for pen-susceptible strains Amox or Pen VK.
Burkholderia (Pseudomonas) pseudomallei (etiology of melioidosis) Can cause primary or secondary skin infection *See NEJM 367:1035, 2012*	Gram-negative	**Initial parenteral rx: Ceftaz** 30–50 mg per kg IV q8h or **IMP** 20 mg per kg IV q8h. Rx minimum 10 days & improving, then po therapy	**Post-parenteral po rx: Adults** *(see Comment for children)*: **TMP-SMX** 5 mg/kg (TMP component) bid + **Doxy** 2 mg/kg bid x 3 mos.	**Children age ≤8 yrs & pregnancy: AM-CL-ER** 1000/62.5, 2 tabs po bid times 20 wks. Even with compliance, relapse rate is 10%. Max. daily ceftazidime dose: 6 gm. For treatment of MDR strains: *Expert Rev Anti-infect Ther 2018,16:87.*
Chlamydia pneumoniae	Chlamydophila pneumoniae	**Azithro** 500 mg on day one then 250 mg qd x 4 days OR **Levo** 750 mg x 5 days	**Doxy** 100 mg q12h x 5 days OR **Clarithro** 500 mg bid x 5 days	Clinical diagnosis, rarely confirmed microbiologically.
Haemophilus influenzae	β-lactamase negative	**AMP** IV, **Amox** po, **TMP-SMX**, **Azithro/Clarithro**, **Doxy.**		25–35% strains β-lactamase positive. ↑ resistance to both TMP-SMX and doxy. *See Table 10A, page 114 for dosages.*
	β-lactamase positive	**Amox-clav**, **O Ceph 2/3**, **P Ceph 3**, **FQ** Dosage: *Table 10A*		
Influenza virus	See *Table 14A, page 186*. Ref: *IDSA Guidelines, CID 68:895, 2019.*			
Klebsiella sp.—ESBL pos. & other coliforms	β-lactamase positive	**IMP** or **MER**; if resistant: **Ceftolo-tazo**, **Ceftaz-avi** or **MER-vabor** *(See footnote[13] for dosing)*		ESBL inactivates all cephalosporins, β-lactam/β-lactamase inhibitor drug activity not predictable; co-resistance to all FQs & often aminoglycosides. Failure of Pip-tazo vs. ESBLs *(JAMA 2018;320:979 & 984).*
Legionella pneumonia	Legionella pneumophila, other legionella species	(**Levo** 750 mg po/IV or **Moxi** 400 mg po/IV) x 7-10 days	**Azithro** 500 mg x1 on day 1 then 250 mg qd for total of 7-10 days	Consider longer courses of therapy for immunocompromised hosts, severe illness. Trend for better outcomes with FQ over macrolide *(JAC 69:2354, 2014).*

 **NOTE: All dosage recommendations are for adults (unless otherwise indicated) and assume normal renal function. § Alternatives consider allergy, PK, compliance, local resistance, cost.*

ANATOMIC SITE/DIAGNOSIS/ MODIFYING CIRCUMSTANCES	ETIOLOGIES (usual)	SUGGESTED REGIMENS*		ADJUNCT DIAGNOSTIC OR THERAPEUTIC MEASURES AND COMMENTS
		PRIMARY	ALTERNATIVE§	
LUNG/Bronchi/Pneumonia/Selected specific therapy after culture results (sputum, blood, pleural fluid, etc.) available. *(continued)*				
Moraxella catarrhalis	93% β-lactamase positive	**Amox-clav**, **O Ceph 2/3**, **P Ceph 2/3**, **Macrolide**[14], **FQ**, **TMP-SMX**. **Doxy** another option. *See Table 10A, page 114 for dosages*		
Mycoplasma pneumoniae	M. pneumoniae	**Doxy** 100 mg q12h x 7-10 days; Peds: Doxy safe regardless of age for rx ≤ 21 days *(AAP Redbook 2018)*.	**Azithro** 500 mg po on day 1 and then 250 mg po once daily for 4 days *(see Comments)* OR **Levo** 750 mg po/IV x 5 days	If Doxy not available, Mino 200 g po/IV x 1 dose, then 100 mg po/IV bid. Increasing prevalence of macrolide resistance so Doxy then Levo are preferred agents for documented mycoplasma infection. Cold agglutinin ass. complications *(JAMA 2018,319:1377)*.
Nocardia pneumonia Expert Help: Wallace Lab (+1) 903-877-7680; CDC (+1) 404-639-3158 Ref: *Medicine 88:250, 2009.*	N. asteroides, N. brasiliensis	**TMP-SMX** 15 mg/kg/day IV/ po in 2-4 divided doses + **Imipenem** 500 mg IV q6h for first 3-4 weeks then **TMP-SMX** 10 mg/kg/day in 2-4 divided doses x 3-6 mos.	**IMP** 500 mg IV q6h + **Amikacin** 7.5 mg/kg IV q12h x 3-4 wks & then po **TMP-SMX**	**Duration:** 3 mos. if immunocompetent; 6 mos. if immunocompromised. **Measure peak sulfonamide levels:** Target is 100-150 mcg/mL 2 hrs post po dose. **Linezolid** active in vitro. In vitro resistance to TMP-SMX may be increasing *(Clin Infect Dis 51:1445, 2010)*, but whether this is associated with worse outcomes is not known.
Pseudomonas aeruginosa	Risk factors: cystic fibrosis, neutropenia, mechanical ventilation, tracheostomy	*Mild, low risk of MDR GNB: Monotherapy:* [**Pip-Tazo**, **Ceftazidime**, **Cefepime**, **IMP**, **MER** or **Aztreonam**] or [**CIP** or **Levo**] *(Dosing in footnote[13])*	*Septic ± high risk for MDR GNB: Combination rx:* [(**Pip-Tazo**, **Ceftaz** or **Cefepime**) + (**Tobra**) or (**CIP** or **Levo**)] or [(**CIP** or **Levo**) + (**Tobra** or **Gent**)] *(Dosing in footnote[13])*	*Known ESBL producer:* MER or **Ceftolo-tazo*** or **Ceftaz-avi*** or **MER-vabor***. *Known KPC producer:* **Ceftaz-avi*** or **MER-vabor**. *Known metallo-type (NDM) carbapenemase producer:* (**Ceftaz-avi*** + **Aztreonam**). * not FDA-approved indication
Q Fever Acute atypical pneumonia. *See MMWR 62 (3):1, 2013.*	Coxiella burnetii	No valvular heart disease: **Doxy** 100 mg po bid x 14 days Doxy safe regardless of age for rx ≤21 days *(AAP Redbook 2018)*	Valvular heart disease: (**Doxy** 100 mg po bid + **hydroxychloroquine** 200 mg tid) x 12 months *See Comment*	In pregnancy: **TMP-SMX DS** 1 tab po bid throughout pregnancy. Even in absence of valvular heart disease, 1% of pts develop endocarditis *(CID 62:537, 2016)*. If hydroxychloroquine intolerant, Doxy + FQ is alternative *(CID 2018,66:719)*.
Staphylococcus aureus Duration of treatment: 2-3 wks if just pneumonia; 6-8 wks if concomitant endocarditis and/or osteomyelitis. *IDSA Guidelines, CID 52 (Feb 1):1, 2011.*	Nafcillin/oxacillin susceptible	**Nafcillin/oxacillin** 2 gm IV q4h	**Vanco** 30-60 mg/kg/d iv in 2-3 divided doses or **Linezolid** 600 mg IV q12h	Adjust dose of vancomycin to achieve target trough concentrations of 15-20 mcg/mL. Some authorities recommend a 25-30 mg/kg loading dose (actual body weight) in severely ill patients *(CID 49:325, 2009)*. Prospective trial for MRSA pneumonia: cure rate with Linezolid (58%), Vanco (47%), p = 0.042; no difference in mortality *(CID 54:621, 2012)*. **Telavancin** 10 mg/kg IV x 60 min q24h another option. Perhaps lower efficacy if CrCl <50mL/min *(AAC 58:2030, 2014)*. Value of negative nasal S. aureus PCR *(CID 67:1, 2018)*.
	MRSA	**Vanco** 15-20 mg/kg q8-12h IV in 2-3 divided doses or **Linezolid** 600 mg IV/po q12h	**Dapto** not an option; pneumonia developed during dapto rx *(CID 49:1286, 2009)*. **Ceftaroline** 600 mg IV q8h	
Stenotrophomonas maltophilia		**TMP-SMX** 15-20 mg/kg/day div q8h (TMP component)	**Mino** 200 mg IV qd *(AAC 63:e00788-19, 2019)*	FQ is an alternative if susceptible in vitro. Rarely may need to use polymyxin combination therapy.
Streptococcus pneumoniae	Pen-susceptible	**AMP** 2 gm IV q6h, **Amox** 1 gm po tid, **Pen G** IV[15], **Doxy**, **O Ceph 2**, **P Ceph 2/3;** may add **Azithro** 500 mg IV/po qd *(JAC 69:1441, 2014)*. *See Table 10A, page 114 for other dosages.* Treat until afebrile, (min. of 5 days) and/or until serum procalcitonin normal.		
	Pen-resistant, high level	**FQs** with enhanced activity: **Gemi**, **Levo**, **Moxi**; **P Ceph 3** (resistance rare); high-dose IV **AMP**; **Vanco** IV—*see Table 5A, page 88 for more data.* If all options not possible (e.g., allergy), **Linezolid** active: 600 mg IV or po q12h. *Dosages Table 10A.* Treat until afebrile, 3-5 days (min. of 5 days). In CAP trial, **Ceftaroline** 600 mg IV q12h superior to Ceftriaxone *(CID 51:641, 2010)*.		

[14] **Macrolide** = Azithromycin, Clarithromycin and Erythromycin.
[15] **IV Pen G dosage:** no meningitis, 2 million units IV q4h. If concomitant meningitis, 4 million units IV q4h.

Abbreviations on page 2. **NOTE: All dosage recommendations are for adults (unless otherwise indicated) and assume normal renal function. § Alternatives consider allergy, PK, compliance, local resistance, cost.*

TABLE 1 (42)

ANATOMIC SITE/DIAGNOSIS/ MODIFYING CIRCUMSTANCES	ETIOLOGIES (usual)	SUGGESTED REGIMENS* PRIMARY	SUGGESTED REGIMENS* ALTERNATIVE§	ADJUNCT DIAGNOSTIC OR THERAPEUTIC MEASURES AND COMMENTS
LUNG/Bronchi/Pneumonia/Selected specific therapy after culture results (sputum, blood, pleural fluid, etc.) available. *(continued)*				
Tularemia **Inhalational tularemia** Ref.: *JAMA 285:2763, 2001 & www.bt.cdc.gov*	Francisella tularemia **Treatment**	(**Streptomycin** 15 mg per kg IV bid) or (**Gent** 5 mg per kg IV qd) times 10 days	**Doxy** 100 mg IV or po bid times 14–21 days or **CIP** 400 mg IV (or 750 mg po) bid times 14–21 days	Pregnancy: *as for non-pregnant adults.* **Tobramycin** should work.
	Postexposure prophylaxis	**Doxy** 100 mg po bid times 14 days	**CIP** 500 mg po bid times 14 days	Pregnancy: *As for non-pregnant adults*
Viral (interstitial) pneumonia suspected *See Influenza, Table 14A, page 186.* Ref: *Chest 133:1221, 2008.*	Consider: **Influenza**, adenovirus, coronavirus (MERS/SARS), hantavirus, metapneumovirus, parainfluenza virus, respiratory syncytial virus	**Oseltamivir** 75 mg po bid for 5 days or **Zanamivir** two 5 mg inhalations twice a day for 5 days.		No known efficacious drugs for adenovirus, coronavirus, hantavirus, metapneumovirus, parainfluenza or RSV. Need travel (MERS/SARS) & exposure (Hanta) history. RSV and human metapneumovirus as serious as influenza in the elderly *(NEJM 352:1749 & 1810, 2005; CID 44:1152 & 1159, 2007).*
Yersinia pestis (Plague) *EID 2017,23:553; MMWR 64:918, 2015*	Y. pestis If aerosolized, suspect bioterror.	(**Gent** 5 mg/kg IV q24h or **Streptomycin** 30 mg/kg/day in 2 div doses) x 10 days	**CIP** 500 mg po bid or 400 mg IV q12h	**Doxy** 200 mg IV q12h x 1 day, then 100 mg po bid x 7-10 days. **Chloro** also effective but potentially toxic. Consider if evidence of plague meningitis.
LUNG—Other Specific Infections				
Aspiration pneumonia/anaerobic lung infection/lung abscess	Anaerobes and viridans group streptococci predominate.	**Clinda** 300-450 mg po tid OR **Amp-sulb** 3 g IV q6h OR **Ceftriaxone** 1 gm IV q24h + **Metro** 500 mg IV q6h OR 1 gm IV q12h	**Moxi** 400 mg po q24h OR **Erta** 1 gm IV q24h	Typically anaerobic infection of the lung: aspiration pneumonitis, necrotizing pneumonia, lung abscess and empyema *(NEJM 380:651, 2019).* Other treatment options: **Pip-Tazo** 3.325 g IV q6h or **Moxi** 400 mg IV/po q24h or **Amox-clav** 875/125 mg. Note: Different from chemical pneumonitis after aspiration of sterile gastric acid *(CID 2018;67:513).*
Chronic pneumonia with fever, night sweats and weight loss	M. tuberculosis, coccidioidomycosis, histoplasmosis	*See Table 11 and Table 12.* For risk associated with TNF inhibitors, *see CID 41(Suppl 3):S187, 2005.*		Risk factors: HIV+, foreign-born, alcoholism, contact with TB, travel into developing countries
Cystic fibrosis **Acute exacerbation of pulmonary symptoms** *BMC Medicine 9:32, 2011* Choice of therapy should be based on results of respiratory cultures.	S. aureus or H. influenzae early in disease; P. aeruginosa later in disease Nontuberculous mycobacteria emerging as an important pathogen *(Semin Respir Crit Care Med 34:124, 2013)*	**For P. aeruginosa:** (Peds doses) **Tobra** 3.3 mg/kg q8h or 12 mg/kg IV q24h. Combine tobra with **Pip-Tazo** 4.5 gm IV q6h **or Ceftaz** 50 mg/kg IV q8h to max of 6 gm per day. If resistant to above, **CIP/ Levo** used if P. aeruginosa susceptible. *See footnote[16] & Comment*	**For S. aureus: (1) MSSA—Oxacillin/Nafcillin** 2 gm IV q4h. **(2) MRSA—Vanco** 15-20 mg/kg (actual wt) IV q8-12h (to achieve target trough concentration of 15-20 µg/mL.	**Cystic Fibrosis Foundation Guidelines:** 1. Combination therapy for P. aeruginosa infection. 2. Once-daily dosing for aminoglycosides. 3. Need more data on continuous infusion beta-lactam therapy. 4. Routine use of steroid not recommended. **Inhalation options** (P. aeruginosa suppression): 1) Nebulized tobra 300 mg bid x 28 days, no rx for 28 days, repeat; 2) Inhaled tobra powder-hand held: 4-28 mg cap bid x 28 days, no rx for 28 days, repeat; Nebulized aztreonam (Cayston): 75 mg tid after pre-dose bronchodilator. Ref: *Med Lett 56:51, 2014.*
	Burkholderia (Pseudomonas) cepacia. Mechanisms of resistance *(Sem Resp Crit Care Med 36:99, 2015)*	**TMP-SMX** 5 mg per kg (TMP) IV q6h Need culture & sens results to guide rx.	**Chloro** 15–20 mg per kg IV/po q6h	**B. cepacia has become a major pathogen.** Patients develop progressive respiratory failure, 62% mortality at 1 yr. **Fail to respond to aminoglycosides,** anti-pseudomonal beta-lactams. Patients with B. cepacia should be isolated from other CF patients.

[16] Other options: (**Tobra** + **Aztreonam** 50 mg per kg IV q8h); (**IMP** 15–25 mg per kg IV q6h + **Tobra**); **CIP commonly used in children**, e.g., **CIP** IV/po + **Ceftaz** IV *(LnID 3:537, 2003).*

Abbreviations on page 2. **NOTE: All dosage recommendations are for adults (unless otherwise indicated) and assume normal renal function. § Alternatives consider allergy, PK, compliance, local resistance, cost.*

TABLE 1 (43)

ANATOMIC SITE/DIAGNOSIS/ MODIFYING CIRCUMSTANCES	ETIOLOGIES (usual)	SUGGESTED REGIMENS* PRIMARY	ALTERNATIVE§	ADJUNCT DIAGNOSTIC OR THERAPEUTIC MEASURES AND COMMENTS
LUNG—Other Specific Infections *(continued)*				
Empyema. *IDSA Treatment Guidelines for Children, CID 53:617, 2011;* exudative pleural effusion criteria *(JAMA 311:2422, 2014).*				
Neonatal	Staph. aureus	*See Pneumonia, neonatal, page 41*		Drainage indicated.
Infants/children (1 month–5 yrs)	Staph. aureus, Strep. pneumoniae, H. influenzae	*See Pneumonia, age 1 month–5 years, page 41*		Drainage indicated.
Child >5 yrs to Adult—Diagnostic thoracentesis; chest tube for empyemas				
Acute, usually parapneumonic *For dosage, see footnote on page 27*	Strep. pneumoniae, Group A strep	**Cefotaxime** or **Ceftriaxone** *(Dosage, see footnote[9] page 27)*	**Vanco**	Tissue Plasminogen Activator (10 mg) + DNase (5 mg) bid x 3 days via chest tube improves outcome *(NEJM 365:518, 2011).*
	Staph. aureus: Check for MRSA	**Nafcillin/Oxacillin** if MSSA	**Vanco** or **Linezolid** if MRSA.	Usually complication of S. aureus pneumonia &/or bacteremia.
	H. influenzae	**Ceftriaxone**	**TMP-SMX** or **Amp-sulb**	Pleomorphic Gm-neg. bacilli. ↑ resistance to TMP-SMX.
Subacute/chronic	Anaerobic strep, Strep. milleri, Bacteroides sp., Enterobacteriaceae, M. tuberculosis	**Clinda** 450–900 mg IV q8h + **Ceftriaxone**	**Cefoxitin** or **IMP** or **Pip-tazo** or **Amp-sulb** *(Dosage, see footnote[9] page 27)*	Intrapleural tissue plasminogen activator (t-PA) 10 mg + DNase 5 mg via chest tube twice daily for 3 days improved fluid drainage, reduced frequency of surgery, and reduced duration of the hospital stay; neither agent effective alone *(N Engl J Med 365:518, 2011).* Pro/con debate: *Chest 145:14, 17, 20, 2014.* Pleural biopsy with culture for mycobacteria and histology if TBc suspected.
Human immunodeficiency virus infection (HIV+):				
CD4 T-lymphocytes <200 per mm³ or clinical AIDS Dry cough, progressive dyspnea, & diffuse infiltrate **Prednisone first if suspect pneumocystis** *(see Comment)*	Pneumocystis jirovecii (PJP or PCP) most likely; also MTB, fungi, Kaposi's sarcoma, & lymphoma **NOTE:** AIDS pts may develop pneumonia due to DRSP or other pathogens—*see below*	*Rx listed here is for* **severe** *pneumocystis; see Table 11A, page 141 for po regimens for* **mild** *disease.* **Prednisone 1st** *(see Comment),* **then:** **TMP-SMX** [IV: 15 mg per kg per day div q8h (TMP component) or po: 2 DS tabs q8h], total of 21 days	(**Clinda** 600 mg IV q8h + **Primaquine** 30 mg po q24h) or (**pentamidine isethionate** 4 mg per kg per day IV) times 21 days. *See Comment*	**Diagnosis (induced sputum or bronchial wash) for:** histology or monoclonal antibody strains or PCR. **Prednisone 40 mg bid po times 5 days then 40 mg q24h po times 5 days then 20 mg q24h po times 11 days is indicated with PCP should be given at initiation of anti-PCP rx; don't wait until pt's condition deteriorates.** If PCP studies negative, consider bacterial pneumonia, TBc, cocci, histo, crypto, Kaposi's sarcoma or lymphoma. **Pentamidine not active vs. bacterial pathogens.**
CD4 T-lymphocytes normal Acute onset, purulent sputum & pulmonary infiltrates ± pleuritic pain. **Isolate pt until TBc excluded: Adults**	Strep. pneumoniae, H. influenzae, aerobic Gm-neg. bacilli (including P. aeruginosa), Legionella rare, MTB.	**Ceftriaxone** 1 gm IV q24h (over age 65 1 gm IV q24h) + **Azithro**. Could use **Levo,** or **Moxi** IV as alternative *(see Comment)*		For suspected bacterial pneumonia, other regimens for CAP also are options.
LYMPH NODES (approaches below apply to lymphadenitis without an obvious primary source)				
Lymphadenitis, acute				
Generalized	Etiologies: EBV, early HIV infection, syphilis, toxoplasma, tularemia, Lyme disease, sarcoid, lymphoma, systemic lupus erythematosus, **Kikuchi-Fujimoto** disease and others. For differential diagnosis of fever and lymphadenopathy *see NEJM 369:2333, 2013.*			
By Region:				
Cervical—*see cat-scratch disease (CSD)*	CSD (B. henselae), Grp A strep, Staph. aureus, anaerobes, MTB (scrofula), M. avium, M. scrofulaceum, M. malmoense, toxo, tularemia		History & physical exam directs evaluation. If nodes fluctuant, aspirate and base rx on Gram & acid-fast stains. **Kikuchi-Fujimoto** disease causes fever and benign self-limited adenopathy; the etiology is unknown *(Blood 129:917, 2017).*	

Abbreviations on page 2. **NOTE: All dosage recommendations are for adults (unless otherwise indicated) and assume normal renal function. § Alternatives consider allergy, PK, compliance, local resistance, cost.*

TABLE 1 (44)

ANATOMIC SITE/DIAGNOSIS/ MODIFYING CIRCUMSTANCES	ETIOLOGIES (usual)	SUGGESTED REGIMENS*		ADJUNCT DIAGNOSTIC OR THERAPEUTIC MEASURES AND COMMENTS
		PRIMARY	ALTERNATIVE§	
LYMPH NODES/Lymphadenitis, acute/By Region *(continued)*				
Inguinal				
Sexually transmitted	HSV, chancroid, syphilis, LGV			
Not sexually transmitted	GAS, SA, tularemia, CSD, Y. pestis (plague)		Consider bubonic plague & glandular tularemia.	
Axillary	GAS, SA, CSD, tularemia, Y. pestis, sporotrichosis		Consider bubonic plague & glandular tularemia.	
Extremity, with associated nodular lymphangitis	Sporotrichosis, leishmania, Nocardia brasiliensis, Mycobacterium marinum, Mycobacterium chelonae, tularemia		Treatment varies with specific etiology	A distinctive form of lymphangitis characterized by subcutaneous swellings along inflamed lymphatic channels. Primary site of skin invasion usually present; regional adenopathy variable.
Nocardia lymphadenitis & skin abscesses	N. asteroides, N. brasiliensis	**TMP-SMX** 5-10 mg/kg/day based on TMP IV/po div in 2-4 doses	**Sulfisoxazole** 2 gm po qid or **Minocycline** 100-200 mg po bid.	**Duration:** 3 mos. if immunocompetent; 6 mos. if immunocompromised. **Linezolid:** 600 mg po bid reported effective *(Ann Pharmacother 41:1694, 2007)*.
By Pathogen:				
Cat-scratch disease—immunocompetent patient Axillary/epitrochlear nodes 46%, neck 26%, inguinal 17% *(Int J Antimicrob Agts 44:16, 2014)*	Bartonella henselae	Adult: **Azithro** 500 mg po x 1, then 250 mg/day x 4 days. **Peds** (<45.5 kg): **Azithro** sol'n 10 mg/kg x 1, then 5 mg/kg per day x 4 days.	Adult: **Clarithro** 500 mg po bid or **RIF** 300 mg po bid or **TMP-SMX** DS 1 tab po bid or **CIP** 500 mg po bid (duration at least 10 days)	**Dx:** Antibody titer; PCR increasingly available. **Hepatosplenic, CNS or Retinal infection:** (**Doxy** 100 mg po bid + **RIF** 300 mg po bid) x 4-6 wks. Needle drainage of suppurative node(s) provides patient comfort.
Bubonic plague *(see also, plague pneumonia)* *Ref: MMWR 64:918, 2015*	Yersinia pestis	(**Streptomycin** 30 mg/kg/day IV in 2 div doses or **Gentamicin** 5 mg/kg/day IV single dose) x 10 days	[**Levo** 500 mg IV/po once daily or **CIP** 500 mg po (or 400 mg IV) q12h] x 10 days or **Moxi** 400 mg IV/po q24h x 10-14 days	**Doxy** 200 mg IV/po bid x 1 day, then 100 mg IV/po bid x 10 days another option. FQs effective in animals & small case series *(EID 2017,23:553)*. Peds dose 4.4 mg/kg/day div bid safe regardless of age for rx ≤21 days *(AAP Redbook 2018)*.
MOUTH				
Aphthous stomatitis, recurrent	Etiology unknown	Topical steroids (Kenalog in Orabase) may ↓ pain and swelling		
Actinomycosis: "Lumpy jaw" after dental or jaw trauma	Actinomyces israelii	**AMP** 200 mg/kg/day in 3-4 divided doses x 2-6 wks then **Pen VK** 2-4 gm/day in 4 divided doses x 6-12 mo	(**Ceftriaxone** 2 gm IV q24h or **Clinda** 600-900 mg IV q8h or **Doxy** 100 mg IV/po bid) x 4-6 wks, then **Pen VK** 2-4 gm/d x 6-12 mos	**NOTE:** Metro not active vs. actinomyces. Recommendations for a 2-6 week run-in IV therapy prior to oral therapy are traditional and empirical. There are case reports of successful treatment with oral therapy preceded by much shorter durations of IV therapy, as little as 3 days, or no IV therapy at all *(Chest 128:2211, 2005)*, particularly for less severe disease. Durations shorter than 3 months may also be effective in less bulky disease.
Buccal cellulitis Children <5 yrs	H. influenzae	**Ceftriaxone** 50 mg/kg IV q24h	**Amox-clav** 45-90 mg/kg po div bid or **TMP-SMX** 8-12 mg/kg (TMP comp) IV/po div bid	With Hib immunization, invasive H. influenzae infections have ↓ by 95%. Now occurring in infants prior to immunization.
Candida Stomatitis ("Thrush")	C. albicans	**Fluconazole**	Echinocandin	*See Table 11, page 132.*
Dental (Tooth) abscess	Aerobic & anaerobic Strep sp.	Mild: **Amox-clav** 875/125 mg po bid	Severe: **Pip-tazo** 3.375 gm IV q6h	Surgical drainage / debridement. If Pen-allergic: **Clinda** 600 mg IV q6-8h
Herpetic stomatitis	Herpes simplex virus 1 & 2	*See Table 14A*		
Submandibular space infection, bilateral (Ludwig's angina)	Oral anaerobes, facultative streptococci, S. aureus (rare)	**Pip-tazo** or (**Pen G** IV + **Metro** IV)	**Clinda** 600 mg IV q6-8h (for Pen-allergic pt)	**Ensure adequate airway** and early surgical debridement. Add Vanco IV if gram-positive cocci on gram stain. Look for dental infection.
Ulcerative gingivitis (Vincent's angina or Trench mouth)	Oral anaerobes + vitamin deficiency	**Pen G** 4 million units IV q4h or **Metro** 500 mg IV q6h	**Clinda** 600 mg IV q8h	Replete vitamins (A-D). Can mimic scurvy. Severe form is NOMA (Cancrum oris) *(Ln 368:147, 2006)*

 **NOTE: All dosage recommendations are for adults (unless otherwise indicated) and assume normal renal function. § Alternatives consider allergy, PK, compliance, local resistance, cost.*

TABLE 1 (45)

ANATOMIC SITE/DIAGNOSIS/ MODIFYING CIRCUMSTANCES	ETIOLOGIES (usual)	SUGGESTED REGIMENS*		ADJUNCT DIAGNOSTIC OR THERAPEUTIC MEASURES AND COMMENTS
		PRIMARY	ALTERNATIVE§	
MUSCLE				
"Gas gangrene" Contaminated traumatic wound. Can be spontaneous without trauma.	C. perfringens, other histotoxic Clostridium sp.	(**Clinda** 900 mg IV q8h) + (**Pen G** 24 million units/day div. q4–6h IV)		Susceptibility of C. tertium to penicillins and metronidazole is variable; resistance to clindamycin and 3GCs is common, so vanco or metro (500 mg q8h) recommended. IMP or MER expected to have activity in vitro against Clostridium spp.
Pyomyositis	Staph. aureus, Group A strep, (rarely Gm-neg. bacilli), variety of anaerobic organisms	(**Nafcillin** or **Oxacillin** 2 gm IV q4h) or **Cefazolin** 2 gm IV q8h if **MSSA**	**Vanco** 15-20 mg/kg q8-12h if **MRSA**	In immunocompromised or if otherwise suspected, add gram-negative and/or anaerobic coverage. Evaluate for drainage of abscesses.
PANCREAS				
Acute alcoholic (without necrosis) (idiopathic) pancreatitis	Not bacterial	None No necrosis on CT	1–9% become infected but prospective studies show no advantage of prophylactic antimicrobials. Observe for pancreatic abscesses or necrosis which require therapy.	
Post-necrotizing pancreatitis; infected pseudocyst; pancreatic abscess	Enterobacteriaceae, enterococci, S. aureus, S. epidermidis, anaerobes, candida	Need culture of abscess/infected pseudocyst to direct therapy; **Pip-tazo** is reasonable empiric therapy		Can often get specimen by fine-needle aspiration. **Moxi**, **MER**, **IMP**, **ERTA** are all options *(AAC 56:6434, 2012)*.
Antimicrobial prophylaxis, necrotizing pancreatitis	As above	Patients with necrotizing pancreatitis who develop gas in the area of necrosis, rising inflammatory markers or persistent fever may be suspected of having infected pancreatic necrosis and would be candidates for antibiotic therapy. Meta-analysis: initiation of antibiotics within 72 hrs of sx onset reduced infected pancreatic necrosis *(J Hepatobil Pancreat Sci 2015;22:316)*.		
PAROTID GLAND				
"Hot" tender parotid swelling	S. aureus, S. pyogenes, oral flora, & aerobic Gm-neg. bacilli (rare), mumps, rarely enteroviruses/ influenza; parainfluenza: **Nafcillin/Oxacillin** 2 gm IV q4h or cefazolin 2 gm IV q8h if MSSA; **Vanco** if MRSA; **Metro** or **Clinda** for anaerobes			Predisposing factors: stone(s) in Stensen's duct, dehydration. Therapy depends on ID of specific etiologic organism.
"Cold" non-tender parotid swelling	Granulomatous disease (e.g., mycobacteria, fungi, sarcoidosis, Sjögren's syndrome), drugs (iodides, et al.), diabetes, cirrhosis, tumors			History/lab results may narrow differential; may need biopsy for diagnosis.
PERITONEUM/PERITONITIS:				
Primary (Spontaneous) Bacterial Peritonitis (SBP) Dx: Pos culture & ≥250 PMN/mcL of ascites fluid Ref: *Aliment Pharmacol Ther 2015,41:1116*	E. coli 33% Other enterobacteriaceae 11% P. aeruginosa 1% Gm+ cocci 40% Strept sp 15% Staph sp 18% Enterococci 9%	**Community-acquired: low risk of MDR GNB, VRE:** **Pip-tazo** 3.375 gm IV q6h or **Ceftriaxone** 2 gm IV q24h or (if beta lactam allergy) **CIP** 400 mg IV q12h *(J Hepatol 60:1310, 2014)*	**Nosocomial: high risk of MDR GNB, VRE:** **MER** 1 gm IV q8h + **Dapto** 6 mg/kg IV q24h **Note:** In random controlled trial, combination superior to Ceftaz alone *(Hepatology 63:1299, 2016)*	**Diagnosis of SBP:** For microbiologic dx: inoculate 10mL of ascitic fluid into one aerobic and one anaerobic blood culture bottles; yield better if inoculate 2 aerobic and 2 anaerobic bottles. *Comment:* for VRE, may need higher doses of Dapto, eg 8-10 mg/kg per day. **Secondary prophylaxis:** Norfloxacin 400 mg po daily or CIP 500 mg po daily until transplantation or liver function improves to compensated state. In RCT, CIP 750 mg po once weekly as effective as Norflox 400 mg po daily *(Am J Gastroenterol 2018;113:1167)*.
		• Average duration of rx 5 days but varies with severity of infection • To protect renal function: on day 1 & day 3 give IV albumin 1.5 gm/kg		
Prophylaxis after UGI (Variceal) bleeding		Hospitalized pts: **Ceftriaxone** 1 gm, IV once daily x 7 days or **Norfloxacin** 400 mg po bid x 7 days or **CIP** 500 mg po bid x 7 days		
Prevention of SBP *(Amer J Gastro 104:993, 2009)*:				
Cirrhosis & ascites *(Aliment Pharmacol Ther 2015,41:1116)* *For prevention after UGI bleeding, see Liver, page 39*		**CIP** 500 mg/day *(J Hepatol 2008,48:774)*		**TMP-SMX** ↓ peritonitis or spontaneous bacteremia from 27% to 3% *(AnIM 122:595, 1995)*. Ref. for CIP: *Hepatology 22:1171, 1995*.

 **NOTE: All dosage recommendations are for adults (unless otherwise indicated) and assume normal renal function. § Alternatives consider allergy, PK, compliance, local resistance, cost.*

TABLE 1 (46)

ANATOMIC SITE/DIAGNOSIS/ MODIFYING CIRCUMSTANCES	ETIOLOGIES (usual)	SUGGESTED REGIMENS*		ADJUNCT DIAGNOSTIC OR THERAPEUTIC MEASURES AND COMMENTS
		PRIMARY	ALTERNATIVE§	
PERITONEUM/PERITONITIS *(continued)*				
Secondary (bowel perforation, ruptured appendix, ruptured diverticula) Ref: *CID 50:133, 2010 (IDSA Guidelines)* **Antifungal rx?** No need if successful uncomplicated 1st surgery for viscus perforation. Treat for candida if: pure culture from abdomen or blood. In controlled study, no benefit from preemptive rx to prevent invasive candidiasis *(CID 61:1671, 2015)*. **Pediatric appendicitis.** In retrospective review, **Ceftriaxone** 50 mg/kg (max 2 gm) once daily + **Metro** 30 mg/kg (max 1500 mg) once daily as effective as **Erta** *(JPIDS 2017,6:57)*	Enterobacteriaceae, Bacteroides sp., enterococci, P. aeruginosa (3-15%). C. albicans *(see Comment)* If VRE documented, dapto may work *(Int J Antimicrob Agents 32:369, 2008)*. *See Table 5A* for other options for treatment of VRE.	**Mild-moderate disease—Inpatient—parenteral rx:** (e.g., focal periappendiceal peritonitis, peridiverticular abscess). **Usually need surgery for source control**. **Pip-tazo** 3.375 gm IV q6h or 4.5 gm IV q8h or 4-hr infusion of 3.375 gm q8h **OR Erta** 1 gm IV q24h **OR Moxi** 400 mg IV q24h **Severe life-threatening disease—ICU patient: Surgery for source control +** **IMP** 500 mg IV q6h or **MER** 1 gm IV q8h or **Dori** 500 mg IV q8h (1-hr infusion) or (**Ceftolozane-tazobactam** 1.5 gm IV q8h + **Metro** 500 mg q8h) or (**Ceftaz-avi** 2.5 gm IV over 2 hrs q8h + **Metro** 500 mg q8h) **Concomitant surgical management important.**	[(**CIP** 400 mg IV q12h or **Levo** 750 mg IV q24h) + (**Metro** 1 gm IV q12h)] or (**CFP** 2 gm q12h + **Metro**) **NOTE:** avoid tigecycline unless no other alternative due to increased mortality risk (FDA warning) [**AMP** + **Metro** + (**CIP** 400 mg IV q8h or **Levo** 750 mg IV q24h)] **OR** [**AMP** 2 gm IV q6h + **Metro** 500 mg IV q6h + **aminoglycoside** *(see Table 10C, page 128)*]	Must "cover" both Gm-neg. aerobic & Gm-neg. anaerobic bacteria. Empiric coverage of MRSA, enterococci and candida not necessary unless culture indicates infection. Cover enterococci if valvular heart disease. **Drugs active only vs. anaerobic Gm-neg. bacilli:** Metro. **Drugs active only vs. aerobic Gm-neg. bacilli:** aminoglycosides, P Ceph 2/3/4, Aztreonam, AP Pen, CIP, Levo, Ceftolozane-tazo, Ceftaz-avibactam. **Drugs active vs. both aerobic/anaerobic Gm-neg. bacteria:** Pip-tazo, DORI, IMP, MER, tigecycline, eravacycline. Increasing resistance of Bacteroides species *(Anaerobe 17:147, 2013; AAC 56:1247, 2012) to:* **Cefoxitin** / **Cefotetan** / **Clindamycin** **% Resistant**: 5-30 / 17-87 / 19-35 Essentially no resistance of Bacteroides to: **Metro, Pip-tazo, Carbapenems.** Case report of B. fragilis resistant to all drugs except minocycline, tigecycline & linezolid *(MMWR 62:694, 2013)*. **Ertapenem** not active vs. P. aeruginosa/Acinetobacter species. If absence of ongoing fecal contamination, **aerobic/anaerobic culture** of peritoneal exudate/abscess may be of help in guiding specific therapy. Less need for aminoglycosides. **With severe pen allergy,** can "cover" Gm-neg. aerobes with **CIP** or **Aztreonam. Remember Dori/IMP/MER are β-lactams.** IMP dose increased to 1 gm q6h if suspect P. aeruginosa and pt. is critically ill. Resistance to Moxi increasing. *See CID 59:698, 2014* (suscept. of anaerobic bacteria). Recent data suggest that short course antibiotic Rx (approx 4 days) may be sufficient where there is adequate source control of complicated intra-abdominal infections *(NEJM 372:21, 2015)*.
Abdominal actinomycosis	A. Israelii and rarely others	**AMP** 200 mg/kg/day in 3-4 divided doses x 4-6 wks then **Pen VK** 2-4 gm/day in 4 divided doses x 6-12 mo	**Doxy** or **Ceftriaxone** or **Clinda**	Presents as mass +/- fistula tract after abdominal surgery, e.g., for ruptured appendix. Can use IV Pen G instead of AMP: 10-20 million units/day IV x 4-6 wks.
Associated with chronic ambulatory peritoneal dialysis (Abdominal pain, cloudy dialysate, dialysate WBC >100 cell/μL with >50% neutrophils; normal = <8 cells/μL. Ref: *Perit Dial Int 30:393, 2010.)*	Gm+ 45%, Gm- 15%, Multiple 1%, Fungi 2%, MTB 0.1% *(Perit Dial Int 24:424, 2004)*.	**Empiric therapy:** Need activity vs. MRSA **(Vanco)** & aerobic gram-negative bacilli (**Ceftaz**, **CFP**, **Carbapenem**, **CIP**, **Aztreonam**, **Gent**). Add **Fluconazole** if gram stain shows yeast. Use intraperitoneal dosing, unless bacteremia (rare). For bacteremia, IV dosing. For dosing detail, *see Table 19, page 255*.		**For diagnosis:** concentrate several hundred mL of removed dialysis fluid by centrifugation. Gram stain concentrate and then inject into aerobic/anaerobic blood culture bottles. A positive Gram stain will guide initial therapy. If culture shows Staph. epidermidis and no S. aureus, good chance of "saving" dialysis catheter; **if multiple Gm-neg. bacilli cultured, consider catheter-induced bowel perforation and need for catheter removal.** *See Perit Dialysis Int 29:5, 2009.* Other indications for catheter removal: relapsing/refractory peritonitis, fungal peritonitis, catheter tunnel infection.

 **NOTE: All dosage recommendations are for adults (unless otherwise indicated) and assume normal renal function. § Alternatives consider allergy, PK, compliance, local resistance, cost.*

TABLE 1 (47)

ANATOMIC SITE/DIAGNOSIS/ MODIFYING CIRCUMSTANCES	ETIOLOGIES (usual)	SUGGESTED REGIMENS*		ADJUNCT DIAGNOSTIC OR THERAPEUTIC MEASURES AND COMMENTS
		PRIMARY	ALTERNATIVE§	
PHARYNX				
Pharyngitis/Tonsillitis: "Strept throat"				
Exudative or Diffuse Erythema				
Associated cough, rhinorrhea, hoarseness and/or oral ulcers suggest viral etiology. IDSA Guidelines on Group A Strep: *CID 55:1279, 2012*. Pros & cons of diagnostics *(JCM 2016,54:2413)* Even with rapid detection of S. pyogenes, probably still need back-up culture if rapid test is negative *(AJM 2016,54:2413)*. 2 POC PCR (NAAT) assays for GpA strep FDA approved: COBAS Strept A, Alere Strept A. Superior to antigen detection *(JCM 2018;56:e01310)*.	Group A, C, G Strep.; EBV; Primary HIV; *N. gonorrhea*; Respiratory viruses. Student health clinic pts: F. necrophorum found in 20%, Gp A Strep in 10% *(AnIM 162:241, 311 & 876, 2015)*. In another study, *F. necrophorum* in 13.5% (age 14-20 yrs) *(JCM 2017,55:1147)*	**For Strep pharyngitis (adult):** (**Pen V** OR **Benzathine Pen**) OR **Cefdinir** OR **Cefpodoxime**). **If suspect F. necrophorum: Amox-clav** OR **Clinda** Peds: **Pen V** or **Amox** *Doses in footnote*[17].	**For Strep pharyngitis: Clinda** OR **Azithro** OR **Clarithro. If suspect F. necrophorum: Metro; Resistant to macrolides** *Doses in footnote*[17].	**Dx: Rapid Strep test**. If rapid test neg., do culture *(CID 59:643, 2014)*. No need for post-treatment rapid strep test or culture. **Complications of Strep pharyngitis**: 1. Acute rheumatic fever – follows Grp A *S. pyogenes* infection, rare after Grp C/G infection. *See footnote*[18]. For prevention, start treatment within 9 days of onset of symptoms. 2. Children age <7 yrs at risk for post-streptococcal glomerulonephritis. 3. Pediatric autoimmune neuropsychiatric disorder associated with Grp A Strep (PANDAS) infection. 4. Peritonsillar abscess; Suppurative phlebitis are potential complications.
		FQs, tetracyclines & TMP-SMX not recommended due to resistance, clinical failures *(JCM 2012;50:4067)*		
	Gonococcal pharyngitis	**Ceftriaxone** 250 mg IM x 1 dose + **Azithro** 1 gm po x 1 dose	FQs not recommended due to resistance	Not effective for pharyngeal GC: spectinomycin, cefixime, cefpodoxime and cefuroxime. Ref: *MMWR 61:590, 2012. See MMWR 64(RR-03):1, 2015 for most recent CDC STD guidelines.*
	Proven *S. pyogenes* recurrence or documented relapse	**Cefdinir** OR **Cefpodoxime**	**Amox-clav** OR **Clinda**	*Doses in footnote*[17]. Prospective study favors Amox-clav *(JAC 1989,24:227)*
	Grp A infections: 6 in 1 yr; 4 in 2 consecutive yrs	Benefit of tonsillectomy unclear *(Peds 2017,139:e20163490)*		Hard to distinguish true Grp A Strep infection from chronic Grp A Strep carriage and/or repeat viral infections.
Peritonsillar abscess – Sometimes a serious complication of exudative pharyngitis ("Quinsy") *(JAC 68:1941, 2013)*	**F. necrophorum** (44%) *(JCM 2018;56:e00487-18)* Grp A Strep (33%) Grp C/G Strep (9%) S. anginosus grp	Surgical drainage plus **Pip-tazo** 3.375 gm IV q6h or (**Metro** 500 mg IV/po q6-8h+ **Ceftriaxone** 2 gm IV q24h)	Pen allergic: **Clinda** 600-900 mg IV q6-8h	**Avoid macrolides: Fusobacterium is resistant.** Reports of beta-lactamase production by oral anaerobes *(Anaerobe 9:105, 2003)*. *See jugular vein suppurative phlebitis, page 52.* Etiologies ref: *Eur J Clin Micro Infect Dis 2015;34:549*. Culture results may allow de-escalation to **Amp-sulb** 3 gm IV q6h.
Other complications	*See parapharyngeal space infection and jugular vein suppurative phlebitis (see next page)*			

[17] **Treatment of Group A, C & G strep: Treatment durations are from approved package inserts. Subsequent studies indicate efficacy of shorter treatment courses. All po unless otherwise indicated.**

PEDS DOSAGE; Benzathine penicillin 25,000 units per kg IM to max. 1.2 million units; **Pen V** 250 mg bid or tid x 10d (wt < 27kg); **Amox** 50 mg/kg po once daily (max 1000 mg) x 10 days; **Amox-clav** 45 mg per kg per day div. q12h x 10 days; **Cephalexin** 20 mg/kg/dose bid (max 500 mg/dose) x 10 days; **Cefuroxime axetil** 20 mg per kg per day div. bid x 5 days; **Cefpodoxime proxetil** 10 mg per kg div. bid x 5 days; **Cefdinir** 7 mg per kg q12h x 5 days or 14 mg per kg q24h x 10 days; **Cefprozil** 15 mg per kg per day div. bid x 10 days; **Cefadroxil** 30 mg/kg once daily (max 1 gm/day) x 10 days; **Clarithro** 15 mg per kg per day div. bid or 250 mg qid x 10 days; **Azithro** 12 mg per kg once daily x 5 days; clinda 20–30 mg per kg per day div. q8h x 10 days.

ADULT DOSAGE; Benzathine penicillin 1.2 million units IM x 1; **Pen V** 500 mg po bid x 10 days; **Cefditoren** 200 mg bid x 10 days; **Cefuroxime axetil** 250 mg bid x 4 days; **Cefpodoxime proxetil** 100 mg bid x 5 days; **Cefdinir** 300 mg q12h x 5 days or 600 mg q24h x 5 days; **Cefditoren** 200 mg bid; **Cefprozil** 500 mg q24h x 10 days; **NOTE:** All **O Ceph 2** drugs approved for 10-day rx of strep pharyngitis; increasing number of studies show efficacy of 4–6 days; **Clarithro** 250 mg bid x 10 days; **Azithro** 500 mg x 1 and then 250 mg q24h x 4 days or 500 mg q24h x 3 days; Clinda 300 mg po tid x 10 days.

[18] Primary rationale for therapy is eradication of Group A strep (GAS) and prevention of acute rheumatic fever (ARF). Benzathine penicillin G has been shown in clinical trials to ↓ rate of ARF from 2.8 to 0.2%. This was associated with clearance of GAS on pharyngeal cultures (CID 19:1110, 1994). Subsequent studies have been based on cultures, not actual prevention of ARF. Treatment decreases duration of symptoms.

Abbreviations on page 2. **NOTE: All dosage recommendations are for adults (unless otherwise indicated) and assume normal renal function. § Alternatives consider allergy, PK, compliance, local resistance, cost.*

TABLE 1 (48)

ANATOMIC SITE/DIAGNOSIS/ MODIFYING CIRCUMSTANCES	ETIOLOGIES (usual)	SUGGESTED REGIMENS*		ADJUNCT DIAGNOSTIC OR THERAPEUTIC MEASURES AND COMMENTS
		PRIMARY	ALTERNATIVE§	
PHARYNX/Pharyngitis/Tonsillitis/Exudative or Diffuse Erythema *(continued)*				
Membranous pharyngitis: due to **Diphtheria** Respiratory isolation, nasal & pharyngeal cultures (special media), obtain antitoxin. **Place pt in respiratory droplet isolation**.	*C. diphtheriae* (human to human), *C. ulcerans* and *C. pseudotuberculosis* (animal to human) (rare)	**Treatment: antibiotics + antitoxin** **Antibiotic therapy: Erythro** 500 mg IV qid OR **Pen G** 50,000 units/kg (max 1.2 million units) IV q12h. Can switch to **Pen VK** 250 mg po qid when able. Treat for 14 days	**Diphtheria antitoxin:** Horse serum. Obtain from CDC, +1 404-639-2889. Do scratch test before IV therapy. Dose depends on stage of illness: <48hrs: 20,000-40,000 units; if NP membranes: 40,000-60,000 units; >3 days & bull neck: 80,000-120,000 units	**Ensure adequate airway.** EKG & cardiac enzymes. F/U cultures 2 wks post-treatment to document cure. Then, diphtheria toxoid immunization. Culture contacts; treat contacts with either single dose of **Pen G** IM: 600,000 units if age <6 yrs, 1.2 million units if age ≥6 yrs. If Pen-allergic, **Erythro** 500 mg po qid x 7-10 days. Assess immunization status of close contacts: toxoid vaccine as indicated. In vitro, C. diphtheriae suscept. to clarithro, azithro, clinda, FQs, TMP/SMX.
Vesicular, ulcerative pharyngitis (viral)	Coxsackie A9, B1-5, ECHO (multiple types), Enterovirus 71, Herpes simplex 1,2	Antibacterial agents not indicated. For HSV-1, 2: **acyclovir** 400 mg tid po x 10 days.	HIV: **Famciclovir** 250 mg po tid x 7-10 days or **Valacyclovir** 1000 mg po bid x 7-10 days	Small vesicles posterior pharynx suggests enterovirus. Viruses are most common etiology of acute pharyngitis. **Suspect viral if concurrent conjunctivitis, coryza, cough, skin rash, hoarseness.**
Epiglottitis (Supraglottis): Concern in life-threatening obstruction of the airway				
Children	H. influenzae (rare), S. pyogenes, S. pneumoniae, S. aureus (includes MRSA), viruses	**Peds dosage:** (**Cefotaxime** 50 mg per kg IV q8h or **Ceftriaxone** 50 mg per kg IV q24h) + **Vanco**	**Peds dosage: Levo** 10 mg/kg IV q24h + **Clinda** 7.5 mg/kg IV q6h	Have tracheostomy set "at bedside". **Levo** use in children is justified as emergency empiric therapy in pts with severe beta-lactam allergy. *Ref: Ped Clin No Amer 53:215, 2006.* Use of steroids is controversial; do not recommend.
Adults	Group A strep, H. influenzae (rare) & many others	Same regimens as for children. **Adult dosage:** *See footnote*[19]		
Parapharyngeal space infection [Spaces include: sublingual, submandibular (Ludwig's angina) *(see page 48)* lateral pharyngeal, retropharyngeal, pretracheal & descending mediastinitis]				
Poor dental hygiene, dental extractions, foreign bodies (e.g., toothpicks, fish bones) Refs: *Infection 2016,44:77; Otol Head Neck Surg 2016,155:155*	Polymicrobic: S. aureus, Strep sp., anaerobes, Eikenella corrodens. Anaerobes outnumber aerobes 10:1.	**Ceftriaxone** 2 gm IV q24h + **Metro** 500 mg IV q8h	**Pip-tazo** 3.375 gm IV q6h or **Amp-sulb** 3 gm IV q6h	Close observation of airway, 1/3 require intubation. MRI or CT to identify abscess; **surgical drainage. Metro** may be given 1 gm IV q12h. Complications: infection of carotid (rupture possible) & jugular vein phlebitis.
Jugular vein suppurative phlebitis (Lemierre's syndrome) *LnID 12:808, 2012.*	Fusobacterium necrophorum in vast majority *(JCM 2018;56:e00487-18)*	**Pip-tazo** 4.5 gm IV q8h or **IMP** 500 mg IV q6h or (**Metro** 500 mg po/IV q8h + **Ceftriaxone** 2 gm IV once daily)	**Clinda** 600–900 mg IV q8h. **Avoid macrolides: fusobacterium is resistant**	Emboli: pulmonary and systemic common. Erosion into carotid artery can occur. Lemierre described F. necrophorum in 1936; other anaerobes & Gm-positive cocci are less common etiologies of suppurative phlebitis post-pharyngitis.
Laryngitis (hoarseness)	Viral (90%)	Not indicated		

[19] Parapharyngeal space infection: **Ceftriaxone** 2 gm IV q24h; **Cefotaxime** 2 gm IV q4–8h; **Pip-tazo** 3.375 gm IV q6h or 4-hr infusion of 3.375 gm q8h; **TMP-SMX** 8–10 mg per kg per day (based on TMP component) div q6h, q8h, or q12h; **Clinda** 600-900 mg IV q6-8h; **Levo** 750 mg IV q24h; **Vanco** 15 mg/kg IV q12h.

Abbreviations on page 2. **NOTE: All dosage recommendations are for adults (unless otherwise indicated) and assume normal renal function. § Alternatives consider allergy, PK, compliance, local resistance, cost.*

ANATOMIC SITE/DIAGNOSIS/ MODIFYING CIRCUMSTANCES	ETIOLOGIES (usual)	SUGGESTED REGIMENS*		ADJUNCT DIAGNOSTIC OR THERAPEUTIC MEASURES AND COMMENTS
		PRIMARY	ALTERNATIVE§	
SINUSES, PARANASAL				
Sinusitis, acute *Guidelines: Pediatrics 132:e262 & 284, 2013 (American Academy of Pediatrics); Otolaryngol Head Neck Surg 2015,152 (Suppl 2):S1*				
Treatment goals: • Speed resolution • Prevent bacterial complications *(see Comment)* • Prevent chronic sinusitis • Avoid unnecessary use of antibiotics Discussion of when to start antibacterial rx *(AnIM 2017,166:201)*	S. pneumonia 33% H. influenza 32% M. catarrhalis 9% Anaerobes 6% Grp A strep 2% Viruses 15-18% S. aureus 10% *(see Comment)*	Most common: obstruction of sinus ostia by inflammation from virus or allergy. Treatment: Saline irrigation **Antibiotics for bacterial sinusitis if:** 1) fever, pain, purulent nasal discharge; 2) still symptomatic after 10 days with no antibiotic; 3) clinical failure despite antibiotic therapy *No penicillin allergy* **Peds: Amox** 90 mg/kg/day divided q12h or **Amox-clav** suspension 90 mg/kg/day (Amox comp) divided q12h. Treat for 10-14 days **Adult: Amox-clav** 1000/62.5- 2 tabs po bid x 5-7 days	*Penicillin allergy* **Peds (if anaphylaxis): Clinda** 30-40 mg/kg/day divided tid or qid x 10-14 days *(see Comment)* **Peds (no anaphylaxis): Cefpodoxime** 10 mg/kg/day po div q12h **Adult (if anaphylaxis): Levo** or **Doxy**. **Adult (no anaphylaxis): Cefpodoxime** 200 mg po bid	**Treatment:** • Clinda: Haemophilus & Moraxella sp. are resistant; may need 2nd drug • Duration of rx: 5-7 days *(IDSA Guidelines)*, 10-14 days *(Amer Acad Ped Guidelines)* • Adjunctive rx: 1) do not use topical decongestant for >3 days; 2) no definite benefit from nasal steroids & antihistamines; 3) saline irrigation may help • Avoid macrolides & TMP-SMX due to resistance • Empiric rx does not target S. aureus: incidence same in pts & controls *(CID 45:e121, 2007)* Potential complications: transient hyposmia, orbital infection, epidural abscess, brain abscess, meningitis, cavernous sinus thrombosis. For other adult drugs and doses, *see footnote*[20].
Clinical failure after 3 days	As above; consider diagnostic tap/aspirate	**Mild/Mod. Disease: AM-CL-ER** OR (**Cefpodoxime**, **Cefprozil**, or **Cefdinir** *Treat 5-10 days. Adult doses in footnote*[20]	**Severe Disease: Gati**[NUS]**, Gemi, Levo, Moxi**	Severe/hospitalized: **Amp-sulb** 3 gm IV q6h or **Ceftriaxone** 1-2 gm IV q24h or **Levo** 750 mg IV/po q24h. If no response in 48 hrs, CT sinus & surgical consult.
Diabetes mellitus with acute ketoacidosis; neutropenia; deferoxamine rx: Mucormycosis	Rhizopus sp., (mucor), aspergillus	*See Table 11, pages 131 & 140.*		
Hospitalized + nasotracheal or nasogastric intubation	Gm-neg. bacilli 47% (pseudomonas, acinetobacter, E. coli common), Gm+ (S. aureus) 35%, yeasts 18%. Polymicrobial in 80%	Remove nasotracheal tube: if fever persists and ENT available, recommend sinus aspiration for C/S & S. aureus PCR prior to empiric therapy **IMP** 0.5 gm IV q6h or **MER** 1 gm IV q8h. Add **Vanco** for MRSA if Gram stain suggestive.	(**Ceftaz** 2 gm IV q8h + **vanco**) or (**CFP** 2 gm IV q12h + **Vanco**).	After 7 days of nasotracheal or nasogastric tubes, 95% have x-ray "sinusitis" (fluid in sinuses), but on transnasal puncture only 38% culture + *(AJRCCM 150:776, 1994)*. For pts requiring mechanical ventilation with nasotracheal tube for ≥1 wk, bacterial sinusitis occurs in <10% *(CID 27:851, 1998)*. May need fluconazole if yeast on Gram stain of sinus aspirate.
Sinusitis, chronic Adults **Defined:** (drainage, blockage, facial pain, ↓ sense of smell) + (Polyps, purulence or abnormal endoscopy or sinus CT scan: *JAMA 314:926, 2015)*	Multifactorial inflammation of upper airways	Standard maintenance therapy: Saline irrigation + topical corticosteroids	Intermittent/Rescue therapy: For symptomatic nasal polyps: oral steroid x 1-3 wks. For polyps + purulence: **Doxy** 200 mg po x 1 dose, then 100 mg po once daily x 20 days	Leukotriene antagonists considered only for pts with nasal polyps. No antihistamines unless clearly allergic sinusitis. Some suggest >12 wks of macrolide rx; data only somewhat supportive; worry about AEs.

[20] **Adult doses for sinusitis (all oral): AM-CL-ER** 2000/125 mg bid, **amox high-dose (HD)** 1 gm tid, **Clarithro** 500 mg bid or **Clarithro ext. release** 1 gm q24h, **Doxy** 100 mg bid, **respiratory FQs** (**Gati** 400 mg q24h[NUS] due to hypo/hyperglycemia; **Gemi** 320 mg q24h *(not FDA indication but should work)*, **Levo** 750 mg q24h x 5 days, **Moxi** 400 mg q24h); **O Ceph** (**Cefdinir** 300 mg q12h or 600 mg q24h, **Cefpodoxime** 200 mg bid, **Cefprozil** 250-500 mg bid, **Cefuroxime** 500 mg bid), **TMP-SMX** 1 double-strength (TMP 160 mg) bid (results after 3- and 10-day rx similar).

Abbreviations on page 2. **NOTE: All dosage recommendations are for adults (unless otherwise indicated) and assume normal renal function. § Alternatives consider allergy, PK, compliance, local resistance, cost.*

TABLE 1 (50)

ANATOMIC SITE/DIAGNOSIS/ MODIFYING CIRCUMSTANCES	ETIOLOGIES (usual)	SUGGESTED REGIMENS* PRIMARY	ALTERNATIVE§	ADJUNCT DIAGNOSTIC OR THERAPEUTIC MEASURES AND COMMENTS
SKIN *See IDSA Guideline: CID 59:147, 2014.*				
Acne vulgaris *(NEJM 379:343, 2018; Med Lett 61:43, 2019).* **Dermatology consult recommended.** ***BP = benzoyl peroxide; TR = topical retinoid; AB = antibiotic***				
	Mild (all topical therapy)	BP or TR or (BP + TR) or topical (BP + AB)	Add TR or BP if not used. Consider topical **Dapsone**	• TR as monotherapy for comedonal acne or with topical AB for mixed or inflammatory acne • **Clinda** & **Erythro** are recommended topical AB • Only use systemic AB if moderate or severe acne that is resistant to topical therapy • Try to limit systemic AB use to 3 mos • Oral isotretinoin should be restricted to severe nodular acne, recalcitrant acne or acne that causes psychosocial distress and/or scarring
	Moderate (topical or combined topical + oral therapy)	Topical combination therapy: (BP + AB + TR) OR (BP + AB) or (BP + TR) OR Oral/topical combination therapy: (Oral AB + TR + BP + topical AB)	Change combination as in Primary or (if female) add oral contraceptive or oral spironolactone to combination	
	Severe (oral antibiotic + topical therapy and maybe oral retinoid)	(Oral AB + topical combination therapy: BP + AB + retinoid) OR (Oral AB + oral isotretinoin)	Consider different oral AB or (if female) add oral contraceptive or oral spironolactone.	
Acne rosacea Ref: *NEJM 2017;377:1754*	Skin mite: Demadex folliculorum *(Arch Derm 146:896, 2010)*	For Erythema stage: generic **Metro** gel or cream bid x 8-12 weeks	Papulopustular: **Ivermectin (Soolantra)** 1% cream once daily x 8-12 weeks (Expensive)	Systemic oral therapy reserved for severe disease, e.g., **Doxy** 40 mg (low dose) once daily +/- **isotretinoin** 0.1-0.5 mg/kg/d (low dose) x 6-8 mos. Many other therapy options, *see NEJM 2017;377:1754.*
Anthrax, cutaneous **To report bioterrorism event: 770-488-7100;** **For info: www.bt.cdc.gov** Treat as inhalation anthrax if systemic illness. Refs: *AJRCCM 184:1333, 2011* (Review); *CID 59:147, 2014* (Clinical Prac Guideline); Pediatrics 133:e1411, 2014.	B. anthracis Spores are introduced into/ under the skin by contact with infected animals/animal products. *See Lung, page 44.*	**Adults: CIP** 500 mg po q12h or **Doxy** 10 mg po q12h. **Peds: CIP** 15 mg/kg (max dose 500 mg) po q12h or for pen-susceptible strain **Amox** 25 mg/kg (max dose 1 gm) po q8h For bioterrorism exposure, 3-dose series of Biothrax Anthrax Vaccine Adsorbed is indicated.		1. Duration of therapy 60 days for bioterrorism event because of potential inhalational exposure and 7-10 days for naturally acquired disease. 2. Consider alternative to Doxy for pregnancy. 3. Alternatives for adults: Levo 750 mg q24h or Moxi 400 mg q24h or Clinda 600 mg q8h or for pen-susceptible strains Amox 1 gm q8h or Pen VK 500 mg q6h 4. Alternatives for children: Doxy 2.2 mg/kg (max dose 100 mg) q12h (tooth staining likely with 60-day regimen age <8 years) or Clindamycin 10 mg/kg (max dose 600 mg) q8h or Levo 8 mg/kg q12h (max dose 250 mg) if <50 kg and 500 mg q24h if >50 kg
Bacillary angiomatosis: For other Bartonella infections, *see Cat-scratch disease lymphadenitis, page 48, and Bartonella systemic infections, page 61*				
In immunocompromised (HIV-1, bone marrow transplant) patients	Bartonella henselae and quintana	**Clarithro** 500 mg po bid or ext. release 1 gm po q24h or **Azithro** 250 mg po q24h *(see Comment)*	**Erythro** 500 mg po qid or **Doxy** 100 mg po bid or (**Doxy** 100 mg po bid + **RIF** 300 mg po bid)	For AIDS pts, continue suppressive therapy until HIV treated and CD >200 cells/μL for 6 mos. **Drugs to avoid:** TMP-SMX, CIP, Pen, cephalosporins.

 **NOTE: All dosage recommendations are for adults (unless otherwise indicated) and assume normal renal function. § Alternatives consider allergy, PK, compliance, local resistance, cost.*

TABLE 1 (51)

ANATOMIC SITE/DIAGNOSIS/ MODIFYING CIRCUMSTANCES	ETIOLOGIES (usual)	SUGGESTED REGIMENS*		ADJUNCT DIAGNOSTIC OR THERAPEUTIC MEASURES AND COMMENTS
		PRIMARY	ALTERNATIVE§	
SKIN *(continued)*				
Bite: Remember tetanus prophylaxis— *See Table 20B, page 257 for rabies prophylaxis.* Review: *CMR 24:231, 2011.* **Avoid primary wound closure.**				
Alligator *(Alligator mississippiensis)*	Gram negatives including Aeromonas hydrophila, Clostridia sp.	Severe wound: Surgical debridement + (**CIP** 400 mg IV /750 mg po bid or **Levo** 750 mg IV qd) + **Amp-sulb** 3 gm q6h; **OR Pip-Tazo** 4.5 g m IV q8h	Severe wound: Surgical debridement + (**TMP-SMX** 8-10 mg/kg/day IV div q6h or q8h + **Amp-sulb** 3 gm q6h or **Cefepime** 2 gm IV q8h + **Metro** 500 mg q8h)	Oral flora of American alligator isolated: Aeromonas hydrophila and other gram-negatives, and anaerobes including Clostridium spp *(S Med J 82:262, 1989).*
Bat, raccoon, skunk	Strep & staph from skin; rabies	**Amox-clav** 875/125 mg po bid or 500/125 mg po tid	**Doxy** 100 mg po bid	In Americas, **anti-rabies rx indicated:** rabies immune globulin + vaccine. *(See Table 20B, page 257)*
Bear	S. aureus, coagulase-negative staph, viridans streptococci, Enterobacteriaceae, Aeromonas, B. cereus, Neisseria spp, E. durans *(Clin Microbiol Rev 24: 231, 2011)*	**Pip-tazo** 4.5 gm IV q8h	**Vanco** IV (trough 15-20 mcg/mL) + [**Cefepime** 2 gm IV OR **CIP** 400 mg IV q8-12h] + **Metro** 500 mg q8h OR **Amox-clav** 875 mg po bid + **CIP** 500-750 mg po bid.	Injuries often result in hospital level care. Infection with Mycobacterium fortuitum reported *(J Clin Micro 43: 1009, 2005).* Rabies occurs in bears *(MMWR 48: 761, 1999).*
Camel	S. aureus, Streptococcus spp, P. aeruginosa, Other Gm-neg bacilli	**Pip-tazo** 4.5 gm q8h	**Cephalexin** 500 mg po qid + **CIP** 750 mg po bid	*See EJCMID 18:918, 1999.* Rabies can occur in camels *(PLoS Negl Trop Dis. 2016; 10(9): e0004890).*
Cat: 80% get infected, culture & treat empirically. Cat-scratch disease: *page 48*	**Pasteurella multocida**, Streptococci, Staph. aureus, Neisseria, Moraxella	**Amox-clav** 875/125 mg po bid 1000/62.5 mg 2 tabs po bid	**Cefuroxime axetil** 0.5 gm po q12h or **Doxy** 100 mg po bid. **Do not use cephalexin.** Sens. to FQs in vitro.	**P. multocida resistant to dicloxacillin, cephalexin, clinda; many strains resistant to erythro** (most sensitive to azithro but no clinical data). P. multocida infection develops within 24 hrs. Observe for osteomyelitis. If culture + for only P. multocida, can switch to pen G IV or pen VK po. *See Dog Bite*
Catfish sting	Toxins (pain may respond to immersion in hot water as tolerated) Evaluate for retained foreign body (spine) May become secondarily infected	**Doxy** 100 mg po bid + **Amox-clav** 875/125 mg po bid		Toxin injury presents as immediate pain, erythema, edema; resembles strep cellulitis. May become infected with marine organisms or staphylococci *(CID 14: 689, 1992).*
Dog: Only 5% get infected; treat only if bite severe or bad co-morbidity (e.g. diabetes).	**Pasteurella canis**, S. aureus, Streptococci, Fusobacterium sp., Capnocytophaga canimorsus	**Amox-clav** 875/125 mg po bid or 1000/62.5 mg 2 tabs po bid	Adult: **Clinda** 300 mg po q6h + **FQ** Child: **Clinda** + **TMP-SMX**	Consider anti-rabies prophylaxis: rabies immune globulin + vaccine *(see Table 20B).* Capnocytophaga in splenectomized pts may cause local eschar, sepsis with DIC. **P. canis resistant to diclox, cephalexin, clinda and erythro;** sensitive to Ceftriaxone, cefuroxime, cefpodoxime and FQs.
Horse	Actinobacillus, Pasteurella, Enteric Gram negative bacilli, S aureus, streptococci, anaerobes	**Amox-clav** 875/125 mg po bid	**Doxy** 100 mg po bid	Debridement often needed. IV antibiotics may be needed for severe wounds. Strep. equi meningitis and brain abscess reported *(Lancet 376: 1194, 2010)*

Abbreviations on page 2. **NOTE: All dosage recommendations are for adults (unless otherwise indicated) and assume normal renal function. § Alternatives consider allergy, PK, compliance, local resistance, cost.*

TABLE 1 (52)

ANATOMIC SITE/DIAGNOSIS/ MODIFYING CIRCUMSTANCES	ETIOLOGIES (usual)	SUGGESTED REGIMENS*		ADJUNCT DIAGNOSTIC OR THERAPEUTIC MEASURES AND COMMENTS
		PRIMARY	ALTERNATIVE§	
SKIN/Bite *(continued)*				
Human For bacteriology, *see CID 37:1481, 2003*	Viridans strep 100%, Staph epidermidis 53%, corynebacterium 41%, **Staph. aureus 29%, eikenella 15%,** bacteroides 82%, peptostrep 26%	**Early** (not yet infected): **Amox-clav** 875/125 mg po bid times 5 days. **Later:** Signs of infection (usually in 3–24 hrs): (**Amp-sulb** 1.5 gm IV q6h or **Cefoxitin** 2 gm IV q8h) or (**Pip-tazo** 3.375 gm IV q6h or 4.5 gm q8h or 4-hr infusion of 3.375 gm q8h). Pen allergy: **Clinda** + (either **CIP** or **TMP-SMX**)		**Cleaning, irrigation and debridement most important.** For clenched fist injuries, x-rays should be obtained. Bites inflicted by hospitalized pts, consider aerobic Gm-neg. bacilli. **Eikenella resistant to clinda, nafcillin/ oxacillin, metro, P Ceph 1, and erythro; susceptible to FQs and TMP-SMX.**
Komodo dragon	Staphylococcus spp, Bacillus spp, Aeromonas, Pseudomonas spp, Enterobacteriaceae, Burkholderia, anaerobes	**Amox-clav** 875 mg po bid plus **CIP** 750 po bid	**Pip-tazo** 4.5 gm IV q8h	Microbiology: see *CMR 24: 231, 2011.* Also have toxic venom *(PNAS 106: 8969, 2009).*
Leech (Medicinal) *(Ln 381:1686, 2013)*	Aeromonas hydrophila	**CIP** (400 mg IV or 750 mg po) bid + **Doxy** 100 mg IV/po bid	**TMP-SMX DS** 1 tab po bid	Aeromonas in GI tract of leeches. Some use prophylactic antibiotics when leeches used medicinally.
Pig (swine)	Polymicrobic: Gm+ cocci, Gm-neg. bacilli, anaerobes, Pasteurella sp., Actinobacillus suis	**Amox-clav** 875/125 mg po bid	**P Ceph 3** or **Amp-sulb** or **IMP**	Information limited but infection is common and serious *(Ln 348:888, 1996).* Pigs may be colonized with MRSA *(Clin Microbiol Rev 24: 231, 2011).* Potential pathogens include Streptococcus suis leading to meningitis *(NEJM 354: 1325, 2006; Rinsho Shinkeigaku 53:732, 2013)*
Prairie dog	Monkeypox	*See Table 14A, page 187.* No rx recommended		Tularemia and bubonic plague reported after prairie dog bites.
Primate, Monkey, non-human *See Table 14A, Herpes simiae.*	Herpesvirus simiae	**Valacyclovir** (PEP) or **Acyclovir** or **Ganciclovir**		From macaques, risk of infection with herpes B virus; rare but potentially fatal encephalitis/myelitis *(CID 35: 1191, 2002).* Potential risk of rabies. Bacteria similar to human bites *(CID 24: 231, 2011)*; for deep bites, can use antibiotics as for human bites.
Rat	Spirillum minus & Streptobacillus moniliformis	**Amox-clav** 875/125 mg po bid	**Doxy** 100 mg po bid	Anti-rabies rx not indicated. Causes rat bite fever (Streptobacillus moniliformis): Pen G or doxy, alternatively erythro or clinda.
Seal	Marine mycoplasma	**Tetracycline** or **Doxy** for 2-4 wks		Can take weeks to appear after bite. Disseminated disease reported *(CID 62:491, 2016).* Differential includes sealpox, resembling Orf *(Br J Derm 152: 791, 2005)* and other bacteria: Bisgaardia hudsonensis *(J Infect 63: 86, 2011)* and Streptococcus halichoeri *(J Clin Microbiol 54: 739, 2016).*
Snake: pit viper (Ref.: *NEJM 347:347, 2002*)	Pseudomonas sp., Enterobacteriaceae, Staph. aureus and epidermidis, Clostridium sp.		**Primary therapy is antivenom**. Tetanus prophylaxis indicated. No need for antibiotic prophylaxis *(Am J Med 2018;131:1367).* **Pip/Tazo** for empirical therapy of infected wound. Adjust per culture results *(Emerg Clin N Amer 35: 339, 2017).*	
Spider bite: Most necrotic ulcers attributed to spiders are probably due to another cause, e.g., cutaneous anthrax *(Ln 364:549, 2004)* or **MRSA infection** (spider bite painful; anthrax not painful.)				
Widow (Latrodectus)	Not infectious	None	May be confused with "acute abdomen". Diazepam or calcium gluconate helpful to control pain, muscle spasm. Tetanus prophylaxis.	
Brown recluse (Loxosceles) *NEJM 352:700, 2005*	Not infectious. Overdiagnosed! Spider distribution limited to S. Central & desert SW of US	Bite usually self-limited & self-healing. No therapy of proven efficacy.	**Dapsone** 50 mg po q24h often used despite marginal supportive data	Dapsone causes hemolysis (check for G6PD deficiency). Can cause hepatitis; baseline & weekly liver panels suggested.
Swan	P aeruginosa	**CIP** 750 mg po bid		Case report of P aeruginosa infection *(Lancet 350: 340, 1997).* However, other aquatic organisms or host skin organisms have potential to cause infection.
Tasmanian devil	Pasteurella multocida *(CID 14: 1266, 1992)*	Treat as cat bite		15% of P multocida from devils were TMP-SMX resistant *(Lett Appl Microbiol 62: 237, 2016)*

Abbreviations on page 2. **NOTE: All dosage recommendations are for adults (unless otherwise indicated) and assume normal renal function. § Alternatives consider allergy, PK, compliance, local resistance, cost.*

TABLE 1 (53)

ANATOMIC SITE/DIAGNOSIS/ MODIFYING CIRCUMSTANCES	ETIOLOGIES (usual)	SUGGESTED REGIMENS*		ADJUNCT DIAGNOSTIC OR THERAPEUTIC MEASURES AND COMMENTS
		PRIMARY	ALTERNATIVE§	
SKIN *(continued)*				
Boils—Furunculosis				
Active lesions *See Table 6, page 90*	Staph. aureus, both MSSA & MRSA *IDSA Guidelines: CID 59:147, 2014*	**Boils and abscesses** uncomplicated patient (e.g., no immunosuppression) **I&D** + **TMP/SMX** 1 DS (2 DS for BMI >40) bid or **I&D** + **Clinda** 300 mg tid equally efficacious *(see NEJM 372:1093, 2015, NEJM 2016,374:823, and NEJM 376:2545, 2017)* **Incision and Drainage mainstay of therapy!**		Other options: **Doxy** 100 mg po bid or **Minocycline** 100 mg po bid for 5-10 days; **Fusidic acid**NUS 250-500 mg po q8-12h ± **RIF**; **Cephalexin** 500 mg po tid-qid or **Dicloxacillin** 500 mg po tid-qid, only in low prevalence setting for MRSA. Also: **Dalbavancin** 1.5 gm IV x 1 or **Oritavancin** 1200 mg IV x 1. If dx uncertainty or for assessing adequacy of I&D, ultrasound is helpful *(NEJM 370:1039, 2014)*. **NOTE: needle aspiration is inadequate.**
To lessen number of furuncle recurrences --decolonization *For surgical prophylaxis, see Table 15B, page 220.*	MSSA & MRSA. *IDSA Guidelines, CID 59:e10, 2014*	7-day therapy: **Chlorhexidine** (2%) washes daily; 2% **Mupirocin ointment** anterior nares 2x daily + (**RIF** 300 mg bid + **Doxy** 100 mg bid).	**Mupirocin ointment** in anterior nares bid x 7 days + **Chlorhexidine** (2%) washes daily x 7 days + (**TMP-SMX DS** 1 tab po bid + **RIF** 300 mg po bid) x 7 days	Optimal regimen uncertain. Can substitute bleach baths for chlorhexidine *(Inf Control Hosp Epidemiol 32:872, 2011) but only modest effect (CID 58:679, 2014)*. In vitro resistance of mupirocin & retapamulin roughly 10% *(AAC 58:2878, 2014)*. One review found mupirocin resistance ranging from 1-81% *(JAC 70:2681, 2015)*.
Burns. Overall management: ISBI Practice Guideline (Burns): *Burns 2016,42:953.*				
Initial wound care Use burn unit, if available Topical rx options *(NEJM 359:1037, 2008; Clin Plastic Surg 36:597, 2009)*	**Not infected** Prophylaxis for potential pathogens: Gm-pos cocci Gm-neg bacilli Candida	Early excision & wound closure. Variety of skin grafts/substitutes. Shower hydrotherapy. Topical antimicrobials	**Silver sulfadiazine** cream 1% applied 1-2 x daily. Minimal pain. Transient reversible neutropenia due to margination in burn – not marrow toxicity	Mafenide acetate cream is an alternative but painful to apply. Anti-tetanus prophylaxis indicated. **Severe burn pt on ventilator:** prophylactic Amp-sulb or Cefazolin may reduce mortality *(CID 62:60 & 67, 2016)*.
Burn wound sepsis	Strep. pyogenes, Enterobacter sp., S. aureus, S. epidermidis, E. faecalis, E. coli, P. aeruginosa. Fungi (rare). Herpesvirus (rare).	**Vanco** high dose to rapidly achieve trough concentration of 15-20 µg/mL + (**MER** 1 gm IV q8h or **Cefepime** 2 gm IV q8h) + **Fluconazole** 6 mg/kg IV qd *See Comments for alternatives*		Vanco allergic/intolerant: **Dapto** 6-10 mg/kg IV qd IgE mediated allergy to beta lactams: **Aztreonam** 2 gm IV q6h. ESBL pos: use a carbapenem; carbapenemase-producer: **Ceftaz-avi or MER-vabor** *(See Table 5B)*
Cellulitis, erysipelas: NOTE: Consider diseases that masquerade as cellulitis, e.g., stasis dermatitis *(Clev Clin J Med 79:547, 2012)*				
Extremities, non-diabetic *For diabetes, see below.* Practice guidelines: *CID 59:147, 2014.* **NOTE:** stasis dermatitis can masquerade as erysipelas *(J Am Acad Derm 2015,73:70)*	Streptococcus sp., Groups A, B, C & G. Staph. aureus, including MRSA (but rare). Strept sp: No purulence Staph sp: Purulence. Etiologic study *(OFID, doi 10.1093 OFID/OFV181)*	**Inpatients: Elevate legs.** **Pen G** 1–2 million units IV q6h or **Cefazolin** 1 gm IV q8h. If **Pen allergic** (if not IgE-mediated): **Cefazolin**. If IgE mediated: **Vanco** 15 mg/kg IV q12h. When afebrile: **Pen VK** 500 mg po qid ac & hs. Total therapy: 10 days.	**Outpatient: Elevate legs.** **Pen VK** 500 mg po qid ac & hs or **Cephalexin** 500 mg qid x 7-10 days. **Pen-allergic: Azithro** 500 mg po x 1 dose, then 250 mg po once daily x 4 days (total 5 days). Rarely, **Linezolid** 600 mg po bid or **Tedizolid** 200 mg po q24h or **Delaflox** 450 mg po q12h x 5-14 days.	• Erysipelas: elevation, IV antibiotic, treat T. pedis if present, if no purulence, no need for culture. • If unsure as to presence of deep abscess, bedside ultrasound can help. If present: furunculosis (boils) • **TMP-SMX** 1 DS bid OR **Clinda** 300 mg tid effective for uncomplicated cellulitis in non-diabetic outpatients *(NEJM 372:2460, 2015)* • **Oritavancin** 1200 mg IV x1 OR **Dalbavancin** 1.5 gm IV x 1 also effective for outpatient therapy of more severe infections in patients who might otherwise be admitted to the hospital *(see NEJM 370:2180, 2014, NEJM 370:2169, 2014)*. • No benefit of adding TMP-SMX to Cephalexin for MRSA coverage *(JAMA 317:2088, 2017)*.
Facial, adult (erysipelas)	Strep. sp. (Grp A, B, C & G), Staph. aureus (to include MRSA), S. pneumo	**Vanco** 15 mg/kg (actual wt) IV q8-12h (to achieve target trough concentration of 15-20 µg/mL x 7-10 days	**Dapto** 4 mg/kg IV q 24h or **Linezolid** 600 mg IV q 12h. Treat 7-10 days if not bacteremic.	**Choice of empiric therapy must have activity vs. S. aureus**. S. aureus erysipelas of face can mimic streptococcal erysipelas of an extremity. Forced to treat empirically for MRSA until in vitro susceptibilities available.

 **NOTE: All dosage recommendations are for adults (unless otherwise indicated) and assume normal renal function. § Alternatives consider allergy, PK, compliance, local resistance, cost.*

TABLE 1 (54)

ANATOMIC SITE/DIAGNOSIS/ MODIFYING CIRCUMSTANCES	ETIOLOGIES (usual)	SUGGESTED REGIMENS*		ADJUNCT DIAGNOSTIC OR THERAPEUTIC MEASURES AND COMMENTS
		PRIMARY	ALTERNATIVE§	
SKIN *(continued)*				
Diabetes mellitus and erysipelas *(See Foot, "Diabetic", page 18)*	Strep. sp. (Grp A, B, C & G), Staph. aureus, Enterobacteriaceae; Anaerobes	**Early mild: TMP-SMX-DS** 1-2 tabs po bid + (**Pen VK** 500 mg po qid or **Cephalexin** 500 mg po qid). **For severe disease: IMP**, **MER**, **Erta** or **Dori** IV + (**Linezolid** 600 mg IV/po bid or **vanco** IV or **dapto** 4 mg/kg IV q 24h). *Dosage, page 18, Diabetic foot*		Prompt surgical debridement indicated to rule out necrotizing fasciitis and to obtain cultures. If septic, consider x-ray of extremity to demonstrate gas. **Prognosis dependent on blood supply: assess arteries.** *See diabetic foot, page 18.* For severe disease, use regimen that targets both aerobic gram-neg bacilli & MRSA. Caution re hyperkalemia with TMP-SMX in those with reduced renal function or concomitant drugs causing hyperkalemia.
Erysipelas 2° to lymphedema (congenital = Milroy's disease); post-breast surgery with lymph node dissection	Streptococcus sp., Groups A, C, G	**Benzathine pen G** 1.2 million units IM q4 wks or **Pen VK** 500 mg po bid or **Azithro** 250 mg po qd		Indicated only if pt is having frequent episodes of cellulitis. Benefit in controlled clinical trial *(NEJM 368:1695, 2013)*.
Erythema multiforme	H. simplex type 1, mycoplasma, Strep. pyogenes, drugs (sulfonamides, phenytoin, penicillins)			Treat underlying disorder / Remove offending drug; symptomatic Rx.
Erythema nodosum	Sarcoidosis, inflammatory bowel disease, MTB, coccidioidomycosis, yersinia, sulfonamides, Whipple's disease.			**Rx: NSAIDs; glucocorticoids** if refractory. Identify and treat precipitant disease if possible.
Erythrasma	Corynebacterium minutissimum	Localized infection: **Topical Clinda** 2-3 x daily x 7-14 days	Widespread infection: **Clarithro** 500 mg po bid or **Erythro** 250 mg po bid) x 14 days	Dx: Coral red fluorescence with Wood's lamp. If infection recurs, prophylactic bathing with anti-bacterial soap or wash with benzyl peroxide. One-time dose of Clari 1 gm po reported to be effective *(Intl J Derm 52:516, 2013; J Derm Treatm 24:70, 2013)*. **Clarithro** 1 gm po x 1 reported to be effective. Mupirocin 2% ointment x 2-4 weeks reported to be effective.
Folliculitis	S. aureus, candida, P. aeruginosa common	Usually self-limited, no Rx needed. Could use topical mupirocin for Staph and topical antifungal for Candida.		
Furunculosis	Staph. aureus	*See Boils, page 57*		
Hemorrhagic bullous lesions				
Hx of sea water-contaminated abrasion or eating raw seafood in cirrhotic pt.	**Vibrio vulnificus**	**Ceftriaxone** 2 gm IV q24h + (**Doxy** or **Minocycline**) 100 mg po/IV bid. Peds: Doxy 4.4 mg/kg/day div bid (safe regardless of age for rx ≤21 days) *(AAP Redbook 2018)*	**CIP** 750 mg po bid or 400 mg IV bid OR **Levo** 750 mg IV q24h	Wound infection in healthy hosts, but bacteremia mostly in cirrhotics or use of TNF-inhibitors. Pathogenesis: Exposure to contaminated seawater. Can cause necrotizing fasciitis. Surgical debridement needed. Ref: *NEJM 2016,375:1780.*
Herpes zoster (shingles): *See Table 14A*				

Abbreviations on page 2. **NOTE: All dosage recommendations are for adults (unless otherwise indicated) and assume normal renal function. § Alternatives consider allergy, PK, compliance, local resistance, cost.*

TABLE 1 (55)

ANATOMIC SITE/DIAGNOSIS/ MODIFYING CIRCUMSTANCES	ETIOLOGIES (usual)	SUGGESTED REGIMENS*		ADJUNCT DIAGNOSTIC OR THERAPEUTIC MEASURES AND COMMENTS
		PRIMARY	ALTERNATIVE§	
SKIN *(continued)*				
Impetigo—*See CID 59:147, 2014.*				
"Honey-crust" lesions (non-bullous). Ecthyma is closely related. Causes "punched out" skin lesions.	**Group A strep impetigo** (rarely Strept. sp. Groups B, C or G); crusted lesions can be Staph. aureus + streptococci. Staph. aureus may be secondary colonizer.	Few lesions: (**Mupirocin** ointment 2% tid or **fusidic acid** cream[NUS] 2%, OR **retapamulin** ointment, 1% bid. Treat for 5 days	Numerous lesions: **Pen VK** 250-500 mg po q6h x 5 days or **Benzathine Pen** 600,000 units IM x 1 or **TMP-SMX** po x 3-5 days *(Lancet 384:2132, 2014)*	Topical rx: OTC ointments (bacitracin, neomycin, polymyxin B not as effective as prescription ointments. For mild disease, topical rx as good as po antibiotics *(Cochrane Database Syst Rev CD003261, 2012)*. **Ecthyma:** Infection deeper into epidermis than impetigo. May need parenteral penicillin. Military outbreaks reported: *CID 48: 1213 & 1220, 2009 (good images)*.
Bullous (if ruptured, thin "varnish-like" crust)	**Staph. aureus** MSSA & MRSA: strains that produce exfoliative toxin A.	**For MSSA:** po therapy with **Diclox**, **Oxacillin**, **Cephalexin**, **Amox-clav**, **Clinda**, **TMP-SMX-DS**, OR **Mupirocin** ointment OR **Retapamulin** ointment	**For MRSA: Mupirocin** ointment OR po therapy with, **TMP-SMX-DS, Minocycline, Doxy, Clinda.** Treat for 7 days	
		For dosages, see Table 10A		
Infected wound, extremity —Post-trauma *(for bites, see page 55; for post-operative, see below)*— **Gram stain negative**				
Mild to moderate; uncomplicated Debride wound, if necessary.	Polymicrobic: S. aureus (MSSA & MRSA), aerobic & anaerobic strep, Enterobacteriaceae, C. perfringens, C. tetani; if water exposure, Pseudomonas sp., Aeromonas sp.	**Clinda** 300-450 mg po tid	**Minocycline** 100 mg po bid or **linezolid** 600 mg po bid	**Culture & sensitivity, check Gram stain. Tetanus toxoid if indicated.** **Mild infection:** Suggested drugs focus on S. aureus & Strep species. If suspect Gm-neg. bacilli, add **AM-CL-ER** 1000/62.5 two tabs po bid. If MRSA is erythro-resistant, may have inducible resistance to clinda. **Fever—sepsis:** Another alternative is **Linezolid** 600 mg IV/po q12h. If Gm-neg. bacilli & severe pen allergy, **CIP or Levo**
Febrile with sepsis—hospitalized Debride wound, if necessary.		[**Pip-tazo** or **Dori**[NAI] OR **IMP** or **MER** or **Erta** *(Dosage, page 27)*] + **Vanco** 15-20 mg/kg q8-12h	(**Vanco** 15-20 mg/kg IV q8-12h OR **Dapto** 6 mg/kg IV q 24h OR **Ceftaroline** 600 mg IV q12h OR **Telavancin** 10 mg/kg IV q24h) + (**CIP** 400 mg IV q12h (q8h if P. aeruginosa) OR **Levo** 750 mg IV q24h)	
Infected wound, post-operative—Gram stain negative: for Gram stain positive cocci – *see below*				
Surgery not involving GI or female genital tract				
Without sepsis (mild, afebrile)	Staph. aureus, Group A, B, C or G strep sp.	**Clinda** 300–450 mg po tid		Check Gram stain of exudate. If Gm-neg. bacilli, **add** β-lactam/β-lactamase inhibitor: **AM-CL-ER** po or (**ERTA** or **Pip-tazo**) IV. *Dosage on page 27.*
With sepsis (severe, febrile)		**Vanco** 15-20 mg/kg (actual wt) IV q8-12h (to achieve target trough concentration of 15-20 µg/mL	**Dapto** 4 mg per kg IV q24h or **telavancin** 10 mg/kg IV q24h	
Surgery involving GI tract (includes oropharynx, esophagus) or female genital tract—fever, neutrophilia	MSSA/MRSA, coliforms, bacteroides & other anaerobes	[**Pip-tazo** or (**P Ceph 3** + **Metro**) or **Dori** or **Erta** or **IMP** or **MER**] + (**Vanco** 1 gm IV q12h or **Dapto** 6 mg/kg IV q 24h) **if severely ill.** **Mild infection: AM-CL-ER** 1000/62.5 mg 2 tabs po bid + **TMP-SMX-DS** 1-2 tabs po bid if Gm+ cocci on Gram stain. *Dosages Table 10A & footnote 23, page 66.*		For all treatment options, *see Peritonitis, page 49.* Most important: Drain wound & get cultures. Can sub **Linezolid** for vanco. Can sub **CIP or Levo** for β-lactams if local susceptibility permits.
Meleney's synergistic gangrene	*See Necrotizing Fasciitis, page 60*			

Abbreviations on page 2. **NOTE: All dosage recommendations are for adults (unless otherwise indicated) and assume normal renal function. § Alternatives consider allergy, PK, compliance, local resistance, cost.*

TABLE 1 (56)

ANATOMIC SITE/DIAGNOSIS/ MODIFYING CIRCUMSTANCES	ETIOLOGIES (usual)	SUGGESTED REGIMENS* PRIMARY	ALTERNATIVE§	ADJUNCT DIAGNOSTIC OR THERAPEUTIC MEASURES AND COMMENTS
SKIN/Infected wound, post-operative—Gram stain negative *(continued)*				
Infected wound, post-op, febrile patient— Positive gram stain: Gram-positive cocci in clusters	S. aureus, possibly MRSA	**Do culture & sensitivity; open & drain wound** **Oral: TMP-SMX-DS** 1 tab po bid or **Clinda** 300–450 mg po tid *(see Comment)*	**IV: Vanco** 15-20 mg/kg q8-12h or **Dapto** 4-6 mg/kg IV q24h or **Ceftaroline** 600 mg IV q12h or **Telavancin** 10 mg/kg IV q24h	Need culture & sensitivity to verify MRSA. Other po options for CA-MRSA include **minocycline** 100 mg po q12h or **Doxy** 100 mg po bid or **linezolid** 600 mg po q12h. If MRSA clinda-sensitive but erythro-resistant, watch out for inducible clinda resistance. Dalbavancin and oritavancin recently FDA approved for treatment of acute bacterial skin and skin structure infections are single dose options for parenteral out-patient therapy.
Necrotizing fasciitis ("flesh-eating bacteria") Reviews: *Infect Dis Clin N Amer 2017;31:497; NEJM 2017,377:2253.*				
Post-surgery, trauma, or streptococcal skin infections *See Gas gangrene, page 49, & Toxic shock, page 68.* Refs: *NEJM 2017,377:2253;* IDSA Guidelines: *CID 2014,59:e10*	**5 types:** (1) Strep sp., Grp A, C, G; (2) Clostridia sp.; (3) polymicrobic: aerobic + anaerobic (if S. aureus + anaerobic strep = Meleney's synergistic gangrene); (4) MRSA; (5) *V. vulnificus*; (6) Klebsiella sp.; (7) Aeromonas sp.	*For treatment of clostridia, see Muscle, gas gangrene, page 49.* The terminology of **polymicrobic** wound infections is not precise: Meleney's synergistic gangrene, Fournier's gangrene, necrotizing fasciitis have common pathophysiology. **All require prompt surgical debridement** + antibiotics. Dx of necrotizing fasciitis req incision & probing of fascial plane. **Need Gram stain/culture** to determine if etiology is strep, clostridia, polymicrobial, or S. aureus. **Treatment: Pen G** if strep or clostridia; **IMP** or **MER** if polymicrobial, add **Vanco OR Dapto** if MRSA suspected. **NOTE: If strep necrotizing fasciitis**, treat with **penicillin** & **clinda** (900 mg IV q6h); **if clostridia ± gas gangrene**, add clinda to penicillin *(see page 49)*. ***See toxic shock syndrome, streptococcal,*** *page 68.* IVIG not recommended.		
Puncture wound—nail, toothpick	Through tennis shoe: P. aeruginosa	Local debridement to remove foreign body & tetanus prophylaxis; no antibiotic therapy.		Osteomyelitis evolves in only 1–2% of plantar puncture wounds. Consider x-ray if chance of radio-opaque foreign body.
Staphylococcal scalded skin syndrome Ref.: *PIDJ 19:819, 2000*	Toxin-producing S. aureus	**Nafcillin/Oxacillin** 2 gm IV q4h (children: 150 mg/kg/ day div. q6h) x 5–7 days for MSSA; **Vanco** 15-20 mg/kg q8-12h (children 40–60 mg/kg/day div. q6h) for MRSA		Toxin causes **intraepidermal split** and positive Nikolsky sign. Biopsy differentiates: drugs cause epidermal/dermal split, **called toxic epidermal necrolysis—**more serious.
Ulcerated skin lesions: Differential Dx	Consider: anthrax, tularemia, P. aeruginosa (ecthyma gangrenosum), plague, blastomycosis, spider (rarely), mucormycosis, mycobacteria, leishmania, YAWS, arterial insufficiency, venous stasis, and others.			
Ulcerated skin: venous/arterial insufficiency; pressure with secondary infection (infected decubiti) Care of non-healing, non-infected ulcers *(AnIM 162:359, 2015).*	Polymicrobic: Streptococcus sp. (Groups A, C, G), enterococci, anaerobic strep, Enterobacteriaceae, Pseudomonas sp., Bacteroides sp., Staph. aureus	Severe local or possible bacteremia: **MER** 1 gm IV q8h or **Pip-tazo** 4.5 gm q6-8h. If Gm-pos cocci on gram stain, add **Vanco** 1 gm q12h. Surgery: debridement, deep cultures & wound coverage. Sacral osteo *(CID 68:358, 2019)*	(**Levo** 750 mg po/IV + **Metro** 500 mg po/IV) q8h or **CFP** 1-2 gm IV q8-12h. If Gm-pos cocci on gram stain, add **Vanco** 1 gm q12h.	• If ulcer clinically inflamed, treat IV with no topical rx. If not clinically inflamed, consider debridement, removal of foreign body, lessening direct pressure for weight-bearing limbs & leg elevation (if no arterial insufficiency). • Society of Vascular Surgery guidelines recommend against routine use of topical antimicrobials *(J Vasc Surg 60 (2 Suppl): 3S, 2014).* • Silver sulfadiazine 1% cream: insufficient evidence. • **Chlorhexidine & povidone iodine may harm "granulation tissue"–Avoid.** If not inflamed, healing improved on air bed, protein supplement, radiant heat, electrical stimulation *(AnIM 159:39, 2013).*
Whirlpool: (Hot Tub) folliculitis	Pseudomonas aeruginosa	Usually self-limited, treatment not indicated		Decontaminate hot tub: drain and chlorinate. Also associated with exfoliative beauty aids (loofah sponges).
Whirlpool: Nail Salon, soft tissue infection	Mycobacterium (fortuitum or chelonae)	**Minocycline**, **Doxy** or **CIP**		For more serious or progressive infection see recommendations for M. fortuitum.
SPLEEN. For post-splenectomy prophylaxis, *see Table 15A, page 218; for Septic Shock Post-Splenectomy, see Table 1, page 68. Vaccines: CID 58:309, 2014.*				
Splenic abscess				
Endocarditis, bacteremia	Staph. aureus, streptococci	**Nafcillin/Oxacillin** 2 gm IV q4h or **Cefazolin** 2 gm IV q8h if MSSA	**Vanco** 15-20 mg/kg IV q8-12h (target trough concentration of 15-20 μg/mL).	Burkholderia (Pseudomonas) pseudomallei is common cause of splenic abscess in SE Asia. Presents with fever and LUQ pain. Usual treatment is antimicrobial therapy and splenectomy.

 **NOTE: All dosage recommendations are for adults (unless otherwise indicated) and assume normal renal function. § Alternatives consider allergy, PK, compliance, local resistance, cost.*

TABLE 1 (57)

ANATOMIC SITE/DIAGNOSIS/ MODIFYING CIRCUMSTANCES	ETIOLOGIES (usual)	SUGGESTED REGIMENS*		ADJUNCT DIAGNOSTIC OR THERAPEUTIC MEASURES AND COMMENTS
		PRIMARY	ALTERNATIVE§	
SPLEEN/Splenic abscess *(continued)*				
Contiguous from intra-abdominal site	Polymicrobic	*Treat as Peritonitis, secondary, page 49*		
Immunocompromised	Candida sp.	**Amphotericin B**	**Fluconazole, caspofungin**	*See Candida, Table 11*
SYSTEMIC SYNDROMES (FEBRILE/NON-FEBRILE) Spread by infected TICK, FLEA, or LICE				
Epidemiologic history crucial. **Babesiosis, Lyme disease, & Anaplasma (Ehrlichiosis)** have same reservoir & tick vector.				
Babesiosis: *see JAMA 315:1767, 2016.* Do not treat if asymptomatic, young, has spleen, and immunocompetent; can be fatal in lymphoma pts.	Etiol.: B. microti et al. Vector: Usually Ixodes ticks Host: White-footed mouse & others	[(**Atovaquone** 750 mg po q12h) + (**Azithro** 600 mg po day 1, then 500-1000 mg per day) times 7-10 days]. If severe infection [**Clinda** 1.2 gm IV bid or 600 mg po tid times 7 days + **Quinine** 650 mg po tid times 7 days. **Ped. dosage: Clinda** 20–40 mg per kg per day and **quinine** 25 mg per kg per day]. **Exchange transfusion**-*See Comment*		**Seven diseases where pathogen visible in peripheral blood smear:** African/ American trypanosomiasis; babesia; bartonellosis; filariasis; malaria; relapsing fever. **Dx:** Giemsa-stained blood smear; antibody test available. PCR if available. **Rx: Exchange transfusions successful adjunct if used early, in severe disease.** May need treatment for 6 or more wks if immunocompromised. Look for Lyme and/or Anaplasma co-infection.
Bartonella infections: Treatment review: *Int J Antimicrob Agts 44:16, 2014.*				
Bacteremia, asymptomatic	B. quintana, B. henselae	**Doxy** 100 mg po/IV bid x 4 wks + **Gent** 1 mg/kg qhs x 1st 2 wks		Rule out endocarditis. Found in homeless, alcoholics, esp. if lice/leg pain. Often missed since asymptomatic.
Cat-scratch disease	B. henselae	**Azithro** 500 mg po x 1 dose, then 250 mg/day po x 4 days. For symptomatic only--*see Lymphadenitis, page 48:* usually lymphadenitis, hepatitis, splenitis, FUO, neuroretinitis, transverse myelitis, oculoglandular syndrome.		
Bacillary angiomatosis; Peliosis hepatis—AIDS	B. henselae, B. quintana	**Uncomplicated:** **Erythro** 500 mg po qid, **Azithro** 500 mg po qd or **Doxy** 100 mg po bid x 3 months or longer. Regardless of CD4 count, DC therapy after 3-4 mos. & observe. If no relapse, no suppressive rx. If relapse, **Doxy**, **Azithro** or **Erythro** x 3 mos. Stop when CD4 >200 x 6 mos.	**Complicated (CNS involvement):** **Doxy** 100 mg IV/po bid + **RIF** 300 mg po bid	**Do not use:** TMP-SMX, CIP, Pen, Ceph. **Manifestations of Bartonella infections:** **HIV/AIDS:** Bacillary angiomatosis; Bacillary peliosis; Bacteremia/endocarditis/FUO **Immunocompetent:** Bacteremia/endocarditis/FUO/ encephalitis; Cat scratch cisease; Vertebral osteo; Trench fever; Parinaud's oculoglandular syndrome
Endocarditis *(see page 30)* *Int J Antimicrob Agts 44:16, 2014*	B. henselae, B. quintana	Surgical removal of infected valve *If suspect endocarditis:* **Ceftriaxone** 2 gm IV once daily x 6 weeks + **Gent** 1 mg/ kg IV q8h x 14 days + **Doxy** 100 mg IV/po bid x 6 wks	*If proven endocarditis:* **Doxy** 100 mg IV/po bid x 6 wks + **Gent** 1 mg/kg IV q8h x 11 days	**Gentamicin toxicity:** If Gent toxicity, substitute Rifampin 300 mg IV/po bid x 14 days. Role of valve removal surgery to cure unclear. Presents as SBE. Diagnosis: ECHO, serology & PCR of resected heart valve. **Note:** Empiric Ceftriaxone for possible endocarditis due to Strept. sp. while awaiting blood culture results.
Oroya fever (acute) & Verruga peruana (chronic) (South American Bartonellosis)	B. bacilliformis; *AAC 48:192, 2014; Pediatrics 128:e1034, 2011*	**Oroya fever:** (Adult) (**CIP** 500 mg po bid + **Ceftriaxone** 1 gm IV once daily) x 14 days OR (**Chloro** 50-75 mg/kg/day IV/po in 4 div doses + **Ceftriaxone** 1 gm IV once daily) x 14 days	**Verruga peruana:** (Adult) **Azithro** 500 mg po once daily x 7 days OR **CIP** 500 mg po bid x 7-10 days	**Oroya fever** (Pregnancy): **Amox-clav** 1000/62.5 mg po bid. Oroya fever, severe infection (Child): (**CIP** or **Chloro**) + **Ceftriaxone** **Verruga peruana** (Child): **Azithro** 10 mg/kg po once daily x 7 days or **CIP** 20 mg/kg po in 2 div doses x 14 days
Trench fever (FUO)	B. quintana	No endocarditis: **Doxy** 100 mg po bid x 4 wks + **Gent** 3 mg/kg once daily for 1st 2 wks of therapy *(AAC 48:1921, 2004).*		Vector is body louse. Do not use: TMP-SMX, FQs, cefazolin or Pen. If endocarditis, need longer rx. *See Emerg ID 2:217, 2006).*

Abbreviations on page 2. *NOTE: All dosage recommendations are for adults (unless otherwise indicated) and assume normal renal function. § Alternatives consider allergy, PK, compliance, local resistance, cost.*

TABLE 1 (58)

ANATOMIC SITE/DIAGNOSIS/ MODIFYING CIRCUMSTANCES	ETIOLOGIES (usual)	SUGGESTED REGIMENS*		ADJUNCT DIAGNOSTIC OR THERAPEUTIC MEASURES AND COMMENTS
		PRIMARY	ALTERNATIVE§	
SYSTEMIC SYNDROMES (FEBRILE/NON-FEBRILE)/Spread by infected TICK, FLEA, or LICE *(continued)*				
Ehrlichiosis[21]. CDC def. is one of: (1) 4x ↑ IFA antibody, (2) detection of Ehrlichia DNA in blood or CSF by PCR, (3) visible morulae in WBC and IFA ≥1:64. New species in WI, MN *(NEJM 365:422, 2011)*.				
Human monocytic ehrlichiosis (HME) *CID 45(Suppl 1):S1, 2007*	Ehrlichia chaffeensis (Lone Star tick is vector)	**Doxy** 100 mg po/IV bid x 7–10 days *(Peds, see footnote[22])*	**Tetracycline** 500 mg po qid x 7–10 days. No current rec. for children or pregnancy	30 states: mostly SE of line from NJ to Ill. to Missouri to Oklahoma to Texas. History of outdoor activity and tick exposure. April-Sept. Fever, rash (36%), leukopenia and thrombocytopenia. Blood smears no help. PCR for early dx.
Human Anaplasmosis (formerly known as Human granulocytic ehrlichiosis) *MMWR 65:1, 2016; JAMA 315:1767, 2016*	Anaplasma (Ehrlichia) phagocytophilum (Ixodes sp. ticks are vector). Dog variant is Ehrlichia ewingii	**Doxy** 100 mg bid po or IV x 7–14 days *(Peds, see footnote[22])*	**Tetracycline** 500 mg po qid x 7–14 days. Not in children or pregnancy. **Chloro** is an alternative.	Upper Midwest, NE, West Coast & Europe. H/O tick exposure. April-Sept. Febrile flu-like illness after outdoor activity. No rash. Leukopenia/ thrombocytopenia common. **Dx:** PCR best; blood smear insensitive *(Am J Trop Med Hyg 93:66, 2015)*. **Rx:** RIF active in vitro *(IDCNA 22:433, 2008)* but worry about resistance developing. Minocycline should work if doxy not available.
Lyme Disease NOTE: Think about concomitant tick-borne disease—e.g., babesiosis, anaplasmosis and ehrlichiosis. **Guidelines:** *CID 51:1, 2010; NEJM 370:1724, 2014; JAMA 315:1767, 2016.*				
Bite by ixodes-infected tick in an endemic area -- **Postexposure prophylaxis**	Borrelia burgdorferi **IDSA guidelines:** *CID 51:1, 2010* Rarely, Borrelia mayonii *(Int J Syst Evol Microbiol 2016; 66:4878)*	**If endemic area,** if nymphal partially engorged deer tick: **Doxy** 200 mg po x 1 dose with food *(Peds, see footnote[22])*	**If not endemic area,** not engorged, not deer tick: No treatment	Prophylaxis study in endemic area: erythema migrans developed in 3% of the control group and 0.4% doxy group *(NEJM 345:79 & 133, 2001)*. Can substitute **Minocycline** for Doxy, if Doxy is unavailable.
Early (erythema migrans) Serologic tests negative	Western blot diagnostic criteria: **IgM**—Need 2 of 3 positive of kilodaltons (KD): 23, 39, 41	**Doxy** 100 mg po bid or **Amoxicillin** 500 mg po tid or **cefuroxime axetil** 500 mg po bid. All regimens x 14–21 days. (10 days as effective as 20: *AnIM 138:697, 2003*). **Azithro** 500 mg per day x 7-10 days. *(Peds dosing, see Comments and footnote[22])*		High rate of clinical failure with azithro & erythro *(Drugs 57:157, 1999)*. **Peds** (all po for 14–21 days): **Amox** 50 mg per kg per day in 3 div. doses or **Cefuroxime axetil** 30 mg per kg per day in 2 div. doses or **Azithro** 10 mg/kg (max 500 mg) per day for 7-10 days. Lesions usually homogenous--not target-like *(AnIM 136:423, 2002)*.
Carditis *See Comment*	**IgG**—Need 5 of 10 positive of KD: 18, 21, 28, 30, 39, 41, 45, 58, 66, 93	(**Ceftriaxone** 2 gm IV q24h) or (**Cefotaxime** 2 gm IV q4h) or (**Pen G** 3 million units IV q4h) x 14–21 days	**Doxy** *(see Comments)* 100 mg po bid x *(Peds, see footnote[22])* 14–21 days or **Amoxicillin** 500 mg po tid x 14–21 days.	First degree AV block: Oral regimen. Generally self-limited. High degree AV block (PR >0.3 sec.): IV therapy—permanent pacemaker not necessary, but temporary pacing in 39% *(CID 59:996, 2014)*.
Facial nerve paralysis (isolated finding, early)	Interest in 2 tier diagnostic approach: 1) standard Lyme ELISA & if positive; 2) C6 peptide ELISA. Better sensitivity/specificity.	(**Doxy** 100 mg po bid) *(Peds, see footnote[22])* or (**Amoxicillin** 500 mg po) tid x 14–21 days	**Ceftriaxone** 2 gm IV q24h x 14–21 days	LP suggested excluding central neurologic disease. If LP neg., oral regimen OK. If abnormal or not done, suggest parenteral Ceftriaxone.
Meningitis, encephalitis *For encephalopathy, see Comment*	Guidance on diagnostics: *EID 22:1169, 2016; JAMA 2018;320:636; CID 2018;66:1133.*	**Ceftriaxone** 2 gm IV q24h x 14–28 days	(**Pen G** 20 million units IV q24h in div. dose) or (**Cefotaxime** 2 gm IV q8h) x 14–28 days	Encephalopathy: memory difficulty, depression, somnolence, or headache, CSF abnormalities. 89% had objective CSF abnormalities. No compelling evidence that prolonged treatment has any benefit in post-Lyme syndrome *(NEJM 374:1209, 2016)*.
Arthritis		(**Doxy** 100 mg po bid) *(Peds, see footnote[22])* or (**Amoxicillin** 500 mg po tid) x 28 days	(**Ceftriaxone** 2 gm IV q24h) or (**Pen G** 20–24 million units per day IV) x 14–28 days	Start with 1 mo of therapy; if only partial response, treat for a second mo.
Pregnancy		**Amoxicillin** 500 mg po tid x 21 days.	**If pen. allergic:** (**Azithro** 500 mg po q24h x 7–10 days) or (**Erythro** 500 mg po qid x 14–21 days). Choice should not include doxy.	

[21] In endemic area (New York), high % of both adult ticks and nymphs were jointly infected with both Anaplasma (HGE) and B. burgdorferi *(NEJM 337:49, 1997)*.
[22] Important Note: Use of **Doxycycline** in children is considered safe regardless of of age for treatment duration of ≤21 days. Pediatric dose: 4.4 mg/kg/day divided bid *(AAP Redbook 2018)*.

 **NOTE: All dosage recommendations are for adults (unless otherwise indicated) and assume normal renal function. § Alternatives consider allergy, PK, compliance, local resistance, cost.*

TABLE 1 (59)

ANATOMIC SITE/DIAGNOSIS/ MODIFYING CIRCUMSTANCES	ETIOLOGIES (usual)	SUGGESTED REGIMENS*		ADJUNCT DIAGNOSTIC OR THERAPEUTIC MEASURES AND COMMENTS
		PRIMARY	ALTERNATIVE§	
SYSTEMIC SYNDROMES (FEBRILE/NON-FEBRILE)/Spread by infected TICK, FLEA, or LICE/Lyme Disease *(continued)*				
Post-Lyme Disease Syndromes		None indicated		No benefit from rx *(AJM 126:665, 2013; CID 51:1, 2010; AAC 58:6701, 2014; NEJM 345:85, 2001)*. Constructive review: *CID 58:1267, 2014.*
Plague, bacteremic *(see also Bubonic plague and plague pneumonia)*	Yersinia pestis	(**Streptomycin** 30 mg/kg/day IV in 2 div doses OR **Gentamicin** 5 mg/kg/day IV single dose) x 10 days	[**Levo** 500 mg IV/po once daily or **CIP** 500 mg po (or 400 mg IV) q12h] x 10 days or **Moxi** 400 mg IV/po q24h x 10-14 days	**Doxy** 200 mg IV/po bid x 1 day, then 100 mg IV/po bid x 7-10 days another option. FQs effective in animals & small case series *(EID 2017,23:553)*.
Relapsing fever				
Louse-borne (LBRF)	*Borrelia recurrentis* Reservoir: human Vector: Louse pediculus humanus	**Tetracycline** 500 mg IV/po x 1 dose or **Doxy** 100 mg IV/po x 1 dose *(Peds, see footnote[22])*	**Erythro** 500 mg IV/po x 1 dose	Jarisch-Herxheimer (fever, ↑ pulse, ↑ resp., ↓ blood pressure) in most patients (occurs in ~2 hrs). Not prevented by prior steroids. **Dx: Examine peripheral blood smear during fever for spirochetes.** Can relapse up to 10 times.
Tick-borne (TBRF)	No Amer: *B. hermsii, B. turicata;* Africa: *B. hispanica, B. crocidurae, B. duttonii;* Russia: *B. miyamoto* *(see Comment)*	**Doxy** 100 mg po bid x 7-10 days *(Peds, see footnote[22])*	**Erythro** 500 mg po qid x 7-10 days	Jarisch-Herxheimer reaction may occur. Postexposure **Doxy** pre-emptive therapy highly effective *(NEJM 355:148, 2006)*. B. miyamoto: Dx by ref lab serum PCR. Fever, headache, thrombocytopenia & tick exposure (NE USA). Seems to respond to Doxy, Azithro, Ceftriaxone *(AnIM 163:91 & 141, 2015; NEJM 373:468, 2015)*. Resistant to Amox *(Am J Med 132:136, 2019)*.
Rickettsial diseases *(MMWR 65(RR-2):1, 2016)*.				
Spotted fevers (NOTE: Rickettsial pox not included)				
Rocky Mountain spotted fever (RMSF) *(LnID 8:143, 2008 and MMWR 55 (RR-4), 2007)*	R. rickettsii (Dermacentor tick vector)	**Doxy** 100 mg po/IV bid x 7 days or x 2 days after temp. normal. Some suggest loading dose: 200 mg IV/po q 12h x 3 days, then 100 mg po bid	**Pregnancy: Chloro** 50 mg/kg/day in 4 div doses. If cannot obtain Chloro, alternative is **Doxy**	Fever, rash (88%), petechiae 40–50%. **Rash spreads from distal extremities to trunk.** Rash in <50% pts in 1st 72 hrs. Dx: Immunohistology on skin biopsy; confirmation with antibody titers. Highest incidence in SE and South Central states; also seen in Oklahoma, S. Dakota, Montana. Cases reported from 42 U.S. states. **NOTE: Only 3–18% of pts present with fever, rash, and hx of tick exposure; many early deaths in children & empiric doxy reasonable** *(MMWR 49: 885, 2000)*.
NOTE: Can mimic ehrlichiosis. Pattern of rash important—*see Comment*				
Other spotted fevers, e.g., Rickettsial pox, African tick bite fever, R. parkeri	At least 8 species on 6 continents *(CID 45 (Suppl 1) S39, 2007)*.	**Doxy** 100 mg po bid x 7 days *(Peds, see footnote[22])*	**Chloro** 500 mg po/IV qid x 7 days Children age < 8 yrs: **Azithro** or **Clarithro** *(if mild disease)*	Clinical diagnosis suggested by: 1) fever, intense myalgia, headache; 2) exposure to mites or ticks; 3) localized eschar (tache noire) or rash. Definitive Dx: PCR of blood, skin biopsy or sequential antibody tests.
Typhus group—Consider in returning travelers with fever				
Louse-borne: epidemic typhus Ref: *LnID 8:417, 2008.*	R. prowazekii (vector is body or head louse)	**Doxy** 100 mg IV/po bid x 7 days; single 200 mg dose 95% effective. *(Peds, see footnote[22])*	**Chloro** 500 mg IV/po qid x 5 days	**Brill-Zinsser disease** *(Ln 357:1198, 2001)* is a relapse of typhus acquired during WWII. Truncal rash (64%) spreads centrifugally—opposite of RMSF. Louse borne typhus is a winter disease. Diagnosis by serology. R. prowazekii found in flying squirrels in SE US. Delouse clothing of infected pt.

 **NOTE: All dosage recommendations are for adults (unless otherwise indicated) and assume normal renal function. § Alternatives consider allergy, PK, compliance, local resistance, cost.*

TABLE 1 (60)

ANATOMIC SITE/DIAGNOSIS/ MODIFYING CIRCUMSTANCES	ETIOLOGIES (usual)	SUGGESTED REGIMENS*		ADJUNCT DIAGNOSTIC OR THERAPEUTIC MEASURES AND COMMENTS
		PRIMARY	ALTERNATIVE§	
SYSTEMIC SYNDROMES (FEBRILE/NON-FEBRILE)/Spread by infected TICK, FLEA, or LICE/Rickettsial diseases *(continued)*				
Murine typhus (cat flea typhus): *EID 14:1019, 2008.*	R. typhi (rat reservoir and flea vector): *CID 46:913, 2008*	**Doxy** 100 mg IV/po bid x 7 days *(Peds, see footnote[22])*	**Chloro** 500 mg IV/po qid x 5 days	Rash in 20-54%, not diagnostic. Without treatment most pts recover in 2 wks. Faster recovery with treatment. Dx based on suspicion; confirmed serologically. Azithro failure *(CID 68:738, 2019)*.
Scrub typhus *(World J Crit Care 4:244, 2015)*	O. tsutsugamushi [rodent reservoir; vector is larval stage of mites (chiggers)]	**Doxy** 100 mg po/IV bid x 7 days. In pregnancy: **Azithro** 500 mg po x one dose	**Chloro** 500 mg po/IV qid x 7 days	Asian rim of Pacific. Confirm with serology. If Doxy resistance suspected, (**RIF** 600 mg po qd or **Azithro** 500 mg po qd) x 5 days *(CID 2018:67:600)*.
Tularemia, typhoidal type Ref. **bioterrorism**: *see JAMA 285:2763, 2001; ID Clin No Amer 22:489, 2008; MMWR 58:744, 2009.*	Francisella tularensis. (Vector depends on geography: ticks, biting flies, mosquitoes identified). Direct inoculation of wounds.	Moderate/severe: [(**Gent** or **Tobra** 5 mg per kg per day div. q8h IV) or (**Streptomycin** 10 mg/kg IV/IM q12h)] x 10 days	Mild: [**CIP** 400 mg IV (or 750 mg po) bid or **Doxy** 100 mg IV/po bid] x 14-21 days *(Peds, see footnote[22])*	Diagnosis: Culture on cysteine-enriched media & serology. Dangerous in the lab. Hematogenous meningitis is a complication: treatment is **Streptomycin** + **Chloro** 50-100 mg/kg/day IV in 4 divided doses *(Arch Neurol 66:523, 2009)*.
Other Zoonotic Systemic Bacterial Febrile Illnesses (not spread by fleas, lice or ticks): Obtain careful epidemiologic history				
Brucellosis				
Refs: *NEJM 352:2325, 2005; CID 46:426, 2008; MMWR 57:603, 2008; BMJ 336:701, 2008; PLoS One 7:e32090, 2012.*	B. abortus–cattle B. suis–swine B. melitensis–goats B. canis–dogs	**Non focal disease:** [**Doxy** 100 mg po bid x 6 wks + **Gent** 5 mg/kg once daily for 1st 7 days	(**Doxy** 100 mg po bid + **RIF** 600-900 mg po once daily) x 6 wks. Less optimal: **CIP** 500 mg po bid + (**Doxy** or **RIF**) x 6 wks	Bone involvement, esp. sacroiliitis in 20-30%. **Neurobrucellosis:** Usually meningitis. 1% of all pts with brucellosis. Role of corticosteroids unclear; not recommended. **Endocarditis:** Rare but most common cause of death. Need surgery + antimicrobials. **Pregnancy:** TMP-SMX may cause kernicterus if given during last week of pregnancy.
		Spondylitis, Sacroiliitis: [**Doxy** + **Gent** (as above) + **RIF**] x min 3 mos	(**CIP** 750 mg po bid + **RIF** 600-900 mg po once daily) x min 3 mos	
		Neurobrucellosis: [**Doxy** + **RIF** (as above) + **Ceftriaxone** 2 gm IV q12h until CSF returned to normal *(AAC 56:1523, 2012)*		
		Endocarditis: Surgery + **[(RIF** + **Doxy** + **TMP-SMX)** x 45 days to 6 mos + **Gent** for 2-4 wks *(CID 56:1407, 2013)*		
		Pregnancy: Not much data. **RIF** 900 mg po once daily x 6 wks	**RIF** 900 mg po once daily + **TMP-SMX** 5 mg/kg (TMP comp) po bid x 4 wks	
Leptospirosis *(Curr Topics Micro Immunol 387:65, 2015)*	Leptospira—in urine of domestic livestock, dogs, small rodents	**Severe illness: Pen G** 1.5 million units IV q6h or **Ceftriaxone** 2 gm q24h. Duration: 7 days	**Mild illness: Doxy** 100 mg IV/po q12h *(Peds, see footnote[22])* or **Amox** 500 mg po tid x 7 days or **Azithro** 1 gm po x 1, then 500 mg po once daily x 2 days	**Severity varies**. Varies from mild anicteric illness to severe icteric disease (Weil's disease) with renal failure and myocarditis. AST/ALT do not exceed 5x normal. Jarisch-Herxheimer reaction can occur post-Pen therapy.

 **NOTE: All dosage recommendations are for adults (unless otherwise indicated) and assume normal renal function. § Alternatives consider allergy, PK, compliance, local resistance, cost.*

TABLE 1 (61)

ANATOMIC SITE/DIAGNOSIS/ MODIFYING CIRCUMSTANCES	ETIOLOGIES (usual)	SUGGESTED REGIMENS* PRIMARY	SUGGESTED REGIMENS* ALTERNATIVE§	ADJUNCT DIAGNOSTIC OR THERAPEUTIC MEASURES AND COMMENTS
SYSTEMIC SYNDROMES (FEBRILE/NON-FEBRILE)/Other Zoonotic Systemic Bacterial Febrile Illnesses *(continued)*				
Salmonella bacteremia other than S. typhi–non-typhoidal)	Salmonella enteritidis— a variety of serotypes from animal sources	If NOT acquired in Asia: (**CIP** 400 mg IV q12h or **Levo** 750 mg po once daily) x 14 days *(See Comment)*	If acquired in Asia: **Ceftriaxone** 2 gm IV q24h or **Azithro** 1 gm po x 1 dose, then 500 mg po once daily x 5-7 days. Do NOT use FQs until susceptibility determined. *(See Comment)*	In vitro resistance to nalidixic acid indicates relative resistance to FQs. Bacteremia can infect any organ/tissue: look for infection of atherosclerotic aorta, osteomyelitis in sickle cell pts. Rx duration range 14 days (immunocompetent) to ≥6 wks if mycotic aneurism or endocarditis. Alternative, if susceptible: **TMP-SMX** 8-10 mg/kg/day (TMP comp) divided q8h. CLSI has established new interpretive breakpoints for susceptibility to Ciprofloxacin: susceptible strains, MIC <0.06 µg/mL *(CID 55:1107, 2012)*.
Miscellaneous Systemic Febrile Syndromes				
Fever in Returning Travelers Etiology by geographic exposure & clinical syndrome *(AnIM 158:456, 2013)*.	Dengue (Flavivirus)	Supportive care; *see Table 14A, page 178*		Average incubation period 4 days; serodiagnosis.
	Malaria (Plasmodia sp)	Diagnosis: peripheral blood smear		*See Table 13A, page 162*
	Typhoid (Salmonella sp)	*See Table 1, page 65.*		Average incubation 7-14 days; diarrhea in 45%.
Kawasaki syndrome 6 weeks to 12 yrs of age, peak at 1 yr of age; 85% below age 5. Tongue image *(NEJM 373:467, 2015)*	Self-limited vasculitis with ↑ temp., rash, conjunctivitis, strawberry tongue, cervical adenitis, red hands/feet & coronary artery aneurysms	**IVIG** 2 gm per kg over 8-12 hrs x 1 + **ASA** 20-25 mg per kg qid THEN **ASA** 3–5 mg per kg per day po q24h times 6–8 wks	If still febrile after 1st dose of IVIG, some give 2nd dose. In Japan: **IVIG** + prednisolone 2 mg/kg/day. Continue steroid until CRP normal for 15 days *(Lancet 379:1571, 2012)*.	IV gamma globulin (2 gm per kg over 10 hrs) in pts rx before 10th day of illness ↓ coronary artery lesions. See *Table 14A, page 188* for IVIG adverse effects. In children, wait until 11+ months after IVIG before giving live virus vaccines. Ref: *Circulation 135:e927, 2017.*
Rheumatic Fever, acute Ref.: *Ln 366:155, 2005*	Post-Group A strep pharyngitis (not Group B, C, or G)	(1) Symptom relief: **ASA** 80–100 mg per kg per day in children; 4–8 gm per day in adults. (2) Eradicate Group A strep: **Pen** times 10 days *(see Pharyngitis, page 51)*. (3) Start prophylaxis: *see below*		
Prophylaxis				
Primary prophylaxis: Treat S. pyogenes pharyngitis	**Benzathine pen G** 1.2 million units IM *(see Pharyngitis, page 51)*		**Penicillin** for 10 days prevents rheumatic fever even when started 7–9 days after onset of illness *(see page 51)*. **Alternative: Penicillin V** 250 mg po bid or **Sulfadiazine (sulfisoxazole)** 1 gm po q24h or **Erythro** 250 mg po bid.	
Secondary prophylaxis (previous documented rheumatic fever)	**Benzathine pen G** 1.2 million units IM q3–4 wks *(AAC 58:6735, 2014)*.		**Duration?** No carditis: 5 yrs or until age 21, whichever is longer; carditis without residual heart disease: 10 since last attack; carditis with residual valvular disease: 10 yrs since last episode or until age 40 whichever is longer *(J Am Coll Cardiol 63 :e57, 2014)*.	
Typhoidal syndrome (typhoid fever, enteric fever) FQ resistance increasing in infected travelers *(BMC Infect DIs 15:212, 2015)*	Salmonella typhi, S. paratyphi A, B, C & S. choleraesuis. **NOTE: In vitro resistance to nalidixic acid predicts clinical failure of CIP (FQs).** Do not use empiric FQs if Asia-acquired infection. Need susceptibility results.	**If NOT acquired in Asia:** (**CIP** 400 mg IV q12h or **Levo** 750 mg po/IV q24h) x 7-14 days. *(See Comment)*	**If acquired in Asia:** (**Ceftriaxone** 2 gm IV daily x 7-14 d) or (**Azithro** 1 gm po x 1 dose, then 500 mg po daily x 7 days) or (**Chloro** 500 mg po/IV q6h x 14 d) *(See Comment)*	**Dexamethasone: Use in severely ill pts: 1st dose just prior to antibiotic, 3 mg/kg IV, then 1 mg/kg q6h x 8 doses.** **Complications:** perforation of terminal ileum &/or cecum, osteo, septic arthritis, **mycotic aneurysm**, meningitis, hematogenous pneumonia. Failure of MER in pt with *S. enterica* strain producing ESBLs and resistant to FQs & azithro responded to addition of fosfomycin IV *(CID 2017;65:1754)*
		Peds: Azithro 10 mg/kg once daily x 7 days *(AAC 51:819, 2007)*.		

Abbreviations on page 2. *NOTE: All dosage recommendations are for adults (unless otherwise indicated) and assume normal renal function. § Alternatives consider allergy, PK, compliance, local resistance, cost.*

TABLE 1 (62)

ANATOMIC SITE/DIAGNOSIS/ MODIFYING CIRCUMSTANCES	ETIOLOGIES (usual)	SUGGESTED REGIMENS*		ADJUNCT DIAGNOSTIC OR THERAPEUTIC MEASURES AND COMMENTS
		PRIMARY	ALTERNATIVE§	
SYSTEMIC SYNDROMES (FEBRILE/NON-FEBRILE) *(continued)*				
Sepsis: Following suggested **empiric** therapy assumes pt is bacteremic; mimicked by viral, fungal, rickettsial infections and pancreatitis *(Intensive Care Med. 2017;43:304).*				
Neonatal—early onset Age <7 days	Group B strep, E. coli, klebsiella, enterobacter, Staph. aureus (uncommon), listeria (rare in U.S.)	**AMP** 150 mg/kg/day IV div q8h + **Cefotaxime** 100 mg/kg/day div q12h ± **Gent** 5 mg/kg q 24 h or 2.5 mg/kg q8h IV or IM (if meningitis, consider increasing to **AMP** 200 mg/kg/day IV div q6h and **Cefotaxime** 150 mg/kg/day div q8h)		Blood cultures are key but only 5–10% of febrile infants have bacterial infection. Discontinue antibiotics after 72 hrs if cultures and course do not support diagnosis. In Spain, listeria predominates; in S. America, salmonella. If Grp B Strep infection + severe beta-lactam allergy, alternatives include: erythro & clinda; report of clinda resistance at 38% & erythro resistance at 51% *(AAC 56:739, 2012).*
Neonatal—late onset Age >7 days	As above + H. influenzae & S. epidermidis	**AMP** 200-300 mg/kg/day IV q6h + **Cefotaxime** 75 mg/kg q8h ± **Gent** 5 mg/kg q24h IV or IM	(**AMP** 200 mg/kg/day IV div q6h + **Ceftriaxone** 75-100 mg/kg IV q24h) or **AMP** 200 mg/kg/day IV div q6 + **Gent** 5 mg/kg/day div once daily or q8h IV or IM.	**If MRSA is a concern**, add **Vanco** 15 mg/kg IV q12h (Wt < 2000 gm). *See also Comment (early onset).*
Child; not neutropenic	Strep. pneumoniae, meningococci, Staph. aureus (MSSA & MRSA), H. influenzae now rare	(**Cefotaxime** 50 mg/kg IV q8h or **Ceftriaxone** 100 mg/kg IV q24h) + **Vanco** 15 mg/kg IV q6h	**Aztreonam** 7.5 mg/kg IV q6h + **Linezolid**	Major concerns are S. pneumoniae & community-associated MRSA. Coverage for Gm-neg. bacilli included but H. influenzae infection now rare. Meningococcemia mortality remains high *(Ln 356:961, 2000).*
Adult; not neutropenic; NO HYPOTENSION but LIFE-THREATENING!—*For Septic shock, see page 68*				**Sepsis**: life-threatening organ dysfunction (identified by an acute change in SOFA (Sequential [Sepsis-Related] Organ Failure Assessment) score ≥2 points) caused by a dysregulated host response to infection. **Septic shock**: sepsis accompanied by circulatory and cellular/metabolic abnormalities sufficient to substantially increase mortality (see *JAMA 2017; 317:847; JAMA 2017; 317:267).* For patients in septic shock unresponsive to volume resuscitation, requiring on-going vasopressor therapy to maintain systolic BP > 90 mm Hg or MAP > 65 mm Hg consider hydrocortisone 50 mg IV q6h + fludrocortisone 50 mcg once daily via NG tube *(NEJM 2018; 378:797, 809, 860 [editorial]).* Note: Pip-tazo inferior to MER vs. ceftriaxone-resistant E. coli/K. pneumo *(JAMA 2018;320:979 & 984).*
Source unclear—consider primary bacteremia, intra-abdominal or skin source. May be **Life-threatening.** Survival greater with quicker, effective empiric antibiotic Rx *(NEJM 2017; 376:2235).*	Aerobic Gm-neg. bacilli; S. aureus; streptococci; others	[(**IMP** or **MER**) + **Vanco**] OR (**Pip-tazo** + **Vanco**) If ESBL and/or carbapenemase-producing GNB. Empiric options pending clarification of clinical syndrome and culture results: **Low prevalence of resistance: Vanco + Pip-tazo** **If high prevalence of resistance,** *see Table 5B, page 89* for treatment options *Dosages in footnote*[23]	(**Dapto** 6 mg/kg IV q24h) + (**Cefepime** or **Pip-tazo**)	
If suspect biliary source *(see Gallbladder page 18)*	Enterococci + aerobic Gm-neg. bacilli	**Pip-tazo** (Do not use if ESBL producer)	**Ceftriaxone** + **Metro** or (**CIP** or **Levo**) + **Metro** *Dosages–footnote*[23]	If enterococci a concern, add ampicillin or vanco to metro regimens
If community-acquired pneumonia with severe sepsis or septic shock *(see page 42 and following pages)*	**S. pneumoniae; MRSA, Legionella, Gm-neg. bacillus, others**	(**Levo** or **Moxi**) + (**Pip-tazo**) + **Vanco**	**Aztreonam** + (**Levo** or **Moxi**) + **Linezolid**	Many categories of CAP, *see material beginning at page 42.* Suggestions based on most severe CAP, e.g., MRSA after influenza or Klebsiella pneumonia in an alcoholic.
If illicit use IV drugs	S. aureus	Include **Vanco** to cover MRSA.		

[23] **P Ceph 3** (**Cefotaxime** 2 gm IV q8h, use q4h if life-threatening; **Ceftizoxime** 2 gm IV q4h; **Ceftriaxone** 2 gm IV q12h), **Pip-tazo** 3.375 gm IV q4h or 4-hr infusion of 3.375 gm q8h, **Aminoglycosides** *(see Table 10C, page 128)*, **AMP** 200 mg/kg/day divided q6h, **Clinda** 900 mg IV q8h, **IMP** 0.5 gm IV q6h, **MER** 1 gm IV q8h, **Erta** 1 gm IV q24h, **Dori** 500 mg IV q8h (1-hr infusion), **Nafcillin/Oxacillin** 2 gm IV q4h, **Aztreonam** 2 gm IV q8h, **Metro** 1 gm loading dose then 0.5 gm q6h or 1 gm IV q12h, **Vanco** loading dose 25-30 mg/kg IV, then 15-20 mg/kg IV q8-12h (dose in obese pt, *see Table 17C, page 252*), **Ceftazidime** 2 gm IV q8h, [Cefepime 2 gm IV q12h (q8h if neutropenic), **Cefpirome**[NUS] 2 gm IV q12h], **CIP** 400 mg IV q12h, **Levo** 750 mg IV q24h, **Linezolid** 600 mg IV q12h.

Abbreviations on page 2. **NOTE: All dosage recommendations are for adults (unless otherwise indicated) and assume normal renal function. § Alternatives consider allergy, PK, compliance, local resistance, cost.*

ANATOMIC SITE/DIAGNOSIS/ MODIFYING CIRCUMSTANCES	ETIOLOGIES (usual)	SUGGESTED REGIMENS*		ADJUNCT DIAGNOSTIC OR THERAPEUTIC MEASURES AND COMMENTS
		PRIMARY	ALTERNATIVE§	
SYSTEMIC SYNDROMES (FEBRILE/NON-FEBRILE)/Sepsis/Adult; not neutropenic *(continued)*				
If suspect intra-abdominal source	Mixture aerobic & anaerobic Gm-neg. bacilli	*See secondary peritonitis, page 50.*		
If petechial rash	Meningococcemia	**Ceftriaxone** 2 gm IV q12h (until sure no meningitis); consider Rocky Mountain spotted fever—*see page 63*		
If suspect urinary source, e.g. pyelonephritis	Aerobic Gm-neg. bacilli & enterococci	*See pyelonephritis, page 37.* Prefer a carbapenem for patients with severe sepsis or septic shock to cover ESBL producers.		
Neutropenia: Child or Adult (absolute PMN count <500 per mm³) in cancer and transplant patients. Guidelines (inpatient): *CID 2011,52:427*; (outpatient): *J Clin Oncol doi:10.1200/JCO.2017.77.6211.*				
Prophylaxis *(J Clin Oncol 31:794, 2013)*				
Post-chemotherapy—impending neutropenia	Pneumocystis (PCP), Viridans strep	In patients expected to have PMN <100 for >7 days consider Levo 500-750 mg po q24h. Acute leukemics undergoing intensive induction consider addition of Fluc 400 mg q24h. In patients with AML or MDS who have prolonged neutropenia, consider Posa instead at 200 mg TID *(N Engl J Med 356:348, 2007)*. Safe & effective during induction rx for acute lymphoblastic leukemia (ALL) *(CID 2017,65:1790)*		
Post allogeneic stem cell transplant	Aerobic Gm-neg bacilli, ↑ risk pneumocystis, herpes viruses, candida aspergillus	**TMP-SMX** (vs. PCP) + **Acyclovir** (vs. HSV/VZV)+ **pre-emptive** monitoring for **CMV** + **Posaconazole** (vs. mold)		In autologous HCT, not active prophylaxis nor CMV screening is recommended. Fluc OK with TMP-SMX and acyclovir.
Empiric therapy—febrile neutropenia (≥38.3°C for >1 hr or sustained >38°C and absolute neutrophil count <500 cells/µL) (IDSA Guidelines: *CID 52:427, 2012*). *(Outpatients: J CLin Oncol doi:10.1200/JCO 2017.77.6211.)*				
Low-risk adults Anticipate <7 days neutropenia, no co-morb, can take po meds	Aerobic Gm-neg bacilli, Viridans strep	**CIP** 750 mg po bid + **Amox-clav** 875 /125 mg po bid. Treat until absolute neutrophil count >1000 cells/µL	Treat as outpatients with 24/7 access to inpatient care if: no focal findings, no hypotension, no COPD, no fungal infection, no dehydration, age range 16-60 yrs; motivated and compliant pts & family. If pen allergy: can substitute **Clinda** 300 mg po qid for Amox-clav	
High-risk adults and children (Anticipate >7 days profound neutropenia, active co-morbidities)	**Aerobic Gm-neg. bacilli; to include P. aeruginosa; cephalosporin-resistant viridans strep; MRSA**	**Empiric therapy:** **CFP**, **IMP**, **MER**, **Dori**, or **PIP-TZ**. Consider addition of **Vanco** as below. *Dosages: See footnote on page 66* **Include empiric Vanco if:** Suspected CLABSI, severe mucositis, SSTI, PNA, or hypotension	**Combination therapy:** If pt has severe sepsis/shock, consider add **Tobra** + **Vanco** + **Echinocandin**	Increasing resistance of viridans streptococci to penicillins, cephalosporins & FQs *(CID 34:1469 & 1524, 2002)*. **What if severe IgE-mediated β-lactam allergy?** Aztreonam plus Tobra. Work-up should include blood, urine, CXR with additional testing based on symptoms. Low threshold for CT scan. If cultures remain neg, but pt afebrile, treat until absolute neutrophil count ≥500 cells/µL. **Note**: Pip-tazo inferior to MER vs. ceftriaxone-resistant E. coli/K. pneumo *(JAMA 2018;320:979 & 984)*.
Persistent fever and neutropenia after 5 days of empiric antibacterial therapy—*see CID 52:427, 2011.*				
	Candida species, aspergillus, VRE, resistant GNB	Add either (**Caspofungin** 70 mg IV day 1, then 50 mg IV q24h or **Micafungin** 100 mg IV q24h or **Anidulafungin** 200 mg IV x 1 dose, then 100 mg IV q24h) **OR Voriconazole** 6 mg per kg IV q12h times 2 doses, then 4 mg per kg IV q12h		Conventional **Ampho B** causes more fever & nephrotoxicity & lower efficacy than lipid-based ampho B; both **Caspofungin** & **Voriconazole** better tolerated & perhaps more efficacious than lipid-based Ampho B *(NEJM 346:225, 2002 & 351:1391 & 1445, 2005)*.

 **NOTE: All dosage recommendations are for adults (unless otherwise indicated) and assume normal renal function. § Alternatives consider allergy, PK, compliance, local resistance, cost.*

TABLE 1 (64)

ANATOMIC SITE/DIAGNOSIS/ MODIFYING CIRCUMSTANCES	ETIOLOGIES (usual)	SUGGESTED REGIMENS*		ADJUNCT DIAGNOSTIC OR THERAPEUTIC MEASURES AND COMMENTS
		PRIMARY	ALTERNATIVE§	
SYSTEMIC SYNDROMES (FEBRILE/NON-FEBRILE)/Sepsis *(continued)*				
Shock syndromes				
Septic shock: Fever & hypotension **Bacteremic shock, endotoxin shock** *Goals:* *1. Effective antibiotics* *2. Fluid resuscitation* *3. Vasoactive drugs, if needed* *4. Source control* *(Intensive Care Med 2017;43:304; JAMA 2017;317:267 & 847)*	Bacteremia with aerobic Gm-neg. bacteria or Gm+ cocci	Lower mortality with **sepsis treatment "bundle"** *(NEJM 2017,376:2235, 2282)* • Blood cultures & serum lactate • Initiate effective antibiotic therapy: o No clear source & MDR GNB are rare: **Pip-tazo** + **Vanco** o No clear source but high prevalence of MDR GNB: if suscept, **MER** or **IMP** • IV crystalloid: 20-40 mL/kg for hypotension or elevated lactate *(NEJM 2018;378:829 & 862)* • If hypotensive after fluids, nor-epinephrine • Attempt to identify & correct source of bacteremia • Monitor lactate & central venous O_2 sat (target ≥70%) • Transfuse if hematocrit <30% *(NEJM 371:1381, 2014)* • *See Comment* for continuation		• For septic shock unresponsive to volume resuscitation and requiring on-going vasopressor therapy to maintain systolic BP > 90 mm Hg or MAP > 65 mm Hg consider hydrocortisone 50 mg IV q6h + fludrocortisone 50 mcg once daily via NG tube *(N Engl J Med 2018; 378:797, 809, and 860 [editorial])*. • Insulin Rx: Current target is glucose level of 140-180 mg/dL. Attempts at tight control (80-110 mg/dL) resulted in excessive hypoglycemia. • Impact of early effective antibiotic therapy *(NEJM 2017,376:2235)* • Bacteremia due to carbapenemase-producing K. pneumoniae: **Ceftaz-avi** or **MER-vabor**. • Shock associated with leaky capillaries which results in increased volume of drug distribution. Hence, need loading dose of antibiotics and, early in treatment, larger maintenance doses *(AAC 59:2995, 2015)*.
Septic shock: post-splenectomy or functional asplenia Asplenic pt care: *Chest 2016, 150:1394*	S. pneumoniae, N. meningitidis, H. influenzae, Capnocytophaga (DF-2)	No dog bite: **Ceftriaxone** 2 gm IV q24h (↑ to 2 gm q12h if meningitis) Post-dog bite: (**Pip-tazo** 3.375 gm IV q6h OR **MER** 1 gm IV q8h) OR **Clinda** 900 mg IV q8h	No dog bite: (**Levo** 750 mg or **Moxi** 400 mg) once IV q24h	Howell-Jolly bodies in peripheral blood smear confirm absence of functional spleen. Often results in **symmetrical peripheral gangrene of digits** due to severe DIC. For prophylaxis, *see Table 15A, page 218*. Vaccines: *CID 58:309, 2014*.
Toxic shock syndrome, Clostridium sordellii				
Clinical picture: shock, capillary leak, hemoconcentration, leukemoid reaction, afebrile	Clostridium sordellii–hemorrhagic & lethal toxins	Fluids, aq. **Pen G** 18–20 million units per day div. q4–6h + **Clinda** 900 mg IV q8h. **Surgical debridement is key.**	Occurs in variety of settings that produce anaerobic tissue, e.g., illicit drug use, post-partum. Several deaths reported after use of abortifacient regimen of mifepristone (RU486) & misoprostol. *(NEJM 363:2540, 2010)*.	
Toxic shock syndrome, staphylococcal				
Colonization by toxin-producing Staph. aureus of: vagina (tampon-assoc.), surgical/traumatic wounds, endometrium, burns	Staph. aureus (toxic shock toxin-mediated)	(**Nafcillin/Oxacillin** 2 gm IV q4h) or (if MRSA, **Vanco** 15-20 mg/kg q8-12h) + **Clinda** 600-900 mg IV q8h	(**Cefazolin** 1–2 gm IV q8h) or (if MRSA, **Vanco** 15-20 mg/kg q8-12h OR **Dapto** 6 mg/kg IV q24h) **Clinda** 600-900 mg IV q8h	Benefit of adjunctive IVIG unclear but may be reasonable for patients with persistent hypotension. Rationale for Clinda is inhibition of toxin production; Linezolid also an option to inhibit toxin production.

 **NOTE: All dosage recommendations are for adults (unless otherwise indicated) and assume normal renal function. § Alternatives consider allergy, PK, compliance, local resistance, cost.*

ANATOMIC SITE/DIAGNOSIS/ MODIFYING CIRCUMSTANCES	ETIOLOGIES (usual)	SUGGESTED REGIMENS*		ADJUNCT DIAGNOSTIC OR THERAPEUTIC MEASURES AND COMMENTS
		PRIMARY	ALTERNATIVE§	
SYSTEMIC SYNDROMES (FEBRILE/NON-FEBRILE)/Sepsis/Shock syndromes *(continued)*				
Toxic shock syndrome, streptococcal. NOTE: For Necrotizing fasciitis without toxic shock, *see page 60*. Ref: *NEJM 2017,377:2253.*				
Associated with **invasive disease**, i.e., erysipelas, necrotizing fasciitis; secondary strep infection of varicella. Secondary household contact TSS cases reported.	Group A, B, C, & G Strep. pyogenes, Group B strep ref: *EID 15:223, 2009.*	(**Pen G** 24 million units per day IV in div. doses) + (**Clinda** 900 mg IV q8h)	**Ceftriaxone** 2 gm IV q24h + **Clinda** 900 mg IV q8h	**Definition:** Isolation of Group A strep, hypotension and ≥2 of: renal impairment, coagulopathy, liver involvement, ARDS, generalized rash, soft tissue necrosis. Associated with invasive disease. **Surgery usually required.** Clinda added to decrease toxin production. **Adjunctive IVIG** (1 gm/kg on day 1, 0.5 gm/kg on days 2 and 3) may be of benefit *(CID 2018;67:1434) (meta-analysis).*
		Prospective observational study *(CID 59:358, 366 & 851, 2014)* indicates: • Clinda decreases mortality • High incidence of secondary cases in household contacts		
Toxin-Mediated Syndromes—no fever unless complicated				
Botulism *(CID. 2017;66(suppl_1):S11. As **biologic weapon:** https://www.cdc.gov/botulism/index.html)*				
	Clostridium botulinum	For all types: Follow vital capacity; other supportive care		**Equine antitoxin:** Contact the local or state health department (1-800-222-1222) or CDC (1-770-488-7100) or for infant botulism 1-510-231-7600. **Antimicrobials:** May make infant botulism worse. Untested in wound botulism. When used, pen G 10–20 million units per day usual dose. If complications (pneumonia, UTI) occur, avoid ant microbials with assoc. neuromuscular blockade, i.e., aminoglycosides, tetracycline, polymyxins. **Differential dx:** Guillain-Barré, myasthenia gravis, tick paralysis, organophosphate toxicity, West Nile virus. EMG can help.
Food-borne Dyspnea at presentation bad sign *(CID 43:1247, 2006)*	Less common: C. barati, C. butyricum	If no ileus, purge GI tract	Heptavalent equine serum antitoxin—CDC *(see Comment)*	
Infant (Adult intestinal botulism is rare variant: *EIN 18:1, 2012*).	Submit blood, wound tissue, and/or implicated food (as pertinent) for mouse toxin bioassay.	Age < 1 year: Human botulinum immunoglobulin. Age > 1 year: Equine serum heptavalent botulinum antitoxin. DO NOT WAIT FOR LAB CONFIRMATION TO TREAT SUSPECTED CASES	**No antibiotics;** may lyse C. botulinum in gut and ↑ load of toxin	
Wound		Debridement & anaerobic cultures. No proven value of local antitoxin. Role of antibiotics untested.	Trivalent equine antitoxin	Wound botulism associated with injection drug use. Mouse bioassay failed to detect toxin in 1/3 of patients *(CID 48:1669, 2009).*
Tetanus: Trismus, generalized muscle rigidity, muscle spasm Ref: *AnIM 154:329, 2011.*	C. tetani–production of tetanospasmin toxin	**Six treatment steps:** 1. Urgent endotracheal intubation to protect the airway. Laryngeal spasm is common. Early tracheostomy. 2. Eliminate reflex spasms with diazepam, 20 mg/kg/day IV or midazolam. Reports of benefit combining diazepam with magnesium sulfate *(Ln 368:1436, 2006)*. Worst cases: need neuromuscular blockade with vecuronium. 3. Neutralize toxin: Human hyperimmune globulin IM; start tetanus immunization–no immunity from clinical tetanus. 4. Surgically debride infected source tissue. Start antibiotic: (**Pen G** 3 million units IV q4h or **Doxy** 100 mg IV q12h or **Metro** 1000 mg IV q12h) x 7-10 days. 5. Avoid light as may precipitate muscle spasms. 6. Use beta blockers, e.g., short acting esmolol, to control sympathetic hyperactivity.		

 **NOTE: All dosage recommendations are for adults (unless otherwise indicated) and assume normal renal function. § Alternatives consider allergy, PK, compliance, local resistance, cost.*

TABLE 1 (66)

ANATOMIC SITE/DIAGNOSIS/ MODIFYING CIRCUMSTANCES	ETIOLOGIES (usual)	SUGGESTED REGIMENS* PRIMARY	ALTERNATIVE§	ADJUNCT DIAGNOSTIC OR THERAPEUTIC MEASURES AND COMMENTS
VASCULAR				
Catheter Related Blood Stream Infections (CRBSI). Ref: *Infect Dis Clin No Amer 2018 Dec;32(4):765-787*				
Tunneled & non-tunneled central venous catheters (CVC), including peripherally-inserted central catheters (PICC). For management of peripheral IV, midline, arterial & hemodialysis catheters, see *Infect Dis Clin No Amer 2018 Dec;32(4):765-787*. **Diagnosis:** concomitant blood cultures from CVC & peripheral vein. A differential time to positive (DTP) of ≥2 hr favors infection of the CVC.	If suspect Gm+ bacteria: empiric rx for MSSA, MRSA, MRSE	**Vanco**	**Dapto**	Recommend in all clinical settings due to high prevalence of MSSA, MRSA & MRSE
	If suspect Gm-neg bacteria, e.g., femoral line, neutropenic	Not critically ill: **Cefepime** or **Pip-tazo** Critically ill: **MER** or **IMP**		
	Empiric rx if high risk of candidemia, e.g., prolonged antibiotic therapy, post-transplant neutropenia, hyperalimentation	**Micafungin** or **Caspofungin**	**Isavuconazole**	
	S. epidermidis in blood: MSSE or MRSE (most often)	IF no attempt to salvage catheter; remove catheter. For MRSE: **Vanco** or **Dapto** For MSSE: **Cefazolin** IF attempt to salvage catheter. Antibiotic as above + antibiotic lock therapy (ALT) x 10-14 days. *(See Comment)*		Antibiotic lock therapy (ALT) not FDA approved. Several options, but prefer sol'n of Minocycline 5 mg + EDTA 30 mg/mL in 25% alcohol. See *AAC 2016;60:3426*. Catheter "dwell" time of a minimum 2-4 hrs/day.
	S. aureus or S. lugdunensis in blood; attempts at salvage therapy not recommended	Remove catheter. For MSSA: (**Nafcillin/Oxacillin**) or **Cefazolin** x 2-6 wks For MRSA: **Vanco** or **Dapto** x 2-6 wks		If bacteremia for >72 hrs after catheter removal, TEE 5-7 days after diagnosis of bacteremia. New CVC: after removal of infected CVC, new blood cultures for 48-72 hrs.
	Enterococcus sp. In blood.	Specific antibiotic rx based on culture ID & susceptibility testing If short term CVC: remove & treat for 7-14 days. If long term CVC: can attempt salvage with combination IV antibiotic + ALT x 10-14 days		TEE if bacteremia persists longer than 72 hrs after start of antibiotic therapy or patient has a prosthetic heart valve.
	Aerobic Gm-neg bacilli (GNB) in blood *(See Comment)*	Mono- or combination therapy for *P. aeruginosa* (or other MDR bacteria). Remove catheter. Can attempt to salvage catheter with systemic antibiotic + ALT x 10-14 days		If gram positive bacilli (GPB) in blood, maybe Leuconostoc sp. or Lactobacillus sp. Both are Vanco resistant but sensitive to **Pen G**, **AMP** or **Clinda**.
	Candida sp. In blood	Remove CVC. **Micafungin**	Remove CVC. **Fluconazole** unless *C. krusei*, then **Isavuconazole**	
Prevention of Catheter-Related Blood Stream Infection				
At Time of Catheter Insertion	1. Maximum sterile barrier precaution 2. Skin prep with 0.5% chlorohexidine and alcohol 3. Use subclavian vein if possible; try to avoid femoral vein/artery			
Post Catheter Insertion	1. Remove CVC as soon as possible 2. Scrub the hub of the catheter with alcohol or alcoholic chlorohexidine 3. Patient bathing with chlorohexidine 4. Change site dressing weekly if transparent or semi-transparent; every 2 days if gauze dressing			
Emerging Prevention Methods	1. Antimicrobial-coated catheters 2. Chlorohexidine impregnated dressings 3. Antibiotic impregnated needles and connectors 4. Catheter lock solutions *(CID 2014;59:1741)*			

 **NOTE: All dosage recommendations are for adults (unless otherwise indicated) and assume normal renal function. § Alternatives consider allergy, PK, compliance, local resistance, cost.*

TABLE 1 (67)

ANATOMIC SITE/DIAGNOSIS/ MODIFYING CIRCUMSTANCES	ETIOLOGIES (usual)	SUGGESTED REGIMENS*		ADJUNCT DIAGNOSTIC OR THERAPEUTIC MEASURES AND COMMENTS
		PRIMARY	ALTERNATIVE§	
VASCULAR/Catheter Related Blood Stream Infections (CRBSI) *(continued)*				
Mycotic aneurysm	S. aureus (28-71%), S. epidermidis, Salmonella sp. (15-24%), M.TBc, S. pneumonia, many others	**Vanco** (dose sufficient to achieve trough level of 15-20 µg/mL) + (**Ceftriaxone** or **Pip-tazo** or **CIP**) **Treatment is combination of antibiotic + surgical resection with revascularization.**	**Dapto** could be substituted for Vanco. For GNB: **Cefepime** or **Carbapenems**	Report of success with Ceftaroline with surgery for mycotic aneurysm due to VISA S aureus resistant to daptomycin *(BMJ Case Rep 2015: PMID 25833910)*. Best diagnostic imaging: CT angiogram. Blood cultures positive in 50-85%. **De-escalate to specific therapy when culture results known.** Treatment duration varies but usually 6 wks from date of definitive surgery.
Suppurative (Septic) Thrombophlebitis				
Cranial dural sinus:				
Cavernous Sinus CN III, IV, V (branches V1/V2), VI at risk (Note: V1 and V2, numbers are subscript)	S. aureus (70%) Streptococcus sp. Anaerobes (rare) Mucormycosis (diabetes)	[**Vanco** (dose for trough conc of 15-20 µg/mL) + **Ceftriaxone** 2 gm IV q12h], add **Metro** 500 mg IV q8h if dental/sinus source	(**Dapto** 8-12 mg/kg IV q24h OR **Linezolid** 600 mg IV q12h), add **Metro** 500 mg IV q8h if dental/sinus source	• Diagnosis: CT or MRI • Treatment: 1) obtain specimen for culture; 2) empiric antibiotics; 3) may need adjunctive surgery; 4) heparin until afebrile, then coumadin for several weeks
Lateral Sinus: Complication of otitis media/mastoiditis (pathogens similar to otitis media)	Polymicrobial (often) Aerobes, e.g., Proteus sp, E. coli S. aureus P. aeruginosa B. fragilis Other GNB	**Cefepime** 2 gm IV q8h + **Metro** 500 mg IV q8h + **Vanco** (dose for trough conc of 15-20 µg/mL)	**MER** 2 gm IV q8h + **Linezolid** 600 mg IV q12h	• Diagnosis: CT or MRI • Treatment: 1) consider radical mastoidectomy; 2) obtain cultures; 3) antibiotics; 4) anticoagulation controversial • Prognosis: favorable
Superior Sagittal Sinus: Complication of bacterial meningitis or bacterial frontal sinusitis. Treat as for meningitis	S. pneumoniae N. meningitides H. influenzae (rare) S. aureus (very rare)	**Ceftriaxone** 2 gm IV q12h + **Vanco** (trough conc of 15-20 µg/mL) + **Dexamethasone**	**MER** 2 gm IV q8h + **Vanco** (trough conc of 15-20 µg/mL) + **Dexamethasone**	• Diagnosis: MRI • Prognosis: bad; causes cortical vein thrombosis, hemorrhagic infarcts and brainstem herniation. • Anticoagulants not recommended

 **NOTE: All dosage recommendations are for adults (unless otherwise indicated) and assume normal renal function. § Alternatives consider allergy, PK, compliance, local resistance, cost.*

TABLE 1 (68)

ANATOMIC SITE/DIAGNOSIS/ MODIFYING CIRCUMSTANCES	ETIOLOGIES (usual)	SUGGESTED REGIMENS*		ADJUNCT DIAGNOSTIC OR THERAPEUTIC MEASURES AND COMMENTS
		PRIMARY	ALTERNATIVE§	
VASCULAR/Suppurative (Septic) Thrombophlebitis *(continued)*				
Jugular Vein, Lemierre's Syndrome: Complication of pharyngitis, tonsillitis, dental infection, EBV. Ref: *NEJM 371:2018, 2015.*	Fusobacterium necrophorum (anaerobe) Less often: Other Fusobacterium S. pyogenes Bacteroides sp.	(**Pip-tazo** 3.375 gm IV q6h OR **Amp-sulb** 3 gm IV q6h) x 4 weeks	[**IMP** 500 mg IV q6h OR (**Metro** 500 mg IV q8h + **Ceftriaxone** 2 gm IV once daily)] x 4 weeks. Another option: **Clinda** 600-900 mg IV q8h	• Diagnosis: Preceding pharyngitis and antibiotics therapy, persistent fever and pulmonary emboli • Imaging: Hi-res CT scan • Role of anticoagulants unclear
Pelvic Vein: Includes ovarian vein and deep pelvic vein phlebitis	Aerobic gram-neg bacilli Streptococcus sp. Anaerobes	Antibiotics + anticoagulation (heparin, then coumadin) *Low prevalence of MDR GNB:* **Pip-tazo** 3.375 gm IV q6h or 4.5 gm IV q8h OR (**Ceftriaxone** 2 gm IV once daily + **Metro** 500 mg IV q8h)	*High prevalence of MDR GNB:* **MER** 1 gm IV q8h. If severe beta-lactam allergy: (**CIP** 400 mg IV q12h + **Metro** 500 mg IV q8h)	• Diagnosis: ovarian vein infection presents 1 week post-partum with fever & local pain; deep pelvic vein presents 3-5 days post-delivery with fever but no local pain. CT or MRI may help. • Treat until afebrile for 48 hrs & WBC normal • Coumadin for 6 weeks
Portal Vein (Pylephlebitis): Complication of diverticulitis, appendicitis and (rarely) other intra-abdominal infection	Aerobic gram-neg bacilli: E. coli, Klebsiella & Proteus most common Other: aerobic/anaerobic streptococci, B. fragilis, Clostridia	*Low prevalence of MDR GNB* (<20%): **Pip-tazo** 4.5 gm IV q8h OR (**CIP** 400 mg IV q12h + **Metro** 500 mg IV q8h)	*High prevalence of MDR GNB* (≥20%): If ESBL producer: **Meropenem** 1-2 gm IV q8h. If carbapenemase producer: **MER-vabor** 4 gm IV over 3 hrs q8h. If not KPC (MBL): **Ceftaz-avi** + **Aztreonam**	• Diagnosis: Pain, fever, neutrophilia in pt with intra-abdominal infection. Abdominal CT scan • Pyogenic liver abscess is a complication • No anticoagulants unless hypercoagulable disease (neoplasm) • Surgery on vein not indicated

TABLE 2 – RECOMMENDED ANTIMICROBIAL AGENTS AGAINST SELECTED BACTERIA

BACTERIAL SPECIES	ANTIMICROBIAL AGENT *(See page 2 for abbreviations)*		
	RECOMMENDED	ALTERNATIVE	ALSO EFFECTIVE[1] (COMMENTS)
Achromobacter xylosoxidans spp xylosoxidans (formerly Alcaligenes)	IMP, MER, DORI (no DORI for pneumonia)	TMP-SMX. Some strains susc. to ceftaz, Pip-tazo	Resistant to aminoglycosides, most cephalosporins & FQs. Ref: *Ann Amer Thor Soc 12:252, 2015*
Acinetobacter calcoaceticus—baumannii complex	If suscept: IMP or MER. For MDR strains: Polymyxin B + (IMP or MER) + Amp-sulb	Amp-sulb used for activity of sulbactam	Resistant to aminoglycosides, FQs. Minocycline, effective against many strains *(CID 51:79, 2010)*
Actinomyces israelii	AMP or Pen G	Doxy, Ceftriaxone	Clindamycin, Erythro
Aerococcus urinae (cystitis)	Amox or Nitrofurantoin	Fosfomycin (A. urinae only); CIP (if susceptible)	Susceptible to Pen G. Frequently resistant to FQs. Increased Ceftriaxone MICs. Generally resistant to TMP-SMX
Aeromonas hydrophila & other sp.	CIP or Levo	TMP-SMX or (P Ceph 3, 4)	*See AAC 56:1110, 2012.*
Arcanobacterium haemolyticum	Azithro	Pen G, Ceftriaxone, Vancomycin, and many other agents	Resistance to TMP-SMX *(AAC 38: 142, 1994)*. Resistance to Levofloxacin, Clindamycin reported *(J Med Microbiol 64: 369, 2015)*
Bacillus anthracis (anthrax): inhalation	*See Table 1, page 44.*		
Bacillus cereus, B. subtilis	Vancomycin, Clinda	FQ, IMP	
Bacteroides sp., B. fragilis & others	Metronidazole or Pip-tazo	DORI, ERTA, IMP, MER, Amox-clav	Increasing resistance to: Clinda, Cefoxitin, Cefotetan, Moxi. Ref: *CID 59:698, 2014.*
Bartonella henselae, quintana *See Table 1, pages 32, 48, 54, 61*	Varies with disease entity & immune status. Active: Azithro, Clarithro, Erythro, Doxy & in combination: RIF, Gent, Ceftriaxone. Not active: CIP, TMP-SMX, Pen, most cephalosporins, Aztreonam.		
Bordetella pertussis	Azithro or clarithro	TMP-SMX	*See PIDJ 31:78, 2012.*
Borrelia burgdorferi, B. afzelii, B. garinii (Lyme & relapsing fever)	See specific disease entity		
Brucella sp.	Drugs & duration vary with localization or non-localization. *See specific disease entities. PLoS One 7:e32090, 2012.*		
Burkholderia cepacia	TMP-SMX or MER or CIP	Minocycline or chloramphenicol	Multiple mechanisms of resistance. Need culture & sensitivity to guide therapy *(Sem Resp Crit Care Med 36:99, 2015)*
Burkholderia pseudomallei *Curr Opin Infect Dis 23:554, 2010; CID 41:1105, 2005*	Initially, IV Ceftaz or IMP or MER, then po (TMP-SMX + Doxy x 3 mos) *(AAC 49:4010, 2005)*. One study showed TMP-SMX alone was non-inferior to combination with Doxy *(Lancet 383: 807, 2014)*		(Thai, 12–80% strains resist to TMP-SMX). FQ not very active in vitro. Amox-clav possible alternative to TMP-SMX *(Int J Antimicrob Agents 43: 310, 2014)*.
Campylobacter jejuni	Azithro	Erythro or CIP	TMP-SMX, Pen & cephalosporins not active.
Campylobacter fetus	Gentamicin	IMP or Ceftriaxone	AMP, Chloramphenicol
Capnocytophaga ochracea (DF-1)	Dog bite: Clinda or Amox-clav	Septic shock, post-splenectomy: Pip-tazo, Clinda, IMP, DORI, MER	FQ activity variable; aminoglycosides, TMP-SMX & Polymyxins have limited activity. *LN ID 9:439, 2009.*
Capnocytophaga canimorsus (DF-2)	Dog bite: Amox-clav, Pip-tazo, CFP		
Chlamydophila pneumoniae	Doxy	Azithro, FQ	Clarithro
Chlamydia trachomatis	Doxy or Azithro	Erythro	
Citrobacter diversus (koseri), C. freundii	Life threatening illness: IMP, MER, DORI	Non-life threatening illness: CIP or Gent	Emergence of resistance: *AAC 52:995, 2007.*
Clostridium (Clostridioides) difficile	Mild illness: Vanco (po)	Moderate/severe illness: Vanco (po) or Fidaxomicin *(CID 51:1306, 2010)*.	*See also Table 1, page 20 re severity of disease.*
Clostridium perfringens	Pen G ± clindamycin	Doxy	Erythro, Chloramphenicol, Cefazolin, Cefoxitin, Pip-tazo, Carbapenems
Clostridium tetani	Metronidazole	Doxy	Role of antibiotics unclear.
Corynebacterium diphtheriae	Erythro + antitoxin	Pen G + antitoxin	RIF reported effective *(CID 27:845, 1998)*
Corynebacterium jeikeium	Vancomycin	Daptomycin (Resistance reported, *JCM 47: 2328, 2009*)	Most strains are resistant to pen and Erythro *(Clin Microbiol Inf 2: 209, 1996)*
Corynebacterium minutissimum	Clinda 1% lotion	Clarithro or Erythro	Causes erythrasma

TABLE 2 (2)

BACTERIAL SPECIES	ANTIMICROBIAL AGENT *(See page 2 for abbreviations)*		
	RECOMMENDED	**ALTERNATIVE**	**ALSO EFFECTIVE[1] (COMMENTS)**
Coxiella burnetii (Q fever) acute disease *(CID 52:1431, 2011).*	Doxy, FQ *(see Table 1, page 33)*	Erythro, Azithro, Clarithro	Endocarditis: Doxy + hydroxychloroquine *(JID 188:1322, 2003; LnID 3:709, 2003; LnID 10:527, 2010).*
chronic disease, e.g., endocarditis	Doxy + hydroxy chloroquine	TMP-SMX, Chloro	
Ehrlichia chaffeensis Ehrlichia ewingii Anaplasma phagocytophilum	Doxy	Rifampin (no large studies)	Chloro not effective. In severe infections, consider doxycycline desensitization if allergic *(MMWR 65(2): 1, 2016).*
Eikenella corrodens	Amox-clav, IV Pen G	TMP-SMX, FQ	Resistant to Clinda, Cephalexin, Erythro, Metro, Diclox
Elizabethkingia meningoseptica (formerly Chryseobacterium)	Levo or TMP-SMX	CIP, Minocycline	Resistant to Pen, cephalosporins, carbapenems, aminoglycosides, Vanco *(JCM 44:1181, 2006)*
Enterobacter species	Recommended agents vary with clinical setting and degree and mechanism of resistance.		
Enterococcus faecalis	Highly resistant. *See Table 5A, page 88*		
Enterococcus faecium	Highly resistant. *See Table 5A, page 88*		
Erysipelothrix rhusiopathiae	Penicillin G or amox	P Ceph 3, FQ	IMP, Pip-tazo (vancomycin, APAG, TMP-SMX resistant)
Escherichia coli	Can be highly resistant. Treatment varies with degree & mechanism of resistance, *see Table 5B.*		
Francisella tularensis (tularemia) *See Table 1, page 46*	Gentamicin, Tobramycin, or Streptomycin	Mild infection: Doxy or CIP	Chloramphenicol, RIF. Doxy/chloro bacteriostatic → relapses *CID 53:e133, 2011.*
Fusobacterium necrophorum	Metro, Ceftriaxone, Pip-tazo	IMP, MER, Clinda	Resistant to macrolides
Gardnerella vaginalis (bacterial vaginosis)	Metronidazole or Tinidazole	Clindamycin	*See Table 1, page 28 for dosage*
Helicobacter pylori	*See Table 1, page 23*		Drugs effective in vitro often fail in vivo.
Haemophilus aphrophilus (Aggregatibacter aphrophilus)	Ceftriaxone	CIP or Levo	Resistant to Vanco, Clinda, Methicillin
Haemophilus ducreyi (chancroid)	Azithro or Ceftriaxone	Erythro, CIP	Most strains resistant to Tetracycline, Amox, TMP-SMX
Haemophilus influenzae Meningitis, epiglottitis & other life-threatening illness	Cefotaxime, Ceftriaxone	AMP if susceptible and β-lactamase neg, FQs	Chloramphenicol rarely used due to hematotoxicity.
non-life-threatening illness	Amox-clav, O Ceph 2/3		Azithro, Clarithro, Telithro
Klebsiella ozaenae/ rhinoscleromatis	CIP	Levo	*Acta Otolaryngol 131:440, 2010.*
Klebsiella species	Treatment varies with degree & mechanism of resistance, *see Table 5B.*		
Lactobacillus species	Pen G or AMP	Clindamycin	**May be resistant to vancomycin**
Legionella sp.	Levo or Moxi	Azithro, Doxy	
Leptospira interrogans	Mild: Doxy or Amox	Severe: Pen G or ceftriaxone	
Leuconostoc	Pen G or AMP	Clinda	**NOTE: Resistant to vancomycin**
Listeria monocytogenes	AMP ± Gent for synergy	TMP-SMX	Erythro, penicillin G (high dose); APAG may be synergistic with ß-lactams. **Cephalosporin-resistant!**
Moraxella (Branhamella) catarrhalis	Amox-clav or O Ceph 2/3, TMP-SMX	Azithro, Clarithro, Dirithromycin, Telithro	Erythro, Doxy, FQs
Morganella sp. (need in vitro susceptibility)	Recommendations vary with clinical syndrome, frequency & mechanism of resistance		
Mycoplasma pneumoniae	Doxy	Azithro, Minocycline	Clindamycin & ß lactams NOT effective. Increasing macrolide resistance *(JAC 68:506, 2013; AAC 58:1034, 2014).*
Neisseria gonorrhoeae (gonococcus)	Ceftriaxone,	Azithro (high dose)	FQs and oral cephalosporins no longer recommended: high levels of resistance.
Neisseria meningitidis (meningococcus)	Ceftriaxone	Pen G, MER, Chloro	(Chloro less effective than other alternatives: *see JAC 70:979, 2015*)
Nocardia asteroides or **Nocardia brasiliensis**	TMP-SMX + IMP	Linezolid	Amikacin + (IMP or ceftriaxone or Cefotaxime) *(AAC 58:795, 2014).*
Pasteurella multocida	Pen G, AMP, Amox, Amox-clav, Cefuroxime, Cefpodoxime	Doxy, Levo, Moxi, TMP-SMX	Resistant to Cephalexin, Oxacillin, Clindamycin, Erythro, Vanco. Rare beta-lactamase-producing isolates have been reported *(EJCMID 20: 210, 2001).*
Peptoniphilus sp. (Peptostreptococcus)	Pen G	Metronidazole	Some clinda resistance *(Clin Micro Infect 2014,20:0857)*

TABLE 2 (3)

BACTERIAL SPECIES	ANTIMICROBIAL AGENT *(See page 2 for abbreviations)*		
	RECOMMENDED	**ALTERNATIVE**	**ALSO EFFECTIVE[1] (COMMENTS)**
Plesiomonas shigelloides	CIP	TMP-SMX	Amox-clav, Ceftriaxone & Chloro active. Resistant to: Amp, Tetra, aminoglycosides
Propionibacterium (now Cutibacterium) acnes (not acne)	Penicillin, Ceftriaxone	Vanco, Dapto, Linezolid	May be resistant to Metro.
Proteus sp, **Providencia sp**, (Need in vitro susceptibility)	Recommended drugs vary with clinical setting and frequency & mechanism of resistance.		
Pseudomonas aeruginosa	Can be highly resistant. Treatment varies with degree & mech. of resist., *see Table 5B*		
Rhodococcus (C. equi)	Customary to use combination Rx. Choose 2 from: Azithro, Levo, or Rif *(Lancet ID 10:350, 2010)*.	(Vanco or IMP) + (Azithro, Levo or RIF)	Vancomycin active in vitro; intracellular location may impair efficacy *(CID 34:1379, 2002)*. Avoid Pen, Cephalosporins, Clinda, Tetra, TMP-SMX.
Rickettsia species (includes spotted fevers)	Doxy	Chloramphenicol (in pregnancy)	*See specific infections* (*Table 1*). *(MMWR 65(RR-2):1, 2016)*
Salmonella typhi *(CID 50:241, 2010; AAC 54:5201, 2010; BMC ID 51:37, 2005)*	If FQ & nalidixic acid susceptible: CIP	Ceftriaxone, Cefixime, Azithro, Chloro	Concomitant steroids in severely ill. Watch for relapse (1-6%) & ileal perforation. Chloro less effective than other alternatives: *see JAC 70:979, 2015)*.
Serratia marcescens	If no in vitro resistance: Pip-tazo, CIP, LEVO, Gent	If in vitro resistance due to ESBL: Carbapenem	Avoid extended spectrum Ceph if possible See specific syndrome if MDR documented.
Shigella sp.	FQ or azithro	Ceftriaxone is alternative; TMP-SMX depends on susceptibility.	
Staph. aureus, methicillin-susceptible	Oxacillin/Nafcillin	P Ceph 1, Vanco, Teicoplanin[NUS], Clinda, Ceftaroline	ERTA, IMP, MER, Amox-clav, FQ, Pip-tazo, Linezolid, Dapto, Telavancin.
Staph. aureus, methicillin-resistant (health-care associated) *IDSA Guidelines: CID 52 (Feb 1):1, 2011.*	Vancomycin	Teicoplanin[NUS], Linezolid, Daptomycin, Telavancin, Ceftaroline	Fusidic acid[NUS]. >60% CIP-resistant in U.S. (Fosfomycin + RIF). *See Table 6, page 90.*
Staph. aureus, methicillin-resistant [community- associated (CA-MRSA)]	(TMP-SMX or Doxy or Mino)	Clinda (if D-test neg—*see Table 5A & 6)*.	CA-MRSA usually not multiply-resistant. Oft resist. to Erythro & Variably to FQ. Vanco, Teico[NUS], Telavancin, Dapto, Ceftaroline can be used in pts requiring hospitalization *(see Table 6, page 90)*.
	Vanco or Teico[NUS]	Linezolid or Dapto	
Staph. epidermidis	MSSE: oxacillin, nafcillin, cefazolin MRSE: Vancomycin	Dapto, linezolid	Rifampin (if Susceptible) often used with (FQ or TMP-SMX) for infections assoc with prostheses.
Staph. haemolyticus	If Oxa-susceptible: oxacillin, nafcillin, cefazolin If Oxa-resistant: Vancomycin	Dapto, linezolid	For UTI: TMP-SMX, nitrofurantoin, oral ceph, FQ may be active.
Staph. lugdunensis	If Oxa-susceptible: oxacillin, nafcillin, cefazolin If Oxa-resistant: Vancomycin	Pen G if pen-susceptible. Daptomycin, linezolid. If Oxa-susc: oral ceph or Amox-clav.	Approx 52% susceptible to Pen G and 95% to oxacillin; high rates of susc to doxy or TMP-SMX *(JCM 55: 585, 2017)*.
Staph. saprophyticus (UTI)	Oral cephalosporin or Amox-clav	FQ	Almost always methicillin-susceptible
Stenotrophomonas (Xanthomonas, Pseudo-monas) maltophilia	TMP-SMX	Minocycline *(Diag Micro Infect Dis 85:352, 2016; JAC 2016,71:1071)*	FQ (if in vitro suscept) *(AAC 2014,58:176)*
Streptobacillus moniliformis	Penicillin G	Doxy	Maybe Erythro, Clinda, Ceftriaxone
Streptococcus anginosus group	Penicillin	Vanco or Ceftriaxone	Avoid FQs; macrolide resistance emerging
Streptococcus pneumoniae penicillin-susceptible	Penicillin G, Amox	Multiple agents effective, e.g., Ceph 2/3, Clinda	If meningitis, higher dose, *see Table 1, page 11.*
penicillin resistant (MIC ≥2.0)	Vanco, Levo, Ceftriaxone, Ceftaroline, Amox (HD), Linezolid		
Streptococcus pyogenes, (Grp A), **Streptococcus sp** (Grp B, C, G). Erysipelas, bacteremia, TSS	Penicillin G, cephalosporin	Clinda, vanco, dapto, linezolid	For TSS, necrotizing fasciitis: Pen G+Clinda. Avoid FQ, TMP-SMX, tetracyclines. Pockets of macrolide/clinda resistance *(JCM 49: 439, 2011)*.
Tropheryma whipplei	Doxy + Hydroxychloroquine	Ceftriaxone or Mero, then TMP-SMX	Clinical failures with TMP-SMX

TABLE 2 (4)

BACTERIAL SPECIES	ANTIMICROBIAL AGENT *(See page 2 for abbreviations)*		
	RECOMMENDED	**ALTERNATIVE**	**ALSO EFFECTIVE[1] (COMMENTS)**
Vibrio cholerae	Azithro	CIP, Doxy	Rehydration salts primary therapy. Vaccine available.
Vibrio parahaemolyticus	Doxy	Azithro, CIP	If bacteremic, treat as for V. vulnificus
Vibrio vulnificus, alginolyticus, damsela	Doxy + Ceftriaxone	Levo	*CID 52:788, 2011*
Yersinia enterocolitica	Ceftriaxone if bacteremic, CIP otherwise	TMP-SMX	CIP resistance *(JAC 53: 1068, 2004)*; also resistance to Pen, Amp, 1st gen Cephs, Erythro.
Yersinia pestis (plague)	Streptomycin or Gent	Doxy or (CIP, Levo, Moxi)	Levo, Moxi. CDC advice for treatment and prevention (https://www.cdc.gov/plague/healthcare/clinicians.html).

[1] Agents are more variable in effectiveness than "Recommended" or "Alternative". Selection of "Alternative" or "Also Effective" based on in vitro susceptibility testing, pharmacokinetics, host factors such as auditory, renal, hepatic function, & cost.

TABLE 3 – SUGGESTED DURATION OF ANTIBIOTIC THERAPY FOR SELECTED CLINICAL SYNDROMES IN IMMUNOCOMPETENT PATIENTS

Overview of variables affecting duration of therapy

Variables involved in duration of therapy are summarized in Curr Opin Infect Dis 2015,28:170 and include:

- PK/PD of antibiotic used, e.g., long tissue half-life of Azithro
- Identified pathogen (etiology)
- Host factors, e.g., neutropenic, HIV
- Severity of infection, e.g., cystitis vs. bacteremia
- Severity of host inflammatory response as measured by biomarkers, e.g., serum procalcitonin

Due to these many variables, it is usually not possible to recommend a definite duration except where there is a single pathogen in a healthy person, e.g., E. coli cystitis or Legionella pneumonia. For most situations, need to individualize duration until the patient is clinically stable and biomarkers have normalized.

CLINICAL SITUATION		DURATION OF THERAPY (Days)
SITE	**CLINICAL DIAGNOSIS**	
Bacteremia	Bacteremia with removable focus (no endocarditis)	Variable, see catheter-related bacteremia
Bone	Osteomyelitis, adult; acute adult; chronic child; acute; staph. and enterobacteriaceae child; acute; strep, meningococci, haemophilus	**42-56** Until ESR normal (often >3 months) **21-28** until ESR normal **14-21**
Ear	Otitis media with effusion	<2 yrs: **10**; ≥2 yrs: **5-7**
Endocardium	Infective endocarditis, native valve: Viridans strep Enterococci Staph. aureus	**14 or 28** *(See Table 1, page 30)* **28 or 42** *(See Table 1, page 31)* **14** (R-sided only) or **28** *(See Table 1, page 31)*
GI *Also see Table 1*	Bacillary dysentery (shigellosis)/traveler's diarrhea	single dose, up to **3** days if no response
	Typhoid fever (S. typhi): Azithro Ceftriaxone FQ Chloramphenicol	**5-7** (children/adolescents) **7-14** [Short course ↑ effective *(AAC 44:450, 2000)*] **7-10** **14**
	Helicobacter pylori	**14** days now preferred
	Pseudomembranous enterocolitis (C. difficile)	**10**
Genital	Pelvic inflammatory disease	**14**
Heart	Pericarditis (purulent)	**28** or until resolution of S&S and biomarkers normalize
Joint	Septic arthritis (non-gonococcal): Adult Infant/child	**14-28** **10-14** (Response varies, stop when resolution of S&S and biomarkers normalize).
	Gonococcal arthritis/disseminated GC infection	**7** *(See Table 1, page 25)*
Kidney	Cystitis, acute	**3** (FQ or TMP-SMX) **5** (nitrofurantoin) **1** (fosfomycin)
	Pyelonephritis	**7** (CIP) **5** (Levo 750 mg)
Intra-abdominal	Peritonitis, secondary	**4-7** (with source control) *(Pharmacother 38:674, 2018)*
Lung *(Pharmacother 38:674, 2018)*	Pneumonia, pneumococcal Community-acquired pneumonia	**5-7** days or fall of serum procalcitonin by 80% or ≤ 0.25 ng/mL
	Pneumonia, enterobacteriaceae or pseudomonal	**14-21, often up to 42** (variable, until biomarkers normalize)
	Pneumonia, staphylococcal	**21-28** (variable, until biomarkers normalize)
	Pneumocystis pneumonia (PCP) in AIDS	**21**
	Other immunocompromised	**14**
	Legionella, mycoplasma, chlamydia	**5-14** days depending on severity of illness, up to 21 in immunocompromised
	Lung abscess	Usually **28-42**, but variable
Meninges	N. meningitidis H. influenzae S. pneumoniae Listeria meningoencephalitis, gp B strep, coliforms	**7** **7** **10-14** **21** (longer in immunocompromised)
	Child: relapses seldom occur until 3 or more days post-rx.	
Multiple systems	Brucellosis *(See Table 1, page 64)*	**42** (depends on site of infection)
	Tularemia *(See Table 1, pages 48, 64)*	**7-21** depending on severity
Muscle	Gas gangrene (clostridial)	**10** but depends on severity
Pharynx	Group A strep pharyngitis *Also see Pharyngitis, Table 1, page 51*	**10** (Pen VK), **5** (O Ceph 2/3, Azithro) *(PIDJ 36:507, 2017)*
	Diphtheria (membranous) Carrier	**14** (Pen G, Erythro) **1 dose** (Pen G), **7-10** (Erythro)
Prostate	Chronic prostatitis	**30-90** (TMP-SMX), **28-42** (FQ)
Sinuses	Acute bacterial sinusitis (usually viral etiology)	**5**
Skin	Cellulitis, erysipelas	**Until 3 days after acute inflamm disappears**
Systemic	Lyme disease	*See Table 1, page 62.*
	Rocky Mountain spotted fever *(See Table 1, page 63)*	**Until afebrile 2 days**
UTI (duration depends on antimicrobial and clinical status)	Cystitis, uncomplicated female	**3-7**
	Cystitis, uncomplicated male	**7**
	Cystitis, complicated	**7-14**
	Pyelonephritis	**5-7**

TABLE 4A – ANTIBACTERIAL ACTIVITY SPECTRA

The data provided are intended to serve as a general guide to antibacterial usefulness based on treatment guidelines and recommendations, in vitro activity, predominant patterns of susceptibility or resistance and/or demonstrated clinical effectiveness. **Variability in resistance patterns due to regional differences or as a consequent of clinical setting (e.g., community-onset vs. ICU-acquired infection) should be taken into account when using this table because activities of certain agents can differ significantly from what is shown in the table,** which are by necessity based on aggregate information. We have revised and expanded the color / symbol key to provide a more descriptive categorization of the table data.

++ = Recommended: Agent is a first line therapy: reliably active in vitro, clinically effective, guideline recommended, recommended as a first-line agent or acceptable alternative agent in the Sanford Guide

+ = Active: Agent is a potential alternative agent (active in vitro, possesses class activity comparable to known effective agents or a therapeutically interchangeable agents and hence likely to be clinically effective, but second line due to overly broad spectrum, toxicity, limited clinical experience, or paucity of direct evidence of effectiveness)

± = Variable: Variable activity such that the agent, although clinically effective in some settings or types of infections is not reliably effective in others, or should be used in combination with another agent, and/or its efficacy is limited by resistance which has been associated with treatment failure

0 = Not recommended: Agent is a poor alternative to other agents because resistance to likely to be present or occur, due to poor drug penetration to site of infection or an unfavorable toxicity profile, or limited or anecdotal clinical data to support effectiveness

? = Insufficient Data to recommend use

NA = No activity: Agent has no activity against this pathogen

	Penicillins												Carbapenems							Fluoroquinolone									Parenteral Cephalosporins													
	Penicillin G	Penicillin VK	Nafcillin	Oxacillin	Cloxacillin	Flucloxacillin	Dicloxacillin	Ampicillin	Amoxicillin	Amox-Clav	Amp-Sulb	Pip-Tazo	Doripenem	Ertapenem	Imp-cilastatin	Imp-cila-rele	Meropenem	Mero-Vabor	Aztreonam	Ciprofloxacin	Delafloxacin	Ofloxacin	Levofloxacin	Moxifloxacin	Norfloxacin	Prulifloxacin	Gemifloxacin	Gatifloxacin	Cefazolin	Cefotetan	Cefoxitin	Cefuroxime	Cefotaxime	Ceftizoxime	Ceftriaxone	Ceftazidime	Cefepime	Ceftaz-Avibac	Ceftaroline	Ceftobiprole	Ceftol-Tazo	Cefiderocol
Aerobic gram-pos cocci																																										
E. faecalis (S)	++	0	0	0	0	0	0	++	++	+	+	+	±	±	+	+	±	±	0	±	+	±	+	+	+	±	+	+	0	0	0	0	0	0	±	0	0	0	0	0	0	0
E. faecium (S)	±	0	0	0	0	0	0	±	±	±	±	±	0	0	0	0	0	0	0	0	0	0	0	±	0	0	±	±	0	0	0	0	0	0	0	0	0	0	0	0	0	0
E. faecalis (VRE)	±	0	0	0	0	0	0	±	±	±	±	±	0	0	0	0	0	0	0	0	0	0	0	0	0	0	0	0	0	0	0	0	0	0	0	0	0	0	0	0	0	0
E. faecium (VRE)	±	0	0	0	0	0	0	±	±	±	±	±	0	0	0	0	0	0	0	0	0	0	0	0	0	0	0	0	0	0	0	0	0	0	0	0	0	0	0	0	0	0
S. aureus MSSA	±	±	++	++	++	++	++	±	±	+	+	+	+	+	+	+	+	+	0	0	+	+	+	+	0	0	+	+	++	+	+	+	+	+	+	±	+	±	+	+	?	0
S. aureus HA-MRSA	0	0	0	0	0	0	0	0	0	0	0	0	0	0	0	0	0	0	0	0	+	0	0	0	0	0	0	0	0	0	0	0	0	0	0	0	0	0	+	+	0	0
S. aureus CA-MRSA	0	0	0	0	0	0	0	0	0	0	0	0	0	0	0	0	0	0	0	0	+	±	±	±	0	0	±	±	0	0	0	0	0	0	0	0	0	0	+	+	0	0
Staph coag-neg (S)	±	±	++	++	++	++	++	±	±	+	+	+	+	+	+	+	+	+	0	+	+	+	+	+	0	+	+	+	++	?	?	+	?	?	?	?	?	?	+	+	?	0
Staph coag-neg (R)	0	0	0	0	0	0	0	0	0	0	0	0	0	0	0	0	0	0	0	0	+	0	±	±	0	0	0	0	0	0	0	0	0	0	0	0	0	0	+	+	0	0
S. epidermidis (R)	0	0	0	0	0	0	0	0	0	0	0	0	0	0	0	0	0	0	0	0	+	0	±	±	0	0	0	0	0	0	0	0	0	0	0	0	0	0	+	+	0	0
S. epidermidis (S)	±	±	++	++	++	++	++	±	±	+	+	+	+	+	+	+	+	+	0	+	+	+	+	+	0	+	+	+	++	+	+	+	+	+	+	?	+	?	+	+	?	0
S. lugdunensis	±	±	++	++	++	++	++	±	±	+	+	+	+	+	+	+	+	+	0	0	+	+	+	+	0	0	+	+	++	+	+	+	+	+	+	?	+	?	+	+	?	0
S. saprophyticus	±	±	+	+	+	+	+	±	±	++	+	+	+	+	+	+	+	+	0	+	+	+	+	+	0	+	+	+	++	+	+	+	+	+	+	?	+	?	+	+	?	0
S. anginosus grp	++	++	+	+	+	+	+	+	+	+	+	+	+	+	+	+	+	+	0	±	+	±	±	±	0	±	±	±	+	+	+	+	+	+	+	+	+	+	+	+	+	0
Strep. pyogenes (A)	++	++	+	+	+	+	+	+	+	+	+	+	+	+	+	+	+	+	0	±	+	±	±	±	0	±	±	±	+	+	+	+	+	+	+	+	+	+	+	+	+	0
Strep. agalactiae (B)	++	++	+	+	+	+	+	+	+	+	+	+	+	+	+	+	+	+	0	±	+	±	±	±	0	±	±	±	+	+	+	+	+	+	+	+	+	+	+	+	+	0

TABLE 4A (2)

	Penicillins												Carbapenems						
	Penicillin G	Penicillin VK	Nafcillin	Oxacillin	Cloxacillin	Flucloxacillin	Dicloxacillin	Ampicillin	Amoxicillin	Amox-Clav	Amp-Sulb	Pip-Tazo	Doripenem	Ertapenem	Imp-cilastatin	Imp-cila-rele	Meropenem	Mero-Vabor	Aztreonam
Aerobic gram-pos cocci *(continued)*																			
Strep. gp C, F, G	++	++	+	+	+	+	+	+	+	+	+	+	+	+	+	+	+	+	0
Strep. pneumoniae	++	++	+	+	+	+	+	+	+	+	+	+	+	+	+	+	+	+	0
Viridans Strep.	±	±	±	±	±	±	±	±	±	±	±	±	+	+	+	+	+	+	0
Aerobic gram-pos bacilli																			
Arcanobacter. sp	+	+	?	?	?	?	?	+	+	+	+	+	+	+	+	+	+	+	0
C. diphtheriae	++	++	0	0	0	0	0	+	+	+	+	+	?	?	?	?	?	?	0
C. jeikeium	0	0	0	0	0	0	0	0	0	0	0	0	0	0	0	0	0	0	0
L. monocytogenes	+	0	0	0	0	0	0	++	+	+	+	+	?	?	?	?	±	±	0
Nocardia sp.	0	0	0	0	0	0	0	0	0	±	?	?	?	0	++	++	+	+	0
Aerobic GNB - Enteric																			
Aeromonas sp.	0	0	0	0	0	0	0	0	0	±	±	+	+	+	+	+	+	+	+
C. jejuni	0	0	0	0	0	0	0	0	0	+	0	0	+	+	+	+	+	+	?
Citrobacter sp.	0	0	0	0	0	0	0	0	0	0	0	++	+	+	+	+	++	+	±
C. koseri	0	0	0	0	0	0	0	0	0	0	0	++	+	+	+	+	++	+	±
E. aerogenes	0	0	0	0	0	0	0	0	0	0	0	+	+	+	+	+	+	+	+
E. cloacae	0	0	0	0	0	0	0	0	0	0	0	+	+	+	+	+	+	+	+
E. coli (S)	0	0	0	0	0	0	0	±	±	+	+	+	+	+	+	+	+	+	+
E. coli, Klebs ESBL	0	0	0	0	0	0	0	0	0	0	0	0	+	+	++	+	++	+	0
E. coli, Klebs KPC	0	0	0	0	0	0	0	0	0	0	0	0	0	0	0	+	0	++	0
E. coli, Klebs MBL	0	0	0	0	0	0	0	0	0	0	0	0	0	0	0	0	0	0	±
Enterics CRE, NOS	0	0	0	0	0	0	0	0	0	0	0	0	0	0	0	±	0	±	0
K. oxytoca	0	0	0	0	0	0	0	0	0	+	+	+	+	+	+	+	+	+	+
K. pneumoniae (S)	0	0	0	0	0	0	0	0	0	+	+	+	+	+	+	+	+	+	+
Morganella sp.	0	0	0	0	0	0	0	0	0	0	0	+	+	+	±	±	+	+	+
P. mirabilis	0	0	0	0	0	0	0	+	+	+	+	+	+	+	±	±	+	+	+
P. vulgaris	0	0	0	0	0	0	0	0	0	+	+	+	+	+	±	±	+	+	+
Providencia sp.	0	0	0	0	0	0	0	0	0	0	0	+	++	++	±	±	++	+	+

	Fluoroquinolone									Parenteral Cephalosporins													
	Ciprofloxacin	Delafloxacin	Ofloxacin	Levofloxacin	Moxifloxacin	Norfloxacin	Prulifloxacin	Gemifloxacin	Gatifloxacin	Cefazolin	Cefotetan	Cefoxitin	Cefuroxime	Cefotaxime	Ceftizoxime	Ceftriaxone	Ceftazidime	Cefepime	Ceftaz-Avibac	Ceftaroline	Ceftobiprole	Ceftol-Tazo	Cefiderocol
Aerobic gram-pos cocci *(continued)*																							
Strep. gp C, F, G	±	+	±	±	±	0	±	±	±	+	+	+	+	+	+	+	+	+	+	+	+	+	0
Strep. pneumoniae	±	+	±	+	+	0	±	+	+	+	+	+	+	+	+	+	+	+	+	+	+	+	0
Viridans Strep.	0	+	0	+	+	0	0	+	+	+	+	+	+	++	+	++	±	+	±	+	+	+	0
Aerobic gram-pos bacilli																							
Arcanobacter. sp	+	?	+	+	+	0	+	+	+	+	+	+	+	+	+	+	+	+	+	+	+	?	0
C. diphtheriae	?	?	?	?	?	0	?	?	?	?	?	?	?	?	?	?	?	?	?	?	?	?	0
C. jeikeium	0	?	0	0	±	0	0	±	0	0	0	0	0	0	0	0	0	0	0	0	0	0	0
L. monocytogenes	0	+	0	+	+	0	0	+	+	0	0	0	0	0	0	0	0	0	0	0	0	0	0
Nocardia sp.	0	?	0	0	0	0	0	0	0	0	0	0	0	±	0	±	0	0	0	0	0	0	0
Aerobic GNB - Enteric																							
Aeromonas sp.	+	+	+	+	+	0	+	+	+	0	0	0	?	+	+	+	+	+	+	?	?	?	?
C. jejuni	+	+	+	+	+	0	+	+	+	0	0	0	0	0	0	0	0	0	0	0	0	0	?
Citrobacter sp.	+	+	+	+	+	+	+	+	+	0	0	0	0	±	±	±	±	++	+	+	+	+	+
C. koseri	+	+	+	+	+	+	+	+	+	0	0	0	0	±	±	±	±	++	+	+	+	+	+
E. aerogenes	+	+	+	+	+	+	+	+	+	0	0	0	0	0	0	0	0	+	+	0	0	+	+
E. cloacae	+	+	+	+	+	+	+	+	+	0	0	0	0	0	0	0	0	+	+	0	0	+	+
E. coli (S)	+	+	+	+	+	+	+	+	+	+	+	+	+	+	+	+	+	+	+	+	+	+	+
E. coli, Klebs ESBL	±	±	±	±	±	±	±	±	±	0	±	±	0	0	0	0	0	0	+	0	0	+	+
E. coli, Klebs KPC	0	0	0	0	0	0	0	0	0	0	0	0	0	0	0	0	0	0	++	0	0	0	+
E. coli, Klebs MBL	±	0	0	±	0	0	±	0	0	0	0	0	0	0	0	0	0	0	0	0	0	0	+
Enterics CRE, NOS	0	0	0	0	0	0	0	0	0	0	0	0	0	0	0	0	0	0	±	0	0	0	?
K. oxytoca	+	+	+	+	+	+	+	+	+	+	+	+	+	+	+	+	+	+	+	+	+	+	+
K. pneumoniae (S)	+	+	+	+	+	+	+	+	+	+	+	+	+	+	+	+	+	+	+	+	+	+	+
Morganella sp.	+	+	+	+	?	+	+	?	?	0	+	+	0	+	+	+	+	++	+	+	+	+	+
P. mirabilis	+	+	+	+	+	+	+	+	+	+	+	+	+	+	+	+	+	+	+	+	+	+	+
P. vulgaris	+	+	+	+	+	+	+	+	+	0	+	+	+	+	+	+	+	+	+	?	?	+	+
Providencia sp.	+	+	+	+	+	+	+	?	?	0	+	+	0	+	+	+	+	+	+	?	?	+	+

TABLE 4A (3)

	Penicillins												Carbapenems						
	Penicillin G	Penicillin VK	Nafcillin	Oxacillin	Cloxacillin	Flucloxacillin	Dicloxacillin	Ampicillin	Amoxicillin	Amox-Clav	Amp-Sulb	Pip-Tazo	Doripenem	Ertapenem	Imp-cilastatin	Imp-cila-rele	Meropenem	Mero-Vabor	Aztreonam
Aerobic GNB - Enteric *(continued)*																			
Salmonella sp.	0	0	0	0	0	0	0	±	±	+	+	+	+	+	+	+	+	+	+
Serratia sp.	0	0	0	0	0	0	0	0	0	0	0	+	+	+	+	+	+	+	+
Shigella sp.	0	0	0	0	0	0	0	0	0	+	+	+	+	+	+	+	+	+	+
Y. enterocolitica	0	0	0	0	0	0	0	0	0	±	±	+	+	?	+	+	+	+	+
Aerobic GNB - Non-enteric																			
Bartonella sp.	0	0	0	0	0	0	0	0	0	0	0	0	0	0	0	0	0	0	0
B. pertussis	0	0	0	0	0	0	0	0	0	0	0	0	0	0	0	0	0	0	0
B. burgdorferi	+	0	0	0	0	0	0	++	++	+	+	0	0	0	0	0	0	0	0
Brucella sp.	0	0	0	0	0	0	0	0	0	0	0	0	0	0	0	0	0	0	0
Capnocytophaga	±	±	0	0	0	0	0	±	±	++	+	++	+	?	+	+	+	+	0
C. burnetii	0	0	0	0	0	0	0	0	0	0	0	0	0	0	0	0	0	0	0
Ehrlichia, Anaplas	0	0	0	0	0	0	0	0	0	0	0	0	0	0	0	0	0	0	0
Eikenella sp	±	±	0	0	0	0	0	±	±	+	+	+	+	+	+	+	+	+	?
F. tularensis	0	0	0	0	0	0	0	0	0	0	0	0	0	0	0	0	0	0	0
H. ducreyi	0	0	0	0	0	0	0	0	0	0	0	0	?	?	?	?	?	?	?
H. influenzae	0	0	0	0	0	0	0	±	±	++	++	+	+	+	+	+	+	+	+
Kingella sp.	+	+	0	0	0	0	0	+	+	+	+	+	+	+	+	+	+	+	?
K. granulomatis	0	0	0	0	0	0	0	0	0	0	0	0	0	0	0	0	0	0	0
Legionella sp.	0	0	0	0	0	0	0	0	0	0	0	0	0	0	0	0	0	0	0
Leptospira sp.	++	0	0	0	0	0	0	+	+	+	+	+	+	+	+	+	+	+	+
M. catarrhalis	0	0	0	0	0	0	0	0	0	++	+	+	+	+	+	+	+	+	+
N. gonorrhoeae	0	0	0	0	0	0	0	0	0	0	0	0	+	+	+	+	+	+	+
N. meningitidis	+	0	0	0	0	0	0	++	++	0	0	+	+	+	+	+	+	+	+
P. multocida	++	++	0	0	0	0	0	++	++	++	++	+	+	+	+	+	+	+	+
R. rickettsii	0	0	0	0	0	0	0	0	0	0	0	0	0	0	0	0	0	0	0
T. pallidum	++	0	0	0	0	0	0	0	0	0	0	0	0	0	0	0	0	0	0
V. cholera	0	0	0	0	0	0	0	0	0	0	0	0	0	0	0	0	0	0	0
V. parahaemolyticus	0	0	0	0	0	0	0	0	0	0	0	0	?	?	?	?	?	?	?

	Fluoroquinolone									Parenteral Cephalosporins													
	Ciprofloxacin	Delafloxacin	Ofloxacin	Levofloxacin	Moxifloxacin	Norfloxacin	Prulifloxacin	Gemifloxacin	Gatifloxacin	Cefazolin	Cefotetan	Cefoxitin	Cefuroxime	Cefotaxime	Ceftizoxime	Ceftriaxone	Ceftazidime	Cefepime	Ceftaz-Avibac	Ceftaroline	Ceftobiprole	Ceftol-Tazo	Cefiderocol
Aerobic GNB - Enteric *(continued)*																							
Salmonella sp.	+	+	+	+	+	0	+	+	+	0	?	?	?	+	+	+	+	+	+	?	?	?	?
Serratia sp.	+	+	+	+	+	0	+	+	+	0	+	0	0	+	+	+	+	+	+	?	?	+	+
Shigella sp.	++	+	+	++	+	0	++	+	+	0	?	?	?	+	+	+	+	+	+	?	?	?	?
Y. enterocolitica	++	+	+	++	+	0	++	?	+	0	±	±	±	++	+	++	±	++	?	?	?	?	0
Aerobic GNB - Non-enteric																							
Bartonella sp.	0	0	0	0	0	0	0	0	0	0	0	0	0	0	0	0	0	0	0	0	0	0	0
B. pertussis	?	?	?	?	?	0	?	?	?	0	0	0	0	0	0	0	0	0	0	0	0	0	0
B. burgdorferi	0	0	0	0	0	0	0	0	0	0	0	0	+	+	0	++	0	0	0	0	0	0	0
Brucella sp.	+	?	?	?	?	0	+	?	?	0	0	0	0	0	0	0	0	0	0	0	0	0	0
Capnocytophaga	±	?	±	±	?	0	±	?	?	0	0	0	0	+	?	+	+	+	+	0	0	0	0
C. burnetii	+	?	+	+	+	0	+	+	+	0	0	0	0	0	0	0	0	0	0	0	0	0	0
Ehrlichia, Anaplas	?	?	?	?	?	0	?	0	0	0	0	0	0	0	0	0	0	0	0	0	0	0	0
Eikenella sp	+	?	+	+	?	0	+	?	?	0	?	+	0	+	?	+	?	?	?	?	?	?	0
F. tularensis	++	?	?	?	?	0	++	?	?	0	0	0	0	0	0	0	0	0	0	0	0	0	0
H. ducreyi	++	?	?	+	?	0	++	?	?	0	0	0	0	0	0	++	0	?	0	0	0	0	0
H. influenzae	+	+	+	++	++	0	+	+	+	0	+	+	+	++	+	++	+	+	+	+	+	+	0
Kingella sp.	+	+	+	++	?	0	+	?	?	+	+	+	+	+	+	++	+	+	+	+	+	+	0
K. granulomatis	++	?	?	?	?	0	++	?	?	0	0	+	0	0	0	+	0	0	0	0	0	0	0
Legionella sp.	++	+	++	++	++	0	++	+	+	0	0	0	0	0	0	0	0	0	0	0	0	0	0
Leptospira sp.	+	+	+	+	+	0	+	+	+	?	?	?	?	++	?	++	?	+	+	?	?	?	0
M. catarrhalis	+	+	+	+	+	0	+	+	+	0	+	±	+	+	+	+	+	+	+	+	+	+	0
N. gonorrhoeae	±	?	±	±	0	0	±	+	0	±	±	±	0	±	±	++	?	+	?	?	?	?	0
N. meningitidis	?	?	?	?	?	0	?	?	?	0	0	0	+	+	+	++	+	+	+	?	?	?	0
P. multocida	+	+	+	+	+	0	+	+	+	0	?	?	+	+	+	+	?	+	?	+	+	+	0
R. rickettsii	±	?	±	±	±	0	±	?	?	0	0	0	0	0	0	0	0	0	0	0	0	0	0
T. pallidum	0	0	0	0	0	0	0	0	0	0	0	0	0	0	0	+	0	0	0	0	0	0	0
V. cholera	+	?	?	?	?	0	+	?	?	0	0	0	0	0	0	0	0	0	0	0	0	0	0
V. parahaemolyticus	+	?	+	+	?	0	+	?	?	0	0	0	0	+	+	+	+	+	+	?	?	?	0

TABLE 4A (4)

	Penicillins												Carbapenems							Fluoroquinolone									Parenteral Cephalosporins													
	Penicillin G	Penicillin VK	Nafcillin	Oxacillin	Cloxacillin	Flucloxacillin	Dicloxacillin	Ampicillin	Amoxicillin	Amox-Clav	Amp-Sulb	Pip-Tazo	Doripenem	Ertapenem	Imp-cilastatin	Imp-cila-rele	Meropenem	Mero-Vabor	Aztreonam	Ciprofloxacin	Delafloxacin	Ofloxacin	Levofloxacin	Moxifloxacin	Norfloxacin	Prulifloxacin	Gemifloxacin	Gatifloxacin	Cefazolin	Cefotetan	Cefoxitin	Cefuroxime	Cefotaxime	Ceftizoxime	Ceftriaxone	Ceftazidime	Cefepime	Ceftaz-Avibac	Ceftaroline	Ceftobiprole	Ceftol-Tazo	Cefiderocol
Aerobic GNB - Non-enteric *(continued)*																																										
V. vulnificus	0	0	0	0	0	0	0	0	0	0	0	0	?	?	?	?	?	?	?	+	?	+	+	?	0	+	?	?	0	0	0	0	+	+	+	+	+	+	?	?	?	0
Y. pestis	0	0	0	0	0	0	0	0	0	0	0	0	0	0	0	0	0	0	0	+	?	?	?	?	0	+	?	?	0	0	0	0	0	0	0	0	0	0	0	0	0	0
Aerobic GNB non-fermenter																																										
A. baumannii	0	0	0	0	0	0	0	0	0	0	±	±	+	0	±	±	±	±	0	±	?	±	±	±	0	±	?	?	0	0	0	0	0	0	±	±	±	?	?	?	±	+
B. cepacia	0	0	0	0	0	0	0	0	0	0	0	0	±	0	±	±	±	±	0	0	0	0	0	0	0	0	0	0	0	0	0	0	0	0	0	±	±	+	0	0	+	+
P. aeruginosa	0	0	0	0	0	0	0	0	0	0	0	+	+	0	+	+	+	+	+	+	+	0	+	0	0	+	0	0	0	0	0	0	0	0	0	+	+	+	0	0	+	+
S. maltophilia	0	0	0	0	0	0	0	0	0	0	0	0	0	0	0	0	0	0	0	0	?	0	±	±	0	0	?	?	0	0	0	0	0	0	0	±	0	±	0	0	0	+
Aerobic - cell wall-deficient																																										
C. trachomatis	0	0	0	0	0	0	0	+	+	0	0	0	0	0	0	0	0	0	0	0	?	++	++	+	0	0	+	+	0	0	0	0	0	0	0	0	0	0	0	0	0	0
Chlamydophila sp.	0	0	0	0	0	0	0	0	0	0	0	0	0	0	0	0	0	0	0	+	?	+	+	+	0	+	+	+	0	0	0	0	0	0	0	0	0	0	0	0	0	0
M. genitalium	0	0	0	0	0	0	0	0	0	0	0	0	0	0	0	0	0	0	0	0	?	0	±	++	0	0	?	+	0	0	0	0	0	0	0	0	0	0	0	0	0	0
M. pneumoniae	0	0	0	0	0	0	0	0	0	0	0	0	0	0	0	0	0	0	0	+	?	+	++	++	0	+	+	+	0	0	0	0	0	0	0	0	0	0	0	0	0	0
U. urealyticum	0	0	0	0	0	0	0	0	0	0	0	0	0	0	0	0	0	0	0	+	?	+	+	+	0	+	?	?	0	0	0	0	0	0	0	0	0	0	0	0	0	0
Anaerobic GNB																																										
B. fragilis	0	0	0	0	0	0	0	0	0	++	+	++	+	++	++	+	++	+	0	0	+	0	0	±	0	0	0	0	0	±	±	0	0	+	0	0	0	0	0	0	+	0
F. necrophorum	±	±	0	0	0	0	0	±	±	+	+	+	+	+	+	+	+	+	0	0	?	0	0	?	0	0	?	?	0	+	+	?	+	?	+	?	?	?	?	?	?	0
P. melaninogenica	±	±	0	0	0	0	0	±	±	+	+	+	+	+	+	+	+	+	0	0	?	0	±	+	0	0	?	?	0	+	+	?	?	?	?	?	?	?	?	?	+	0
Anaerobic gram-positive																																										
Actinomyces sp.	++	++	0	0	0	0	0	++	++	+	+	+	+	+	+	+	+	+	0	0	?	0	?	?	0	0	?	?	0	?	+	0	+	+	+	?	?	?	?	?	?	0
C. difficile	0	0	0	0	0	0	0	0	0	0	0	0	0	0	0	0	0	0	0	0	0	0	0	0	0	0	0	0	0	0	0	0	0	0	0	0	0	0	0	0	0	0
Clostridium sp.	++	+	0	0	0	0	0	+	+	+	+	+	+	+	+	+	+	+	0	0	+	0	0	0	0	0	0	0	0	+	+	?	+	+	+	?	?	?	?	?	?	0
P. acnes	++	+	?	?	?	?	?	+	+	+	+	+	+	+	+	+	+	+	0	±	0	±	±	±	0	±	?	?	+	+	+	+	+	+	++	+	+	+	+	+	+	0
Peptostreptococci	++	++	0	0	0	0	0	++	++	+	+	+	+	+	+	+	+	+	0	0	+	0	+	+	0	0	?	+	+	+	+	+	+	+	+	+	+	+	+	+	+	0

TABLE 4A (5)

	Oral Cephalosporins										Aminoglyco			
	Cefadroxil	Cephalexin	Cefaclor	Cefprozil	Cefurox-Axe	Cefixime	Ceftibuten	Cefpodoxime	Cefdinir	Cefditoren	Gentamicin	Tobramycin	Amikacin	Plazomicin
Aerobic gram-pos cocci														
E. faecalis (S)	0	0	0	0	0	0	0	0	0	0	±	0	0	0
E. faecium (S)	0	0	0	0	0	0	0	0	0	0	±	0	0	0
E. faecalis (VRE)	0	0	0	0	0	0	0	0	0	0	±	0	0	0
E. faecium (VRE)	0	0	0	0	0	0	0	0	0	0	±	0	0	0
S. aureus MSSA	+	+	+	+	+	0	0	+	+	+	±	?	?	0
S. aureus HA-MRSA	0	0	0	0	0	0	0	0	0	0	±	?	?	0
S. aureus CA-MRSA	0	0	0	0	0	0	0	0	0	0	±	?	?	0
Staph coag-neg (S)	?	?	?	?	?	0	0	?	?	?	±	?	?	0
Staph coag-neg (R)	0	0	0	0	0	0	0	0	0	0	±	?	?	0
S. epidermidis (R)	0	0	0	0	0	0	0	0	0	0	±	?	?	0
S. epidermidis (S)	+	+	+	+	+	0	0	+	+	+	±	?	?	0
S. lugdunensis	+	+	+	+	+	?	?	+	+	+	±	?	?	0
S. saprophyticus	++	++	++	+	+	?	?	+	+	+	0	0	0	0
S. anginosus grp	+	+	+	+	+	+	+	+	+	+	±	?	?	0
Strep. pyogenes (A)	+	+	+	+	+	+	+	+	+	+	±	0	0	0
Strep. agalactiae (B)	+	+	+	+	+	+	+	+	+	+	±	0	0	0
Strep. gp C, F, G	+	+	+	+	+	+	+	+	+	+	±	0	0	0
Strep. pneumoniae	+	+	+	+	+	+	+	+	+	+	0	0	0	0
Viridans Strep.	+	+	+	0	+	+	0	+	+	+	±	0	0	0
Aerobic gram-pos bacilli														
Arcanobacter. sp	+	+	+	+	+	+	+	+	+	?	?	?	?	0
C. diphtheriae	?	?	?	?	?	?	?	?	?	?	0	0	0	0
C. jeikeium	0	0	0	0	0	0	0	0	0	0	0	0	0	0
L. monocytogenes	0	0	0	0	0	0	0	0	0	0	±	?	?	0
Nocardia sp.	0	0	0	0	0	0	0	0	0	0	0	0	++	0

			Macrolides				Tetracyclines					
	Chloramphen	Clindamycin	Erythromycin	Azithromycin	Clarithromycin	Telithromycin	Doxycycline	Eravacycline	Minocycline	Omadacycline	Tetracycline	Tigecycline
Aerobic gram-pos cocci												
E. faecalis (S)	±	0	0	0	0	0	±	+	±	+	±	+
E. faecium (S)	±	0	0	0	0	0	±	+	±	+	±	+
E. faecalis (VRE)	±	0	0	0	0	0	±	±	±	±	±	±
E. faecium (VRE)	±	0	0	0	0	0	±	±	±	±	±	±
S. aureus MSSA	+	+	±	±	±	+	+	+	+	+	+	+
S. aureus HA-MRSA	+	±	0	0	0	±	+	+	+	+	±	+
S. aureus CA-MRSA	+	+	0	0	0	±	+	+	+	+	±	+
Staph coag-neg (S)	+	+	±	±	±	+	+	+	+	+	+	+
Staph coag-neg (R)	+	±	0	0	0	±	±	+	±	+	±	+
S. epidermidis (R)	+	±	0	0	0	±	±	+	±	+	±	+
S. epidermidis (S)	+	+	+	+	+	+	+	+	+	+	+	+
S. lugdunensis	+	+	+	+	+	+	+	+	+	+	+	+
S. saprophyticus	+	+	±	±	±	?	+	+	+	+	+	+
S. anginosus grp	+	+	±	±	±	+	±	+	±	+	±	+
Strep. pyogenes (A)	+	+	±	±	±	+	?	+	?	+	?	+
Strep. agalactiae (B)	+	+	±	±	±	+	?	+	?	+	?	+
Strep. gp C, F, G	+	+	±	±	±	+	?	+	?	+	?	+
Strep. pneumoniae	+	+	±	±	±	+	±	+	±	+	±	+
Viridans Strep.	+	±	±	±	±	+	±	+	±	+	±	+
Aerobic gram-pos bacilli												
Arcanobacter. sp	?	++	++	++	++	+	++	+	+	+	+	+
C. diphtheriae	0	+	++	+	+	?	?	0	?	0	?	0
C. jeikeium	0	0	0	0	0	0	?	+	?	+	?	+
L. monocytogenes	0	0	0	0	0	0	0	0	0	0	0	0
Nocardia sp.	0	0	0	?	?	?	?	?	±	?	0	?

	Glyco/Lipo						Ox-lid		Poly			Other							
	Daptomycin	Vancomycin	Teicoplanin	Telavancin	Oritavancin	Dalbavancin	Linezolid	Tedizolid	Polymyxin B	Colistin	Lefamulin	Fusidic Acid	Rif (comb)	TMP-SMX	Nitrofurantoin	Fosfomycin (IV)	Fosfomycin (po)	Metronidazole	Quinu-Dalfo, Pristina
Aerobic gram-pos cocci																			
E. faecalis (S)	+	++	++	+	+	+	+	+	0	0	0	±	±	0	+	±	±	0	0
E. faecium (S)	+	±	±	±	+	±	++	+	0	0	0	±	±	0	+	±	±	0	+
E. faecalis (VRE)	+	0	0	±	+	0	++	+	0	0	0	0	±	0	+	±	±	0	0
E. faecium (VRE)	+	0	0	±	+	0	++	+	0	0	0	0	±	0	+	±	±	0	+
S. aureus MSSA	+	+	+	+	+	+	+	+	0	0	+	+	±	+	0	+	0	0	+
S. aureus HA-MRSA	++	++	++	+	+	+	++	+	0	0	+	+	±	+	0	+	0	0	+
S. aureus CA-MRSA	++	++	++	+	+	+	+	+	0	0	+	+	±	+	0	+	0	0	+
Staph coag-neg (S)	+	+	+	+	+	+	+	+	0	0	0	+	±	+	0	+	0	0	+
Staph coag-neg (R)	++	++	++	+	+	+	++	+	0	0	0	+	±	+	0	±	0	0	+
S. epidermidis (R)	++	++	++	+	+	+	++	+	0	0	0	+	±	+	0	±	0	0	+
S. epidermidis (S)	+	+	+	+	+	+	+	+	0	0	0	+	±	+	0	+	0	0	+
S. lugdunensis	+	+	+	+	+	+	+	+	0	0	0	+	±	+	0	0	0	0	+
S. saprophyticus	+	+	+	+	?	?	0	0	0	0	0	0	0	+	+	±	±	0	0
S. anginosus grp	0	+	+	+	+	+	+	+	0	0	+	?	0	0	0	0	0	0	+
Strep. pyogenes (A)	+	+	+	+	+	+	+	+	0	0	+	?	0	±	0	+	0	0	+
Strep. agalactiae (B)	+	+	+	+	+	+	+	+	0	0	+	?	0	±	0	+	0	0	+
Strep. gp C, F, G	+	+	+	+	+	+	+	+	0	0	?	?	0	±	0	+	0	0	+
Strep. pneumoniae	±	+	+	+	?	?	+	+	0	0	+	?	0	±	0	+	0	0	+
Viridans Strep.	0	++	++	+	+	+	+	+	0	0	+	?	0	?	0	0	0	0	+
Aerobic gram-pos bacilli																			
Arcanobacter. sp	+	++	+	+	?	?	+	?	0	0	0	0	0	0	0	0	0	0	+
C. diphtheriae	0	0	0	0	0	0	0	0	0	0	0	0	0	0	0	0	0	0	0
C. jeikeium	+	++	+	+	0	0	+	?	0	0	0	0	0	0	0	0	0	0	0
L. monocytogenes	0	0	0	0	0	0	+	?	0	0	0	0	0	+	0	0	0	0	0
Nocardia sp.	0	0	0	0	0	0	+	?	0	0	0	0	0	++	0	0	0	0	0

TABLE 4A (6)

	Oral Cephalosporins									
	Cefadroxil	Cephalexin	Cefaclor	Cefprozil	Cefurox-Axe	Cefixime	Ceftibuten	Cefpodoxime	Cefdinir	Cefditoren
Aerobic GNB - Enteric										
Aeromonas sp.	?	0	?	?	?	?	?	?	?	?
C. jejuni	0	0	0	0	0	0	0	0	0	0
C. freundii	0	0	0	0	0	+	+	+	+	?
C. koseri	0	0	0	0	0	+	+	+	+	?
E. aerogenes	0	0	0	0	0	0	0	0	0	0
E. cloacae	0	0	0	0	0	0	0	0	0	0
E. coli (S)	±	±	±	+	+	+	+	+	+	?
E. coli, Klebs ESBL	0	0	0	0	0	0	0	0	0	0
E. coli, Klebs KPC	0	0	0	0	0	0	0	0	0	0
E. coli, Klebs MBL	0	0	0	0	0	0	0	0	0	0
Enterics CRE, NOS	0	0	0	0	0	0	0	0	0	0
K. oxytoca	±	±	±	+	+	+	+	+	+	?
K. pneumoniae (S)	±	±	±	+	+	+	+	+	+	?
Morganella sp.	0	0	0	0	0	0	0	0	0	0
P. mirabilis	+	+	+	+	+	+	+	+	+	?
P. vulgaris	0	0	0	0	0	+	+	+	?	?
Providencia sp.	0	0	0	0	0	+	+	+	?	?
Salmonella sp.	0	0	0	0	0	+	+	+	+	?
Serratia sp.	0	0	0	0	0	+	0	0	0	0
Shigella sp.	0	0	0	0	0	+	+	+	+	?
Y. enterocolitica	0	0	0	0	0	+	+	?	?	?
Aerobic GNB - Non-enteric										
Bartonella sp.	0	0	0	0	0	0	0	0	0	0
B. pertussis	0	0	0	0	0	0	0	0	0	0
B. burgdorferi	0	0	0	0	++	0	0	0	0	0
Brucella sp.	0	0	0	0	0	0	0	0	0	0

	Aminoglyco						Macrolides			
	Gentamicin	Tobramycin	Amikacin	Plazomicin	Chloramphen	Clindamycin	Erythromycin	Azithromycin	Clarithromycin	Telithromycin
Aerobic GNB - Enteric										
Aeromonas sp.	+	+	+	?	+	0	0	0	0	0
C. jejuni	+	+	+	?	?	?	++	++	+	0
C. freundii	+	+	+	+	?	0	0	0	0	0
C. koseri	+	+	+	+	?	0	0	0	0	0
E. aerogenes	+	+	+	+	0	0	0	0	0	0
E. cloacae	+	+	+	+	0	0	0	0	0	0
E. coli (S)	+	+	+	+	+	0	0	±	0	0
E. coli, Klebs ESBL	±	±	±	++	±	0	0	0	0	0
E. coli, Klebs KPC	±	±	±	++	0	0	0	0	0	0
E. coli, Klebs MBL	±	±	±	++	0	0	0	0	0	0
Enterics CRE, NOS	±	±	±	++	0	0	0	0	0	0
K. oxytoca	+	+	+	+	+	0	0	0	0	0
K. pneumoniae (S)	+	+	+	+	+	0	0	0	0	0
Morganella sp.	+	+	+	+	?	0	0	0	0	0
P. mirabilis	+	+	+	+	?	0	0	0	0	0
P. vulgaris	+	+	+	+	±	0	0	0	0	0
Providencia sp.	±	±	+	+	?	0	0	0	0	0
Salmonella sp.	+	+	+	?	+	0	0	+	0	0
Serratia sp.	+	+	+	+	0	0	0	0	0	0
Shigella sp.	+	+	+	?	+	0	0	+	0	0
Y. enterocolitica	+	+	+	?	0	0	0	0	0	0
Aerobic GNB - Non-enteric										
Bartonella sp.	++	0	0	0	0	0	+	++	++	?
B. pertussis	0	0	0	0	0	0	+	++	++	?
B. burgdorferi	0	0	0	0	0	0	+	+	+	?
Brucella sp.	+	?	?	0	+	0	0	0	0	0

	Tetracyclines						Glyco/Lipo					
	Doxycycline	Eravacycline	Minocycline	Omadacycline	Tetracycline	Tigecycline	Daptomycin	Vancomycin	Teicoplanin	Telavancin	Oritavancin	Dalbavancin
Aerobic GNB - Enteric												
Aeromonas sp.	+	+	+	+	0	+	0	0	0	0	0	0
C. jejuni	±	?	±	?	±	?	0	0	0	0	0	0
C. freundii	0	+	0	+	0	+	0	0	0	0	0	0
C. koseri	0	+	0	+	0	+	0	0	0	0	0	0
E. aerogenes	0	+	0	+	0	+	0	0	0	0	0	0
E. cloacae	0	+	0	+	0	+	0	0	0	0	0	0
E. coli (S)	±	+	±	+	±	+	0	0	0	0	0	0
E. coli, Klebs ESBL	0	+	0	+	0	+	0	0	0	0	0	0
E. coli, Klebs KPC	0	+	0	+	0	+	0	0	0	0	0	0
E. coli, Klebs MBL	0	+	0	+	0	+	0	0	0	0	0	0
Enterics CRE, NOS	0	+	0	+	0	+	0	0	0	0	0	0
K. oxytoca	0	+	±	+	0	+	0	0	0	0	0	0
K. pneumoniae (S)	0	+	±	+	0	+	0	0	0	0	0	0
Morganella sp.	0	0	0	0	0	0	0	0	0	0	0	0
P. mirabilis	0	0	0	0	0	0	0	0	0	0	0	0
P. vulgaris	0	0	0	0	0	0	0	0	0	0	0	0
Providencia sp.	0	0	0	0	0	0	0	0	0	0	0	0
Salmonella sp.	±	+	±	+	0	+	0	0	0	0	0	0
Serratia sp.	0	+	0	+	0	+	0	0	0	0	0	0
Shigella sp.	±	+	±	+	0	+	0	0	0	0	0	0
Y. enterocolitica	+	?	?	?	?	?	0	0	0	0	0	0
Aerobic GNB - Non-enteric												
Bartonella sp.	++	?	+	?	+	?	0	0	0	0	0	0
B. pertussis	?	0	?	0	?	0	0	0	0	0	0	0
B. burgdorferi	++	?	+	?	+	?	0	0	0	0	0	0
Brucella sp.	+	?	+	?	+	?	0	0	0	0	0	0

	Ox-lid		Poly			Other							
	Linezolid	Tedizolid	Polymyxin B	Colistin	Lefamulin	Fusidic Acid	Rif (comb)	TMP-SMX	Nitrofurantoin	Fosfomycin (IV)	Fosfomycin (po)	Metronidazole	Quinu-Dalfo, Pristina
Aerobic GNB - Enteric													
Aeromonas sp.	0	0	+	+	0	0	0	+	0	?	0	0	0
C. jejuni	0	0	0	0	0	0	0	0	0	0	0	0	0
C. freundii	0	0	+	+	0	0	0	±	±	+	+	0	0
C. koseri	0	0	+	+	0	0	0	±	±	+	+	0	0
E. aerogenes	0	0	+	+	0	0	0	+	±	±	±	0	0
E. cloacae	0	0	+	+	0	0	0	+	±	±	±	0	0
E. coli (S)	0	0	+	+	0	0	0	±	+	+	+	0	0
E. coli, Klebs ESBL	0	0	+	+	0	0	0	±	±	+	+	0	0
E. coli, Klebs KPC	0	0	+	+	0	0	0	±	±	±	±	0	0
E. coli, Klebs MBL	0	0	+	+	0	0	0	0	0	±	±	0	0
Enterics CRE, NOS	0	0	+	+	0	0	0	±	±	±	±	0	0
K. oxytoca	0	0	+	+	0	0	0	±	+	±	±	0	0
K. pneumoniae (S)	0	0	+	+	0	0	0	±	+	±	±	0	0
Morganella sp.	0	0	0	0	0	0	0	±	0	0	0	0	0
P. mirabilis	0	0	0	0	0	0	0	±	0	+	+	0	0
P. vulgaris	0	0	0	0	0	0	0	±	0	±	±	0	0
Providencia sp.	0	0	0	0	0	0	0	±	0	+	+	0	0
Salmonella sp.	0	0	0	0	0	0	0	±	0	0	0	0	0
Serratia sp.	0	0	0	0	0	0	0	+	0	±	±	0	0
Shigella sp.	0	0	0	0	0	0	0	±	0	0	0	0	0
Y. enterocolitica	0	0	0	0	0	0	0	+	0	0	0	0	0
Aerobic GNB - Non-enteric													
Bartonella sp.	0	0	0	0	0	0	±	0	0	0	0	0	0
B. pertussis	0	0	0	0	0	0	0	+	0	0	0	0	0
B. burgdorferi	0	0	0	0	0	0	0	0	0	0	0	0	0
Brucella sp.	0	0	0	0	0	0	±	+	0	0	0	0	0

TABLE 4A (7)

	Oral Cephalosporins										Aminoglyco						Macrolides				Tetracyclines						Glyco/Lipo						Ox-lid		Poly			Other							
	Cefadroxil	Cephalexin	Cefaclor	Cefprozil	Cefurox-Axe	Cefixime	Ceftibuten	Cefpodoxime	Cefdinir	Cefditoren	Gentamicin	Tobramycin	Amikacin	Plazomicin	Chloramphen	Clindamycin	Erythromycin	Azithromycin	Clarithromycin	Telithromycin	Doxycycline	Eravacycline	Minocycline	Omadacycline	Tetracycline	Tigecycline	Daptomycin	Vancomycin	Teicoplanin	Telavancin	Oritavancin	Dalbavancin	Linezolid	Tedizolid	Polymyxin B	Colistin	Lefamulin	Fusidic Acid	Rif (comb)	TMP-SMX	Nitrofurantoin	Fosfomycin (IV)	Fosfomycin (po)	Metronidazole	Quinu-Dalfo, Pristina
Aerobic GNB - Non-enteric *(continued)*																																													
Capnocytophaga	0	0	0	0	0	0	0	0	0	0	±	±	±	0	+	++	?	?	?	?	+	?	+	?	+	?	0	0	0	0	0	0	0	0	0	0	0	0	0	±	0	0	0	0	0
C. burnetii	0	0	0	0	0	0	0	0	0	0	0	0	0	0	+	0	+	+	+	?	++	?	+	?	+	?	0	0	0	0	0	0	0	0	0	0	0	0	±	+	0	0	0	0	0
Ehrlichia, Anaplas	0	0	0	0	0	0	0	0	0	0	0	0	0	0	±	0	0	0	0	0	++	?	+	?	+	?	0	0	0	0	0	0	0	0	0	0	0	0	±	0	0	0	0	0	0
Eikenella sp	0	0	0	?	0	?	?	?	?	?	±	0	0	0	+	0	0	0	0	0	+	?	+	?	+	?	0	0	0	0	0	0	0	0	0	0	0	0	0	0	0	0	0	0	0
F. tularensis	0	0	0	0	0	0	0	0	0	0	++	+	?	0	+	?	0	?	?	?	++	?	+	?	+	?	0	0	0	0	0	0	0	0	0	0	0	0	0	0	0	0	0	0	0
H. ducreyi	0	0	0	0	0	0	0	0	0	0	0	0	0	0	0	0	++	++	?	?	0	0	0	0	0	0	0	0	0	0	0	0	0	0	0	0	0	0	0	0	0	0	0	0	0
H. influenzae	0	0	±	+	+	+	+	+	+	+	0	0	0	0	+	0	0	+	+	+	+	+	+	+	+	+	0	0	0	0	0	0	0	0	0	0	+	0	0	+	0	+	0	0	0
Kingella sp.	0	0	0	+	0	+	+	+	+	+	+	0	0	0	+	0	0	?	?	?	+	+	+	+	+	+	0	0	0	0	0	0	0	0	0	0	0	0	0	+	0	0	0	0	0
K. granulomatis	0	0	0	0	0	0	0	0	0	0	+	?	?	0	+	0	++	++	+	0	++	?	+	?	+	?	0	0	0	0	0	0	0	0	0	0	0	0	0	++	0	0	0	0	0
Legionella sp.	0	0	0	0	0	0	0	0	0	0	0	0	0	0	0	0	++	++	++	+	+	+	+	+	+	+	0	0	0	0	0	0	0	0	0	0	+	0	±	+	0	0	0	0	0
Leptospira sp.	?	?	?	?	?	?	?	?	?	?	0	0	0	0	+	0	+	++	+	?	++	?	+	?	+	?	0	0	0	0	0	0	0	0	0	0	0	0	0	?	0	0	0	0	0
M. catarrhalis	0	0	±	+	+	+	+	+	+	+	0	0	0	0	0	0	+	+	+	+	+	?	+	?	+	?	0	0	0	0	0	0	0	0	0	0	+	0	0	+	0	0	0	0	0
N. gonorrhoeae	0	0	0	0	0	+	0	+	0	0	0	0	0	0	0	0	0	+	0	0	±	?	±	?	±	?	0	0	0	0	0	0	0	0	0	0	0	0	0	0	0	0	0	0	0
N. meningitidis	0	0	0	0	0	0	0	0	0	0	0	0	0	0	+	0	0	0	0	0	0	0	0	0	0	0	0	0	0	0	0	0	0	0	0	0	0	0	0	0	0	0	0	0	0
P. multocida	?	0	0	?	+	+	?	+	+	?	±	±	±	0	?	0	0	+	0	0	+	+	+	+	+	+	0	0	0	0	0	0	0	0	0	0	0	0	0	+	0	0	0	0	0
R. rickettsii	0	0	0	0	0	0	0	0	0	0	0	0	0	0	+	0	0	0	±	0	++	?	+	?	+	?	0	0	0	0	0	0	0	0	0	0	0	0	0	0	0	0	0	0	0
T. pallidum	0	0	0	0	0	0	0	0	0	0	0	0	0	0	0	0	0	+	0	0	+	?	?	?	+	?	0	0	0	0	0	0	0	0	0	0	0	0	0	0	0	0	0	0	0
V. cholera	0	0	0	0	0	0	0	0	0	0	0	0	0	0	0	0	+	+	?	?	+	?	+	?	+	?	0	0	0	0	0	0	0	0	0	0	0	0	0	0	0	0	0	0	0
V. parahaemolyticus	0	0	0	0	0	0	0	0	0	0	?	?	?	0	+	?	?	+	0	0	+	?	?	?	+	?	0	0	0	0	0	0	0	0	0	0	0	0	0	?	0	0	0	0	0
V. vulnificus	0	0	0	0	0	0	0	0	0	0	?	?	?	0	+	0	0	?	0	0	+	?	+	?	+	?	0	0	0	0	0	0	0	0	0	0	0	0	0	?	0	0	0	0	0
Y. pestis	0	0	0	0	0	0	0	0	0	0	+	?	?	0	+	0	0	0	0	0	+	?	+	?	+	?	0	0	0	0	0	0	0	0	0	0	0	0	0	+	0	0	0	0	0
Aerobic GNB non-fermenter																																													
A. baumannii	0	0	0	0	0	0	0	0	0	0	0	0	±	0	0	0	0	0	0	0	0	+	±	+	±	+	0	0	0	0	0	0	0	0	+	+	0	0	0	±	0	0	0	0	0
B. cepacia	0	0	0	0	0	0	±	0	0	0	0	0	0	0	±	0	0	0	0	0	0	0	±	0	±	0	0	0	0	0	0	0	0	0	0	0	0	0	0	±	0	0	0	0	0
P. aeruginosa	0	0	0	0	0	0	0	0	0	0	+	+	+	±	0	0	0	0	0	0	0	0	0	0	0	0	0	0	0	0	0	0	0	0	+	+	0	0	0	0	0	±	±	0	0
S. maltophilia	0	0	0	0	0	0	0	0	0	0	0	0	0	0	+	0	0	0	0	0	+	+	+	+	0	+	0	0	0	0	0	0	0	0	+	+	0	0	0	++	0	0	0	0	0

TABLE 4A (8)

	Oral Cephalosporins										Aminoglyco			
	Cefadroxil	Cephalexin	Cefaclor	Cefprozil	Cefurox-Axe	Cefixime	Ceftibuten	Cefpodoxime	Cefdinir	Cefditoren	Gentamicin	Tobramycin	Amikacin	Plazomicin
Aerobic - cell wall-deficient														
C. trachomatis	0	0	0	0	0	0	0	0	0	0	0	0	0	0
Chlamydophila sp.	0	0	0	0	0	0	0	0	0	0	0	0	0	0
M. genitalium	0	0	0	0	0	0	0	0	0	0	0	0	0	0
M. pneumoniae	0	0	0	0	0	0	0	0	0	0	0	0	0	0
U. urealyticum	0	0	0	0	0	0	0	0	0	0	0	0	0	0
Anaerobic GNB														
B. fragilis	0	0	0	0	0	0	0	0	0	0	0	0	0	0
F. necrophorum	?	?	?	?	?	?	?	?	?	?	0	0	0	0
P. melaninogenica	?	?	?	?	?	?	?	?	?	?	0	0	0	0
Anaerobic gram-positive														
Actinomyces sp.	?	?	?	?	?	?	?	?	?	?	0	0	0	0
C. difficile	0	0	0	0	0	0	0	0	0	0	0	0	0	0
Clostridium sp.	?	?	?	?	?	?	?	?	?	?	0	0	0	0
P. acnes	+	0	+	+	+	+	+	?	?	?	+	?	?	0
Peptostreptococci	+	+	+	+	+	+	+	+	?	?	0	0	0	0

			Macrolides				Tetracyclines					
	Chloramphen	Clindamycin	Erythromycin	Azithromycin	Clarithromycin	Telithromycin	Doxycycline	Eravacycline	Minocycline	Omadacycline	Tetracycline	Tigecycline
Aerobic - cell wall-deficient												
C. trachomatis	0	0	+	++	+	?	++	0	+	0	+	0
Chlamydophila sp.	+	0	+	+	+	+	++	+	+	+	+	+
M. genitalium	0	0	?	++	?	?	±	?	±	?	±	?
M. pneumoniae	0	0	±	±	±	±	++	+	++	+	++	+
U. urealyticum	0	0	++	++	+	?	++	?	+	?	+	?
Anaerobic GNB												
B. fragilis	+	0	0	0	0	0	±	+	±	+	±	+
F. necrophorum	+	+	0	0	0	0	+	+	+	+	+	+
P. melaninogenica	+	+	±	±	±	0	+	+	+	+	+	+
Anaerobic gram-positive												
Actinomyces sp.	+	++	++	+	+	?	+	?	+	?	+	?
C. difficile	0	0	0	0	0	0	0	0	0	0	0	0
Clostridium sp.	+	+	+	+	+	?	+	+	+	+	+	+
P. acnes	+	±	±	±	±	?	+	+	+	+	+	+
Peptostreptococci	+	+	±	±	±	?	+	+	+	+	+	+

	Glyco/Lipo						Ox-lid		Poly			Other							
	Daptomycin	Vancomycin	Teicoplanin	Telavancin	Oritavancin	Dalbavancin	Linezolid	Tedizolid	Polymyxin B	Colistin	Lefamulin	Fusidic Acid	Rif (comb)	TMP-SMX	Nitrofurantoin	Fosfomycin (IV)	Fosfomycin (po)	Metronidazole	Quinu-Dalfo, Pristina
Aerobic - cell wall-deficient																			
C. trachomatis	0	0	0	0	0	0	0	0	0	0	0	0	0	0	0	0	0	0	0
Chlamydophila sp.	0	0	0	0	0	0	0	0	0	0	+	0	±	0	0	0	0	0	0
M. genitalium	0	0	0	0	0	0	0	0	0	0	0	0	0	0	0	0	0	0	0
M. pneumoniae	0	0	0	0	0	0	0	0	0	0	+	0	0	0	0	0	0	0	0
U. urealyticum	0	0	0	0	0	0	0	0	0	0	0	0	0	0	0	0	0	0	0
Anaerobic GNB																			
B. fragilis	0	0	0	0	0	0	0	0	0	0	0	0	0	0	0	0	0	++	0
F. necrophorum	0	0	0	0	0	0	0	0	0	0	0	0	0	0	0	0	0	++	0
P. melaninogenica	0	0	0	0	0	0	0	0	0	0	0	0	0	0	0	0	0	++	0
Anaerobic gram-positive																			
Actinomyces sp.	0	?	0	?	0	0	+	?	0	0	0	0	0	0	0	0	0	0	0
C. difficile	0	++	0	0	0	0	0	0	0	0	0	0	0	0	0	0	0	+	0
Clostridium sp.	±	+	+	+	+	+	+	0	0	0	0	0	0	0	0	0	0	+	0
P. acnes	+	+	+	+	+	+	0	0	0	0	0	0	0	±	0	0	0	0	0
Peptostreptococci	+	+	+	+	+	+	+	?	0	0	0	0	0	0	0	+	0	±	0

TABLE 4B - ANTIFUNGAL ACTIVITY SPECTRA

	Antifungal Drugs								
	Fluconazole	Itraconazole	Voriconazole	Posaconazole	Isavuconazonium sulfate	Anidulafungin	Caspofungin	Micafungin	Amphotericin B
Fungi									
Aspergillus fumigatus	0	±	++	+	++	±	±	±	+
Aspergillus terreus	0	±	++	+	++	±	±	±	0
Aspergillus flavus	0	±	++	+	++	±	±	±	+
Candida albicans	++	+	+	+	+	++	++	++	+
Candida auris	0	±	±	±	±	+	+	+	±
Candida dubliniensis	++	+	+	+	+	++	++	++	++
Candida glabrata	±	±	±	±	±	++	++	++	++
Candida guilliermondii	++	++	++	++	+	++	++	++	++
Candida krusei	0	0	+	+	+	++	++	++	++
Candida lusitaniae	++	+	+	+	+	++	++	++	0
Candida parapsilosis	++	+	+	+	+	+	+	+	++
Candida tropicalis	++	+	+	+	+	++	++	++	++
Cryptococcus sp.	++	+	+	+	+	0	0	0	++
Dematiaceous molds	0	++	++	+	+	±	±	±	+
Fusarium sp.	0	±	±	±	±	0	0	0	±
Mucormycosis	0	0	0	+	+	0	0	0	++
Scedo apiospermum	0	0	+	±	±	0	0	0	0
Scedo (Lomentospora) prolificans	0	0	0	0	0	0	0	0	0
Trichosporon spp.	±	+	+	+	+	0	0	0	+
Dimorphic Fungi									
Blastomyces	±	++	+	+	+	0	0	0	++
Coccidioides	++	++	+	+	+	0	0	0	++
Histoplasma	±	++	+	+	+	0	0	0	++
Sporothrix	±	++	+	+	+	0	0	0	++

TABLE 4C – ANTIVIRAL ACTIVITY SPECTRA

	Viruses													
	Adenovirus	BK Virus	Cytomegalovirus	Hepatitis B	Hepatitis C	Herpes simplex	HPV	Influenza A	Influenza B	JC Virus / PML	RSV	Smallpox	Monkeypox	Varicella-zoster
Hepatitis B														
Adefovir	NA	NA	NA	+	NA	NA	NA	NA	NA	NA	NA	NA	NA	NA
Emtricitabine	NA	NA	NA	±	NA	NA	NA	NA	NA	NA	NA	NA	NA	NA
Entecavir	NA	NA	NA	++	NA	NA	NA	NA	NA	NA	NA	NA	NA	NA
Lamivudine	NA	NA	NA	±	NA	NA	NA	NA	NA	NA	NA	NA	NA	NA
Telbivudine	NA	NA	NA	±	NA	NA	NA	NA	NA	NA	NA	NA	NA	NA
Tenofovir (TDF and TAF)	NA	NA	NA	++	NA	±	NA	NA	NA	NA	NA	NA	NA	NA
Hepatitis C														
Daclatasvir	NA	NA	NA	NA	++	NA	NA	NA	NA	NA	NA	NA	NA	NA
Dasabuvir	NA	NA	NA	NA	++	NA	NA	NA	NA	NA	NA	NA	NA	NA
Elbasvir	NA	NA	NA	NA	++	NA	NA	NA	NA	NA	NA	NA	NA	NA
Glecaprevir	NA	NA	NA	NA	++	NA	NA	NA	NA	NA	NA	NA	NA	NA
Grazoprevir	NA	NA	NA	NA	++	NA	NA	NA	NA	NA	NA	NA	NA	NA
Interferon alfa, peg	NA	NA	NA	++	+	NA	NA	NA	NA	NA	NA	NA	NA	NA
Ledipasvir	NA	NA	NA	NA	++	NA	NA	NA	NA	NA	NA	NA	NA	NA
Ombitasvir	NA	NA	NA	NA	++	NA	NA	NA	NA	NA	NA	NA	NA	NA
Paritaprevir	NA	NA	NA	NA	++	NA	NA	NA	NA	NA	NA	NA	NA	NA
Pibrentasvir	NA	NA	NA	NA	++	NA	NA	NA	NA	NA	NA	NA	NA	NA
Ribavirin	±	NA	NA	0	+	NA	NA	NA	NA	NA	±	NA	NA	NA
Simeprevir	NA	NA	NA	NA	+	NA	NA	NA	NA	NA	NA	NA	NA	NA
Sofosbuvir	NA	NA	NA	NA	++	NA	NA	NA	NA	NA	NA	NA	NA	NA
Velpatasvir	NA	NA	NA	NA	++	NA	NA	NA	NA	NA	NA	NA	NA	NA
Voxilaprevir	NA	NA	NA	NA	++	NA	NA	NA	NA	NA	NA	NA	NA	NA
Influenza														
Amantadine	NA	NA	NA	NA	NA	NA	NA	0	0	NA	NA	NA	NA	NA
Baloxavir	NA	NA	NA	NA	NA	NA	NA	+	+	NA	NA	NA	NA	NA
Oseltamivir	NA	NA	NA	NA	NA	NA	NA	++	++	NA	NA	NA	NA	NA
Peramivir	NA	NA	NA	NA	NA	NA	NA	+	+	NA	NA	NA	NA	NA
Rimantadine	NA	NA	NA	NA	NA	NA	NA	0	0	NA	NA	NA	NA	NA
Zanamivir	NA	NA	NA	NA	NA	NA	NA	++	++	NA	NA	NA	NA	NA
Herpes, CMV, VZV, misc.														
Acyclovir	NA	NA	0	NA	NA	++	NA	NA	NA	NA	NA	NA	NA	+
Cidofovir	+	+	++	NA	NA	+	NA	NA	NA	+	NA	+	+	+
Famciclovir	NA	NA	0	NA	NA	++	NA	NA	NA	NA	NA	NA	NA	+
Foscarnet	NA	NA	++	NA	NA	+	NA	NA	NA	NA	NA	NA	NA	+
Ganciclovir	±	NA	++	NA	NA	+	NA	NA	NA	NA	NA	NA	NA	+
Letermovir	NA	NA	++	NA	NA	NA	NA	NA	NA	NA	NA	NA	NA	NA
Valacyclovir	NA	NA	0	NA	NA	++	NA	NA	NA	NA	NA	NA	NA	++
Valganciclovir	±	NA	++	NA	NA	+	NA	NA	NA	NA	NA	NA	NA	+
Pox Viruses														
Tecovirimat	NA	NA	NA	NA	NA	NA	NA	NA	NA	NA	NA	+	+	NA
Topical Agents														
Imiquimod	NA	NA	NA	NA	NA	NA	++	NA	NA	NA	NA	NA	NA	NA
Penciclovir	NA	NA	0	NA	NA	+	NA	NA	NA	NA	NA	NA	NA	0
Podofilox	NA	NA	NA	NA	NA	NA	++	NA	NA	NA	NA	NA	NA	NA
Sinecatechins	NA	NA	NA	NA	NA	NA	+	NA	NA	NA	NA	NA	NA	NA
Trifluridine	NA	NA	NA	NA	NA	+	NA	NA	NA	NA	NA	NA	NA	NA

TABLE 5A – TREATMENT OPTIONS FOR SYSTEMIC INFECTION DUE TO MULTI-DRUG RESISTANT GRAM-POSITIVE BACTERIA

ORGANISM	RESISTANT TO	PRIMARY TREATMENT OPTIONS	ALTERNATIVE TREATMENT OPTIONS	COMMENTS
Enterococcus faecium; Enterococcus faecalis (Consultation suggested) For review of VRE treatment: *Infect Dis Clin North Am 30:415, 2016.*	Vancomycin (VRE), Ampicillin, Penicillin G, Gentamicin (high level resistance)	**E. faecium**, systemic infection, bacteremia: **Dapto** 10-12 mg/kg IV q24h + (**AMP** 2 gm IV q4h OR **Ceftaroline** 600 mg IV q8h). Less desirable alternatives: [**Linezolid** 600 mg po/IV q12h OR **Quinupristin-Dalfopristin** 7.5 mg/kg IV (central line)] ± **AMP** 2 gm IV q4h Note: Quinu-dalfo for E. faecium only	**E. faecalis**: Resistance to AMP or Pen rare. If no resistance: **AMP** 2 gm IV q4h + **Ceftriaxone** 2 gm IV q12h. If Pen-resistant due to beta-lactamase: **Dapto** 8-12 mg/kg IV q12h + **Amp-sulb** 3 gm IV q6h.	**Addition of a beta lactam to Dapto reverses Dapto resistance & impedes development of resistance.** *E. faecalis* rarely resistance to penicillins. Linezolid 600 mg IV/po bid an alternative to Dapto for the treatment of VRE bacteremia, systemic infection, but data are conflicting as to which is better *(CID 61:871, 2015 and CID 61:879, 2015).* Dapto dose > 9 mg/kg is associated with lower mortality in treatment of VRE bacteremia *(CID 64:1026, 2017).* Linezolid should be used for treatment of VRE infections if Dapto MIC > 4 μg/ml.
Staphylococcus aureus *(See Table 6 for more details)*	Vancomycin (VISA or VRSA) and all beta lactams (except Ceftaroline)	**Dapto** 6-12 mg/kg IV q24h or (**Dapto** 6-12 mg/kg IV q24h + **Ceftaroline** 600 mg IV q8h) *(AAC 56:5296, 2012).*	**Telavancin** 10 mg/kg IV q24h or **Linezolid** 600 mg IV/po q12h	**Confirm dapto susceptibility** as VISA strains may be non-susceptible. If prior vanco therapy (or persistent infection on vanco) there is significant chance of developing resistance to dapto *(JAC 66:1696, 2011).* Addition of an anti-staphylococcal beta-lactam (nafcillin or oxacillin) may restore susceptibility against Dapto-resistant MRSA *(AAC 54:3161, 2010).* Combination of Dapto + Oxacillin has been successful in clearing refractory MRSA bacteremia *(CID 53:158, 2011)*; Dapto + Ceftaroline may also be effective.
Streptococcus pneumoniae	Penicillin G (MIC ≥4 μg/mL)	If no meningitis: **Ceftriaxone** 2 gm IV once daily OR **Ceftaroline** 600 mg IV q12h OR **Linezolid** 600 mg IV/po q12h	Meningitis: **Vanco** 15 mg/kg IV q8h OR **MER** 2 gm IV q8h	Ceftriaxone 2 gm IV q12h should also work for meningitis for strains with Ceftriaxone MIC ≤ 0.5 mcg/mL.

TABLE 5B: TREATMENT OPTIONS FOR SYSTEMIC INFECTION DUE TO CULTURE-IDENTIFIED MULTI-DRUG RESISTANT GRAM-NEGATIVE BACILLI

Many of the treatment options for extensively drug resistant GNB are not FDA approved indications (NAI). Suggested options are based on a combination of in vitro data, animal models, observational studies or clinical trials for selected pathogens. For dosing, see specific topics in *Table 1* or drug listings in *Table 10A*.

ORGANISM	RESISTANT TO	PRIMARY TREATMENT OPTIONS	ALTERNATIVE TREATMENT OPTIONS	COMMENTS
Acinetobacter calcoaceticus—baumannii complex	All beta-lactams (except Sulbactam), AG, FQ, TMP-SMX	*If susceptible*: **Cefepime**, **Ceftazidime**, **Amp-sulb** *If MDR & suscept*: **MER** or **IMP**	*If critically ill*: **MER** + **Amp-sulb** + **Polymyxin B** (**Colistin** if UTI) Check suscept. to **AMK** & **Minocycline**	Colistin + RIF and Colistin + MER failed in clinical trials *(CID 57:349, 2013; LnID 18:391, 2018)*. In vitro suscept *(AAC 63:e01154-19, 2019)*. Cefiderocol active in vitro.
Extended spectrum beta lactamase (ESBL) produced by E. coli, K. pneumoniae, Enterobacteriaceae, P. aeruginosa	All cephalosporins, FQ, AG, TMP-SMX	**MER** or **IMP**	**Ceftolo-tazo***, **Ceftaz-avi***, **MER-vabor***	Pip-tazo discordance: even if sensitive in vitro, may fail clinically. Pip-Tazo failed in a clinical trial vs. MER in ceftriaxone-resistant E. coli/K. pneumo *(JAMA 2018;320:979 & 984)*. For UTI: Nitrofurantoin, Fosfomycin.
OXA-48 producing Enterobacteriaceae	All penicillins, FQ, AG, TMP-SMX	*If sensitive*: **Cefepime**, **Ceftazidime**	*If critically ill*: **Ceftaz-avi** + **Aztreonam**	More common in areas bordering the Mediterranean Sea *(Clin Micro Rev 2014;27:241)*.
KPC (serine carbapenemase) producing Enterobacteriaceae	All penicillins, cephalosporins, Aztreonam, carbapenems, FQ, AG, TMP-SMX	**Ceftaz-avi***, **MER-vabor**, **IMP-relebactam**	None proven effective: ID consultation	MER + polymyxin failed in controlled clinical trial *(LnID 2018,18:391)*. Check Plazomicin susceptibility.
Metallo-carbapenemase producing GNB	All beta lactams (except Aztreonam), FQ, AG, TMP-SMX	**Ceftaz-avi*** + **Aztreonam**	None proven effective: ID consultation	
Stenotrophomonas maltophilia	All beta lactams, FQ, AG	**TMP-SMX**	*If susceptible in vitro*: **FQ**, **Minocycline**	Ticar-clav no longer available. Ref: *Sem Resp CCM 36:99, 2015*

* Not FDA-approved indication

TABLE 6 – SUGGESTED MANAGEMENT OF SUSPECTED OR CULTURE-POSITIVE METHICILLIN-RESISTANT S. AUREUS INFECTIONS

IDSA Guidelines: *CID 52 (Feb 1):1, 2011.*

NOTE: Distinction between community and hospital strains of MRSA blurring.

CLINICAL ILLNESS	ABSCESS, NO IMMUNOSUPPRESSION, OUT-PATIENT CARE	PNEUMONIA	BACTEREMIA OR POSSIBLE ENDOCARDITIS OR BACTEREMIC SHOCK	TREATMENT FAILURE *(See footnote[2])*
Management *Drug doses in footnote[1].*	**TMP/SMX** 1 DS (2 DS if BMI >40) po bid OR **Clinda** 300 mg (450 mg for BMI >40) po tid *(NEJM 372:1093, 2015).* For larger abscesses, multiple lesions or systemic inflammatory response: **I&D** + (**Oritavancin** 1500 mg x 1 or **Dalbavancin** 1000 mg x 1 than 500 mg x 1 a wk later) an option for outpatient management of sicker patients with more extensive infection who might otherwise be admitted *(see NEJM 370:2180, 2014, NEJM 370:2169, 2014).*	**Vanco** IV or **Linezolid** IV	**Vanco** 15-20 mg/kg IV q8-12h. Confirm adequate vanco troughs of 15-20 μg/mL Switch to alternative regimen if **Vanco** MIC >2 μg/mL. If patient has slow response to vanco, consider alternative therapy. **Dapto** 8-12 mg/kg q24h.	**Dapto** 8-12 mg/kg IV q24h; confirm in vitro susceptibility as prior vanco therapy may select for daptomycin non-susceptibility (MIC >1 μg/mL) & some VISA strains are daptomycin non-susceptible. **Use combination therapy for bacteremia or endocarditis:** dapto + beta-lactam combination therapy [**Dapto** 8-12 mg/kg IV q24h + (**Nafcillin/Oxacillin** 2 gm IV q4h OR **Ceftaroline** 600 mg IV q8h) appears effective against MRSA strains as salvage therapy even if non-susceptible to dapto *(Int J Antimicrob Agents, 42:450, 2013, AAC 54:3161, 2010, AAC 56:6192, 2013).* **Ceftaroline** 600 mg IV q8h *(AAC 61:e02015, 2017, Am J Health Syst Pharm. 74:201, 2017).* **Linezolid** 600 mg IV/po q12h (Linezolid is bacteriostatic and should not be used as a single agent in suspected endovascular infection). **Telavancin** 10 mg/kg q24h IV *(CID 52:31, 2011; AAC 58:2030, 2014).*
Comments	**Fusidic acid** 500 mg tid (where available) + **RIF** also an option; do not use rifampin alone as resistance rapidly emerges. Patients not responding after 2-3 days should be evaluated for complicated infection and switched to **Vancomycin**.	Prospective study of **Linezolid** vs **Vanco** showed slightly higher cure rate with Linezolid, no difference in mortality *(CID 54:621, 2012).*	TMP-SMX **NOT** recommended in bacteremic pts; inferior to Vanco *(BMJ 350:2219, 2015).* Adjunctive rifampin did not improve outcomes in patients with *S. aureus* bacteremia *(Lancet 391:668, 2018).*	

[1] **Clindamycin:** 300 mg po tid. **Daptomycin:** 6 mg/kg IV q24h is the standard, FDA-approved dose for bacteremia and endocarditis but 8-12 mg/kg q24h is recommended by some and for treatment failures. **Doxycycline or Minocycline:** 100 mg po bid. **Linezolid:** 600 mg po/IV bid. **Quinupristin-Dalfopristin (Q-D):** 7.5 mg per /kg IV q8h via central line. **Rifampin:** Long serum half-life justifies dosing 600 mg po q24h; however, frequency of nausea less with 300 mg po bid. **TMP-SMX-DS:** Standard dose 8–10 mg per kg per day. For 70 kg person = 700 mg TMP component per day. **TMP-SMX** contains 160 mg TMP and 800 mg SMX. The dose for treatment of CA-MRSA skin and soft tissue infections (SSTI) is 1 DS tablet twice daily. **Vancomycin:** 1 gm IV q12h; up to 45-60 mg/kg/day in divided doses may be required to achieve target trough concentrations of 15-20 mcg/mL recommended for serious infections.

[2] The median duration of bacteremia in endocarditis is 7-9 days in patients treated with vancomycin *(AnIM 115:674, 1991).* Longer duration of bacteremia, greater likelihood of endocarditis *(JID 190:1140, 2004).* Definition of failure unclear. Clinical response should be factored in. **Unsatisfactory clinical response especially if blood cultures remain positive >4 days.**

TABLE 7 – ANTIBIOTIC HYPERSENSITIVITY REACTIONS & DRUG DESENSITIZATION METHODS

Penicillin. Oral route (Pen VK) preferred. 1/3 pts develop transient reaction, usually mild. **Perform in ICU setting. Discontinue β-blockers. Have IV line, epinephrine, ECG, spirometer available.** Desensitization works as long as pt is receiving Pen; allergy returns after discontinuance. History of Steven-Johnson, exfoliative dermatitis, erythroderma are contraindications. Skin testing for evaluation of Pen allergy: Testing with major determinant (benzyl Pen polylysine) and minor determinants has negative predictive value (97-99%). Risk of systemic reaction to skin testing <1% *(Ann Allergy Asth Immunol 106:1, 2011)*. General refs: *CID 58:1140, 2014*.

- **Method:** Prepare dilutions using **Pen-VK** oral soln, 250 mg/5mL. Administer each dose @ 15 min intervals in 30 mL water/flavored bev. After Step 14 observe pt for 30 min, then give full therapeutic dose by route of choice. Ref: *Allergy, Prin & Prac, Mosby, 1993, pg. 1726.*

Step	Dilution (mg/mL)	mL Administered	Dose/Step		Cumulative Dose Given	
			mg	units	mg	units
1	0.5	0.1	0.05	80	0.05	80
2	0.5	0.2	0.1	160	0.15	240
3	0.5	0.4	0.2	320	0.35	560
4	0.5	0.8	0.4	640	0.75	1,200
5	0.5	1.6	0.8	1,280	1.55	2,480
6	0.5	3.2	1.6	2,560	3.15	5,040
7	0.5	6.4	3.2	5,120	6.35	10,160
8	5	1.2	6	9,600	12.35	19,760
9	5	2.4	12	19,200	24.35	38,960
10	5	4.8	24	38,400	48.35	77,360
11	50	1	50	80,000	98.35	157,360
12	50	2	100	160,000	198.35	317,360
13	50	4	200	320,000	398.35	637,360
14	50	8	400	640,000	798.35	1,277,360

TMP-SMX. Perform in hospital/clinic. Refs: *CID 20:849, 1995; AIDS 5:311, 1991.*

- **Method:** Use **TMP-SMX** oral susp, (40 mg TMP/200 mg SMX)/5 mL. Take with 6 oz water after each dose. Corticosteroids, antihistaminics NOT used.

Hour	Dose (TMP/SMX) (mg)
0	0.004/0.02
1	0.04/0.2
2	0.4/2
3	4/20
4	40/200
5	160/800

Penicillin. Parenteral (Pen G) route. Follow procedures/notes under Oral (Pen-VK) route. Ref: Allergy, Prin & Prac, Mosby, 1993, pg. 1726.

- **Method:** Administer **Pen G** IM, IV or sc as follows:

Step	Dilution (units/mL)	mL Administered	Dose/Step (units)	Cumulative Dose Given (units)
1	100	0.2	20	20
2		0.4	40	60
3		0.8	80	140
4	1,000	0.2	200	340
5		0.4	400	740
6		0.8	800	1,540
7	10,000	0.2	2,000	3,540
8		0.4	4,000	7,540
9		0.8	8,000	15,540
10	100,000	0.2	20,000	35,540
11		0.4	40,000	75,540
12		0.8	80,000	155,540
13	1,000,000	0.2	200,000	355,540
14		0.4	400,000	755,540
15		0.8	800,000	1,555,540

Ceftriaxone. Ref: *Allergol Immunopathol (Madr) 37:105, 2009.*

- **Method:** Infuse **Ceftriaxone** IV @ 20 min intervals as follows:

Day	Dose (mg)
1	0.001, then 0.01, then 0.1, then 1
2	1, then 5, then 10, then 50
3	100, then 250, then 500
4	1000

Desensitization Methods for Other Drugs (References)

- **Ceftazidime.** *Curr Opin All Clin Immunol 6(6): 476, 2006.*
- **Ceftaroline.** *Open Forum Infect Dis 2:1, 2015.*
- **Clindamycin.** *J Allergy Clin Immunol Pract 2018 Apr 12 [Epub ahead of print]).*
- **Daptomycin.** *Ann All Asthma Immun 100:87, 2008.*
- **Doxycycline.** *ID Cases 11:70, 2018; Ann Allergy Asthma Immunol 111:73, 2013.*
- **Entecavir.** *Ann Allergy Asthma Immunol 2019 June 22 [Epub ahead of print].*
- **Flucloxacillin.** *AAC 2018 Sept 17 [Epub ahead of print]).*
- **Imipenem-Cilastatin.** *Ann Pharmacother 37:513, 2003.*
- **Liposomal Amphotericin B.** *J Allergy Clin Immunol Pract 5:181, 2017.*
- **Meropenem.** *Ann Pharmacother 37:1424, 2003.*
- **Metronidazole.** *Allergy Rhinol 5:1, 2014.*
- **Valganciclovir.** *Transplantation 98:e50, 2014.*
- **Vancomycin.** *Intern Med 45:317, 2006.*
- General review, including desensitization protocols for **Amp, Cefepime, CIP, Clarithro, Clinda, Dapto, Linezolid, Tobra** *(CID 58:1140, 2014).*

TABLE 7 (2)

Ceftaroline. 12-step IV desensitization protocol. Ref: *Open Forum Infect Dis 2:1, 2015.*

- Method: Cumulative drug infused: 600 mg. Total time required for all 12 steps: 318 minutes.

Step	Conc (mg/mL)	Vol infused (mL)	Infusion duration (min)	Drug infused this step (mg)	Cumulative drug infused (mg)
1	0.0002	5	15	0.001	0.001
2	0.0002	15	15	0.003	0.004
3	0.002	5	15	0.01	0.014
4	0.002	15	15	0.03	0.04
5	0.02	5	15	0.1	0.14
6	0.02	15	15	0.3	0.4
7	0.2	5	15	1	1.4
8	0.2	15	15	3	4.4
9	2	5	15	10	14.4
10	2	15	15	30	44.4
11	2	25	15	50	94.4
12	2	255	153	510	604.4

Valganciclovir. 12-step oral desensitization protocol. Ref: *Transplantation 98:e50, 2014.*

- Method: Administer doses at 15-minute intervals; entire protocol takes 165 minutes. Cumulative dose administered: 453.6 mg

Step	Drug administered this step (mg)	Cumulative drug administered (mg)
1	0.1	0.1
2	0.2	0.3
3	0.4	0.7
4	0.8	1.5
5	1.6	3.1
6	3.5	6.6
7	7	13.6
8	14	27.6
9	28	55.6
10	58	113.6
11	115	228.6
12	225	453.6

TABLE 8 – PREGNANCY RISK AND SAFETY IN LACTATION

Drug	Risk Category (Old)	Use during Lactation
Antibacterials		
Amikacin	D	Probably safe, monitor infant for GI toxicity
Azithromycin	B	Safe, monitor infant for GI toxicity
Aztreonam	B	Safe, monitor infant for GI toxicity
Cefiderocol	No human data, nontoxic in animals	No data
Cephalosporins	B	Safe, monitor infant for GI toxicity
Chloramphenicol	C	Avoid use
Ciprofloxacin	C	Avoid breastfeeding for 3-4 hrs after a dose, monitor infant for GI toxicity
Clarithromycin	C	Safe, monitor for GI toxicity
Clindamycin	B	Avoid use if possible, otherwise monitor infant for GI toxicity
Colistin (polymyxin E)	C	Probably safe with monitoring, but data limited
Dalbavancin	C	Probably safe with monitoring, but no data available
Daptomycin	B	Probably safe with monitoring, but data limited
Delafloxacin	No human data, nontoxic in animals	No data
Doripenem	B	Probably safe with monitoring, but no data available
Doxycycline	D	Short-term use safe, monitor infant for GI toxicity
Eravacycline	Avoid during 2nd and 3rd trimesters	Avoid breastfeeding during treatment and for 4 days after last dose
Ertapenem	B	Safe
Erythromycin	B	Safe
Fidaxomicin	B	Probably safe
Fosfomycin	B	Probably safe with monitoring
Fusidic acid	-	Safety not established
Gatifloxacin	C	Short-term use safe
Gemifloxacin	C	Short-term use safe
Gentamicin	D	Probably safe
Imipenem - Cilastatin	C	Safe, monitor infant for GI toxicity
Imipenem - Cilastatin - Relebactam	Insufficient data in humans, evidence of embryofetal toxicity in animals	Safety not established, avoid use
Isepamicin	D	Safety not established, avoid use
Lefamulin	May cause fetal harm based on toxicity in animal studies	Avoid use; pump & discard milk during and 2 days post-rx
Levofloxacin	C	Avoid breastfeeding for 4-6 hrs after a dose, monitor infant for GI toxicity
Linezolid	C	Probably safe with monitoring. Systemic exposure is low: in one pt, breast milk linezolid conc were 3.5-12.2 µg/mL and the infant's serum conc was <0.2 µg/mL *(JAC 72:2677, 2017)*.
Meropenem	B	Probably safe with monitoring, but no data available
Meropenem-Vaborbactam	Humans ND, toxic in animals	Probably safe with monitoring, but no data available
Metronidazole	B	Data and opinions conflict; best to avoid
Minocycline	D	Short-term use safe, monitor infant for GI toxicity
Moxifloxacin	C	Short-term use safe, monitor infant for GI toxicity; avoid if possible
Netilmicin	D	Safety not established
Nitrofurantoin	B	Avoid if infant <8 days of age
Ofloxacin	C	Avoid breastfeeding for 4-6 hrs after a dose, monitor infant for GI toxicity
Omadacycline	Avoid during 2nd and 3rd trimesters	Avoid breastfeeding during treatment and for 4 days after last dose
Oritavancin	C	Probably safe with monitoring, but no data available; avoid if possible
Penicillins	B	Safe, monitor infant for GI toxicity
Plazomicin	No data	No data
Polymyxin B	C	Topical administration safe (no data with systemic use)
Quinupristin/ Dalfopristin	B	Probably safe with monitoring, but no data available; avoid if possible
Rifaximin	C	Probably safe with monitoring, but no data available; avoid if possible
Sarecycline	Do not use (risk of fetal harm, tooth discoloration, inhibition of bone growth)	No data; avoid use
Streptomycin	D	Probably safe, monitor infant for GI toxicity
Tedizolid	C	Probably safe with monitoring, but no data available; avoid if possible
Telavancin	C	Probably safe with monitoring, but no data available; avoid if possible
Telithromycin	C	Probably safe with monitoring, but no data available; avoid if possible
Tetracycline	D	Short-term use safe, monitor infant for GI toxicity

TABLE 8 (2)

Drug	Risk Category (Old)	Use during Lactation
Antibacterials *(continued)*		
Tigecycline	D	Safety not established, avoid use
TMP-SMX	C	Risk of kernicterus in premature infants; avoid if infant G6PD-deficient
Tobramycin	D	Probably safe, monitor infant for GI toxicity
Vancomycin	C	Safe with monitoring
Antifungals		
Amphotericin B (all products)	B	Probably safe, but no data available
Anidulafungin	B	Safety not established, avoid use
Caspofungin	C	Probably safe with monitoring, but no data available; avoid if possible
Fluconazole (other regimens)	D	Safe with monitoring
Fluconazole (single dose)	C	Safe with monitoring
Flucytosine	C	Safety not established, avoid use
Griseofulvin	C	Safety not established, avoid use
Isavuconazonium sulfate	C	Avoid use
Itraconazole	C	Little data available, avoid if possible
Ketoconazole	C	Little data available, avoid if possible
Micafungin	C	Safety not established, avoid use
Posaconazole	C	Safety not established, avoid use
Terbinafine	B	Little data available, avoid if possible
Voriconazole	D	Safety not established, avoid use
Antimycobacterials		
Amikacin	D	Probably safe, monitor infant for GI toxicity
Bedaquiline	B	Safety not established, avoid use
Capreomycin	C	Probably safe, monitor infant for GI toxicity
Clofazimine	C	May color breast milk pink; probably safe but avoid if possible
Cycloserine	C	Probably safe
Dapsone	C	Safe
Delamanid	Humans ND, toxic in animals	Safety not established, avoid use
Ethambutol	Safe	Probably safe
Ethionamide	C	Probably safe with monitoring
Isoniazid	C	Safe
Para-aminosalicylic acid	C	Probably safe
Pretomanid	No human data; Increased post-implantation loss in rats	No data
Pyrazinamide	C	Probably safe
Rifabutin	B	Probably safe
Rifampin	C	Probably safe
Rifapentine	C	Probably safe
Streptomycin	D	Probably safe
Thalidomide	X	Safety not established
Antiparasitics		
Albendazole	C	Data limited; one-time dose considered safe by WHO
Artemether/ Lumefantrine	Human data suggest no risk	Data limited; probably safe, particularly if infant weighs at least 5 kg
Atovaquone	C	Data limited; probably safe, particularly if infant weighs at least 5 kg
Atovaquone/Proguanil	C	Data limited; probably safe, particularly if infant weighs at least 5 kg
Benznidazole	Avoid	Safe with monitoring
Chloroquine	C	Probably safe with monitoring, but data limited; avoid if possible
Dapsone	C	Safe, but avoid if infant G6PD-deficient
Eflornithine	C	Probably safe, monitor infant for toxicity
Fexinidazole	No human data; best to avoid in 1st trimester	No data; avoid if possible
Ivermectin	C	Probably safe, monitor infant for toxicity
Mebendazole	C	Probably safe, monitor infant for toxicity
Mefloquine	B	Probably safe, monitor infant for toxicity
Miltefosine	D	Safety not established, avoid use
Moxidectin	Humans: insufficient data Animals: no embryo/ fetal toxicity	Safety not established; avoid use if possible
Nitazoxanide	B	Probably safe with monitoring, but data limited; avoid if possible
Pentamidine	C	Safety not established, avoid use
Praziquantel	B	Probably safe, monitor infant for toxicity

TABLE 8 (3)

Drug	Risk Category (Old)	Use during Lactation
Antiparasitics *(continued)*		
Primaquine	Avoid in pregnancy (risk of hemolysis if fetus G6PD-deficient)	Probably safe, monitor infant for toxicity
Pyrimethamine	C	Safe with monitoring
Quinidine	C	Probably safe, monitor infant for toxicity
Quinine	X	Probably safe, but avoid if infant G6PD-deficient
Secnidazole	No human data, safe in animals	Safety not established, avoid breastfeeding for 96 hours after dose
Sulfadoxine/ Pyrimethamine	C	Little data available, avoid use if possible
Tafenoquine	Not recommended (risk of hemolytic anemia if fetus G6PD-deficient)	Avoid breastfeeding x3 months after dose if infant G6PD-deficient or status unknown
Tinidazole	C	Safety not established, avoid use
Triclabendazole	No human data; no fetal toxicity in rabbits, rats	
Antivirals		
Acyclovir	B	Safe with monitoring
Adefovir	C	Safety not established, avoid use if possible
Amantadine	C	Avoid use
Baloxavir	No human data; safe in animals	Probably safe but no data
Cidofovir	C	Avoid use
Daclatasvir	No human data	Safety not established, avoid use if possible
Entecavir	C	Safety not established, avoid use if possible
Famciclovir	B	Safety not established, avoid use
Foscarnet	C	Safety not established, avoid use
Ganciclovir	C	Safety not established, avoid use
Interferons	C	Probably safe, monitor infant for toxicity
Letermovir	Humans ND, toxic in animals	Safety not established, avoid use
Oseltamivir	C	Probably safe, monitor infant for toxicity
Peramivir	C	Safety not established, avoid use if possible
Ribavirin	X	No data, but probably safe with monitoring
Rimantadine	C	Avoid use
Simeprevir	C (X w/ribavirin)	Safety not established, avoid use if possible
Sofosbuvir	B (X w/ribavirin)	Safety not established, avoid use if possible
Tecovirimat	Humans ND, safe in animals	Safety not established, avoid use if possible
Telbivudine	B	Safety not established, avoid use if possible
Tenofovir AF (Vemlidy)	Humans ND, safe in animals	Safety not established, avoid use if possible
Valacyclovir	B	Safe with monitoring
Valganciclovir	C	Safety not established, avoid use
Zanamivir	C	Probably safe, but no data
Antivirals (hep C combinations)		
Epclusa	Humans ND, safe in animals	Safety not established, avoid if possible
Harvoni	B	Safety not established
Mavyret	Humans ND, safe in animals	Safety not established, avoid use if possible
Technivie	B	Safety not established
Viekira Pak	B	Safety not established
Vosevi	Humans ND, safe in animals	Safety not established, avoid use if possible
Zepatier	Humans ND, safe in animals	Safety not established, avoid if possible
Antiretrovirals (HIV-infected mothers are generally discouraged from breastfeeding their infants. When required, country-specific recommendations should be followed)		
Abacavir	C	
Atazanavir	B	
Darunavir	C	
Darunavir/ritonavir	Avoid in pregnancy (↓ exposure of DRV, RTV)	
Delavirdine	C	
Didanosine	B	
Dolutegravir	B	

TABLE 8 (4)

Drug	Risk Category (Old)	Use during Lactation
Antiretrovirals *(continued)*		
Doravirine	Humans ND, safe in animals	
Efavirenz	D	
Elvitegravir	B	
Emtricitabine	B	
Enfuvirtide	B	
Etravirine	B	
Fosamprenavir	C	
Ibalizumab-uiyk	Human, animals: no data	
Indinavir	C	
Lamivudine	C	
Lopinavir/r	C	
Maraviroc	B	
Nelfinavir	B	
Nevirapine	B	
Raltegravir	Safe in human (based on 400 mg bid dosing only)	
Rilpivirine	B	
Ritonavir	B	
Saquinavir	B	
Stavudine	C	
Tenofovir alafenamide (TAF)	No human data, safe in animals	Safety not established, avoid if possible
Tenofovir disoproxil (TDF)	B	
Tipranavir	C	
Zalcitabine	C	
Zidovudine	C	
Antiretroviral Combinations		
Atripla (EFV-FTC-TAF)	D	
Biktarvy (BIC-FTC-TAF)	Humans ND, safe in animals	
Cimduo (3TC-TDF)	Humans: inadequate data, Animals: toxic in rabbits	
Combivir (3TC-ZDV)	C	
Complera (RPV-FTC-TDF)	B	
Descovy (FTC-TAF)	Humans ND, nontoxic in animals	
Dovato (DTG-3TC)	Avoid in 1st trimester (neural tube defects)	
Epzicom (3TC-ABC)	Humans nontoxic, toxic in animals	
Evotaz (ATV-cobi)	B	
Genvoya (EVG-cobi-FTC-TAF)	Humans: inadequate data Animals: nontoxic	
Juluca (DTG-RPV)	Avoid in 1st trimester (neural tube defects)	
Odefsey (RPV-FTC-TAF)	Humans: inadequate data Animals: nontoxic	
Prezcobix (DRV-cobi)	Avoid in pregnancy due to lower exposures of DRV and cobicistat	
Stribild (EVG-cobi-FTC-TDF)	B	
Symfi, Symfi Lo (EFV-3TC-TDF)	Risk of fetal harm from EFV; avoid in first trimester	
Symtuza (DRV-cobi-FTC-TAF)	Avoid in pregnancy due to lower exposures of DRV and RTV	

TABLE 8 (5)

Drug	Risk Category (Old)	Use during Lactation
Antiretroviral Combinations *(continued)*		
Temixys (3TC-TDF)	Humans: 3TC safe, TDF no data Animals: 3TC embryotoxic, TDF safe	
Triumeq (DTG-3TC-ABC)	Avoid in 1st trimester (neural tube defects)	
Trizivir (ABC-3TC-ZDV)	C	
Truvada (FTC-TDF)	B	

TABLE 9A – SELECTED PHARMACOLOGIC FEATURES OF ANTIMICROBIAL AGENTS

For pharmacodynamics, see Table 9B; for Cytochrome P450 interactions, see Table 9C. Table terminology key at bottom of each page. Additional footnotes at end of Table 9A, page 109.

DRUG	REFERENCE DOSE (SINGLE OR MULTIPLE)	FOOD REC (PO DRUGS)[1]	ORAL ABS (%)	PEAK SERUM CONC[2] (μg/mL)	PROTEIN BINDING (%)	VOLUME OF DISTRIBUTION (Vd)[3]	AVG SERUM T½ (hr)[4]	BILE PEN (%)[5]	CSF/ BLOOD[6] (%)	CSF PENETRATION[7]	AUC[8] (μg*hr/mL)	Tmax (hr)
ANTIBACTERIALS												
Aminoglycosides												
Amik, Gent, Kana, Tobra	*See Table 10C*			*See Table 10C*	0-10	0.26 L/kg	2-3	10-60	0-30	No		
Neomycin	po	Tab/soln ± food	<3	0	ND	ND	ND	ND	ND	ND	ND	ND
Plazomicin	15 mg/kg IV q24h	-	-	51-74 (15 mg/kg SD)	20	18-31 L	3.5	ND	ND	ND	226-257 (SD, 0-∞)	-
Carbapenems												
Doripenem	500 mg IV			23 (SD)	8,1	16.8 L Vss	1	117 (0-611)	ND	ND	36,3	
Ertapenem	1 gm IV			154 (SD)	95	0.12 L/kg Vss	4	10	ND	ND	572,1	
Imipenem-cilastatin	500 mg IV			40 (SD)	15-25	0.27 L/kg	1	minimal	8,5	Possibly[9]	42,2	
Imipenem-cilastatin-relebactam	1.25 gm IV q6h	-	-	Imi 104.3 μM, Rel 64.0 μM (SS)	Imi 20, Cil 40, Rel 22	Imi 24.3, Cil 13.8, Rel 19 L (Vss)	Imi 1, Cil 1, Rel 1.2	Imi minimal	Imi 8.5	Possibly[9]	Imi 573.9, Rel 427.3 μM-hr (24 hr, SS)	-
Meropenem	1 gm IV			49 (SD)	2	0.29 L/kg	1	3-300	≈ 2	Possibly[9]	72,5	
Meropenem/ Vaborbactam	Mer 2 gm/ Vab 2 gm IV q8h			Mer 43.4, Vab 55.6 (SS)	Mer 2, Vab 33	Mer 20.2L, Vab 18.6 L (Vss)	Mer 1.2, Vab 1.7	ND	ND	ND	Mer 138, Vab 196 (8 hr, SS)	
Cephalosporins (IV)												
Cefazolin	1 gm IV			188 (SD)	73-87	0.19 L/kg	1,9	29-300	1-4	No	236	
Cefepime	2 gm IV			164 (SD)	20	18 L Vss	2	10-20	10	Yes	284,8	
Cefiderocol	2 gm IV q8h	-	-	138 (SS)	40-60	18 L	2-3	ND	ND	ND	394.7 (8 hr, SS)	-
Cefotaxime	1 gm IV			100 (SD)	30-51	0.28 L/kg	1,5	15-75	10	Yes	70	
Cefotetan	1 gm IV			158 (SD)	78-91	10.3 L	4,2	2-21			504	
Cefoxitin	1 gm IV			110 (SD)	65-79	16.1 L Vss	0,8	280	3	No		
Ceftaroline	600 mg IV q12h			21.3 (SS)	20	20.3 L Vss	2.7	ND	ND	ND	56.3 (12 hr)	
Ceftazidime/ Avibactam	2.5 gm IV q8h			Ceftaz 90.4, Avi 14.6 (SS)	Ceftaz <10, Avi 5.7-8.2	Ceftaz 17 L, Avi 22.2 L (Vss)	Ceftaz 2.8, Avi 2.7	ND	ND	ND	Ceftaz 291, Avi 38.2 (8 hr)	
Ceftazidime	1 gm IV			69 (SD)	<10	0.24 L/kg Vss	1,9	13-54	20-40	Yes	127	
Ceftizoxime	1 gm IV			60 (SD)	30	0.34 L/kg	1,7	34-82			85	
Ceftobiprole[NUS]	500 mg IV			33-34.2 (SD)	16	18 L Vss	2.9-3.3				116	
Ceftolozane/ Tazobactam	1.5 gm IV q8h			Ceftolo 74.4, Tazo 18 (SS)	Ceftolo 16-21, Tazo 30	Ceftolo 13.5 L, Tazo 18.2 L (Vss)	Ceftolo 3.1, Tazo 1.0	ND	ND	ND	Ceftolo 182, Tazo 25 (8 hr)	

Food Effect (po dosing): **+ food** = take with food, **no food** = take without food, **± food** = take with or without food; **Oral % AB** = % absorbed; **Peak Serum Level: SD** = after single dose, **SS** = steady state after multiple doses; **Volume of Distribution (Vd): V/F** = Vd/oral bioavailability, **Vss** = Vd at steady state, **Vss/F** = Vd at steady state/oral bioavailability; **CSF Penetration:** therapeutic efficacy comment based on dose, usual susceptibility or target organism & penetration into CSF; **AUC** = area under drug concentration curve; **24hr** = AUC 0-24; **Tmax** = time to max plasma concentration.

TABLE 9A (2) *(Footnotes at the end of table)*

DRUG	REFERENCE DOSE (SINGLE OR MULTIPLE)	FOOD REC (PO DRUGS)[1]	ORAL ABS (%)	PEAK SERUM CONC[2] (μg/mL)	PROTEIN BINDING (%)	VOLUME OF DISTRIBUTION (Vd)[3]	AVG SERUM T½ (hr)[4]	BILE PEN (%)[5]	CSF/ BLOOD[6] (%)	CSF PENETRATION[7]	AUC[8] (μg*hr/mL)	Tmax (hr)
ANTIBACTERIALS *(continued)*												
Cephalosporins (IV) *(continued)*												
Ceftriaxone	1 gm IV			150 (SD)	85-95	5.8-13.5 L	8	200-500	8-16	Yes	1006	
Cefuroxime	1.5 gm IV			100 (SD)	33-50	0.19 L/kg Vss	1,5	35-80	17-88	Marginal	150	
Cephalosporins (po)												
Cefaclor	500 mg po	Cap/susp ± food	93	13 (SD)	22-25	0.33 L/kg V/F	0,8	≥60			20,5	0.5-1.0
Cefaclor ER	500 mg po	Tab + food		8.4 (SD)	22-25		0,8	≥60			18,1	2,5
Cefadroxil	500 mg po	Cap/tab/susp ± food	90	16 (SD)	20	0.31 L/kg V/F	1,5	22			47,4	ND
Cefdinir	300 mg po	Cap/susp ± food	25	1.6 (SD)	60-70	0.35 L/kg V/F	1,7				7,1	2,9
Cefditoren pivoxil	400 mg po	Tab + food	16	4 (SD)	88	9.3 L Vss/F	1,6				20	1.5-3.0
Cefixime	400 mg po	Tab/susp ± food	50	3-5 (SD)	65	0.93 L/kg V/F	3,1	800			25,8	4
Cefpodoxime proxetil	200 mg po	Tab + food, Susp ± food	46	2.3 (SD)	40	0.7 L/kg V/F	2,3	115			14,5	2-3
Cefprozil	500 mg po	Tab/susp ± food	95	10.5 (SD)	36	0.23 L/kg Vss/F	1,5				25,7	1,5
Ceftibuten	400 mg po	Cap/susp no food	80	15 (SD)	65	0.21 L/kg V/F	2,4				73,7	2,6
Cefuroxime axetil	250 mg tab po	Susp + food, tab ± food	52	4.1 (SD)	50	0.66 L/kg V/F	1,5				12,9	2,5
Cephalexin	500 mg po	Cap/tab/susp ± food	90	18 (SD)	5-15	0.38 L/kg V/F	1	216			29	1
Monobactams												
Aztreonam	1 gm IV			90 (SD)	56	12.6 L Vss	2	115-405	3-52	ND	271	
Penicillins												
Amox/Clav ER	2 tabs [total 2000/125 mg]	Tab + food	ND	17/2.1 (SD)	18/25	0.36/0.21 (both L/kg)	1.4/1.0	amox 100-3000	ND	ND	71.6/5.3 (0-∞)	1.5/1.03
Amox/Clav	875/125 mg po	Cap/tab/susp ± food	80/ 30-98	11.6/2.2 (SD)	18/25	0.36/0.21 (both L/kg)	1.4/1.0	amox 100-3000	ND	ND	26.8/5.1 (0-∞)	ND
Amoxicillin ER	775 mg po	Tab + food		6.6 (SD)	20		1.2-1.5				29,8	3,1
Amoxicillin	500 mg po	Cap/tab/susp ± food	80	5.5-7.5 (SD)	17	0.36 L/kg	1,2	100-3000	13-14	Yes (IV only)	22	1-2
Amp/Sulb	3 gm IV			109-150/ 48-88 (SD)	28/38	0.29/0.3 (both L/kg)	1.4/1.7	amp 100-3000	ND	ND	120/71 (0-∞)	
Ampicillin	2 gm IV			100 (SD)	18-22	0.29 L/kg	1,2	100-3000	13-14	Yes		
Benzathine Penicillin G	1.2 million units IM			0.15 (SD)								
Cloxacillin[NUS]	500 mg po	Cap no food	50	7.5-14 (SD)	95	0.1 L/kg	0,5					1-1.5
Dicloxacillin	500 mg po	Cap no food	37	10-17 (SD)	98	0.1 L/kg	0,7	5-8	ND	ND	ND	1-1.5
Nafcillin	500 mg IV			30 (SD)	90-94	27.1 L Vss	0.5-1	>100	9-20	Yes w/ high doses	18,1 (0-∞)	

Food Effect (po dosing): + food = take with food, **no food** = take without food, **± food** = take with or without food; **Oral % AB** = % absorbed; **Peak Serum Level: SD** = after single dose, **SS** = steady state after multiple doses; **Volume of Distribution (Vd): V/F** = Vd/oral bioavailability, **Vss** = Vd at steady state, **Vss/F** = Vd at steady state/oral bioavailability; **CSF Penetration:** therapeutic efficacy comment based on dose, usual susceptibility or target organism & penetration into CSF; **AUC** = area under drug concentration curve; **24hr** = AUC 0-24; **Tmax** = time to max plasma concentration.

TABLE 9A (3) *(Footnotes at the end of table)*

DRUG	REFERENCE DOSE (SINGLE OR MULTIPLE)	FOOD REC (PO DRUGS)[1]	ORAL ABS (%)	PEAK SERUM CONC[2] (μg/mL)	PROTEIN BINDING (%)	VOLUME OF DISTRIBUTION (Vd)[3]	AVG SERUM T½ (hr)[4]	BILE PEN (%)[5]	CSF/ BLOOD[6] (%)	CSF PENETRATION[7]	AUC[8] (μg*hr/mL)	Tmax (hr)
ANTIBACTERIALS *(continued)*												
Penicillins *(continued)*												
Oxacillin	500 mg IV	Cap no food	50	43 (SD)	90-94	0.4 L/kg	0.5-0.7	25	10-15	Yes		
Penicillin G	2 million units IV			20 (SD)	65	0.35 L/kg	0,5	500	5-10	Yes: Pen-sens S pneumo		
Penicillin V	500 mg po	Tab/soln no food	60-73	5-6 (SD)	65		0,5					ND
Pip/Tazo	3.375 gm IV			242/24 (SD)	16/48	0.24/0.4 (both L/kg)	1/1	>100	ND	ND	242/25	
Pivmecillinam	400 mg po q12h	Tab ± food	60-70	3 (400 mg SD)	5-10	0.2-0.4 L/kg	1	ND	ND	ND	ND	
Temocillin	2 gm IV	-	-	150-200 (SD)	70-85	0.2 L/kg	4	800-1000	8-15	ND	785 (0-∞)	-
Fluoroquinolones[10]												
Ciprofloxacin	400 mg IV q12h			4.6 (SS)	20-40	2.4 L/kg	4	2800-4500	26	Inadequate for Strep	25.4 (24 hr)	
Ciprofloxacin	500 mg ER po q24h	Tab ± food		1.6 (SS)	20-40	2.4 L/kg	6,6				8 (24 hr)	1-4
Ciprofloxacin	750 mg po q12h	Tab/susp ± food	70	3.6 (SS)	20-40	2.4 L/kg	4	2800-4500			31.6 (24 hr)	1-2
Delafloxacin	300 mg IV or 450 mg po q12h	Tab ± food	59	po 7.45, IV 9.3 (SS)	84	30-48 L Vss	4.2-8.5	ND	ND	ND	po 30.8, IV 23.4 (12 hr)	1
Gemifloxacin	320 mg po q24h	Tab ± food	71	1.6 (SS)	55-73	2-12 L/kg Vss/F	7				9.9 (24 hr)	0.5-2.0
Levofloxacin	750 mg po/IV q24h	Tab ± food, soln no food	99	po 8.6, IV 12.1 (SS)	24-38	244 L Vss	7				po 90.7, IV 108 (24 hr)	po 1.6
Moxifloxacin	400 mg po/IV q24h	Tab ± food	89	4.2-4.6 (SS)	30-50	2.2 L/kg	10-14		>50	Yes *(CID 49:1080, 2009)*	po 48, IV 38 (24 hr)	po 1-3
Norfloxacin	400 mg po q12h	Tab no food	30-40	1.5 (400 mg SD)	10-15	1.7 L/kg	3-4	700	ND	No	6.4 (400 mg	1
Ofloxacin	400 mg po q12h	Tab ± food	98	4.6-6.2 (SS)	32	1-2.5 L/kg	7				82.4 (24 hr)	1-2
Prulifloxacin[NUS]	600 mg po	Tab ± food	ND	1.6 (SD)	45	1231 L	10.6-12.1	ND	negligible		7,3	1
GLYCOPEPTIDES, LIPOGLYCOPEPTIDES, LIPOPEPTIDES												
Dalbavancin	1 gm IV			280-300 (SD)	93-98	0.11 L/kg	147-258	ND	ND	ND	23.443	
Daptomycin	4-6 mg/kg IV q24h			58-99 (SS)	92	0.1 L/kg Vss	8-9		0-8		494-632 (24 hr)	
Oritavancin	1200 mg IV			138 (SD)	85	87.6 L	245 (terminal)	ND	ND	ND	2800 (0-∞)	
Teicoplanin	6 mg/kg IV	-	-	40-50 (SD)	90-95	0.9-1.6 L/kg Vss	70-100	ND	negligible	No	500-600 (0-∞)	-
Telavancin	10 mg/kg IV q24h			108 (SS)	90	0.13 L/kg	8,1	Low			780 (24 hr)	
Vancomycin	1 gm IV q12h			20-50 (SS)	<10-55	0.7 L/kg	4-6		7-14	Need high doses	500-600 if trough 20 (24 hr)	

Food Effect (po dosing): + food = take with food, **no food** = take without food, **± food** = take with or without food; **Oral % AB** = % absorbed; **Peak Serum Level: SD** = after single dose, **SS** = steady state after multiple doses; **Volume of Distribution (Vd): V/F** = Vd/oral bioavailability, **Vss** = Vd at steady state, **Vss/F** = Vd at steady state/oral bioavailability; **CSF Penetration:** therapeutic efficacy comment based on dose, usual susceptibility or target organism & penetration into CSF; **AUC** = area under drug concentration curve; **24hr** = AUC 0-24; **Tmax** = time to max plasma concentration.

TABLE 9A (4) *(Footnotes at the end of table)*

DRUG	REFERENCE DOSE (SINGLE OR MULTIPLE)	FOOD REC (PO DRUGS)[1]	ORAL ABS (%)	PEAK SERUM CONC[2] (μg/mL)	PROTEIN BINDING (%)	VOLUME OF DISTRIBUTION (Vd)[3]	AVG SERUM $T_{1/2}$ (hr)[4]	BILE PEN (%)[5]	CSF/ BLOOD[6] (%)	CSF PENETRATION[7]	AUC[8] (μg*hr/mL)	Tmax (hr)
MACROLIDES, AZALIDES, LINCOSAMIDES, KETOLIDES												
Azithromycin	500 mg IV			3.6 (SD)	7-51	33.3 L/kg	68	High			9.6 (24 hr, pre SS)	
Azithromycin	500 mg po	Tab/susp ± food	37	0.4 (SD)	7-51	31.1 L/kg	68	High			4,3	2,5
Azithromycin ER	2 gm po	Susp no food	≈ 30	0.8 (SD)	7-51	31.1 L/kg	59	High			20	5
Clarithromycin	500 mg po q12h	Tab/susp ± food	50	3-4 (SS)	65-70	4 L/kg	5-7	7000			20 (24 hr)	2.0-2.5
Clarithromycin ER	1 gm ER po q24h	Tab + food	≈ 50	2-3 (SS)	65-70							5-8
Clindamycin	150 mg po	Cap ± food	90	2.5 (SD)	85-94	1.1 L/kg	2,4	250-300		No	ND	0,75
Clindamycin	900 mg IV q8h			14.1 (SS)	85-94	1.1 L/kg	2,4	250-300		No	ND	
Erythromycin base, esters	500 mg po	Tab/susp no food, DR caps ± food	18-45	0.1-2 (SD)	70-74	0.6 L/kg	2-4		2-13	No		delay rel: 3
Erythromycin lactobionate	500 mg IV			3-4 (SD)	70-74	0.6 L/kg	2-4					
Telithromycin	800 mg po q24h	Tab ± food	57	2.3 (SS)	60-70	2.9 L/kg	10	7			12.5 (24 hr)	1
MISCELLANEOUS ANTIBACTERIALS												
Chloramphenicol	1 gm po q6h	Cap ± food	High	18 (SS)	25-50	0.8 L/kg	4,1		45-89	Yes	ND	
Fosfomycin disodium (IV)	12-24 gm/day (divided q8-12h)	-	-	200-400 (4-8 gm IV, SD)	<10	0.3 L/kg	2.0-3.8	ND	20-50	Yes	405-448 (3 gm SD)	-
Fosfomycin tromethamine (po)	3 gm po	Sachet ± food	40	26 (3 gm SD)	<10	136.1 L Vss/F	5.7	ND	20-50	No	145-193 (3 gm SD)	2
Fusidic acid[NUS]	500 mg po	Tab + food	91	30 (SD)	95-99	0.3 L/kg	15	100-200	ND	ND	442 (0-∞)	2-4
Lefamulin	150 mg IV (or 600 mg po) q12h	Tab no food	25	IV 3.6, po 2.24 (SS)	94.8-97.1	86.1 L Vss	8	ND	ND	ND	IV 28.6, po 32.7 (SS, 24 hr)	po 0.88-2
Metronidazole	500 mg IV/po q6h	ER tab no food, tab/cap ± food	100	20-25 (SS)	20	0.6-0.85 L/kg	6-14	100	45-89	ND	560 (24 hr)	ER 6.8, regular 1.6
Pristinamycin	2 gm po	Tab + food	ND	PIA 0.76, PIIA 0.58 (SD)	ND	ND	PIA 4.03, PIIA 2.83	ND	ND	ND	PIA 2.2, PIIA 1.21 (2 gm SD, 0-∞)	PIA 3.25, PIIA 3.08
Quinupristin-dalfopristin	7.5 mg/kg IV q8h			Q 3.2/D 8 (SS)	ND	Q 0.45/D 0.24 (L/kg) Vss	Q 0.85/D 0.7	ND	ND	ND	Q 7.2/D 10.6 (24 hr)	
Rifampin	600 mg po	Cap no food	70-90	7 (SD)	80	0.65 L/kg Vss	1.5-5	10.000	7-56	Yes	40-60 (24 hr)	1.5-2
Rifaximin	200 mg po tid	Tab ± food	<0.4	0.0007-0.002 (SS)	67,5	ND	2-5			No	0,008	1
Secnidazole	2 gm po	Granules ± food	ND	45.4 (SD)	<5	42 L	17	ND	ND	ND	1332 (2 gm SD)	4
TMP/SMX	160/800 mg po q12h	Tab/susp ± food	85	1-2/40-60 (SS)	44/70	100-120 L/ 12-18 L	11/9	100-200	50/40		ND	1-4

Food Effect (po dosing): + food = take with food, **no food** = take without food, **± food** = take with or without food; **Oral % AB** = % absorbed; **Peak Serum Level: SD** = after single dose, **SS** = steady state after multiple doses; **Volume of Distribution (Vd): V/F** = Vd/oral bioavailability, **Vss** = Vd at steady state, **Vss/F** = Vd at steady state/oral bioavailability; **CSF Penetration:** therapeutic efficacy comment based on dose, usual susceptibility or target organism & penetration into CSF; **AUC** = area under drug concentration curve; **24hr** = AUC 0-24; **Tmax** = time to max plasma concentration.

TABLE 9A (5) *(Footnotes at the end of table)*

DRUG	REFERENCE DOSE (SINGLE OR MULTIPLE)	FOOD REC (PO DRUGS)[1]	ORAL ABS (%)	PEAK SERUM CONC[2] (μg/mL)	PROTEIN BINDING (%)	VOLUME OF DISTRIBUTION (Vd)[3]	AVG SERUM T½ (hr)[4]	BILE PEN (%)[5]	CSF/ BLOOD[6] (%)	CSF PENETRATION[7]	AUC[8] (μg*hr/mL)	Tmax (hr)
MISCELLANEOUS ANTIBACTERIALS *(continued)*												
TMP/SMX	160/800 mg IV q8h			9/105 (SS)	44/70	100-120 L/ 12-18 L	11/9	40-70			ND	
Trimethoprim	100 mg po	Tab ± food	80	1 (SD)	44	100-120 L V/F	8-15					1-4
OXAZOLIDINONES												
Linezolid	600 mg po/IV q12h	Tab/susp ± food	100	15-20 (SS)	31	40-50 L Vss	5		60-70	Yes (*AAC 50:3971, 2006*)	po 276, IV 179 (24 hr)	po 1.3
Tedizolid	200 mg po/IV q24h	Tab ± food	91	po 2.2, IV 3.0 (SS)	70-90	67-80 L Vss	12	ND	ND	ND	po 25.6, IV 29.2 (24 hr)	po 3, IV 1.1
POLYMYXINS												
Colistin (Polymyxin E)	150 mg IV			5-7.5 (SD)	≈ 50	0.34 L/kg	colistimethate 1.5-2, Colistin >4	0		No		
Polymyxin B	1.5 mg/kg IV q12h			2.8 (avg conc at SS)	60	ND	4.5-6 (old data)	ND	ND	No	66.9 (24 hr)	
TETRACYCLINES, GLYCYLCYCLINES												
Doxycycline	100 mg po	Tab/cap/susp + food		1.5-2.1 (SD)	93	53-134 L Vss	18	200-3200	26	No	31,7 (0-∞)	2
Eravacycline	1 mg/kg IV q12h	-	-	1.825 (SS)	79-90	321 L (Vss)	20	ND	ND	ND	6.31 (12 hr)	-
Minocycline	200 mg po	Cap/tab ± food	ND	2.0-3.5 (SD)	76	80-114 L Vss	16	200-3200	ND	ND	48,3 (0-∞)	2,1
Omadacycline	100 mg IV (or 300 mg po) q24h	Tab no food	35	IV 2.12, po 0.95 (SS)	20	190 L (Vss)	15.5-16.8	ND	ND	ND	IV 12.14, po 11.16 (24 hr)	po 2.5
Sarecycline	60-150 mg po q24h	Tab ± food	ND	ND	62.5-74.7	91.4-97.0 (Vss)	21-22	ND	ND	ND	ND	1.5-2.0
Tetracycline	250 mg po	Cap no food	ND	1.5-2.2 (SD)	20-65	1.3 L/kg	6-12	200-3200	Poor	No	30 (0-∞)	2-4
Tigecycline	50 mg IV q12h			0.63 (SS)	71-89	7-9 L/kg	42	138	5.9-10.6	No	4.7 (24 hr)	
ANTIFUNGALS												
Benzofuran												
Griseofulvin (ultramicrosize)	250 mg po	Tab + food (high fat)	27-72	0.6-0.67 (SD)	ND	ND	9-24	ND	ND	ND	8.6-9.0 (0-∞)	4
Polyenes												
Ampho B deoxycholate	0.4-0.7 mg/kg IV q24h			0.5-3.5 (SS)		4 L/kg	24		0		17 (24 hr)	
Ampho B lipid complex (ABLC)	5 mg/kg IV q24h			1-2.5 (SS)		131 L/kg	173				14 (24 hr)	
Ampho B liposomal	5 mg/kg IV q24h			83 (SS)		0.1-0.4 L/kg Vss	6,8				555 (24 hr)	
Antimetabolites												
Flucytosine	2.5 gm po	Cap ± food	78-90	30-40 (SD)	ND	0.6 L/kg	3-5		60-100	Yes	ND	2

Food Effect (po dosing): **+ food** = take with food, **no food** = take without food, **± food** = take with or without food; **Oral % AB** = % absorbed; **Peak Serum Level: SD** = after single dose, **SS** = steady state after multiple doses; **Volume of Distribution (Vd): V/F** = Vd/oral bioavailability, **Vss** = Vd at steady state, **Vss/F** = Vd at steady state/oral bioavailability; **CSF Penetration:** therapeutic efficacy comment based on dose, usual susceptibility or target organism & penetration into CSF; **AUC** = area under drug concentration curve; **24hr** = AUC 0-24; **Tmax** = time to max plasma concentration.

TABLE 9A (6) *(Footnotes at the end of table)*

DRUG	REFERENCE DOSE (SINGLE OR MULTIPLE)	FOOD REC (PO DRUGS)[1]	ORAL ABS (%)	PEAK SERUM CONC[2] (µg/mL)	PROTEIN BINDING (%)	VOLUME OF DISTRIBUTION (Vd)[3]	AVG SERUM T½ (hr)[4]	BILE PEN (%)[5]	CSF/ BLOOD[6] (%)	CSF PENETRATION[7]	AUC[8] (µg*hr/mL)	Tmax (hr)
ANTIFUNGALS *(continued)*												
Azoles												
Fluconazole	400-800 mg po/IV	Tab/susp ± food	90	6.7-14 (SD)	10	50 L V/F	20-50		50-94	Yes	140 (8 hr) after 3 mg/kg SD	po: 1-2
Isavuconazonium sulfate (Isavuconazole)	372 mg po/IV q24h (maint)	Cap ± food	98	7.5 (SS)	99	450 L Vss	130	ND	ND	ND	121.4 (24 hr)	2-3
Itraconazole	200 mg oral soln po q24h	Cap/tab + food, soln no food	55+	Itra 2.0, OH-Itra 2.0 (SS)	99,8	796 L	35		0		Itra 29.3, OH-Itra 45.2 (24 hr)	Itra 2.5, OH-Itra 5.3
Ketoconazole	200 mg po	Tab ± food	variable	3.5 (SD)	99	1.2 L/kg	8	ND	<10	No	12	1-2
Posaconazole oral susp	400 mg po bid	Susp + food	ND	0.2-1.0 (200 mg SD)	98-99	226-295 L	20-66	ND	ND	Yes (*JAC 56:745, 2005*)	9.1 (12 hr)	3-5
Posaconazole injection	300 mg IV q24h	-	-	3.3 (SS)	98-99	226-295 L	20-66	ND	ND	Yes (*JAC 56:745, 2005*)	36.1 (24 hr)	1,5
Posaconazole tab	300 mg tab po q24h	Tab + food	54	2.1-2.9 (SS)	98-99	226-295 L	20-66	ND	ND	Yes (*JAC 56:745, 2005*)	37.9 (24 hr)	3-5
Voriconazole	200 mg po q12h	Tab/susp no food	96	3 (SS)	58	4.6 L/kg Vss	variable	ND	22-100	Yes (*CID 37:728, 2003*)	39.8 (24 hr)	1-2
Echinocandins												
Anidulafungin	100 mg IV q24h			7.2 (SS)	>99	30-50 L	26.5			No	112 (24 hr)	
Caspofungin	50 mg IV q24h			8.7 (SS)	97	9.7 L Vss	13	ND		No	87.3 (24 hr)	
Micafungin	100 mg IV q24h			10.1 (SS)	>99	0.39 L/kg	15-17			No	97 (24 hr)	
ANTIMYCOBACTERIALS												
First line, tuberculosis												
Ethambutol	25 mg/kg po	Tab + food	80	2-6 (SD)	10-30	6 L/kg Vss/F	4		10-50	No	29,6	2-4
Isoniazid (INH)	300 mg po	Tab/syrup no food	100	3-5 (SD)	<10	0.6-1.2 L/kg	0.7-4		up to 90	Yes	20,1	1-2
Pyrazinamide	20-25 mg/kg po	Tab ± food	95	30-50 (SD)	5-10		10-16		100	Yes	500	2
Rifabutin	300 mg po	Cap + food	20	0.2-0.6 (SD)	85	9.3 L/kg Vss	32-67	300-500	30-70	ND	4.0 (24 hr)	2.5-4.0
Rifampin	600 mg po	Cap no food	70-90	7 (SD)	80	0.65 L/kg Vss	1.5-5	10.000	7-56	Yes	40-60 (24 hr)	1.5-2
Rifapentine	600 mg po q72h	Tab + food	ND	15 (SS)	98	70 L	13-14	ND	ND	ND	320 (72 hr)	4,8
Streptomycin	15 mg/kg IM			25-50 (SD)	0-10	0.26 L/kg	2,5	10-60	0-30	No		
Second line, tuberculosis												
Amikacin	15 mg/kg IM			25-50 (SD)	0-10	0.26 L/kg	2.5	10-60	0-30	No		
Bedaquiline	400 mg po qd	Tab + food	ND	3.3 (week 2)	>99	≈ 60 x total body water Vss	24-30 (terminal 4-5 mo)	ND	≈ 0	No	22 (24 hr) after 8 wks	5

Food Effect (po dosing): **+ food** = take with food, **no food** = take without food, **± food** = take with or without food; **Oral % AB** = % absorbed; **Peak Serum Level: SD** = after single dose, **SS** = steady state after multiple doses; **Volume of Distribution (Vd): V/F** = Vd/oral bioavailability, **Vss** = Vd at steady state, **Vss/F** = Vd at steady state/oral bioavailability; **CSF Penetration:** therapeutic efficacy comment based on dose, usual susceptibility or target organism & penetration into CSF; **AUC** = area under drug concentration curve; **24hr** = AUC 0-24; **Tmax** = time to max plasma concentration.

TABLE 9A (7) *(Footnotes at the end of table)*

DRUG	REFERENCE DOSE (SINGLE OR MULTIPLE)	FOOD REC (PO DRUGS)[1]	ORAL ABS (%)	PEAK SERUM CONC[2] (μg/mL)	PROTEIN BINDING (%)	VOLUME OF DISTRIBUTION (Vd)[3]	AVG SERUM T½ (hr)[4]	BILE PEN (%)[5]	CSF/ BLOOD[6] (%)	CSF PENETRATION[7]	AUC[8] (μg*hr/mL)	Tmax (hr)
ANTIMYCOBACTERIALS *(continued)*												
Second line, tuberculosis *(continued)*												
Capreomycin	1 gm IM			30 (SD)	ND	0.4 L/kg	2-5	ND	<10	No	ND	1-2
Cycloserine	250 mg po	Cap no food	70-90	4-8 (SD)	<20	0.47 L/kg	10	ND	54-79	Yes	110	1-2
Delamanid	100 mg po q12h	Tab + food	25-47	ND	≥99.5	2100 L V/F	30-38	ND	ND	ND	ND	ND
Ethionamide	250 mg po	Tab ± food	near 100	2.2 (SD)	30	93.5 L	1.9	ND	≈ 100	Yes	7.7 (250 mg SD)	1,5
Kanamycin	15 mg/kg IM			25-50 (SD)	0-10	0.26 L/kg	2,5	10-60	0-30	No		
Para-aminosalicylic acid (PAS)	4 g (granules)po	Granules + food	ND	9-35 (SD)	50-60	0.9-1.4 L/kg V/F	0.75-1.0	ND	10-50	Marginal	108 (4 gm SD, 0-∞)	8
Pretomanid	200 mg po q24h	Tab + food	ND	2.0 (200 mg SD)	86.4	97 L V/F	17.4	ND	ND	ND	53.0 (200 mg SD, 0-∞)	5
ANTIPARASITICS												
Antimalarials												
Artemether/ lumefantrine	4 tabs (80 mg/480 mg)	Tab + food	ND	Art 0.06-0.08, DHA 0.09-0.1, Lum 7.4-9.8 (SD)	Art 95.4, DHA 47-76, Lum 99.7	ND	Art 1.6-2.2, DHA 1.6-2.2, Lum 101-119				Art 0.15-0.26, DHA 0.29, Lum 158-243	Art 1.5-2, Lum 6-8
Artesunate (AS)	120 mg IV	-	-	DHA 2.4 (SD)	AS 62-75, DHA 66-82	AS 0.1-0.3, DHA 0.5-1 L/kg	AS 2-4 min, DHA 0.5-1 hr	ND	ND	ND	DHA 2.1 (SD, 0-∞)	25 min (to DHA)
Atovaquone	750 po bid	Susp + food	47	24 (SS)	99,9	0.6 L/kg Vss	67	ND	<1	No	801 (750 mg x1)	ND
Chloroquine phosphate	300 mg base	Tab + food	90	0.06-0.09 (SD)	55	100-1000 L/kg	45-55 days (terminal)	ND	ND	ND	ND	1-6
Dihydroartemisinin–piperaquine	Varies by body wt	Tab no food	ND	SD: DHA 0.75, PPQ 0.18 (dose?)	DHA 44-93, PPQ >99	DHA 0.8 L/kg, PPQ 730 L/kg	DHA 1, PPQ 22 days	ND	ND	ND	SD: DHA 2 (0-∞), PPQ 1.7 (0-24) (dose?)	DHA 1-2, PPQ 5
Mefloquine	1.25 gm po	Tab + food		0.5-1.2 (SD)	98	20 L/kg	13-24 days					17
Primaquine	30 mg (base) po q24h x14 days	Tab + food	ND	0.18-0.2	ND	3 L/kg	3.7-9.6	ND	ND	ND	1.2-1.6	2-3
Proguanil[11]	100 mg po	Tab + food	ND	ND	75	1600-2600 L V/F	12-21	ND	ND	ND	ND	ND
Quinine sulfate	648 mg po	Cap + food	76-88	3.2 (SD)	69-92	2.5-7.1 L/kg V/F	9.7-12.5	ND	2-7	No	28 (12 hr)	2,8
Tafenoquine	200 mg po	Tab + food	ND	0.15 (SD)	>99.5	1600-2500 L	15 days (terminal)	ND	ND	ND	ND	12-15
ANTIPARASITICS, Other												
Albendazole	400 mg po	Tab + food	Poor	0.5-1.6 (sulfoxide)	70	ND	8-12	ND	ND	ND	ND	2-5 (sulfoxide)

Food Effect (po dosing): + food = take with food, **no food** = take without food, **± food** = take with or without food; **Oral % AB** = % absorbed; **Peak Serum Level: SD** = after single dose, **SS** = steady state after multiple doses; **Volume of Distribution (Vd): V/F** = Vd/oral bioavailability, **Vss** = Vd at steady state, **Vss/F** = Vd at steady state/oral bioavailability; **CSF Penetration:** therapeutic efficacy comment based on dose, usual susceptibility or target organism & penetration into CSF; **AUC** = area under drug concentration curve; **24hr** = AUC 0-24; **Tmax** = time to max plasma concentration.

TABLE 9A (8) *(Footnotes at the end of table)*

DRUG	REFERENCE DOSE (SINGLE OR MULTIPLE)	FOOD REC (PO DRUGS)[1]	ORAL ABS (%)	PEAK SERUM CONC[2] (µg/mL)	PROTEIN BINDING (%)	VOLUME OF DISTRIBUTION (Vd)[3]	AVG SERUM T½ (hr)[4]	BILE PEN (%)[5]	CSF/ BLOOD[6] (%)	CSF PENETRATION[7]	AUC[8] (µg*hr/mL)	Tmax (hr)
ANTIPARASITICS, Other *(continued)*												
Antimony, pentavalent	10-20 mg/kg IM/IV	-	-	7.23-10.5 (10 mg/kg q24h, SS)	ND	approx 260 L (Vss)	elim 2 hr, term 1-3 days	ND	ND	ND	65.4 (10 mg/kg q24h, 0-∞)	IM: 0.5-2
Benznidazole	100 mg po	Tab + food	92	2.2	44	39.2 L V/F	13.3	ND	ND	ND	51.3 (0-Inf)	2.9
Benznidazole (Arg)												
Benznidazole (Bra)												
Dapsone	100 mg po q24h	Tab ± food	70-100	1.1 (SS)	70	1.5 L/kg	10-50	ND	ND	ND	52.6 (24 hr)	2-6
Diethylcarbamazine	6 mg/kg po	Tab + food	80-85	1.93 (SD)	ND	182 L V/F	9	ND	ND	ND	23.8 (0-∞)	1-2
Fexinidazole	1800 mg x4d, 1200 mg x6d	Tab + food	ND	Fex 485, M1 5574, M2 11330 (ng/mL, SS)	Fex 95.4, M1 25.9, M2 41.6	Fex 3768 L (V/F)	Fex 14, M1 15, M2 23	ND	M1 52, M2 31	Yes	Fex 6596, M1 77263 (ng*hr/mL, 0-24)	Fex/M1 2-6, M2 14-24
Ivermectin	12 mg po	Tab no food	60	0.05-0.08 (SD)	93	3-3.5 L/kg	20	ND	ND	No	ND	4
Mebendazole	100 mg po	Tab ± food	<10	Negligible	90-95	1-2 L/kg	3-6	ND	ND	ND	ND	2-4
Miltefosine	50 mg po tid	Cap + food	ND	76 (after 23 days)	95	ND	7-31 days	ND	ND	ND	486 (8hr)	2-8
Moxidectin	8 mg po x1	Tab ± food	ND	0.06 (SD)	ND	2421 L	23 days	ND	ND	ND	2.7-3.4 (0-∞)	4
Nitazoxanide	500 mg po	Tab/susp + food	Susp 70% of tab	Nitazox 9-11, gluc 7.3-10.5 (SD)	Nitazox 99	ND	Nitazox 1.3-1.8	ND	ND	ND	Nitazox 40, gluc 46.5-63.0	Nitazox, gluc: 1-4
Praziquantel	20 mg/kg po	Tab + food	80	0.2-2.0 (SD)		8000 L V/F	0.8-1.5				1,51	1-3
Pentamidine	4 mg/kg IV/IM q24h	-	-	0.6 (SD)	69	200-400 L/kg (Vss)	terminal 11-12 days	ND	ND	ND	0.75 (3 mg/kg IV SD)	IM: 1
Pyrimethamine	25 mg po	Tab ± food	High	0.1-0.3 (SD)	87	3 L/kg	96					2-6
Tinidazole	2 gm po	Tab + food	48	48 (SD)	12	50 L	13	ND	ND	ND	902	1.6
Triclabendazole	10 mg/kg po	Tab + food	ND	Tricla 1.16, sulfoxide 38.6, sulfone 2.29 (µmol/mL, SD)	96.7-98.8	sulfoxide 1 L/kg	Tricla 8, sulfoxide 14, sulfone 11	ND	ND	ND	Tricla 5.72, sulfoxide 386, sulfone 30.5 (µmol*hr/L, SD)	Tricla, sulfoxide: 3-4
ANTIVIRALS (non-HIV)												
Hepatitis B												
Adefovir	10 mg po	Tab ± food	59	0.02 (SD)	≤4	0.37 L/kg Vss	7,5				0,22	1,75
Entecavir	0.5 mg po q24h	Tab/soln no food	100	4.2 ng/mL (SS)	13	>0.6 L/kg V/F	128-149 (terminal)	ND	ND	ND	0.014 (24 hr)	0.5-1.5
Telbivudine	600 mg po q24h	Tab/soln ± food		3.7 (SS)	3,3	>0.6 L/kg V/F	40-49				26.1 (24 hr)	2
Tenofovir AF (Vemlidy)	25 mg po q24h	Tab + food	ND	0.27 (SS)	80	ND	0.51	ND	ND	ND	0.27 (24 hr)	0,48

Food Effect (po dosing): + food = take with food, **no food** = take without food, **± food** = take with or without food; **Oral % AB** = % absorbed; **Peak Serum Level: SD** = after single dose, **SS** = steady state after multiple doses; **Volume of Distribution (Vd): V/F** = Vd/oral bioavailability, **Vss** = Vd at steady state, **Vss/F** = Vd at steady state/oral bioavailability; **CSF Penetration:** therapeutic efficacy comment based on dose, usual susceptibility or target organism & penetration into CSF; **AUC** = area under drug concentration curve; **24hr** = AUC 0-24; **Tmax** = time to max plasma concentration.

TABLE 9A (9) *(Footnotes at the end of table)*

DRUG	REFERENCE DOSE (SINGLE OR MULTIPLE)	FOOD REC (PO DRUGS)[1]	ORAL ABS (%)	PEAK SERUM CONC[2] (µg/mL)	PROTEIN BINDING (%)	VOLUME OF DISTRIBUTION (Vd)[3]	AVG SERUM T½ (hr)[4]	BILE PEN (%)[5]	CSF/ BLOOD[6] (%)	CSF PENETRATION[7]	AUC[8] (µg*hr/mL)	Tmax (hr)
ANTIVIRALS (non-HIV) *(continued)*												
Hepatitis C												
Daclatasvir	60 mg po q24h	Tab ± food	67	0.18 (Cmin, SS)	99	47 Vss	12-15	ND	ND	ND	11 (24 hr)	2
Dasabuvir	250 mg po q12h	Tab + food	ND	0.03-3.1 (10-1200 mg SD)	ND	ND	5-8	ND	ND	ND	ND	3
Elbasvir/ Grazoprevir	(Elba 50 + Grazo 100 mg) q24h	Tab ± food	ND	Elba 0.121, Grazo 0.165 (SS)	Elba >99.9, Grazo >98.8	ND	Elba 24, Grazo 31	ND	ND	ND	Elba 1.92, Grazo 1.42 (24 hr)	Elba 3, Grazo 2
Glecaprevir/ Pibrentasvir (Mavyret)	Gle 300 mg + Pib 120 mg q24h	Tab + food	ND	Gle 0.6, Pib 0.11 (SS)	Gle 97.5, Pib >99.9	ND	Gle 6, Pib 13	ND	ND	ND	Gle 4.8, Pib 1.43 (24 hr)	Gle 5, Pib 5
Ledipasvir/ Sofosbuvir (Harvoni)	90 mg + Sofos 400 g po q24h	Tab ± food	ND	Ledip: 0.3 (SS)	Ledip: >99.8	ND	Ledip: 47	ND	ND	ND	Ledip: 7.3 (24hr)	Ledip: 4-4.5
Ombitasvir (with Paritaprevir/RTV)	25 mg po q24h	Tab + food	ND	0.56 (SS)	ND	ND	28-34	ND	ND	ND	0.53 (24 hr)	4-5
Paritaprevir/RTV (with Ombitasvir)	150 mg (+ RTV 100 mg) po q24h	Tab + food	ND	ND	ND	ND	5,8	ND	ND	ND	ND	4,3
Ribavirin	600 mg po	Tab/cap/soln + food	64	3.7 (SS)	minimal	2825 L V/F	44 (terminal 298)	ND	ND	ND	228 (12 hr)	2
Simeprevir	150 mg po	Cap + food	ND	ND	>99.9	ND	41	ND	ND	ND	57.5 (24 hr)	4-6
Sofosbuvir	400 mg po q24h	Tab ± food	ND	Sofos: 0.6 (SS)	Sofos: 61-65	ND	Sofos: 0.5-0.75	ND	ND	ND	Sofos: 0.9 (24 hr)	0.5-2
Velpatasvir/ Sofosbuvir (Epclusa)	100 mg (+ Sofos 400 mg) po q24h	Tab ± food	ND	Velpat: 0.26 (SS)	Velpat: >99.5	ND	Velpat: 15	ND	ND	ND	Velpat: 2.98 (24 hr)	Velpat: 3
Voxilaprevir/ Velpatasvir/ Sofosbuvir (Vosevi)	Vox 100 + Vel 100 + Sof 400 mg q24h	Tab + food	ND	Vox 0.19, Vel 0.31, Sof 0.68 (SS)	Vox >99, Vel >99, Sof 61-65	ND	Vox 33, Vel 17, Sof 0.5	ND	ND	ND	Vox 2.6, Vel 4.0, Sof 1.7 (24 hr)	Vox 4, Vel 4, Sof 2
Herpesvirus												
Acyclovir	400 mg po bid	Tab/cap/susp ± food	10-20	1.21 (SS)	9-33	0.7 L/kg	2.5-3.5	ND	ND	ND	7.4 (24 hr)	1.5-2
Cidofovir (w/probenecid)	5 mg/kg IV	Probenecid: ± food		19.6 (SD)	<6	0.41 L/kg Vss	2.6 (diphosphate: 17-65)	ND	0	No	40,8	1,1
Famciclovir	500 mg po	Tab ± food	77	3-4 (SD)	<20	1.1 L/kg (Penciclovir)	2-3 (Penciclovir)				8.9 (Penciclovir)	0.9 (Penciclovir)

Food Effect (po dosing): + food = take with food, **no food** = take without food, **± food** = take with or without food; **Oral % AB** = % absorbed; **Peak Serum Level: SD** = after single dose, **SS** = steady state after multiple doses; **Volume of Distribution (Vd): V/F** = Vd/oral bioavailability, **Vss** = Vd at steady state, **Vss/F** = Vd at steady state/oral bioavailability; **CSF Penetration:** therapeutic efficacy comment based on dose, usual susceptibility or target organism & penetration into CSF; **AUC** = area under drug concentration curve; **24hr** = AUC 0-24; **Tmax** = time to max plasma concentration.

TABLE 9A (10) *(Footnotes at the end of table)*

DRUG	REFERENCE DOSE (SINGLE OR MULTIPLE)	FOOD REC (PO DRUGS)[1]	ORAL ABS (%)	PEAK SERUM CONC[2] (µg/mL)	PROTEIN BINDING (%)	VOLUME OF DISTRIBUTION (Vd)[3]	AVG SERUM T½ (hr)[4]	BILE PEN (%)[5]	CSF/ BLOOD[6] (%)	CSF PENETRATION[7]	AUC[8] (µg*hr/mL)	Tmax (hr)
ANTIVIRALS (non-HIV) *(continued)*												
Herpesvirus *(continued)*												
Foscarnet	60 mg/kg IV			155 (SD)	4	0.46 L/kg	3 (terminal 18-88)	No			2195 µM*hr	
Ganciclovir	5 mg/kg IV			8.3 (SD)	1-2	0.7 L/kg Vss	3,5				24,5	
Letermovir	480 mg po/IV q24h	Tab ± food	35-94	13 (po, SS)	99	45.5 L Vss	12	ND	ND	ND	71.5 (po, 24 hr)	0.75-2.25
Valacyclovir	1 gm po	Tab ± food	55	5.6 (SD)	13-18	0.7 L/kg	3				19.5 (Acyclovir)	
Valganciclovir	900 mg po q24h	Tab/soln + food	59	5.6 (SS)	1-2	0.7 L/kg	4				29.1 (Ganciclo)	1-3 (Ganciclo)
Influenza												
Baloxavir marboxil (prodrug)	40 mg po x1	ND	ND	ND	ND	ND	96 (baloxavir acid)	ND	ND	ND	ND	4 (baloxavir acid)
Laninamivir (octanoate=prodrug)	40 mg (prodrug) inhaled x1	-	-	Lan: 0.024 (SD)	Lan: <0.01	ND	Lan 64.7; Lan octanoate 1.8	ND	ND	ND	Lan: 0.745 (0-∞)	Lan: 4
Oseltamivir	75 mg po bid	Cap/susp ± food	75	carboxylate 0.35 (SS)	3	carboxylate 23-26 L	carboxylate 6-10				carboxylate 5.4 (24 hr)	
Peramivir	600 mg IV			46.8 (SD)	<30	12.56 L	20	ND	ND	ND	102.7 (0-∞)	
Rimantadine	100 mg po q12h	Tab ± food	75-93	0.4-0.5 (SS)	40	17-19 L/kg	25				3,5	6
Other non-HIV antivirals												
Tecovirimat	600 mg po q12h	Cap + food	ND	2.11 (SS)	77-82	1030 L (Vz/F)	20	ND	ND	ND	28.8 (24 hr, SS)	4-6
ANTIRETROVIRALS												
NRTIs												
Abacavir (ABC)	600 mg po q24h	Tab/soln ± food	83	4.3 (SS)	50	0.86 L/kg	1,5	20,6	3	36	12 (24 hr)	1,3
Didanosine enteric coated (ddI)	400 mg EC po q24h (pt ≥60 kg)	Cap/soln no food	30-40	ND	<5	308-363 L	1,6	25-40	2	ND	2,6(24 hr)	2
Emtricitabine (FTC)	200 mg po q24h	Cap/soln ± food	cap 93, soln 75	1.8 (SS)	<4	ND	10	39	3	ND	10 (24 hr)	1-2
Lamivudine (3TC)	300 mg po q24h	Tab/soln ± food	86	2.6 (SS)	<36	1.3 L/kg	5-7	18	2	ND	11 (300 mg x1)	ND
Stavudine (d4T)	40 mg po bid (pt ≥60 kg)	Cap/soln ± food	86	0.54 (SS)	<5	46 L	1.2-1.6	3,5	2	20	2.6 (24 hr)	1
Tenofovir alafenamide (TAF)	25 mg po q24h	Tab ± food	ND	0.16 (SS)	80	ND	0.51	ND	ND	ND	0.21 (24hr)	1
Tenofovir disoproxil (TDF)	300 mg po q24h	Tab ± food	39 w/food	0.3 (300 mg x1)	<7	1.2-1.3 L/kg Vss	17	>60	1	ND	2.3 (300 mg x1)	1
Zidovudine (ZDV)	300 mg po bid	Tab/cap/syrup ± food	60	1-2 (300 mg x1)	<38	1.6 L/kg	0.5-3	11	4	2	2.1 (300 mg x1)	0.5-1.5

Food Effect (po dosing): **+ food** = take with food, **no food** = take without food, **± food** = take with or without food; **Oral % AB** = % absorbed; **Peak Serum Level: SD** = after single dose, **SS** = steady state after multiple doses; **Volume of Distribution (Vd): V/F** = Vd/oral bioavailability, **Vss** = Vd at steady state, **Vss/F** = Vd at steady state/oral bioavailability; **CSF Penetration:** therapeutic efficacy comment based on dose, usual susceptibility or target organism & penetration into CSF; **AUC** = area under drug concentration curve; **24hr** = AUC 0-24; **Tmax** = time to max plasma concentration.

TABLE 9A (11) *(Footnotes at the end of table)*

DRUG	REFERENCE DOSE (SINGLE OR MULTIPLE)	FOOD REC (PO DRUGS)[1]	ORAL ABS (%)	PEAK SERUM CONC[2] (μg/mL)	PROTEIN BINDING (%)	VOLUME OF DISTRIBUTION (Vd)[3]	AVG SERUM T½ (hr)[4]	BILE PEN (%)[5]	CSF/ BLOOD[6] (%)	CSF PENETRATION[7]	AUC[8] (μg*hr/mL)	Tmax (hr)
ANTIRETROVIRALS *(continued)*												
NNRTIs												
Delavirdine (DLV)	400 mg po tid	Tab ± food	85	19 (SS)	98	ND	5,8	ND	3	ND	180 μM*hr (24 hr)	1
Doravirine (DOR)	100 mg po qd	Tab ± food	64	0.962 (SS)	76	60.5 L (Vss)	15	ND	ND	ND	16.1 (24 hr)	2
Efavirenz (EFV)	600 mg po q24h	Cap/tab no food	42	4.1 (SS)	99	252 L V/F	40-55	ND	3	ND	184 μM*hr (24 hr)	3-5
Etravirine (ETR)	200 mg po bid	Tab + food	ND	0.3 (SS)	99,9	ND	41	ND	2	ND	9 (24 hr)	2.5-4.0
Nevirapine (NVP)	200 mg po bid	Tab/susp ± food	>90	2 (200 mg x1)	60	1.21 L/kg Vss	25-30	ND	4	63	110 (24 hr)	4
Rilpivirine (RPV)	25 mg po qd	Tab + food	ND	0.1-0.2 (25 mg x1)	99,7	152 L	45-50	ND	ND	ND	2.4 (24 hr)	4-5
PIs												
Atazanavir (ATV)	400 mg po q24h	Cap/powder + food	Good	2.3 (SS)	86	88.3 L V/F	7	ND	2	ND	22.3 (24 hr)	2,5
Cobicistat	150 mg po q24h	Take with food	ND	0.99 (SS)	97-98	ND	4-Mar	ND	ND	ND	7.6 (24 hr)	3.5
Darunavir (DRV)	600 mg (+ RTV 100 mg) po bid	Tab/susp + food	82	3.5 (SS)	95	2 L/kg	15	ND	3	ND	116.8 (24 hr)	2.5-4.0
Fosamprenavir (FPV)	700 mg (+RTV 100 mg) po bid	Tab ± food; susp: adult no, peds +	ND	6 (SS)	90	ND	7,7	ND	3	ND	79.2 (24 hr)	2,5
Indinavir (IDV)	800 mg (+ RTV 100 mg) po bid	Boosted cap + food	65	20.2 μM (SS)	60	ND	1.2-2.0	ND	4	11	249 μM*hr (24 hr)	0,8 (fasting)
Lopinavir/RTV (LPV/r)	400 mg/100 mg po bid	Tab ± food, soln + food	ND	9.6 (SS)	98-99	ND	LPV 5-6	ND	3	ND	LPV 186 (24 hr)	LPV 4
Nelfinavir (NFV)	1250 mg po bid	Tab/powder + food	20-80	3-4 (SS)	98	2-7 L/kg V/F	3.5-5	ND	1	0	53 (24 hr)	ND
Ritonavir (RTV)	Boosting dose varies	Cap/soln + food	65	11.2 (600 mg bid SS)	98-99	0.41 L/kg V/F	3-5	ND	1	ND	121.7 (600 mg soln SD)	soln 2-4
Saquinavir (SQV)	1 gm (+RTV 100 mg) po bid	Tab/cap + food	4 (SQV alone)	0.37 (SS)	97	700 L Vss	1-2	ND	1	ND	29.2 (24 hr)	ND
Tipranavir (TPV)	500 mg (+RTV 200 mg) po bid	Cap/soln + food	Low	47-57 (SS)	99,9	7.7-10 L	5.5-6	ND	1	ND	1600 μM*hr (24 hr)	3
INSTIs												
Bictegravir (BIC)	50 mg q24h (as Biktarvy)	Tab ± food	ND	6.15 (SS)	>99	ND	17,3	ND	ND	ND	102 (24 hr)	2-4
Dolutegravir (DTG)	50 mg po q24h	Tab ± food	ND	3.67 (SS)	>99	17.4 L V/F	14	ND	4	ND	53.6 (24 hr)	2-3
Elvitegravir (EVG)	85-150 mg po q24h	Tab + food	ND	1.2-1.5 (SS)	98-99	ND	8.7 (w/RTV)	ND	ND	ND	18 (24 hr)	4
Raltegravir (RAL)	400 mg po bid	Tab/susp ± food	ND	11.2 μM (SS)	83	287 L Vss/F	9	ND	3	1-53.5	28.7 μM*hr (12 hr)	3

Food Effect (po dosing): + food = take with food, **no food** = take without food, **± food** = take with or without food; **Oral % AB** = % absorbed; **Peak Serum Level: SD** = after single dose, **SS** = steady state after multiple doses; **Volume of Distribution (Vd): V/F** = Vd/oral bioavailability, **Vss** = Vd at steady state, **Vss/F** = Vd at steady state/oral bioavailability; **CSF Penetration:** therapeutic efficacy comment based on dose, usual susceptibility or target organism & penetration into CSF; **AUC** = area under drug concentration curve; **24hr** = AUC 0-24; **Tmax** = time to max plasma concentration.

TABLE 9A (12) *(Footnotes at the end of table)*

DRUG	REFERENCE DOSE (SINGLE OR MULTIPLE)	FOOD REC (PO DRUGS)[1]	ORAL ABS (%)	PEAK SERUM CONC[2] (μg/mL)	PROTEIN BINDING (%)	VOLUME OF DISTRIBUTION (Vd)[3]	AVG SERUM T½ (hr)[4]	BILE PEN (%)[5]	CSF/ BLOOD[6] (%)	CSF PENETRATION[7]	AUC[8] (μg*hr/mL)	Tmax (hr)
ANTIRETROVIRALS *(continued)*												
Fusion, Entry Inhibitors												
Enfuvirtide (ENF, T20)	90 mg sc bid		84 (sc % ab)	5 (SS)	92	5.5 L Vss	3,8	ND	1	ND	97.4 (24 hr)	4-8
Maraviroc (MVC)	300 mg po bid	Tab ± food	33	0.3-0.9 (SS)	76	194 L	14-18	ND	3	ND	3 (24 hr)	0.5-4.0
Monoclonal Antibodies												
Ibalizumab-uiyk	2 gm IV load, then 800 mg IV q2 weeks	ND	ND	ND	ND	4.8 L	Dose-dependent (2.7-64 depending on dose)	ND	ND	ND	ND	ND

1 Refers to adult oral preparations unless otherwise noted; + food = take with food, no food = take without food, ± food = take with or without food
2 SD = after a single dose, SS = at steady state
3 V/F = Vd/oral bioavailability; Vss = Vd at steady state; Vss/F = Vd at steady state/oral bioavailability
4 Assumes CrCl >80 mL/min
5 (Peak concentration in bile/peak concentration in serum) x 100. If blank, no data
6 CSF concentrations with inflammation
7 Judgment based on drug dose and organism susceptibility. CSF concentration ideally ≥10x MIC.
8 AUC = area under serum concentration vs. time curve; 12 hr = AUC 0-12, 24 hr = AUC 0-24
9 Concern over seizure potential
10 Take all oral FQs 2-4 hours before sucralfate or any multivalent cation (calcium, iron, zinc)
11 Given with Atovaquone as Malarone for malaria prophylaxis

TABLE 9B – PHARMACODYNAMICS OF ANTIBACTERIALS*

BACTERIAL KILLING/PERSISTENT EFFECT	DRUGS	THERAPY GOAL	PK/PD MEASUREMENT
Concentration-dependent/Prolonged persistent effect	Aminoglycosides; daptomycin; ketolides; quinolones; metro	High peak serum concentration	24-hr AUC[1]/MIC
Time-dependent/No persistent effect	Penicillins; cephalosporins; carbapenems; monobactams	Long duration of exposure	Time above MIC
Time-dependent/Moderate to long persistent effect	Clindamycin; erythro/azithro/clarithro; linezolid; tetracyclines; vancomycin	Enhanced amount of drug	24-hr AUC[1]/MIC

* Adapted from *Craig, WA: IDC No. Amer 17:479, 2003 & Drusano, G.L.: CID 44:79, 2007*

Food Effect (po dosing): **+ food** = take with food, **no food** = take without food, **± food** = take with or without food; **Oral % AB** = % absorbed; **Peak Serum Level: SD** = after single dose, **SS** = steady state after multiple doses; **Volume of Distribution (Vd): V/F** = Vd/oral bioavailability, **Vss** = Vd at steady state, **Vss/F** = Vd at steady state/oral bioavailability; **CSF Penetration:** therapeutic efficacy comment based on dose, usual susceptibility or target organism & penetration into CSF; **AUC** = area under drug concentration curve; **24hr** = AUC 0-24; **Tmax** = time to max plasma concentration.

TABLE 9C – ENZYME -AND TRANSPORTER- MEDIATED INTERACTIONS OF ANTIMICROBIALS

>50% of all drugs are metabolized by one or more members of the CYP450 enzyme system. The metabolism of a drug that is a substrate of a particular CYP enzyme may be induced (accelerated) by another drug, resulting in under dosing and therapeutic failure. Conversely the metabolism of a drug may be inhibited (slowed) by another drug, resulting in overdosing and toxicity. A drug may act a substrate for more than one enzyme, or it may inhibit or induce multiple enzymes. Inhibition tends to be a relatively quick process related to the dose of the inhibitor, whereas induction occurs more slowly. Risk is amplified when two or more drugs that are enzyme inhibitors or inducers are administered. CYP450 enzymes commonly involved in drug interactions include CYP3A4, CYP2C9/19, CYP1A2, and CYP2D6.

Drug transporter systems may also be involved in drug interactions. Transporters are found in many tissues, such as the kidney and GI tract, and they work to pump drugs into cells (influx) or out of cells (efflux). Examples of important drug transporters systems include P-glycoprotein (PGP), organic anion transporter (OAT), and organic cation transporter (OCT).

Knowledge of these enzymes is useful in understanding clinically relevant drug interactions and can also assist in predicting previously unrecognized interactions. With respect to specific antimicrobials, always check for drug-drug interactions when ordering these inhibitors that may cause elevated serum concentrations: macrolides, ciprofloxacin, metronidazole, TMP-SMX, isoniazid, azole antifungals, antiretrovirals, and anti-HCV drugs. Nafcillin, rifamycins, and certain antiretrovirals are known to induce metabolism and lead to treatment failure. If a drug interaction is recognized and no suitable alternative regimen exists, check serum concentration of the affected drug (if available), adjust dose, and monitor for toxicity. See *Table 22A* for common drug-drug interactions.

DRUG	ISOZYME/TRANSPORTER THAT DRUG IS A SUBSTRATE OF	INHIBITED BY DRUG	INDUCED BY DRUG	IMPACT ON SERUM DRUG CONCENTRATIONS*
Antibacterials				
Azithromycin	PGP	PGP (weak)		mild ↑
Cephalexin	MATE1			No effect expected
Chloramphenicol		2C19, 3A4		↑
Ciprofloxacin		1A2; 3A4 (minor)		↑
Clarithromycin	3A4	3A4, PGP, OAT		↑
Clindamycin	3A4			No effect expected
Dicloxacillin			2C9, 2C19, 3A4	↓
Eravacycline	3A4			No effect expected
Erythromycin	3A4, PGP	3A4, PGP, OAT		↑
Flucloxacillin			3A4?	↓
Fusidic acid	3A4	3A4, BCRP, OATP1B1		↑
Imipenem-cilastatin-relebactam	Rele: OAT3, OAT4, MATE1, MATE2K			No effect expected (VPA interaction different mech)
Lefamulin	3A4	3A4		↑
Levofloxacin		OCT		↑
Meropenem	OAT1, OAT3			No effect expected
Metronidazole		2C9		↑
Nafcillin			2C9 (?), 3A4	↓
Norfloxacin		1A2 (weak)		mild ↑
Omadacycline	PGP			No effect expected
Oritavancin		2C9 (weak), 2C19 (weak)	2D6 (weak), 3A4 (weak)	mild ↑ or ↓
Plazomicin		MATE1, MATE2-K		↑
Pristinamycin		3A4		↑
Quinupristin-Dalfopristin		3A4		↑
Rifampin	PGP, OATP1B1	OAT, OATP1B1	1A2, 2B6, 2C8, 2C9, 2C19, 2D6 (weak), 3A4, PGP	↓

TABLE 9C (2)

DRUG	Substrate	Inhibits	Induces	Impact
Antibacterials *(continued)*				
Rifaximin	3A4, PGP, OAT1A2, OATP1B1/3	PGP		No effect expected
Sarecycline		PGP		↑
Telithromycin		3A4; PGP (?)		↑
Tigecycline	PGP			No effect expected
TMP/SMX	SMX: 2C9 (major), 3A4	TMP: 2C8; SMX: 2C9		↑
Trimethoprim		2C8		↑
Antifungals				
Fluconazole		2C9, 2C19, 3A4		↑
Isavuconazole	3A4	3A4, PGP, OCT2		↑
Itraconazole	3A4	3A4, PGP		↑
Ketoconazole	3A4	3A4, PGP		↑
Posaconazole	PGP	3A4, PGP		↑
Terbinafine		2D6		↑
Voriconazole	2C9, 2C19, 3A4	2C9, 2C19, 3A4		↑
Antimycobacterials (Rifampin listed above)				
Bedaquiline	3A4			No effect expected
Delamanid	3A4			No effect expected
Isoniazid (INH)		2C19, 3A4	2E	↑ or ↓
Pretomanid		OAT3		↑
Rifabutin	3A4		3A4	↓
Rifapentine			2C9, 3A4	↓
Thalidomide	2C19			No effect expected
Antiparasitics				
Artemether/Lumefantrine	3A4 (Art, Lum)	2D6 (Lum)	3A4 (Art)	↑ or ↓
Chloroquine	2C8, 2D6	2D6		↑
Dapsone	3A4			No effect expected
Fexinidazole	1A2, 2B6, 2C19, 2D6 (minor), 3A4/5; also FMO3			
Halofantrine	3A4	2D6		↑
Mefloquine	3A4, PGP	PGP		↑
Praziquantel	3A4			No effect expected
Primaquine	2D6, others?			No effect expected
Proguanil	2C19 (→cycloguanil)			No effect expected
Quinine sulfate	main 3A4, also 1A2, 2C9, 2D6	2D6		↑
Tafenoquine		OCT, MATE1, MATE2K		↑
Tinidazole	3A4			No effect expected
Triclabendazole		2C19		↑

TABLE 9C (3)

DRUG	Substrate	Inhibits	Induces	Impact
Antivirals (Hepatitis B)				
Entecavir	OCT2			↑
Antivirals (Hepatitis C)				
Daclatasvir	3A4, PGP			↑
Dasabuvir	3A4, PGP, OATP1B1	2C8, UGT1A1, OATP1B1, OATP1B3		↑
Elbasvir	CYP3A4, PGP	BCRP		↑
Glecaprevir	PGP, BCRP, OATP1/3	1A2 (weak), 3A4 (weak), PGP, BCRP, OATP1B1/3, UGT1A1 (weak)		↑
Grazoprevir	CYP3A4, PGP, OATP1B1/3	CYP3A4 (weak), BCRP		↑
Ledipasvir	PGP, BCRP	PGP, BCRP		↑
Ombitasvir	3A4, PGP	2C8, UGT1A1		↑
Paritaprevir	2C8, 2D6, 3A4, PGP	UGT1A1, OATP1B1		↑
Pibrentasvir	PGP, BCRP	1A2 (weak), 3A4 (weak), PGP, BCRP, OATP1B1/3, UGT1A1 (weak)		↑
Simeprevir	3A4, PGP, OAT	1A2 (weak), 3A4, PGP, OAT		↑
Sofosbuvir	PGP, BCRP			No effect expected
Velpatasvir	2B6, 2C8, 3A4, PGP, BCRP, OATP1B1/3	PGP, BCRP, OATP1B1/3, OATP2B1		↑
Antivirals (Herpesvirus)				
Cidofovir	OAT1, OAT3			No effect expected
Letermovir	2D6, 3A4, OATP1B1/3	2C8, 3A4, OATP1B1/3	2C9, 2C19, 3A4	↑ or ↓
Antivirals (miscellaneous)				
Tecovirimat	UGT1A1, 1A4	2C8 (weak), 2C19 (weak), BCRP (weak)	3A4 (weak)	↑ or ↓
Antiretrovirals				
Atazanavir	3A4, PGP	1A2, 2C8, 3A4, UGT1A1		↑
Bictegravir (BIC)	3A4, UGT1A1	OCT2, MATE1		↑
Cobicistat (part of Stribild)	2D6, 3A4	2D6, 3A4, PGP, BCRP, OATP1B1, OATP1B3		↑
Darunavir	3A4	3A4		↑
Delavirdine	2D6, 3A4	2C9, 2C19, 3A4		↑
Dolutegravir	3A4, UGT1A1			↑
Doravirine	3A4			No effect expected
Efavirenz	2B6, 3A4	2B6, 2C9, 2C19	2C19, 3A4	↑ or ↓
Elvitegravir (part of Stribild)	CYP3A4, UGT1A1/3	PGP (weak)	2C9 (weak)	mild ↑ or ↓
Etravirine	2C9, 2C19, 3A4	2C9; 2C19 (weak)	3A4	↑ or ↓
Fosamprenavir	3A4	3A4		↑
Indinavir	3A4, PGP	3A4, PGP		↑
Lamivudine	PGP, BCRP, MATE1, MATE2-K, OCT2			No effect expected
Lopinavir	3A4	3A4		↑

TABLE 9C (4)

DRUG	Substrate	Inhibits	Induces	Impact
Antiretrovirals *(continued)*				
Maraviroc	3A4, PGP	2D6		↑
Nelfinavir	2C19, 3A4, PGP	3A4, PGP	3A4 (?)	↑ or ↓
Nevirapine	2B6, 3A4		3A4	↓
Raltegravir	UGT			No effect expected
Rilpivirine	3A4			No effect expected
Ritonavir	3A4, PGP	2D6, 3A4, PGP	1A2, 2B6, 2C9, 3A4 (long term), PGP (long term), UGT	↑ or ↓
Saquinavir	3A4, PGP	3A4, PGP		↑
Tenofovir alafenamide	PGP, BCRP, OATP1B1/3			No effect expected
Tenofovir disoproxil fum	PGP, BCRP			No effect expected
Tipranavir	3A4, PGP	OAT	PGP (weak)	↑ or ↓

***Refers to serum concentrations of companion drugs that may be affected by the listed antimicrobial. ↑=increase, ↓=decrease, blank=no drugs should be affected**

TERMINOLOGY:

BCRP = breast cancer resistance protein
CYP450 nomenclature, e.g. 3A4: 3 = family, A = subfamily, 4 = gene
OAT = organic anion transporter
OATP = organic anion transporter polypeptide
OCT = organic cation transporter
PGP = P-glycoprotein
UGT = uridine diphosphate glucuronosyltransferase

REFERENCES:

Hansten PD, Horn JR. The Top 100 Drug Interactions: A Guide to Patient Management. Freeland (WA): H&H Publications, 2014; primary literature; package inserts.

TABLE 10A – ANTIBIOTIC DOSAGE* AND SIDE-EFFECTS

CLASS, AGENT, GENERIC NAME (TRADE NAME)	USUAL ADULT DOSAGE*	ADVERSE REACTIONS, COMMENTS
NATURAL PENICILLINS		**Allergic reactions a major issue.** 10% of all hospital admissions give history of pen allergy; but only 10% have allergic reaction if given penicillin. Why? Possible reasons: inaccurate history, waning immunity with age, aberrant response during viral illness. If given, **Bicillin C-R IM (procaine Pen + benzathine Pen)** could be reaction to procaine. **Most serious reaction is immediate IgE-mediated anaphylaxis;** incidence only 0.05% but 5-10% fatal. Other IgE-mediated reactions: urticaria, angioedema, laryngeal edema, bronchospasm, abdominal pain with emesis, or hypotension. All appear within 4 hrs. Can form IgE antibody against either the beta-lactam ring or the R-group side chain. **Morbilliform rash after 72 hrs is not IgE-mediated and not serious.** **Serious late allergic reactions:** Coombs-positive hemolytic anemia, neutropenia, thrombocytopenia, serum sickness, interstitial nephritis, hepatitis, eosinophilia, drug fever. **Cross-allergy to cephalosporins and carbapenems** varies from 0-11%. One factor is similarity, or lack of similarity, of side chains. **For pen desensitization,** *see Table 7.* For skin testing, suggest referral to allergist. High **CSF** concentrations cause seizures. Reduce dosage with renal impairment, *see Table 17A.* Allergy refs: *CID 59:1113, 2014; JAC 69:20-43, 2014; CID 58:1140, 2014.*
Benzathine penicillin G (Bicillin L-A)	**600,000–1.2 million units IM q2–4 wks**	
Penicillin G	**Low: 600,000–1.2 million units IM per day** **High: ≥20 million units IV q24h(=12 gm) div q4h**	
Penicillin V (250 & 500 mg caps)	**0.25–0.5 gm po bid, tid, qid before meals & at bedtime.** Pen V preferred over Pen G for oral therapy due to greater acid stability.	
PENICILLINASE-RESISTANT PENICILLINS		
Dicloxacillin (Dynapen) **(250 & 500 mg caps)**	**0.125–0.5 gm po q6h before meals**	Blood levels ~2 times greater than cloxacillin so preferred for po therapy. Hemorrhagic cystitis reported. Acute abdominal pain with GI bleeding without antibiotic-associated colitis also reported. Can impede warfarin.
Flucloxacillin[NUS] (Floxapen, Lutropin, Staphcil)	**0.25–0.5 gm po q6h** **1–2 gm IV q4h**	Cholestatic hepatitis occurs in 1:15,000 exposures: more frequently in age >55 yrs, females and therapy >2 wks duration. Can appear wks after end of therapy and take wks to resolve *(JAC 66:1431, 2011)*. **Recommendation: use only in severe infection.**
Nafcillin (Unipen, Nafcil)	**1–2 gm IV/IM q4h.** Due to >90% protein binding, need 12 gm/day for bacteremia.	Extravasation can result in tissue necrosis. With 200–300 mg per kg per day hypokalemia may occur. **Reversible neutropenia (over 10% with ≥21-day rx, occasionally WBC <1000 per mm³).** Can impede warfarin effect.
Oxacillin (Prostaphlin)	**1–2 gm IV/IM q4h.** Due to >90% protein binding, need 12 gm/day for bacteremia.	**Hepatic dysfunction with ≥12 gm per day.** LFTs usually ↑ 2–24 days after start of rx, reversible. In children, more rash and liver toxicity with oxacillin as compared to nafcillin *(CID 34:50, 2002)*.
AMINOPENICILLINS		
Amoxicillin (Amoxil, Polymox)	**250 mg–1 gm po tid**	IV available in UK & Europe. IV amoxicillin rapidly converted to ampicillin. Rash with infectious mono– *see Ampicillin.* Increased risk of cross-allergenicity with oral cephalosporins with identical side-chains: cefadroxil, cefprozil.
Amoxicillin extended release (Moxatag)	**One 775 mg tab po once daily**	Allergic reactions, C. difficile associated diarrhea, false positive test for urine glucose with clinitest.
Amoxicillin-clavulanate (Augmentin) **Amox-clav extra-strength peds suspension (ES-600)** **AM-CL-ER—extended release adult tabs**	*See Comment for adult products* **Peds Extra-Strength susp.: 600/42.9 per 5 mL. Dose: 90/6.4 mg/kg div bid.** For adult formulations, *see Comments* IV amox-clav available in Europe	With bid regimen, less clavulanate & less diarrhea. In pts with immediate allergic reaction to Amox-clav, ⅓ due to Clav component *(J Allergy Clin Immunol 125:502, 2010)*. **Hepatotoxicity linked to clavulanic acid; Amox-clav causes 13-23% of drug-induced liver injury. Onset delayed. Usually mild; rare liver failure** *(Gastroenterol 148:1340, 2015; NEJM 381:264, 2019)*. **Comparison adult Augmentin dosage regimens:** Augmentin 500/125 1 tab po tid Augmentin 875/125 1 tab po bid Augmentin-XR 1000/62.5 2 tabs po bid
Ampicillin (Principen) (250 & 500 mg caps)	**0.25–0.5 gm po q6h** **50–200 mg/kg IV/day div q6h**	A maculopapular rash occurs (not urticarial), **not true penicillin allergy,** in 65–100% pts with infectious mono, 90% with chronic lymphocytic leukemia, and 15–20% in pts taking allopurinol. EBV-associated rash does not indicate permanent allergy; post-EBV no rash when challenged. Increased risk of true cross-allergenicity with oral cephalosporins with identical side chains: cefaclor, cephalexin, loracarbef.

*NOTE: all dosage recommendations are for adults (unless otherwise indicated) & assume normal renal function.
(See page 2 for abbreviations)

TABLE 10A (2)

CLASS, AGENT, GENERIC NAME (TRADE NAME)	USUAL ADULT DOSAGE*	ADVERSE REACTIONS, COMMENTS
AMINOPENICILLINS *(continued)*		
Ampicillin-sulbactam (Unasyn)	**1.5-3 gm IV q6h. For resistant Acinetobacter, 8 gm Amp/4 gm sulb IV over 4 hr q8h in combination with Meropenem and Polymyxin B.**	Supplied in vials: amp 2 gm, sulbactam 1 gm. Adjust dose for renal insufficiency, *see Table 17A*. For combination regimen dosing (Amp-sulb + MER + Polymyxin B), *see Table 1, page 43*).
ANTIPSEUDOMONAL PENICILLINS		
Piperacillin-tazobactam (Zosyn) Prolonged infusion dosing, *see Comment and Table 10D*. Obesity dosing, *see Table 17C*.	**Favor prolonged infusion:** load with 4.5 gm IV over 30 min, then 4 hrs later start 3.375 gm IV over 4 hrs & repeat q8h. Ties up IV line for 12 of 24 hrs. Old dose (except P. aeruginosa): 3.375 gm IV q6h or 4.5 gm q8h. Old P. aeruginosa dose: 3.375 gm q4h or 4.5 gm q6h.	Prolonged infusion references *(CID 44:357, 2007; AAC 54:460, 2010)*. • Cystic fibrosis + P. aeruginosa infection: 350-450 mg/kg/day div q4-6h For obesity dosing adjustment *see Table 17C, page 252*. Documented drug-induced thrombocytopenia *(J Thrombo Haemostasis 11:169, 2012)*. Reports of greater risk of nephrotoxicity from PIP/TZ + Vancomycin compared with Cefepime + Vancomycin *(AAC 61: e02089-16, 2017; CID 64: 116, 2017)* others find no increased risk *(CID 68:1456, 2019)*.
Temocillin[NUS]	**2 gm IV q12h.**	Semi-synthetic penicillin stable in presence of classical & ESBLs plus AmpC beta-lactamases. Source: *www.eumedica.be*
CARBAPENEMS. Review: *AAC 55:4943, 2011.* **NOTE: Cross allergenicity: In studies of pts with history of Pen-allergy but no confirmatory skin testing, 0-11% had allergic reactions with cephalosporin therapy** *(JAC 54:1155, 2004)*. **In better studies, pts with positive skin tests for Pen allergy were given Carbapenem: no reaction in 99%** *(J Allergy Clin Immunol 124:167, 2009)*. Of 12 pts with IgE-mediated reaction to ceph, 2 suffered rash & 1 an IgE reaction when given a carbapenem *(CID 59:1113, 2014)*. Incidence of carbapenem-resistant GNB highest in Georgia, Maryland & New York *(JAMA 314:1455 & 1479, 2015)*.		
Doripenem (Doribax) Ref: *CID 49:291, 2009. For prolonged infusion dosing, see Table 10D*	Intra-abdominal & complicated UTI: **500 mg IV q8h (1-hr infusion).** For prolonged infusion, *see Table 10D, page 129*. Do not use for pneumonia	Most common adverse reactions (≥5%): Headache, nausea, diarrhea, rash & phlebitis. Seizure reported in post-marketing surveillance. Can lower serum valproic acid levels. Adjust dose if renal impairment. Somewhat more stable in solution than **IMP** or **MER** *(JAC 65:1023, 2010; CID 49:291, 2009)*. FDA safety announcement (01/05/12): Trial of DORI for the treatment of VAP stopped early due to safety concerns. Compared to IMP, patients treated with DORI were observed to have excess mortality and poorer cure rate. **NOTE: DORI is not approved to treat any type of pneumonia; DORI is not approved for doses greater than 500 mg q8h.**
Ertapenem (Invanz)	**1 gm IV/IM q24h.**	**Lidocaine** diluent for IM use; ask about lidocaine allergy. Standard dosage may be inadequate in obesity (BMI ≥40). Reports of DRESS (drug rash eosinophilia systemic symptoms) Syndrome. Visual hallucinations reported *(NZ Med J 122:76, 2009)*. No predictable activity vs. P. aeruginosa.
Imipenem - cilastatin (Primaxin, Tienam) Ref: *JAC 58:916, 2006*	**0.5 gm IV q6h**; for P. aeruginosa: 1 gm q6–8h *(see Comment)*.	For P. aeruginosa, increase dosage to 3 or 4 gm per day div. q8h or q6h. Continuous infusion of carbapenems more efficacious & safer *(AAC 49:1881, 2005)*. **Seizures:** risk of seizure low but greatest with carbapenems. No diff between IMP and MER *(JAC 69:2043, 2014)*. Cilastatin blocks enzymatic degradation of Imipenem in lumen of renal proximal tubule & also prevents tubular toxicity. Compared to MER, more in vitro resistance to IMP vs. Proteus sp., Providencia sp., Morganella sp. *(Can ID Med Micro 2014,25:285)*
Imipenem-cilastatin-relebactam (Recarbrio)	**1.25 gm IV over 30 min q6h** Adjust dose if CrCl < 90 mL/min	**Seizure risk:** avoid concomitant valproic acid or divalproex sodium. C. diff toxin-mediated diarrhea reported. Active vs. KPC-producing GNB.
Meropenem (Merrem)	**0.5–1 gm IV q8h. Up to 2 gm IV q8h for meningitis. Prolonged infusion** in critically ill: If CrCl ≥50: 2 gm (over 3 hr) q8h If CrCl 30-49: 1 gm (over 3 hr) q8h If CrCl 10-29: 1 gm (over 3 hr) q12h *(Inten Care Med 37:632, 2011)*.	**Seizures:** In meta-analysis, risk of seizure low but greatest with carbapenems among beta-lactams. No diff between IMP and MER *(JAC 69:2043, 2014)*. Comments: Does not require a dehydropeptidase inhibitor (cilastatin). Activity vs aerobic gm-neg. slightly ↑ over IMP, activity vs staph & strep slightly ↓; anaerobes: B. ovatus, B. distasonis more resistant to meropenem.

*NOTE: all dosage recommendations are for adults (unless otherwise indicated) & assume normal renal function.

TABLE 10A (3)

CLASS, AGENT, GENERIC NAME (TRADE NAME)	USUAL ADULT DOSAGE*	ADVERSE REACTIONS, COMMENTS
CARBAPENEMS *(continued)*		
Meropenem-vaborbactam (Vabomere)	4 gm (2 gm meropenem + 2 gm vaborbactam) IV q8h infused over 3 hrs (with estimated eGFR >50 mL/min).	Combination of Meropenem with vaborbactam. Vaborbactam inhibits common serine beta-lactamases, ESBLs, KPCs. and AmpC but not metallo-beta-lactamases or oxacillinases with carbapenemase activity. Approved for the the treatment of complicated urinary tract infections in patients age ≥18 years caused by *E. coli, K. pneumoniae, E. cloacae*, and other susceptible aerobic gram-negative bacilli. **Contraindicated:** if known hypersensitivity to meropenem or beta lactams. **AEs:** hypersensitivity reactions, seizure potential, C. diff-associated diarrhea, thrombocytopenia, neuromotor impairment, phlebitis (infusion site), diarrhea, headache. **Major interactions:** valproic acid (concomitant use not recommended), probenecid.
MONOBACTAMS		
Aztreonam (Azactam)	**1 gm q8h–2 gm IV q6h.**	Can be used in pts with allergy to penicillins/cephalosporins with exception of Ceftazidime as **side-chains of Aztreonam and Ceftazidime are identical.** PK/PD *(JAC 2016,71:2704)*.
Aztreonam for Inhalation (Cayston)	**75 mg inhaled tid x 28 days.** Use bronchodilator before each inhalation.	Improves respiratory symptoms in CF pts colonized with P. aeruginosa. Alternative to inhaled Tobra. AEs: bronchospasm, cough, wheezing. So far, no emergence of other resistant pathogens. Ref: *Chest 135:1223, 2009.*
CEPHALOSPORINS (1st parenteral, then oral drugs). NOTE: Prospective data demonstrate correlation between use of cephalosporins (esp. 3rd generation) and ↑ risk of C. difficile toxin-induced diarrhea. May also ↑ risk of colonization with vancomycin-resistant enterococci. *See Oral Cephalosporins, page 118,* **for important note on cross-allergenicity.**		
1st Generation, Parenteral		
Cefazolin (Ancef, Kefzol)	**1-1.5 gm IV/IM q8h, occasionally 2 gm IV q8h for serious infections, e.g., MSSA bacteremia (max. 12 gm/day)**	**Do not give into lateral ventricles—seizures!** No activity vs. MRSA. Very low risk of cross-allergenicity with other cephalosporins or beta-lactams.
2nd Generation, Parenteral (Cephamycins): May be active in vitro vs. ESBL-producing aerobic gram-negative bacilli. Do not use as there are no clinical data for efficacy.		
Cefotetan (Cefotan)	**1–3 gm IV/IM q12h. (max. dose not >6 gm q24h).**	Increasing resistance of B. fragilis, Prevotella bivia, Prevotella disiens (most common in pelvic infections); do not use for intra-abdominal infections. Methylthiotetrazole (MTT) side chain can inhibit vitamin K activation. Avoid alcohol-disulfiram reaction.
Cefoxitin (Mefoxin)	**1 gm q8h–2 gm IV/IM q6-8h.**	Increasing resistance of B. fragilis isolates.
Cefuroxime (Kefurox, Ceftin, Zinacef)	**0.75–1.5 gm IV/IM q8h.**	Improved activity against H. influenzae compared with 1st generation cephalosporins. *See Cefuroxime axetil for oral preparation.*
3rd Generation, Parenteral – Use correlates with incidence of C. difficile toxin diarrhea; most are inactivated by ESBLs and amp C cephalosporinase from aerobic gram-negative bacilli.		
Cefoperazone-Sulbactam[NUS] (Sulperazon)	**Usual dose (Cefoperazone comp) 1–2 gm IV q12h;** if larger doses, do not exceed 4 gm/day of sulbactam.	In SE Asia & elsewhere, used to treat intra-abdominal, biliary, & gyn. infections. Other uses due to broad spectrum of activity. Possible clotting problem due to side-chain.
Cefotaxime (Claforan)	**1 gm q8–12h to 2 gm IV q4h.**	Maximum daily dose: 12 gm; give as 4 gm IV q8h. Similar to ceftriaxone but, unlike ceftriaxone, but requires multiple daily doses.
Ceftizoxime (Cefizox)	From **1-2 gm IV q8-12h** up to **2 gm IV q4h.**	Maximum daily dose: 12 gm; can give as 4 gm IV q8h
Ceftobiprole[NUS] Similar activity to ceftaroline, incl MRSA	**0.5 gm IV over 2 hrs q8h**	Associated with caramel-like taste disturbance. Ref.: *Clin Microbiol Infections 13(Suppl 2):17 & 25, 2007.* Hydrolyzed by ESBL & AmpC cephalosporinase.
Ceftriaxone (Rocephin)	Commonly used IV dosage in adults: **1-2 gm once daily** Purulent meningitis: **2 gm q12h.** Can give **IM** in 1% lidocaine.	**"Pseudocholelithiasis"** 2° to sludge in gallbladder by ultrasound (50%), symptomatic (9%) *(NEJM 322:1821, 1990)*. More likely with ≥2 gm per day with pt on total parenteral nutrition and not eating *(AnIM 115:712, 1991)*. Has led to cholecystectomy *(JID 17:356, 1995)* and gallstone pancreatitis *(Ln 17:662, 1998)*. Can cause drug-induced thrombocytopenia *(J Thrombo & Haemo 2012,11:169)*. Combination of Ceftriaxone & Lansoprazole led to 1.4 x increased risk of increased QTc to >500 msec *(J Am Coll Cardio 2016,68:1756)*. For Ceftriaxone Desensitization, *see Table 7, page 91.*

*NOTE: all dosage recommendations are for adults (unless otherwise indicated) & assume normal renal function.

CLASS, AGENT, GENERIC NAME (TRADE NAME)	USUAL ADULT DOSAGE*	ADVERSE REACTIONS, COMMENTS
CEPHALOSPORINS *(continued)*		
Antipseudomonal		
Cefepime (Maxipime) For obesity dosing, *see Table 17C*	**Usual dose: 1–2 gm IV q8-12h.** **Prolonged infusion dosing:** Initial dose: 15 mg/kg over 30 min, then immediately begin: If CrCl >60: 6 gm (over 24 hr) daily If CrCl 30-60: 4 gm (over 24 hr) daily If CrCl 11-29: 2 gm (over 24 hr) daily	Active vs P. aeruginosa and many strains of Enterobacter, Serratia, C. freundii resistant to Ceftazidime, Cefotaxime, Aztreonam. More active vs MSSA than 3rd generation cephalosporins. Not "porin-dependent". Neutropenia after 14 days rx *(Scand J Infect Dis 42:156, 2010)*. Failures vs. E. cloacae bacteremia with MIC of 4-8 mcg/mL *(AAC 2015,59:7558)*. **FDA Safety warning (June 2012):** risk of non-convulsive status epilepticus, especially in pts with renal insufficiency when doses not adjusted. Seizure activity resolved after drug discontinuation and/or hemodialysis in the majority of pts. Postulated mechanism: binding to GABA receptors *(Scand J Infect Dis 46:272, 2014; Crit Care 17:R264, 2013.*
Cefpirome[NUS] (HR 810)	**1–2 gm IV q12h**	Active against Enterobacteriaceae and aerobic Gram-positive cocci (not enterococci or MRSA). Has activity against some P. aeruginosa. No useful activity against anaerobic bacilli.
Ceftazidime (Fortaz, Tazicef)	**Usual dose: 1–2 gm IV/IM q8–12h.** **Prolonged infusion dosing:** Initial dose: 15 mg/kg over 30 min, then immediately begin: If CrCl >50: 6 gm (over 24 hr) daily If CrCl 31-50: 4 gm (over 24 hr) daily If CrCl 10-30: 2 gm (over 24 hr) daily *(AAC 49:3550, 2005; Infect 37:418, 2009)*.	Often used in healthcare-associated infections, where P. aeruginosa is a consideration. Use may result in ↑ incidence of C. difficile-assoc. diarrhea and/or selection of vancomycin-resistant E. faecium. Risk of cross-allergenicity with aztreonam (same side chain).
Anti-staphylococcal (MRSA)		
Ceftaroline fosamil (Teflaro)	**600 mg IV q12h (5-60 min infusion)** Pneumonia/bacteremia 600 mg IV q8h[NAI]. *See Comment*	**Avid binding to PBP 2a; active vs. MRSA.** Inactivated by Amp C & ESBL enzymes. Approved for MRSA skin and skin structure infections and used for MRSA pneumonia and bacteremia, but not approved indications *(J Infect Chemother 19:42, 2013)*. Active in vitro vs. VISA, VRSA. Refs: *CID 52:1156, 2011.* Used successfully for bacteremia and bone/joint infections, but NAI *(AAC 58:2541, 2014)*. Risk of neutropenia *(JAC 71:2010, 2016; AAC 60: 264, 2016)*.
Anti-ESBL resistant GNB		
Ceftolozane-tazobactam (Zerbaxa) Ref: *CID 2016,63:234*	1.5 gm (1/0.5 gm) IV q8h for gm-neg complicated UTI & complicated intra-abdominal (add Metro 500 mg IV q8h) infection	Infuse over 1 hr. Active vs. P. aeruginosa *(AAC 2017,61:e0046517)* and many gm-neg bacteria producing ESBLs. Cross-reaction in Beta-lactam allergic pts. Decreased efficacy w/ CrCl 30-50 mL/min. Also approved for hospital-acquired & ventilator-associated pneumonia.
Anti-ESBL and Serine-carbapenemase resistant GNB		
Ceftazidime-avibactam (Avycaz) Ref: *CID 2016,63:234; JAC 2016,71:2713*	2.5 gm (2 gm Ceftazidime/0.5 gm avibactam) IV over 2 hrs q8h for gram-negative complicated UTI & add metronidazole 500 mg IV q8h for complicated intra-abdominal infection. Also approved for suscept GNB causing nosocomial pneumonia *(LnID 2017,18:229 & 285)*.	Active against ESBL- & KPC-producing aerobic gm-neg bacilli. No activity vs. GNB-producing metallo-carbapenemases. Decreased efficacy in pts with w/ CrCl 30-50 mL/min (in clinical trials).
Anti-ESBL, Amp C, Serine & Metallo Carbapenemase GNB		
Cefiderocol (Fetroja) See FDA-approved package insert	Adult: 2 gm IV over 3 hrs q8h x 7-14 days Adjust dose for renal impairment (see Table 17A) Peds: no data	Siderophore cephalosporin FDA-approved for treatment of adults with complicated UTI, including pyelonephritis. Stable in vitro in presence of virtually all cephalosporinases and carbapenemases. Reserve for use in pts. With limited or no treatment options. Not active vs. gram positive and anaerobic bacteria. Note: In randomized trial of cefiderocol vs. Best Available Therapy for pneumonia, bacteremia, complicated UTI due to MDR GNB, higher all-cause mortality with Cefiderocol, but not statistically significant.

(See page 2 for abbreviations)

*NOTE: all dosage recommendations are for adults (unless otherwise indicated) & assume normal renal function.

TABLE 10A (5)

CLASS, AGENT, GENERIC NAME (TRADE NAME)	USUAL ADULT DOSAGE*	ADVERSE REACTIONS, COMMENTS
CEPHALOSPORINS *(continued)*		
Oral Cephalosporins		
1st Generation, Oral		**Cross-Allergenicity: Patients with a history of IgE-mediated allergic reactions to penicillin (e.g., bronchospasm anaphylaxis, angioneurotic edema, immediate urticaria) should not receive a cephalosporin.** If the history is a "measles-like" rash to penicillin, available data suggest a 5–10% risk of rash in such patients; there is no enhanced risk of anaphylaxis. • In pts with history of Pen "reaction" and no skin testing, 0.2-8.4% react to a cephalosporin *(Aller Asthma Proc 26:135, 2006)*. If positive Pen G skin test, only 2% given a cephalosporin will react. Can predict with cephalosporin skin testing, but not easily available *(An IM 141:16, 2004; AJM 125:572, 2008)*. • IgE antibodies against either ring structure or side chains; 80% pts lose IgE over 10 yrs post-reaction *(J Aller Clin Immunol 103:918, 1999)*. Amox, Cefadroxil, Cefprozil have similar side chains; Amp, Cefaclor, Cephalexin, Cefadrine have similar side chains. • If Pen/Ceph skin testing not available or clinically no time, proceed with cephalosporin if history does not suggest IgE-mediated reaction, prior reaction more than 10 yrs ago or cephalosporin side chain differs from implicated Pen. Any of the cephalosporins can result in **C. difficile toxin**-mediated diarrhea/enterocolitis. There are **few drug-specific adverse effects, e.g.:** **Cefaclor:** Serum sickness-like reaction 0.1–0.5%--arthralgia, rash, erythema multiforme but no adenopathy, proteinuria or demonstrable immune complexes. **Cefdinir:** Drug-iron complex causes red stools in roughly 1% of pts. **Cefditoren pivoxil:** Hydrolysis yields pivalate. Pivalate absorbed (70%) & becomes pivaloylcarnitine which is renally excreted; 39–63% ↓ **in serum carnitine concentrations.** Carnitine involved in fatty acid (FA) metabolism & FA transport into mitochondria. Effect transient & reversible. Contraindicated in patients with carnitine deficiency or those in whom inborn errors of metabolism might result in clinically significant carnitine deficiency. Also contains caseinate (milk protein); **avoid if milk allergy** (not same as lactose intolerance). Need gastric acid for optimal absorption. **Cefpodoxime:** There are rare reports of acute liver injury, bloody diarrhea, pulmonary infiltrates with eosinophilia. **Cephalexin:** Can cause false-neg. urine dipstick test for leukocytes.
Cefadroxil (Duricef) (500 mg caps, 1 gm tabs)	**0.5–1 gm po q12h.**	
Cephalexin (Keflex) (250 & 500 mg tabs)	**0.25–1 gm po q6h (max 4 gm/day).**	
2nd Generation, Oral		
Cefaclor (Ceclor, Raniclor) (250 & 500 mg caps)	**0.25–0.5 gm po q8h.**	
Cefprozil (Cefzil) (250 & 500 mg tabs)	**0.25–0.5 gm po q12h.**	
Cefuroxime axetil po (Ceftin)	**0.125–0.5 gm po q12h.**	
3rd Generation, Oral		
Cefdinir (Omnicef) (300 mg cap)	**300 mg po q12h or 600 mg q24h.**	
Cefditoren pivoxil (Spectracef)	**400 mg po bid.**	
Cefixime (Suprax) (400 mg tab)	**0.4 gm po q12–24h.**	
Cefpodoxime proxetil (Vantin)	**0.1–0.2 gm po q12h.**	
Ceftibuten (Cedax) (400 mg tab)	**0.4 gm po q24h.**	
AMINOGLYCOSIDES AND RELATED ANTIBIOTICS – *See Table 10C, page 128, and Table 17A, page 237*		
GLYCOPEPTIDES, LIPOGLYCOPEPTIDES, LIPOPEPTIDES		
Dalbavancin (Dalvance)	**1000 mg IV over 30 min; one week later, 500 mg IV over 30 min or 1500 mg IV over 30 min x 1 dose.** Avoid use with saline, drug may precipitate out of solution.	**If CrCl<30**: 750 mg IV initial dose, then one week later 375 mg IV. **Hemodialysis:** Dose as for normal renal function Red man syndrome can occur with rapid infusion. Potential cross-reaction in those with hypersensitivity to other glycopeptides. No activity vs. VRE. Concomitant statins increase risk of myopathy/rhabdo *(CID 67:1356, 2018)*.
Daptomycin (Cubicin) Resistance: *JAC 2018,73:1.* Case series success in treating right- & left-sided endocarditis with higher dose of 8-10 mg/kg/day *(JAC 68:936 & 2921, 2013)*. In retrospective study, better survival in VRE bacteremia if dosed at ≥ 10 mg/kg/day *(CID 2017,64:605)*.	**Skin/soft tissue: 4 mg per kg IV over 2 or 30 minutes q24h** **Bacteremia/right-sided endocarditis: 6 mg per kg IV over 2 or 30 minutes q24h; up to 12 mg/kg IV q24h under study** **Morbid obesity:** base dose on total body weight *(AAC 51:2741, 2007)*, for other dosing recommendations, *see Table 17C , page 252.* Dapto + ceftaroline may work as salvage therapy in pts with refractory MRSA bacteremia *(AAC 57:66, 2013; AAC 56:5296, 2012)*.	**Pneumonia:** Dapto should not be used to treat pneumonia unless hematogenous in origin and is FDA approved for right-sided endocarditis with or without septic embolization/hematogenous pneumonia due to S. aureus. **Dapto Resistance:** Can occur de novo, after or during Vanco therapy, or after or during Dapto therapy *(CID 50(Suppl 1):S10, 2010)*. As Dapto MIC increases, MRSA more susceptible to TMP-SMX, nafcillin, oxacillin *(AAC 54:5187, 2010; CID 53:158, 2011)*. **Potential muscle toxicity:** Suggest weekly CPK; DC dapto if CPK exceeds 10x normal level or if symptoms of myopathy and CPK >1,000. Package insert: stop statins during dapto rx. Dapto interferes with protime reagents & artificially prolongs the PT. *(Blood Coag & Fibrinolysis 19:32, 2008)*. **NOTE:** Dapto well-tolerated at doses up to 12 mg/kg q24h x 14d *(AAC 50:3245, 2006)*. **Immune thrombocytopenia** reported *(AAC 56:6430, 2012)*. Reversible neutropenia with long-term use reported *(CID 56:1353, 2013)*. **Eosinophilic pneumonia**/chronic steroid-dep pneumonia reported *(CID 50:737, 2010; CID 50:e63, 2010)*.

*NOTE: all dosage recommendations are for adults (unless otherwise indicated) & assume normal renal function.

TABLE 10A (6)

CLASS, AGENT, GENERIC NAME (TRADE NAME)	USUAL ADULT DOSAGE*	ADVERSE REACTIONS, COMMENTS
GLYCOPEPTIDES, LIPOGLYCOPEPTIDES, LIPOPEPTIDES *(continued)*		
Oritavancin (Orbactiv) Review: *CID 61:627, 2015*	**1200 mg IV over 3 hr x 1 dose.** Dilute in D5W; do not use saline	Artificially increases PT & INR x 24 hr&aPTT x 48 hr. **Drug-drug interactions with warfarin:** ↑ warfarin serum levels. Acute urticarial has occurred. No dose adjustment for renal or hepatic insuff. Not removed by hemodialysis. In vitro activity vs. VRE *(AAC 56:1639, 2012)*.
Teicoplanin (Targocid) (where available)	**For septic arthritis—maintenance dose 12 mg/kg per day; S. aureus endocarditis— trough serum levels >20 mcg/mL required (12 mg/kg q12h times 3 loading dose, then 12 mg/kg q24h)**	Hypersensitivity: fever (at 3 mg/kg 2.2%, at 24 mg per kg 8.2%), skin reactions 2.4%. Marked ↓ platelets (high dose ≥15 mg per kg per day). Red neck syndrome less common than with vancomycin.
Telavancin (Vibativ) Lipoglycopeptide Ref: *CID 60:787, 2015; CID 61(Suppl 2), 2015*	10 mg/kg IV q24h if CrCl >50 mL/min. Infuse each dose over 1 hr.	**Avoid during pregnancy: teratogenic in animals.** Do pregnancy test before therapy. Adverse events: **dysgeusia (taste) 33%;** nausea 27%; vomiting 14%; headache 14%; ↑ creatinine (3.1%); foamy urine (13%); flushing if infused rapidly. In clin trials, **evidence of renal injury** in 3% telavancin vs. 1% vanco. In practice, renal injury reported in 1/3 of 21 complicated pts *(JAC 67:723, 2012)*. Interferes with PT, aPTT & INR for 18 hrs post-infusion.
Vancomycin (Vancocin) *AAC 60:2601, 2016.* *See Comments for po dose.* Continuous infusion dosing, *see Table 10D* **DRESS:** Drug reaction with eosinophilia and systemic signs/ symptoms. Risk increased with HLA-A* 32:01 *(J Allergy Clin Immun 144:183, 2019)*	**Initial doses based on actual wt, including for obese pts.** Subsequent doses adjusted based on measured trough serum levels. **For critically ill pts, give loading dose of 25-30 mg/kg IV then 15-20 mg/kg IV q8-12h.** Target trough level is 15-20 mg/mL. For individual doses over 1 gm, infuse over 1.5-2 hrs. **Dosing for morbid obesity (BMI ≥40 kg/m2): If CrCl ≥50 mL/min & pt not critically ill:** 30 mg/kg/day divided q8-12h—no dose over 2 gm. Infuse doses of 1 gm or more over 1.5-2 hrs. Check trough levels. **Morbid obesity & critically ill:** Loading dose of 25-30 mg/kg (based on actual wt), then 15-20 mg/kg (actual wt) IV q8-12h. Infuse over 1.5-2 hrs. **Limit maximal single dose to 2 gm.** **Oral tabs for C. difficile:** 125 mg po q6h Generic drug now available	Vanco treatment failure of MRSA bacteremia associated with Vanco trough concentration <15 μg/mL & MIC >1 μg/mL *(CID 52:975, 2011)*. IDSA Guideline supports target trough of 15-20 μg/mL *(CID 52:e18, 2011)*. Pertinent issues: • Max Vanco effect vs. MRSA when ratio of AUC/MIC >400 *(CID 52:975, 2011)*. • MIC values vary with method used, so hard to be sure/compare *(JCM 49:269, 2011)*. • With MRSA Vanco MIC = 1 & Vanco dose >3 gm/day IV, AUC/MIC >400 in 80% with est. risk of nephrotoxicity of 25%. With MIC = 2 & 4 gm/day IV, AUC/MIC >400 in only 57% (nephrotoxicity risk 35%) *(CID 52:969, 2011)*. • Risk of AKI also associated with concomitant Pip-tazo *(AAC 2018;62:e00264)*. • If pt clinically failing Vanco (regardless of MIC or AUC/MIC), consider other drugs active vs. MRSA: Ceftaroline, Daptomycin, Linezolid, Telavancin. *(See Table 5A)*. **Oral vanco for C. difficile colitis: 125 mg po q6h.** Commercial po formulation very expensive. Can compound po vanco from IV formulation (not recommended): 5 g, IV vanco powder + 47.5 mL sterile H2O, 0.2 gm saccharin, 0.05 gm stevia powder, 40 mL glycerin and then enough cherry syrup to yield 100 mL = 50 mg vanco/mL. Oral dose = 2.5 mL q6h po. FDA-approved oral solution (Firvanq) 25/50 mg/mL when reconstituted. Suggest 125 mg/dose. **Intrathecal dose:** 5-10 mg/day (infants); 10-20 mg/day (children & adults) to target CSF concentration of 10-20 mg/mL. **Nephrotoxicity:** Risk increases with dose and duration; reversible *(AAC 57:734, 2013)*. **Red Neck Syndrome:** consequence of rapid infusion with non-specific histamine release. **Other adverse effects:** rash, immune thrombocytopenia *(J Thrombo Haemostasis 11:169, 2012)*, fever, neutropenia, **IgA bullous dermatitis** *(CID 38:442, 2004)*. **Obesity dosing:** Frequent under dosing *(AJM 121:515, 2008)*. For obesity dosing adjustments, *see Table 17C, page 252.* For CrCl calculation for morbidly obese *patient see Table 10C or Am J Health Sys Pharm 66:642, 2009.*
CHLORAMPHENICOL, CLINDAMYCIN(S), ERYTHROMYCIN GROUP, KETOLIDES, OXAZOLIDINONES, QUINUPRISTIN-DALFOPRISTIN		
Chloramphenicol (Chloromycetin)	**50-100 mg/kg/day po/IV div q6h (max 4 gm/day)**	No oral drug distrib in U.S. Hematologic (↓ RBC ~1/3 pts, aplastic anemia 1:21,600 courses). Gray baby syndrome in premature infants, anaphylactoid reactions, optic atrophy or neuropathy (very rare), digital paresthesias, minor disulfiram-like reactions. Recent review suggests Chloro is probably less effective than current alternatives for serious infection: respiratory tract, enteric, meningitis *(JAC 70:979, 2015)*.
Clindamycin (Cleocin)	**0.15–0.45 gm po q6h. 600–900 mg IV/IM q8h.** In obese child, calc dose based on total body wt *(AAC 2017,61:e0201416)*	Based on number of exposed pts, these drugs are the most frequent cause of **C. difficile toxin-mediated diarrhea**. In most severe form can cause pseudomembranous colitis/toxic megacolon. Available as caps, IV sol'n, topical (for acne) & intravaginal suppositories & cream. **Used to inhibit synthesis of toxic shock syndrome toxins.**
Lincomycin (Lincocin)	**0.6 to 1 gm IV q8-12h**	Rarely used. Risk of C difficile. Requires appropriate dilution and infusion time based on dose (see Package Insert).

(See page 2 for abbreviations)

*NOTE: all dosage recommendations are for adults (unless otherwise indicated) & assume normal renal function.

TABLE 10A (7)

CLASS, AGENT, GENERIC NAME (TRADE NAME)	USUAL ADULT DOSAGE*	ADVERSE REACTIONS, COMMENTS
CHLORAMPHENICOL, CLINDAMYCIN(S), ERYTHROMYCIN GROUP, KETOLIDES, OXAZOLIDINONES, QUINUPRISTIN-DALFOPRISTIN *(continued)*		
Erythromycin Group (Review drug interactions before use)		
Azithromycin (Zithromax) **Azithromycin ER** (Zmax)	**po preps:** Tabs 250 & 600 mg. Peds suspension: 100 & 200 mg per 5 mL. Adult ER suspension: 2 gm. Dose varies with indication, *see Table 1*, Acute otitis media *(page 12)*, acute exac. chronic bronchitis *(page 40)*, Comm.-acq. pneumonia *(pages 42–43)*, & sinusitis *(page 53)*. **IV:** 0.5 gm per day.	**Gastroparesis:** Erythro is alt drug for rx of gastroparesis. Initiates peristalsis by binding to motilin receptors & improves gastric emptying for approx 2 wks; then effect lost due to tachyphylaxis. Erythro dose: 1.5-3 mg/kg IV over 45 min q6h or 250 mg po liquid susp bid. Ref: *Gastro Clin NA 2015,44:97*. **Frequent drug-drug interactions:** *see Table 22A page 259*. Major concern is prolonged QT_c interval on EKG. **Prolonged QTc:** Erythro, clarithro & azithro all increase risk of ventricular tachycardia via increase in QTc interval. Can be congenital or acquired *(NEJM 358:169, 2008)*. Caution if positive family history of sudden cardiac death, electrolyte abnormalities or concomitant drugs that prolong QTc. **↑ risk QTc >500 msec! Risk amplified by other drugs** [macrolides, antiarrhythmics, & drug-drug interactions *(see FQs page 122 for list)*]. *www.qtdrugs.org & www.torsades.org*. Ref: *Am J Med 128:1362, 2015*. Cholestatic hepatitis in approx. 1:1000 adults (not children) given E estolate. **Drug-drug interactions of note:** Erythro or clarithro with statins: high statin levels, rhabdomyolysis *(Ann Int Med 158:869, 2013)*; concomitant clarithro & colchicine (gout) can cause fatal colchicine toxicity (pancytopenia, renal failure) *(CID 41:291, 2005)*. Concomitant clarithro & Ca++ channel blockers increase risk of hypotension, kidney injury *(JAMA 310:2544, 2013)*. Hypoglycemia with concomitant sulfonylureas *(JAMA Int Med 174:1605, 2014)*. **Transient reversible tinnitus or deafness** with ≥4 gm per day of erythro IV in pts with renal or hepatic impairment. Reversible sensorineural hearing loss with Azithro *(J Otolaryngol 36:257, 2007)*. Dosages of oral erythro preparations expressed as base equivalents. Variable amounts of erythro esters required to achieve same free erythro serum level. **Azithromycin** reported to exacerbate symptoms of myasthenia gravis. **FDA alerts**: clarithromycin use associated with increased cardio- and cerebro-vascular events; azithromycin use to prevent bronchiolitis obliterans after donor stem cell transplant associated with increased cancer relapse and death.
Erythromycin Base and esters (Erythrocin) IV name: E. lactobionate	**0.25 gm q6h–0.5 gm po/IV q6h: 15–20 mg/kg up to 4 gm q24h. Infuse over 30+ min.**	
Clarithromycin (Biaxin) or clarithro extended release (Biaxin XL)	**0.5 gm po q12h.** **Extended release: Two 0.5 gm tabs po per day.**	
Fidaxomicin (Dificid) (200 mg tab)	**One 200 mg tab po bid x 10 days with or without food**	Approved for C. difficile toxin-mediated diarrhea, including hypervirulent NAP1/B1/027 strains. Minimal GI absorption; high fecal concentrations. Limited activity vs. normal bowel flora. In trial vs. po Vanco, lower relapse rate vs. non-NAP1 strains than Vanco *(NEJM 364:422, 2011)*. Despite absence of GI absorption, 12 pts developed allergic reactions; known macrolide allergy in 3 of 12 *(CID 58:537, 2014)*.
Ketolides: **Telithromycin** (Ketek) *(Med Lett 46:66, 2004; Drug Safety 31:561, 2008)*	**Two 400 mg tabs po q24h.** 300 mg tabs available.	Drug warnings: acute liver failure & serious liver injury post treatment. *(AnIM 144:415, 447, 2006)*. **Uncommon: blurred vision** 2° slow accommodation; may cause exacerbation of **myasthenia gravis (Black Box Warning: Contraindicated in this disorder)**. Liver, eye and myasthenia complications may be due to inhibition of nicotinic acetylcholine receptor at neuromuscular junction *(AAC 54:5399, 2010)*. Potential QT_c prolongation. Several **drug-drug interactions** *(Table 22A, page 259) (NEJM 355:2260, 2006)*. No longer marketed in US.
Tedizolid phosphate (Sivextro) Ref: *CID 61:1315, 2015.*	**200 mg IV/po once daily. Infuse IV over 1 hr.**	**IV dose reconstituted in 250 mL of normal saline;** incompatible with lactated ringers as non-soluble in presence of divalent cations. SST clinical trial result *(JAMA 309:559 & 609, 2013)*. Excreted by liver. No adjustment for renal insufficiency. Weak inhibitor of monoamine oxidase, hence risk of serotonin syndrome, but low risk *(AAC 57:3060, 2013)*. Low risk of thrombocytopenia at therapeutic doses *(AAC 2016,71:2553)*.
Linezolid (Zyvox) (600 mg tab) Review: *JAC 66(Suppl 4):3, 2011*	**po or IV dose: 600 mg q12h.** Available as 600 mg tabs, oral suspension (100 mg per 5 mL), & IV solution. Special populations Refs: Renal insufficiency *(J Infect Chemother 17:70, 2011; AAC 63:e00605, 2019)*; Liver transplant *(CID 42:434, 2006)*; Cystic fibrosis *(AAC 48:281, 2004)*; Burns *(J Burn Care Res 31:207, 2010)*. Obesity: clinical failure with standard dose in 265 kg patient *(Ann Pharmacother 47:e25, 2013)*.	**Reversible myelosuppression:** thrombocytopenia, anemia, & neutropenia reported. Most often after >2 wks of therapy. Increased risk on hemodialysis or peritoneal dialysis *(Int J Antimicrob Ag 36:179, 2010; JAC doi:10.1093/jac/dkv184)* **Lactic acidosis; peripheral neuropathy, optic neuropathy:** After 4 or more wks of therapy. Data consistent with time and dose-dependent inhibition of intramitochondrial protein synthesis *(Pharmacotherapy 27:771, 2007)*. Neuropathy, not reversible. Mitochondrial toxicity *(AAC 2017;61:e00542-17)*. **Inhibitor of monoamine oxidase;** risk of severe hypertension if taken with foods rich in tyramine. Avoid concomitant pseudoephedrine, phenylpropanolamine, and caution with SSRIs[1]. **Serotonin syndrome** (fever, agitation, mental status changes, tremors). Risk with concomitant SSRIs: *(CID 42:1578 and 43:180, 2006)*. Incidence low *(AAC 57:5901, 2013)*. Other: black hairy tongue, acute interstitial nephritis *(IDCP 17:61, 2009)*, teeth staining *(CID 2016,62:617)*. **Rhabdomyolysis:** case probably related to linezolid in a patient receiving linezolid as a component of multi-drug therapy for XDR tuberculosis *(CID 54:1624, 2012)*. **Resistance:** Linezolid resistant S. epidermidis and MRSA due to mutation of the 23S rRNA binding site *(JAC 68:4, 2013)*.

[1] **SSRI** = selective serotonin reuptake inhibitors, e.g., fluoxetine (Prozac).

(See page 2 for abbreviations)

*NOTE: all dosage recommendations are for adults (unless otherwise indicated) & assume normal renal function.

TABLE 10A (8)

CLASS, AGENT, GENERIC NAME (TRADE NAME)	USUAL ADULT DOSAGE*	ADVERSE REACTIONS, COMMENTS
CHLORAMPHENICOL, CLINDAMYCIN(S), ERYTHROMYCIN GROUP, KETOLIDES, OXAZOLIDINONES, QUINUPRISTIN-DALFOPRISTIN *(continued)*		
Quinupristin + Dalfopristin (Synercid) *(CID 36:473, 2003)*	**7.5 mg per kg IV q12h for skin/skin structure infections, infused over 1 hour.** [For previous indication of VRE infection, dose used was 7.5 mg per kg IV q8h]. Give by central line.	Venous irritation (5%); none with central venous line. Asymptomatic ↑ in unconjugated bilirubin. **Arthralgia** 2%–50% *(CID 36:476, 2003)*. **Note:** E. faecium susceptible; E. faecalis resistant. **Drug-drug interactions:** Cyclosporine, nifedipine, midazolam, many more—*see Table 22A*.
TETRACYCLINES		
Doxycycline (Vibramycin, Doryx, Monodox, Adoxa, Periostat) (20, 50, 75, 100 mg tab)	**Adult: 100 mg po/IV q12h; Child (regardless of age): 4.4 mg/kg/day po/IV divided bid x max of 21 days** (considered safe, *AAP Redbook 2018; J Ped 2015;166:1246*).	Similar to other tetracyclines. ↑ nausea on empty stomach. Erosive esophagitis, esp. if taken at bedtime; **take with lots of water.** Phototoxicity & photo-onycholysis occur but less than with tetracycline. Deposition in teeth less than with tetracycline *(JAC 2017;72:2887)*. Can be used in patients with renal failure. Pseudotumor cerebri (intracranial hypertension) can occur. *Comments:* Effective in treatment and prophylaxis for malaria, leptospirosis, typhus fevers.
Eravacycline (Xerava) Activity similar to omadacycline & tigecycline, see *Table 4A*)	1 mg/kg IV infused over 60 min q12h x 4-14 days (increase to 1.5 mg/kg if co-administered with strong CYP3A4 inducer, e.g., RIF). Severe liver disease: 1 mg/kg IV q12h x 1 day, then 1 mg/kg IV q24h.	Approved for complicated intra-abdominal infections in adults. **Warnings**: life-threatening hypersensitivity reactions if known tetracycline allergy; Pregnancy (2nd/3rd trimester) risk of tooth discoloration and bone growth inhibition. **Common AEs**: infusion site reactions, nausea, vomiting.
Minocycline (Minocin, Dynacin) (50, 75, 100 mg cap; 45, 90, 135 mg ext rel tab; IV prep) Contains Mg++. Monitor serum Mg++ levels if renal impairment.	**200 mg po/IV loading dose, then 100 mg po/IV q12h** IV minocycline available.	**Vestibular symptoms** (30–90% in some groups, none in others): vertigo 33%, ataxia 43%, nausea 50%, vomiting 3%, women more frequently than men. Hypersensitivity pneumonitis, reversible, ~34 cases reported *(BMJ 310:1520, 1995)*. Can cause slate-grey **pigmentation** of the skin and other tissues with long-term use. **Intracranial hypertension** can occur. *Comments:* More effective than other tetracyclines vs staph and in prophylaxis of meningococcal disease. P. acnes: many resistant to other tetracyclines, not to mino. Induced autoimmunity reported in children treated for acne *(J Ped 153:314, 2008)*. Active vs Nocardia asteroides, Mycobacterium marinum and many acinetobacter isolates.
Omadacycline (Nuzyra) Activity similar to eravacycline & tigecycline, see *Table 4A*)	**CABP/ABSSSI:** Loading: (IV/po): 200 mg IV infused over 60 min or 100 mg IV infused over 30 min twice on day 1; Maintenance: 100 mg IV infused over 30 min qd or 300 mg po qd. **ABSSSI** (po): Loading: 450 mg po qd days 1 & 2; Maintenance: 300 mg po qd	Duration: 7-14 days. Breastfeeding not recommended during treatment and for 4 days after last dose. Fast for 4 hrs before dosing. No food for 2 hrs after dosing; no dairy products, antacids, multivitamins for 4 hrs after dosing. **Contraindication:** known tetracycline hypersensitivity. **Warnings:** Higher mortality risk in CAP vs. Moxi. Tooth discoloration/enamel dysplasia in 2nd half of pregnancy. Inhibition of bone growth in 2nd/3rd trimesters. AEs: diarrhea, nausea, vomiting, constipation; infusion site reactions; increased AST, ALT, GGT; hypertension; headache; insomnia. Ref: *CID 69:180, 2019*.
Tetracycline, Oxytetracycline (Sumycin) (250, 500 mg cap) *(CID 36:462, 2003)*	**0.25–0.5 gm po q6h, 0.5–1 gm IV q12h**	GI (oxy 19%, tetra 4), anaphylactoid reaction (rare), deposition in teeth, negative N balance, hepatotoxicity, enamel agenesis, pseudotumor cerebri/encephalopathy. Outdated drug: Fanconi syndrome. *See drug-drug interactions, Table 22A.* **Contraindicated in pregnancy, hepatotoxicity in mother, transplacental to fetus.** *Comments:* **Pregnancy:** IV dosage over 2 gm per day may be associated with fatal hepatotoxicity. (Ref: *JAC 66:1431, 2011*).
Tigecycline (Tygacil) Meta-analysis & editorial: *Ln ID 11:804 & 834, 2011.* Also *CID 54:1699 & 1710, 2012.*	**100 mg IV initially, then 50 mg IV q12h with po food, if possible to decrease risk of nausea.** **If severe liver dis. (Child Pugh C):** 100 mg IV initially, then 25 mg IV q12h	Derivative of tetracycline. High incidence of nausea (25%) & vomiting (20%) but only 1% of pts discontinued therapy. Pregnancy Category D. Do not use in children under age 18. Like other tetracyclines, may cause photosensitivity, pseudotumor cerebri, pancreatitis, a catabolic state (elevated BUN) and maybe hyperpigmentation *(CID 45:136, 2007)*. Decreases serum fibrinogen *(AAC 59:1650, 2015)*. **Tetracycline, minocycline & tigecycline** associated with acute pancreatitis *(Int J Antimicrob Agents, 34:486, 2009)*. **Black Box Warning:** In meta-analysis of clinical trials, all cause mortality higher in pts treated with tigecycline (2.5%) vs. 1.8% in comparators. Cause of mortality risk difference of 0.6% (95% CI 0.1, 1.2) not established. Tigecycline should be reserved for use in situations when alternative treatments are not suitable *(FDA MedWatch Sep 27, 2013)*. Poor result due to low serum levels *(AAC 56:1065 & 1466, 2012)*; high doses superior to low doses for *HAP (AAC 57:1756, 2013)*.

*NOTE: all dosage recommendations are for adults (unless otherwise indicated) & assume normal renal function.

TABLE 10A (9)

CLASS, AGENT, GENERIC NAME (TRADE NAME)	USUAL ADULT DOSAGE*	ADVERSE REACTIONS, COMMENTS
FLUOROQUINOLONES (FQs): All can cause false-positive urine drug screen for opiates *(Pharmacother 26:435, 2006)*. Toxicity review*: Drugs Aging 27:193, 2010.*		
Ciprofloxacin (Cipro) and **Ciprofloxacin-extended release** (Cipro XR, Proquin XR) (100, 250, 500, 750 mg tab; 500 mg ext rel tab)	Usual Parenteral Dose: **400 mg IV q12h** For P. aeruginosa: **400-600 mg IV q8h** *(JAC 74:1662, 2019)* Uncomplicated Urethritis/cystitis (Oral) Dose: **250 mg po bid or CIP XR 500 mg po once daily** Other Indications (Oral): **500-750 mg po bid**	FQs are a common precipitant of **C. difficile toxin-mediated diarrhea.** **Children:** No FQ approved for use under age 16 based on joint cartilage injury in immature animals. Articular SEs in children est. at 2–3% *(LnID 3:537, 2003)*. The exception is anthrax. Pathogenesis believed to involve FQ chelation of Mg++ and damaging chondrites *(AAC 51:1022, 2007; Int J Antimicrob Agents 33:194, 2009)*. No evidence of cartilage damage with Levo in children *(Pediatrics 134:e146, 2014)*. **CNS toxicity:** Poorly understood. Varies: lightheadedness, confusion, seizures. Trouble with attention/memory. Peripheral neuropathy occurs: rapid onset, potentially permanent injury. **Gemi skin rash:** Macular rash after 8–10 days of rx. Incidence of rash with ≤5 days of therapy only 1.5%. Frequency highest females, < age 40, treated 14 days (22.6%). In men, < age 40, treated 14 days, frequency 7.7%. Mechanism unclear. Indication to DC therapy. Ref: *Diag Micro Infect Dis 68:140, 2010*. **Hypoglycemia/hyperglycemia (Dysglycemia):** Increased risk, esp. of hypoglycemia in diabetic pts from any of the marketed FQs *(CID 57:971, 2013)*. **Thrombocytopenia** in critically ill *(J Thrombo Haemostasis 11:169, 2012)*. **Opiate screen false-positives:** FQs can cause false-positive urine assay for opiates *(Ann Pharmacotherapy 38:1525, 2004)*. **Photosensitivity:** *See Table 10B, page 127.* **QT_c (corrected QT) interval prolongation:** ↑ QT_c (>500 msec or >60 msec from baseline) is considered possible with any FQ (except Delaflox). ↑ QT_c can lead to torsades de pointes and ventricular fibrillation. Overall risk is 4.7/10,000 person yrs *(CID 55:1457, 2012)*. Risk low with current marketed drugs. Risk ↑ in women, ↓ K^+, ↓ mg^{++}, bradycardia. (Refs.: *CID 43:1603, 2006*). Major problem is ↑ risk with concomitant drugs.
Delafloxacin (Baxdela) 450 mg tablets IV for injection	**300 mg IV q12h infused over 1 hr** **450 mg po q12h** Treat 5-14 days (skin, skin structure), 5-10 days (CAP) Can switch from IV to po during course of rx	
Gatifloxacin (Tequin) (where available) *See comments*	**200–400 mg IV/po q24h**. *(See comment)* Ophthalmic solution (Zymar)	
Gemifloxacin (Factive) (320 mg tab)	**320 mg po q24h**.	
Levofloxacin (Levaquin) (250, 500, 750 mg tab)	**250–750 mg po/IV q24h.** For most indications, 750 mg is preferred dose. po therapy: avoid concomitant dairy products, multivitamins, iron, antacids due to chelation by multivalent cations & interference with absorption. No dose adjustment for morbid obesity.	**Avoid concomitant drugs with potential to prolong QTc such as** *(see www.qtdrugs.org; www.torsades.org)*: (see list below)

Antiarrhythmics:	Anti-Infectives:	Anti-Hypertensives:	CNS Drugs:	Misc:
Amiodarone Disopyramide Dofetilide Flecainide Ibutilide Procainamide Quinidine, quinine Sotalol	Azole antifungals Antimalarials (Artemether-Lumefantrine, Chloroquine, Dihydroartemisinin-Piperaquine, Halofantrine, Mefloquine) Antiretrovirals (Atazanavir, Kaletra, Rilpivirine, Saquinavir) Bedaquiline Delamanid Fluoroquinolones Lefamulin Macrolides (Erythromycin, Clarithromycin, Azithromycin) Pentamidine Pentavalent antimony Peramivir? Telavancin Triclabendazole?	Bepridil Indapamide Isradipine Moexipril Nicardipine	Fluoxetine Haloperidol Phenothiazines Pimozide Quetiapine Risperidone Sertraline Tricyclics Venlafaxine Ziprasidone	Dolasetron Droperidol Fosphenytoin Methadone Naratriptan Ondansetron Salmeterol Sumatriptan Tamoxifen Tizanidine

*NOTE: all dosage recommendations are for adults (unless otherwise indicated) & assume normal renal function.

TABLE 10A (10)

CLASS, AGENT, GENERIC NAME (TRADE NAME)	USUAL ADULT DOSAGE*	ADVERSE REACTIONS, COMMENTS
FLUOROQUINOLONES (FQs) *(continued)*		
Moxifloxacin (Avelox)	**400 mg po/IV q24h.** Note: no need to increase dose for morbid obesity *(JAC 66:2330, 2011).* Ophthalmic solution (Vigamox)	**Tendinopathy:** Over age 60, approx. 2–6% of all Achilles tendon ruptures attributable to use of FQ *(ArIM 163:1801, 2003).* ↑ risk with concomitant steroid, renal disease or post-transplant (heart, lung, kidney) *(CID 36:1404, 2003).* **Chelation:** Risk of chelation of oral FQs by multivalent cations **(Ca++, Mg++, Fe++, Zn++)**. Avoid dairy products, multivitamins *Clin Pharmacokinet 40 (Suppl 1) 33:2001).* **Allergic Reactions:** Rare (1:50,000). IgE-mediated: urticaria, anaphylaxis. 3 pts with Moxi had immediate reactions but tolerated CIP *(Ann Pharmacother 44:740, 2010).* **Myasthenia gravis:** Any of the FQs may exacerbate muscle weakness in pts. with myasthenia gravis. **Retinal detachment:** Inconsistent data. **Carpal tunnel syndrome:** Pharmacoepidemiological study found increased risk of CTS with FQ use *(CID 65: 684, 2017).* **Pseudotumor cerebri:** Significant risk ratio (4-6) reported *(Neurology 2017;89:892).* **Aortic aneurysm tear:** Hazard ratio 1.2-2.9 *(BMJ 360:K678, 2018).*
Ofloxacin (Floxin)	**200–400 mg po bid.** Ophthalmic solution (Ocuflox)	
Prulifloxacin (where available) Ref: *Drugs 64:2221, 2004.*	Tablets: 250 and 600 mg. Usual dose: **600 mg po once daily**	**Contraindications:** persons with celiac disease, pregnancy, nursing mothers, persons with seizure disorder **AEs:** similar to other FQs
PLEUROMUTILINS		
Lefamulin (Xenleta)	Adult: **600 mg po q8h or 150 mg IV q12h** Extend dosing interval if severe hepatic impairment	**AEs:** nausea, vomiting, diarrhea (including C. diff toxin colitis); more frequent with oral dosing. **Pregnancy:** may cause fetal harm; check for pregnancy before use. Breastfeeding safety unknown. **DDI:** Many due to CYP450 transporter interactions. Can increase QTc esp if interaction increases Lefamulin or other drug serum levels.
Retapamulin	Topical agent, *see page 126*	
POLYMYXINS (POLYPEPTIDES) Note: **Proteus sp., Providencia sp, Serratia sp., B. cepacia are intrinsically resistant to polymyxins.** Review: *CID 59:88, 2014.*		
Polymyxin B (Poly-Rx) 1 mg = 10,000 international units **Where available, Polymyxin B preferred over Colistin.**	Doses based on actual body weight. ***LOADING DOSE:*** 2.5 mg/kg IV over 2 hrs. ***MAINTENANCE DOSE:*** 12 hrs later 1.5 mg/kg over 1 hr, then repeat q12h. No dose reduction for renal insufficiency. **Intrathecal therapy for meningitis:** 5 mg/day into CSF x 3-4 days, then 5 mg every other day x 2 or more weeks.	**Adverse effects: Neurologic:** rare, but serious, is neuromuscular blockade; other, circumoral paresthesias, extremity numbness, blurred vision, drowsy, irritable, ataxia; can manifest as respiratory arrest *(Chest 141:515, 2012).* **Renal:** reversible acute tubular necrosis. Renal injury in 42% (Polymyxin B) vs. 60% (Colistin) *(CID 57:1300, 2013).* **Skin:** Hyperpigmentation in 8% of 249 pts *(J Clin Pharm Ther 2017;42:573).* PK study showed no need to reduce dose for renal insufficiency *(CID 57:524, 2013).* **Polymyxin B preferred over Colistin (except for UTI)** *(see Comment under Colistin for discussion).* Combination therapy (polymyxin + carbapenem) failed in controlled clinical trial *(LnID 2018,18:391).*

(See page 2 for abbreviations)

*NOTE: all dosage recommendations are for adults (unless otherwise indicated) & assume normal renal function.

TABLE 10A (11)

CLASS, AGENT, GENERIC NAME (TRADE NAME)	USUAL ADULT DOSAGE*	ADVERSE REACTIONS, COMMENTS
POLYMYXINS (POLYPEPTIDES) *(continued)*		
Colistin, Polymyxin E (Colymycin) Polymyxin E (Colistin) and Polymyxin B are polymyxin class parenteral antibiotics active against multi-drug resistant (MDR) gram negative bacilli, e.g., *A. baumannii, P. aeruginosa, E. coli, K. pneumoniae*. **Resistance issues:** Serratia sp, Proteus sp., Providencia sp., Morganella sp., and B. cepacia are intrinsically resistant to polymyxins. Pan-resistant strains of Enterobacteriaceae, including resistance to colistin mediated by plasmid-encoded gene mcr-1 *(AAC 60: 2443, 2016)* have been identified worldwide. **Colistin is the preferred polymyxin for:** Urinary tract infections (UTIs) & Adjunctive inhalation therapy for pneumonia caused by MDR gram-negative bacilli. For all other indications, Polymyxin B: equivalent efficacy, faster attainment of target serum conc, less inter-patient variability in PK, no dose adjustment for renal impairment and lower risk of renal toxicity *(AAC 60: 2443, 2016; and AAC 2017:61: e02319-16))*	**Formulation and conversion:** Colistin is formulated as a prodrug, colistimethate (CMS). Product vials may be labeled as international units (IU) or mg of prodrug or mg of **colistin base activity (CBA)** of active drug. **Always dose based on the CBA**. *To avoid dosing errors read product labels carefully!* **Conversions** *(CID 2014, 58:139)*: 1 mg CBA = 30,000 IU CMS; 33 mg CBA = 1,000,000 IU CMS; 1 mg CBA = 2.4 mg CMS. Dosing recommendations continue to evolve. At present, there are 3 sets of dosing guidance: **PK Study Group**: creatinine clearance (CrCl)-based dosing *(CID 2017;64:565)*; **European Medicines Agency (EMA)**: CrCl-based dosing *(CID 2016, 62:552)*; **U.S. FDA:** weight- and CrCl-based dosing, as found in the package insert (June 2016). Complicated calculation-based dosing has been replaced by simpler PK-based dosing using CrCl levels as benchmarks. The PK Study Group recommendations use finer divisions between CrCl levels; the EMA recommendations use broader divisions. *See Comments.* For **severe systemic infection** and patients not on dialysis of any kind (Note: for dosing in patients on intermittent hemodialysis or CRRT, see Table 17A): 1. **Loading Dose:** Administer a Colistin loading dose IV, then begin daily maintenance dosing 12 hours later. Loading dose formula: 4 x body weight in kg. Use lower of ideal or actual weight. May result in loading dose > 300 mg CBA. Start daily maintenance dose 12 hrs. later. 2. **Maintenance Dose: Then, Total Daily maintenance dose: Divide daily dose to bid or tid** (from Total Daily maintenance dose table (Comments): Editors prefer PK Study Group). Once daily dosing not recommended due to potential for toxicity and lack of efficacy data. **Other adult dosing:** **Inhaled therapy:** 50-75 mg CBA in 3-4 mL saline via vibrating mesh nebulizer 2-3 times/day: concentration in lung epithelial lining is 100-1000x greater with inhaled dosing vs. IV dosing alone **Meningitis** (intraventricular or intrathecal dose): 10 mg/day x several weeks; intrathecal dose often combined with IV dosing **Pediatric dosing:** **Systemic Infection:** 2.5-5 mg/kg/day in 2-4 divided doses (based on ideal body weight). **Cystic Fibrosis:** 3-8 mg/kg/day in 3 divided doses (based on ideal body weight). **Note: Resistance and allergy issues.** The plasmid-encoded colistin resistance gene, mcr-1, has been found in E. coli and Klebsiella sp. Resistance is due to modification of the lipid A target of the polymyxins. Strains may also produce metallo-carbapenemases, resulting in pan-resistance *(See LnID 2016,16:161; LnID 2016, 16:287; AAC 2016, 60:4420)*. For carbapenem-allergic patients, no clear alternatives for a companion drug with colistin. Combination therapy with Rifampin did not improve clinical response or 30-day mortality in patients with Acinetobacter infections *(CID 2013, 57:349; Epidemiol Infect 2013, 141:1214)*. In vitro and in vivo exposure to polymyxins results in rapid selection of resistant sub-populations. In vitro, minocycline prevented emergence of resistance and augmented Colistin activity but no clinical trial data. Tigecycline may function similarly, but no data.	**Nephrotoxicity** *(Pharmacotherapy 35:28, 2015)*: Reversible acute tubular necrosis due to localization of drug in proximal tubular cells: *AAC 2017; 61:e02319-16*. Depending on criteria, incidence of toxicity varies, average around 25%. Risk factors: length of therapy, daily dose, and cumulative dose; exposure to concomitant nephrotoxins; obesity, diabetes mellitus, age and hypertension. In animal models, high dose ascorbic acid and melatonin prevented toxicity. In critically ill, the benefit of patient salvage may exceed the risk of nephrotoxicity. **Neurotoxicity:** Frequent vertigo, facial paresthesias, abnormal vision, confusion, ataxia. Rarely, neuromuscular blockade results in respiratory failure; may unmask or exacerbate myasthenia gravis. In cystic fibrosis patients, 29% experienced paresthesias, ataxia or both. **Other:** Maybe hyper-pigmentation *(CID 45:136, 2007)*. **Discussion and critiques of current dosing recommendations.** The PK Study Group favors the EMA recommendations over the current (June 2016) U.S. FDA approved dosing *(CID 2016, 62:552)*. The weight- and CrCl-based approach in the FDA approved dosing is more complicated than either the PK Study Group or EMA recommendations. The PK Study Group recommendations are based on PK study of 214 critically ill patients *(CID 2017; 64:565)*. In patients with CrCl >80 mL/min, EMA recommended doses failed to achieve target serum concentration in 66% of patients versus less than 10% in patients with CrCl < 80 mL/min *(CID 2016, 62:552)* due to rapid renal clearance of colistimethate prodrug with less time for conversion of prodrug to active colistin. **Total Daily maintenance dose:** (see table below)

Total Daily maintenance dose:

CrCl (mL/min)	PK Study Group (doses div bid or tid)*	EMA (doses div bid or tid)*	U.S. FDA (Wt - IBW)*
≥90	360 mg/day	300 mg/day	2.5-5 mg/kg/day div 2-4 doses
80 to <90	340 mg/day		
70 to <80	300 mg/day		2.5-3.8 mg/kg/day div 2 doses
60 to <70	275 mg/day		
50 to <60	245 mg/day		
40 to <50	220 mg/day	183-250 mg/day	2.5 mg/kg once daily or div bid
30 to <40	195 mg/day		
20 to <30	175 mg/day	150-183 mg/day	1.5 mg/kg q36h
10 to <20	160 mg/day		
5 to <10	145 mg/day	117 mg/day	N/R
<5	130 mg/day		

* All doses are stated as colistin base activity (CBA) in mg.
IBW = ideal body weight

(See page 2 for abbreviations)

*NOTE: all dosage recommendations are for adults (unless otherwise indicated) & assume normal renal function.

TABLE 10A (12)

CLASS, AGENT, GENERIC NAME (TRADE NAME)	USUAL ADULT DOSAGE*	ADVERSE REACTIONS, COMMENTS
MISCELLANEOUS AGENTS		
Fosfomycin po (Monurol) Fosfomycin tromethamine	Adult: **3 gm po x 1** (uncomplicated UTI) **or 3 gm po q3d x 3** (complicated UTI) **or x 7 days** (prostatitis). Child: **2 gm po x 1** (UTI)	**AEs:** diarrhea (more common than with TMP-SMX or nitrofurantoin), headache. Large sodium load. Active vs. susceptible gram-negative bacilli.
Fosfomycin IV (Ivozfo) Fosfomycin disodium (Available in Canada, Europe, Australia) US: emergency single patient IND from FDA (1-888-300-4374)	Adult: **12-24 gm IV daily div q8-12h** (osteo, complicated UTI, nosocomial pneumonia); **16-24 gm IV daily div q6-8h** (meningitis). Child: *see Table 16*	
Fusidic acid (Fucidin, Taksta) (where available)	**500 mg po/IV tid (Denmark & Canada)** **US: loading dose of 1500 mg po bid x 1 day, then 600 mg po bid**	Activity vs. MRSA of importance. Approved outside the U.S.; currently in U.S. clinical trials. Ref for proposed US regimen: *CID 52 (Suppl 7):S520, 2011.*
Methenamine hippurate (Hiprex, Urex)	**1 gm po bid**	Nausea and vomiting, skin rash or dysuria. Overall ~3%. Methenamine requires (pH ≤ 5.5) urine to liberate formaldehyde. Useful in suppressive therapy after infecting organisms cleared; do not use for pyelonephritis. *Comment:* Do not force fluids; may dilute formaldehyde. Of no value in pts with chronic Foley. If urine pH >5.5, co-administer ascorbic acid (1–2 gm q4h) to acidify the urine; cranberry juice (1200–4000 mL per day) has been used, results ±. Do not use concomitantly with sulfonamides (precipitate), or in presence of renal or severe hepatic dysfunction.
Methenamine mandelate (Mandelamine)	**1 gm po qid**	
Metronidazole (Flagyl) (250, 375, 500 mg tab/cap) Prevotella sp: some resistance *(JAC 2018,73:265).*	Anaerobic infections: **usually IV, 7.5 mg per kg (~500 mg) q6h (not to exceed 4 gm q24h).** With long T½, **can use IV at 15 mg per kg q12h.** If life-threatening, use loading dose of **IV 15 mg per kg. Oral dose: 500 mg qid; extended release tabs** available 750 mg Giardia, amebiasis: *See Table 13*	**Common AEs:** nausea (12%), metallic taste, "furry" tongue. **Avoid alcohol during 48 hrs after last dose to avoid disulfiram reaction (N/V, flushing, tachycardia, dyspnea).** Neurologic AEs with high dose/long Rx: peripheral, autonomic and optic neuropathy. **Aseptic meningitis, encephalopathy, seizures & reversible cerebellar lesion** reported *(NEJM 374:1465, 2016); CID 2017,64:525.* Possible association of po metronidazole with acute pancreatitis *(Clin Epidemiol 10:1573, 2018).* Risk of hypoglycemia with concomitant sulfonylureas. Can use IV sol'n as enema for *C. diff colitis.* **Resistant anaerobic organisms:** Actinomycetes, Peptostreptococci. **Once-daily IV dosing** of 1,500 mg: based on long serum T1/2; standard in Europe *(JAC 19:410, 2007).* **Safe to use in pregnancy** *(Curr Drug Safety 2015,10:170).*
Nitazoxanide	*See Table 13B, page 173*	
Nitrofurantoin Systematic rev: *JAC 70:2456, 2015*	Active UTI: **Furadantin/Macrodantin 50-100 mg po qid x 5-7 days OR Macrobid 100 mg po bid x 5-7 days** Dose for long-term UTI suppression: **50–100 mg at bedtime**	Absorption ↑ with meals. Increased activity in acid urine, much reduced at pH 8 or over. Nausea and vomiting, **peripheral neuropathy,** pancreatitis. **Pulmonary reactions** (with chronic rx): acute ARDS type, **chronic desquamative interstitial pneumonia with fibrosis**. Intrahepatic cholestasis & **hepatitis** similar to chronic active hepatitis. Hemolytic anemia in G6PD deficiency. Drug rash, eosinophilia, systemic symptoms (DRESS) hypersensitivity syndrome reported *(Neth J Med 67:147, 2009).* Should not be used in infants <1 month of age. Birth defects: increased risk reported *(Arch Ped Adolesc Med 163:978, 2009).*
Rifampin (Rimactane, Rifadin) (150, 300 mg cap) **Use in combination only**	**300 mg po/IV bid or 600 mg po/IV qd.** Rapid selection of resistant bacteria if used as monotherapy	Causes orange-brown discoloration of sweat, urine, tears, contact lens. **Many important drug-drug interactions,** *see Table 22A.* Immune complex flu-like syndrome: fever, headache, myalgias, arthralgia--especially with intermittent rx. Drug induced immune thrombocytopenia *(J Thrombosis & Haemostasis 2012,11:169).* Can cause interstitial nephritis. Risk-benefit of adding RIF to standard therapies for S. aureus endocarditis *(AAC 52:2463, 2008).* *See also, Antimycobacterial Agents, Table 12B, page 157.*
Rifamycin (Aemcolo)	Tablets: 194 mg. Adult: **2 tabs bid x 3 days**	Approved for *E. coli* induced traveler's diarrhea; do not use if fever and/or bloody stools.
Rifaximin (Xifaxan) (200, 550 mg tab)	Traveler's diarrhea: **200 mg tab po tid** times 3 days. Hepatic encephalopathy: **550 mg tab po bid.** C. diff diarrhea as "chaser": **400 mg po tid**	For traveler's diarrhea and hepatic encephalopathy *(AAC 54:3618, 2010; NEJM 362:1071, 2010).* In general, adverse events equal to or less than placebo. Monitor INR in those taking warfarin. Systemic exposure may increase with severe hepatic disease or P-glycoprotein inhibitors.

(See page 2 for abbreviations)

*NOTE: all dosage recommendations are for adults (unless otherwise indicated) & assume normal renal function.

TABLE 10A (13)

CLASS, AGENT, GENERIC NAME (TRADE NAME)	USUAL ADULT DOSAGE*	ADVERSE REACTIONS, COMMENTS
MISCELLANEOUS AGENTS *(continued)*		
Secnidazole (Solosec)	2 gm packet (granules): sprinkle on applesauce, yogurt or pudding and consume mixture within 30 min without chewing granules. Follow with glass of water to aid swallowing	Nitroimidazole for treatment of bacterial vaginosis in adults. Vulvo-vaginal candidiasis may develop requiring antifungal therapy. Potential carcinogenicity seen in rodent studies. Avoid chronic use. **AEs:** Vulvo-vaginal candidiasis (≥2%), headache, nausea, dysgeusia, vomiting, diarrhea, abdominal pain, vulvo-vaginal pruritus.
Sulfonamides [e.g., sulfisoxazole (Gantrisin), sulfamethoxazole (Gantanol), (Truxazole), sulfadiazine]	Dose varies with indications. *See Nocardia & Toxoplasmosis*	**CNS:** fever, headache, dizziness; **Derm:** mild rash to life threatening Stevens-Johnson syndrome, toxic epidermal necrolysis *(Brit J Derm 2016,174:1194)*, photosensitivity; **Hem:** agranulocytosis, aplastic anemia; **Cross-allergenicity:** other sulfa drugs, sulfonylureas, diuretics, crystalluria (esp. sulfadiazine-need ≥1500 mL po fluid/day); **Other:** serum sickness, hemolysis if G6PD def, polyarteritis, SLE reported.
Tinidazole (Tindamax)	**Tabs 250, 500 mg. 2 gm po once or once daily depending on indication** (amebiasis, giardiasis, trichomoniasis, bacterial vaginosis)	**Adverse reactions:** metallic taste 3.7%, nausea 3.2%, anorexia/vomiting 1.5%. All higher with multi-day dosing. Avoid alcohol during & for 3 days after last dose; cause disulfiram reaction, flushing, N/V, tachycardia.
Trimethoprim (Trimpex, Proloprim, and others) (100, 200 mg tab)	**100 mg po q12h or 200 mg po q24h.**	**CNS:** drug fever, aseptic meningitis; **Derm:** rash (3-7% at 200 mg/day), phototoxicity, Stevens-Johnson syndrome (rare), toxic epidermal necrolysis (rare); **Renal:** ↑ K+, ↓ Na+, ↑ Cr; Hem: neutropenia, thrombocytopenia, methemoglobinemia. ACE inhibitors & aldactone increase serum K+. Higher incidence & severity when combined. Increased risk of death. *BMJ 2014, 349:g6196*. Mechanism: *JAMA 2015,314:2406*.
Trimethoprim (TMP)-Sulfamethoxazole (SMX) (Bactrim, Septra, Sulfatrim, Cotrimoxazole) Single-strength (SS) is 80 TMP/400 SMX, double-strength (DS) 160 TMP/800 SMX	**Standard po rx: 1 DS tab bid.** **P. jirovecii: IV rx (base on TMP component): standard 8–10 mg per kg IV per day divided q6h, q8h, or q12h.**	Adverse reactions in 10%: GI: nausea, vomiting, anorexia. Skin: Rash, urticaria, photosensitivity. More serious (1–10%): TMP, ACE inhibitors & aldactone increase serum K+. Higher incidence of severity when combined. Increased risk of death *(BMJ 349:g6196, 2014)*. **Stevens-Johnson syndrome & toxic epidermal necrolysis.** Skin reactions may represent toxic metabolites of SMX rather than allergy *(Ann Pharmacotherapy 32:381, 1998)*. Daily ascorbic acid 0.5–1.0 gm may promote detoxification *(JAIDS 36:1041, 2004)*. Risk of **hypoglycemia** with concomitant sulfonylureas. **Sweet's Syndrome** can occur. Hyperkalemia: Both TMP & ACE inhibitors can block renal tubular secretions of K+ & lead to dangerous hyperkalemia *(BMJ 349:g6196, 2014)*. TMP one etiology of **aseptic meningitis.** Report of psychosis during treatment of PCP *(JAC 66:1117, 2011)*. TMP-SMX contains sulfites and may trigger asthma in sulfite-sensitive pts. Frequent drug cause of thrombocytopenia. No cross allergenicity with other sulfonamide non-antibiotic drugs *(NEJM 349:1628, 2003)*. **For TMP-SMX desensitization,** *see Table 7, page 91.*
Topical Antimicrobial Agents Active vs. S. aureus & Strep. pyogenes *(CID 49:1541, 2009)*. **Review of topical antiseptics, antibiotics** *(CID 49:1541, 2009)*.		
Bacitracin (Baciguent)	20% bacitracin zinc ointment, apply 1-5 x/day.	Active vs. staph, strep & clostridium. Contact dermatitis occurs. Available without prescription.
Fusidic acid ointment	**2% ointment, apply tid**	Available in Canada and Europe *(Leo Laboratories)*. Active vs. S. aureus & S. pyogenes.
Mupirocin (Bactroban)	**Skin cream or ointment 2%: Apply tid times 10 days. Nasal ointment 2%: apply bid times 5 days.**	Skin cream: itch, burning, stinging 1–1.5%; Nasal: headache 9%, rhinitis 6%, respiratory congestion 5%. Not active vs. enterococci or gm-neg bacteria. Summary of resistance: *JAC 70:2681, 2015.* If large amounts used in azotemic pts, can accumulate polyethylene glycol *(CID 49:1541, 2009)*.
Polymyxin B—Bacitracin (Polysporin)	5000 units/gm; 400 units/gm. Apply 1-4x/day	Polymyxin active vs. some gm-neg bacteria but not Proteus sp., Serratia sp. or gm-pos bacteria. *See Bacitracin comment above.* Available without prescription.
Polymyxin B—Bacitracin—Neomycin (Neosporin, triple antibiotic ointment (TAO))	5000 units/gm; 400 units/gm; 3.5 mg/gm. Apply 1-3x/day.	*See Bacitracin and polymyxin B comments above.* Neomycin active vs. gm-neg bacteria and staphylococci; not active vs. streptococci. Contact dermatitis incidence 1%; risk of nephro- & oto-toxicity if absorbed. TAO spectrum broader than mupirocin and active mupirocin-resistant strains *(DMID 54:63, 2006)*. Available without prescription.
Retapamulin (Altabax)	1% ointment; apply bid. 5, 10 & 15 gm tubes.	Microbiologic success in 90% S. aureus infections and 97% of S. pyogenes infections *(J Am Acd Derm 55:1003, 2006)*. Package insert says **for MSSA only** (not enough MRSA pts in clinical trials). Active vs. some mupirocin-resistant S. aureus strains. Resistance can occur *(see Clin Microbiol Rev 30: 827, 2017)*.
Silver sulfadiazine	1% cream, apply once or twice daily.	A sulfonamide but the active ingredient is released silver ions. Activity vs. gram-pos & gram-neg bacteria (including P. aeruginosa). Often used to prevent infection in pts with 2nd/3rd degree burns. Rarely, may stain into the skin.

(See page 2 for abbreviations)

*NOTE: all dosage recommendations are for adults (unless otherwise indicated) & assume normal renal function.

TABLE 10B – ANTIMICROBIAL AGENTS ASSOCIATED WITH PHOTOSENSITIVITY

Photosensitivity is classified as either photoallergic (type IV hypersensitivity) or phototoxic (direct tissue injury). Phototoxic reactions are much more common than photoallergic reactions. UVA radiation is most commonly implicated.

The following drugs (listed alphabetically) are known to cause photosensitivity in some individuals. Note that photosensitivity lasts for several days after the last dose of the drug, at least for tetracyclines. There is no intent to indicate relative frequency or severity of reactions. *Drug Saf 2019, 42:827.*

DRUG OR CLASS	COMMENT
Antiparasitic drugs	Pyrimethamine (one report), Quinine (may cross-react with quinidine). Rare reports with Chloroquine. Recent report of phototoxicity with Atovaquone-Proguanil, confirmed by photopatch testing.
Azole antifungals	Voriconazole, Itraconazole, Ketoconazole, (but not Fluconazole). One report of solar urticaria in a patient receiving Terbinafine.
Cefotaxime	Manifested as photodistributed telangiectasia.
Ceftazidime	Increased susceptibility to sunburn observed.
Dapsone	Confirmed by rechallenge and photopatch testing.
Efavirenz	Three reports.
Flucytosine	Two reports.
Fluoroquinolones	The worst offenders have a halogen atom at C-8 of the quinolone nucleus (Lomefloxacin, Sparfloxacin). Recent data suggest that certain other molecular features, such as a large polar group at N-1, can mitigate the effect of the C-8 halogen; thus Delafloxacin seems to be relatively non-phototoxic despite having a chlorine at C-8. After Sparfloxacin, the rank of phototoxic potential among other FQs is Ciprofloxacin>Gemifloxacin>Levofloxacin>Norfloxacin>Ofloxacin. Gatifloxacin and Moxifloxacin have not been linked to phototoxic events to date *(Photochem Photobiol Sci 2018;17:773)*.
Griseofulvin	Not thought to be a potent photosensitizer, although a few old reports exist.
Isoniazid	Confirmed by rechallenge.
Pyrazinamide	Confirmed by rechallenge.
Saquinavir	One report.
Tenofovir disoproxil fumarate	One report, confirmed by histopathology and photopatch testing.
Tetracyclines	Reported with Tetracycline and Doxycycline. Uncommon with Minocycline.
Tigecycline	No reports.
Trimethoprim	Alone and in combination with Sulfamethoxazole.

TABLE 10C – AMINOGLYCOSIDE ONCE DAILY AND MULTIPLE DAILY DOSING REGIMENS

(If estimated CrCl <90 mL/min or if on dialysis, see *Table 17A*, ***page 237*)**

- General Note: dosages are given as **once daily dose (OD)** and **multiple daily doses (MDD).**
- For **calculation of dosing weight in non-obese patients** use **Ideal Body Weight (IBW):**

  Female: 45.5 kg + 2.3 kg per inch over 60 inch height = dosing weight in kg;

  Male: 50 kg + 2.3 kg per inch over 60 inch height = dosing weight in kg.
- **Adjustment for calculation of dosing weight in obese patients** (actual body weight (ABW) is ≥ 30% above IBW): IBW + 0.4 (ABW minus IBW) = adjusted weight *(Pharmacotherapy 27:1081, 2007; CID 25:112, 1997).*
- **If estimated CrCl >90 mL/min, use doses in this table. If CrCl <90 mL/min or if on dialysis, use doses in** *Table 17A*, ***page 237.***

- **For non-obese patients, calculate estimated creatinine clearance (CrCl) as follows:**

$$\frac{(140 \text{ minus age}) \times (\text{IBW in kg})}{72 \times \text{serum creatinine}} = \text{CrCl in ML/min for men. Multiply answer by 0.85 for women (estimated)}$$

- **For morbidly obese patients, calculate estimated creatinine clearance (CrCl) as follows** *(AJM 84:1053, 1988):*

$$\frac{(137 \text{ minus age}) \times [(0.285 \times \text{wt in kg}) + (12.1 \times \text{ht in meters}^2)]}{51 \times \text{serum creatinine}} = \text{CrCl (obese male)}$$

$$\frac{(146 \text{ minus age}) \times [(0.287 \times \text{wt in kg}) + (9.74 \times \text{ht in meters}^2)]}{60 \times \text{serum creatinine}} = \text{CrCl (obese female)}$$

DRUG	MDD AND OD IV REGIMENS/ TARGETED PEAK (P) AND TROUGH (T) SERUM LEVELS	COMMENTS For more data on once-daily dosing, *see AAC 55:2528, 2011 and Table 17A, page 237*
Gentamicin (Garamycin), **Tobramycin** (Nebcin)	MDD: 2 mg per kg load, then 1.7 mg per kg q8h P 4–10 mcg/mL, T 1–2 mcg per mL OD: 5.1 (7 if critically ill) mg per kg q24h P 16–24 mcg per mL, T <1 mcg per mL	**All aminoglycosides have potential to cause tubular necrosis and renal failure, deafness due to cochlear toxicity, vertigo due to damage to vestibular organs, and rarely neuromuscular blockade.** Risk minimal with oral or topical application due to small % absorption unless tissues altered by disease. Risk of nephrotoxicity ↑ with concomitant administration of cyclosporine, vancomycin, ampho B, radiocontrast. Risk of nephrotoxicity ↓ by once-daily dosing method (especially if baseline renal function normal). In general, same factors influence risk of ototoxicity. **NOTE: There is no known method to eliminate risk of aminoglycoside nephro/ototoxicity. Proper rx attempts to ↓ the % risk.** The clinical trial data of OD aminoglycosides have been reviewed extensively by meta-analysis *(CID 24:816, 1997).* **Serum levels:** Collect peak serum level (PSL) exactly 1 hr after the start of the infusion of the 3rd dose. In critically ill pts, PSL after the 1st dose as volume of distribution and renal function may change rapidly. One in 500 patients (Europe) have mitochondrial mutation that predicts cochlear toxicity *(NEJM 360:640 & 642, 2009).* Aspirin supplement (3 gm/day) attenuated risk of cochlear injury from gentamicin *(NEJM 354:1856, 2006).* Vestibular injury usually bilateral & hence no vertigo but imbalance & oscillopsia *(Med J Aust 196:701, 2012).*
Kanamycin (Kantrex), **Amikacin** (Amikin), **Streptomycin**	MDD: 7.5 mg per kg q12h P 15–30 mcg per mL, T 5–10 mcg per mL OD: 15 mg per kg q24h P 56–64 mcg per mL, T <1 mcg per mL	
Netilmicin*	MDD: 2 mg per kg q8h P 4–10 mcg per mL, T 1–2 mcg per mL OD: 6.5 mg per kg q24h P 22–30 mcg per mL, T <1 mcg per mL	
Plazomicin (Zemdri)	OD: 15 mg per kg q24h P: 74 mcg per mL, T: <1 mcg per mL	
Isepamicin*	Only OD: Severe infections 15 mg per kg q24h, less severe 8 mg per kg q24h	
Spectinomycin (Trobicin)*	2 gm IM times 1–gonococcal infections	
Neomycin—oral	Prophylaxis GI surgery: 1 gm po times 3 with erythro, *see Table 15B, page 220* For hepatic coma: 4–12 gm per day po	
Tobramycin—inhaled (Tobi): *See Cystic fibrosis, Table 1, page 46 & Table 10E, page 130.* Adverse effects few: transient voice alteration (13%) and transient tinnitus (3%).		
Paromomycin—oral: *See Entamoeba and Cryptosporidia, Table 13A, page 160.*		

* where available

TABLE 10D – PROLONGED OR CONTINUOUS INFUSION DOSING OF SELECTED ANTIBIOTICS

Prolonged or continuous infusion of beta-lactams is at least as successful as intermittent dosing. Hence, this approach can be part of stewardship programs as supported by recent publications.

Antibiotic stability is a concern. Factors influencing stability include drug concentration, IV infusion diluent *(e.g. NS vs. D5W)*, type of infusion device, and storage temperature *(Ref: P&T 36:723, 2011)*. Portable pumps worn close to the body expose antibiotics to temperatures closer to body temperature (37°C) than to room temperature (around 25°C). Carbapenems are particularly unstable and may require wrapping of infusion pumps in cold packs or frequent changes of infusion bags or cartridges.

A meta-analysis of observational studies found reduced mortality among patients treated with extended or continuous infusion of carbapenems or piperacillin-tazobactam (pooled data) as compared to standard intermittent regimens. The results were similar for extended and continuous regimens when considered separately. There was a mortality benefit with piperacillin-tazobactam but not carbapenems *(CID 56:272, 2013)*. The lower mortality could, at least in part, be due to closer professional supervision engendered by a study environment. On the other hand, a small prospective randomized controlled study of continuous vs. intermittent Pip-Tazo, and meropenem found a higher clinical cure rate and a trend toward lower mortality in the continuous infusion patients *(CID 56:236, 2013)*.

DRUG/METHOD	MINIMUM STABILITY	RECOMMENDED DOSE	COMMENTS
Ampicillin-sulbactam (Prolonged)	@ 37ºC: In NS at 24 hr amp 77%, sulb 93% *(IJAA 6:S31, 1996)* @ 25ºC: 8 hr (NS)* @ 4ºC: 48 hr (NS)* *(amp/sulb conc ≤ 30 mg/15 mg per mL)	12 gm (8 gm amp + 4 gm sulb) IV over 4 hours q8h	Recommended dose is for VAP due to Acinetobacter. High dose found safe and effective in observational studies *(Scand J ID 39:38, 2007; J Infect 56:432, 2008)*. The need for a high-dose prolonged-infusion sulbactam regimen is supported by pharmacodynamic computer simulation studies using serum concentration measurements in healthy volunteers *(AAC 57:3441, 2013)*. Recommended dose is for patients with normal renal function.
Cefepime (Continuous)	@ 37°C: 8 hours @ 25°C: 24 hours @ 4°C: ≥24 hours	Initial dose: 15 mg/kg over 30 min, then immediately begin: • If CrCl >60: 6 gm (over 24 hr) daily • If CrCl 30-60: 4 gm (over 24 hr) daily • If CrCl 11-29: 2 gm (over 24 hr) daily	CrCl adjustments extrapolated from prescribing information, not clinical data. Refs: *JAC 57:1017, 2006; Am. J. Health Syst. Pharm. 68:319, 2011.*
Ceftazidime (Continuous)	@ 37°C: 8 hours @ 25°C: 24 hours @ 4°C: ≥24 hours	Initial dose: 15 mg/kg over 30 min, then immediately begin: • If CrCl >50: 6 gm (over 24 hr) daily • If CrCl 31-50: 4 gm (over 24 hr) daily • If CrCl 10-30: 2 gm (over 24 hr) daily	CrCl adjustments extrapolated from prescribing information, not clinical data. Refs: *Br J Clin Pharmacol 50:184, 2000; IJAA 17:497, 2001; AAC 49:3550, 2005; Infect 37: 418, 2009; JAC 68:900, 2013.* Pyridine, a byproduct of ceftazidime degradation, is a theoretic toxicity concern; minimize risk by limiting daily dose to 6 gm, using NS as the infusion vehicle, keeping ceftazidime concentration ≤3 gm per 100 mL if possible, and maintaining infusion device temperature between 15-22 ºC *(AJHP 2019;76:200)*.
Doripenem (Prolonged)	@ 37°C: 8 hours (in NS) @ 25°C: 24 hours (in NS) @ 4ºC: 24 hours (in NS)	• If CrCl ≥50: 500 mg (over 4 hr) q8h • If CrCl 30-49: 250 mg (over 4 hr) q8h • If CrCl 10-29: 250 mg (over 4 hr) q12h	Based on a single study *(Crit Care Med 36:1089, 2008)*.
Meropenem (Prolonged)	@ 37°C: <4 hours @ 25°C: 4 hours @ 4°C: 24 hours	• If CrCl ≥50: 2 gm (over 3 hr) q8h • If CrCl 30-49: 1 gm (over 3 hr) q8h • If CrCl 10-29: 1 gm (over 3 hr) q12h	Initial 1 gm dose reasonable but not used by most investigators. Ref: *Intens Care Med 37:632, 2011.*
Pip-tazo (Prolonged)	@ 37°C: 24 hours @ 25°C: 24 hours @ 4°C: no data	Initial dose: 4.5 gm over 30 min, then 4 hrs later start: • If CrCl ≥20: 3.375 gm (over 4 hr) q8h • If CrCl <20: 3.375 gm (over 4 hr) q12h	Reasonable to begin first infusion 4 hrs after initial dose. Refs: *CID 44:357, 2007; AAC 54:460, 2010.* *See CID 56:236, 245 & 272, 2013.* In obese patients (>120 kg), may need higher doses: 6.75 gm or even 9 gm (over 4 hrs) q8h to achieve adequate serum levels of tazobactam *(Int J Antimicrob Agts 41:52, 2013)*.
Temocillin	@ 37°C: 24 hours @ 25°C: 24 hours These apply to Temocillin 4 gm/48 mL dilution *(JAC 61:382, 2008)*	Initial dose: 2 gm over 30 min, then immediately begin: • If CrCl >50: 6 gm (over 24 hr) daily • If CrCl 31-50: 3 gm (over 24 hr) daily • If CrCl 10-30: 1.5 gm (over 24 hr) daily • If CrCl <10: 750 mg (over 24 hr) daily CVVH: 750 mg (over 24 hr) daily	CVVH: 750 mg (over 24 hr) daily offers higher probability of reaching desired PK/PD target than conventional q8h dosing. This study not designed to assess clinical efficacy *(JAC 70:891, 2015)*.

TABLE 10D (2)

DRUG/METHOD	MINIMUM STABILITY	RECOMMENDED DOSE	COMMENTS
Vancomycin (Continuous)	@ 37°C: 48 hours @ 25°C: 48 hours @ 4°C: 58 days (at conc 10 µg/mL)	Loading dose of 15-20 mg/kg over 30-60 minutes, then 30 mg/kg by continuous infusion over 24 hrs. No data on pts with renal impairment.	Adjust dose to target plateau concentration of 20-25 µg/mL. Higher plateau concentrations (30-40 µg/mL) achieved with more aggressive dosing increase the risk of nephrotoxicity *(Clin Micro Inf 19:E98, 2013)*. The AUC/MIC ratio is superior to T>MIC for predicting Vancomycin efficacy. Successful treatment of MRSA is associated with a steady-state AUC_{0-24}/MIC of ≥400. Vancomycin administration by continuous infusion is gaining acceptance as a treatment option. Limited clinical data demonstrate no improvement in efficacy over intermittent infusion although target concentrations are more rapidly achieved with less variability *(JAC 68:743, 2013; Ann Pharmacother 47:219, 2013)*. A recent meta-analysis suggests decreased nephrotoxicity compared to intermittent infusion but definitive conclusions are premature *(JAC 67:17, 2012)*. With continuous infusion the AUC_{0-24} can be calculated by multiplying a single concentration measured at state state by 24 *(AAC 62:e02042, 2018)*.

TABLE 10E – INHALATION ANTIBIOTICS

There are many reasons to consider inhaled antibiotics as an adjunct to parenteral therapy: • spectrum of activity that includes MDR GNB • documented high drug concentration in lung epithelial alveolar lining fluid • benefit in animal models of pneumonia • improved drug delivery (nebulizer) systems • Low risk of serious AEs. Refs: *Adv Drug Del Rev 2015,85-65* (review); *Chest 2017, 151:737* (clinical debate). The 2016 IDSA HAP/VAP guidelines suggest augmenting parenteral therapy with inhaled antibiotics, especially for highly resistant bacteria *(CID 2016;63:e61)*.

INHALED DRUG	DELIVERY SYSTEM	DOSE	COMMENT
Aztreonam (Cayston)	Altera vibrating mesh nebulizer	75 mg tid x 28 days (every other month)	Improves pulmonary function, reduces bacterial load, reduces frequency of exacerbations, and improves symptoms in **cystic fibrosis (CF)** pts *(Exp Opin Pharmacother 14:2115, 2013)*. Cost per treatment cycle about $6070.
Colistin (colistimethate) dry powder (EMA approved) Note: Polymyxin B is not used for inhalation due to toxicity to lung epithelial cells *(AAC 2017,61:e02690-16)*	Various *(see Comments)*	Most commonly used: 50-75 mg CBA in 3-4 mL NS via vibrating mesh nebulizer 2-3 times/day	Much variability and confusion in dosing. Nebulized colistimethate (CMS) 1-2 million IU (33-66 mg CBA) effective in **cystic fibrosis** *(Exp Opin Drug Deliv 9:333, 2012)*. Recent review is encouraging *(Expert Rev Anti Infect Ther 13:1237, 2015)*. In-depth PK study in 6 CF patients supportive in that nebulization of colistimethate achieved sputum colistimethate and colistin concentrations higher than those achieved from IV administration *(AAC 58:2570, 2014)*.
Fosfomycin + Tobramycin (FTI) 4:1 wt/wt	eFlow vibrating mesh nebulizer	FTI 160/40 or 80/20 bid x 28 days	Both doses maintained improvements in FEV1 following a 28-day inhaled aztreonam run-in (vs. placebo) in **CF patients** with *P. aeruginosa*; FTI 80/20 better tolerated than 160/40 *(AJRCCM 185:171, 2012)*.
Levofloxacin	eFlow vibrating mesh nebulizer	240 mg bid x 28 days	Reduced sputum density of *P. aeruginosa*, need for other antibiotics, and improved pulmonary function compared to placebo in **CF pts** *(AJRCCM 183:1510, 2011)*.
Liposomal Amikacin (Arikayce)	eFlow vibrating mesh nebulizer (Lamira, PARI Pharma)	590 mg (8.4 mL) once daily	For use as part of a combination regimen for **refractory MAC** in patients with limited or no alternative treatment options. Black box warning: associated with an increased risk of respiratory adverse reactions including hypersensitivity pneumonitis, hemoptysis, bronchospasm, and exacerbation of underlying pulmonary disease.
Tobramycin (TOBI, Bethkis)	PARI LC PLUS jet nebulizer	300 mg bid x 28 days (every other month)	Cost (generic): about $5769 for one treatment cycle.
Tobramycin (TOBI Podhaler)	28 mg dry powder caps	4 caps (112 mg) bid x 28 days (every other month)	Improvement in FEV1 similar to Tobra inhaled solution in **CF patients** with chronic *P. aeruginosa* but more airway irritation with the powder. Cost of one month treatment cycle about $6700 *(Med Lett 56:51, 2014)*.

TABLE 11A – TREATMENT OF FUNGAL INFECTIONS

For Antifungal Activity Spectra, *see Table 4B, page 86*

<table>
<tr><th rowspan="2">TYPE OF INFECTION/ORGANISM/
SITE OF INFECTION</th><th colspan="2">ANTIMICROBIAL AGENTS OF CHOICE</th><th rowspan="2">COMMENTS</th></tr>
<tr><th>PRIMARY</th><th>ALTERNATIVE</th></tr>
<tr><td colspan="4">Aspergillosis (A. fumigatus most common, also A. flavus and others) (See NEJM 360:1870, 2009; Chest 146:1358, 2014). Diagnosis: Chest 156:834, 2019.</td></tr>
<tr><td>Allergic bronchopulmonary aspergillosis (ABPA) Clinical manifestations: wheezing, pulmonary infiltrates, bronchiectasis & fibrosis. Airway colonization assoc. with ↑ blood eosinophils, ↑ serum IgE, ↑ specific serum antibodies.</td><td>Acute asthma attacks associated with ABPA: Corticosteroids</td><td>Rx of ABPA: Itra oral sol'n 200 mg po bid times 16 wks or longer</td><td>Itra decreases number of exacerbations requiring corticosteroids with improved immunological markers, improved lung function & exercise tolerance (CID 63:433, 2016).</td></tr>
<tr><td>Allergic fungal sinusitis: relapsing chronic sinusitis; nasal polyps without bony invasion; asthma, eczema or allergic rhinitis; ↑ IgE levels and isolation of Aspergillus sp. or other dematiaceous sp. (Alternaria, Cladosporium, etc.)</td><td>Rx controversial: systemic corticosteroids + surgical debridement (relapse common).</td><td>For failures try Itra 200 mg po bid times 12 mos or Flu nasal spray.</td><td>Controversial area.</td></tr>
<tr><td>Aspergilloma (fungus ball)</td><td colspan="2">No therapy or surgical resection. Efficacy of antimicrobial agents not proven.</td><td>Aspergillus may complicate pulmonary sequestration.</td></tr>
<tr><td>Invasive, pulmonary (IPA) or extrapulmonary:
Post-transplantation and post-chemotherapy in neutropenic pts (PMN <500 per mm³) but may also present with neutrophil recovery.
Common pneumonia in transplant recipients. Usually a late (≥100 days) complication in allogeneic bone marrow & liver transplantation: High mortality (CID 44:531, 2007).
Typical x-ray/CT lung lesions (halo sign, cavitation, or macronodules) (CID 44:373, 2007).
Galactomannan antigen immunoassay: Detects aspergillus cell wall polysaccharide. Adjunct to diagnosis in neutropenic pts. Serum sens/spec. varies from 21-86% sens/80-92% spec. BAL fluid 60-100% sens/68-100% spec. False neg. if receiving antifungals. False pos. if colonized by aspergillus or infected by Fusarium, histo or blasto (JAMA 2017;318:1175).
Better diagnostic strategy: combination of serum galactomannan & aspergillus PCR (not routinely available) (LnID 13:519, 2013).
Beta D-Glucan: in fungal cell wall. Can detect with immunoassay. Many false positives + low sensitivity (JCM 51:3478, 2013).</td><td colspan="2">Primary therapy (See CID 63:433, 2016):
Vori 6 mg/kg IV q12h on day 1; then either (4 mg/kg IV q12h) or (200 mg po q12h for body weight ≥40 kg, but 100 mg po q12h for body weight <40 kg) (use actual wt). Goal trough (day 4): 1.0–5.5 mg/L associated with improved response rates and reduced adverse effects (Clin Infect Dis 55:1080, 2012).
Verify in vitro susceptibility (CID 68:1463, 2019).

Alternative therapies:
Isavuconazonium sulfate loading dose of 372 mg (equivalent to isavuconazole 200 mg) IV/po q8 x 6 doses then 372 mg IV/po daily
OR
Liposomal Ampho B (LAB) (L-AmB) 3-5 mg/kg/day IV;
OR
Ampho B lipid complex (ABLC) 5 mg/kg/d IV;
OR
Caspo 70 mg/day then 50 mg/day thereafter;
OR
Mica[NAI] 100 mg bid (JAC 64:840, 2009– based on PK/PD study);
OR
Posa[NAI] 200 mg qid, then 400 mg bid after stabilization of disease.

In documented azole-resistant invasive aspergillosis, most experts suggest change to either Liposomal Ampho B or combination of Vori + echinocandin (JID 2017;216(S3):S436)</td><td>Voriconazole more effective than Ampho B. Vori, both a substrate and an inhibitor of CYP2C19, CYP2C9, and CYP3A4, has potential for deleterious drug interactions (e.g., with protease inhibitors). Review concomitant medications. Measure serum level with prolonged therapy or for patients with possible drug-drug interactions. In patients with CrCl <50 mL/min, po may be preferred due to concerns for nephrotoxicity of IV vehicle in renal dysfunction. (Clin Infect Dis 54:913, 2012)
Isavuconazole: (prodrug isavuconazonium sulfate): A randomized control trial of Isavuconazole vs. Voriconazole for invasive aspergillosis demonstrated that Isavuconazole is non-inferior to voriconazole for the treatment of invasive aspergillosis (Ln 2016;387:760).
Ampho B: not recommended except as a lipid formulation, either L-AMB or ABLC. 10 mg/kg and 3 mg/kg doses of L-AMB are equally efficacious with greater toxicity of higher dose (CID 2007; 44:1289–97). One comparative trial found greater toxicity with ABLC than with L-AMB: 34.6% vs 9.4% adverse events and 21.2% vs 2.8% nephrotoxicity (Cancer 112:1282, 2008). Vori preferred as primary therapy.
Posaconazole: 42% response rate in open-label trial of patients refractory/intolerant to conventional therapy (CID 44:2, 2007). Concern for cross-resistance with azole-non-responders. Measurement of serum concentrations advisable.
Caspofungin: ~50% response rate in IPA. Licensed for salvage therapy.
Micafungin: Favorable responses to micafungin as a single agent in 6/12 patients in primary therapy group and 9/22 in the salvage therapy group (J Infect 53: 337, 2006).
Combination therapy: A RCT of Voriconazole plus Anidulafungin vs. Voriconazole alone showed a trend towards reduced mortality in all patients with invasive aspergillosis in the combination therapy arm (Ann Intern Med 162:81, 2015). Subgroup of patients with invasive aspergillosis whose diagnosis was established by radiographic findings and GM positivity had lower mortality with combination therapy. Combination therapy should be strongly considered although further data is needed to determine which patients would benefit the most. Some experts would recommend addition of echinocandin to amphotericin-based regimen or other azoles as well.</td></tr>
</table>

See page 2 for abbreviations. All dosage recommendations are for adults (unless otherwise indicated) and assume normal renal function.

TABLE 11A (2)

TYPE OF INFECTION/ORGANISM/ SITE OF INFECTION	ANTIMICROBIAL AGENTS OF CHOICE		COMMENTS
	PRIMARY	ALTERNATIVE	
Blastomycosis *(CID 46: 1801, 2008)* *(Blastomyces dermatitidis)* Cutaneous, pulmonary or extrapulmonary.	**LAB,** 3-5 mg/kg per day; OR **Ampho B,** 0.7-1 mg/kg per day, for 1-2 weeks, **then Itra** oral sol'n 200 mg tid for 3 days followed by Itra 200 mg bid for 6 -12 months	**Itra** oral sol'n 200 mg tid for 3 days then once or twice per day for 6-12 months for mild to moderate disease; OR **Flu** 400-800 mg per day for those intolerant to Itra	Serum levels of **Itra** should be determined after 2 weeks to ensure adequate drug exposure. Flu less effective than Itra; role of Vori or Posa unclear but active in vitro. Can look for Blastomyces in antigen in urine as aid to diagnosis.
Blastomycosis: CNS disease *(CID 50:797, 2010)*	**LAB** 5 mg/kg per day for 4–6 weeks, followed by **Flu** 800 mg per day	**Itra** oral sol'n 200 mg bid or tid; OR **Vori** 200-400 mg q12h	Flu and Vori have excellent CNS penetration, to counterbalance their slightly reduced activity compared to Itra. Treat for at least 12 months and until CSF has normalized. Monitor serum Itra levels to assure adequate drug concentrations. More favorable outcome with Voriconazole *(CID 50:797, 2010)*.
Candidiasis: Candida is a common cause of nosocomial bloodstream infection. *C. albicans* & non-albicans species show ↓ susceptibility to antifungal agents (esp. fluconazole). In immunocompromised pts where antifungal prophylaxis (esp. fluconazole) is widely used. Oral, esophageal, or vaginal candidiasis is a major manifestation of advanced HIV & represents common AIDS-defining diagnosis. *See CID 62:e1, 2016 for updated IDSA Guidelines.*			
Candidiasis: Bloodstream infection *(C. albicans & C. glabrata)*. Diagnosis: *Chest 156:834, 2019.*			
Bloodstream: non-neutropenic patient Remove all intravascular catheters if possible; replace catheters at a new site (not over a wire). Higher mortality associated with delay in therapy *(CID 43:25, 2006)*. ***Candida auris:*** This is an emerging **multi-drug resistant** Candida species able to cause a wide-range of infections. It can misidentified as *Candida haemulonii* or *Saccharomyces cerevisiae*. Molecular methods are needed to confirm species. Often resistant to azoles and amphotericin, some are also echinocandin resistant *(CID 2018,66:306)*. Multi-drug resistant Candida species *(JID 2017;216(S3):S445)*.	**Capso** 70 mg IV loading dose, then 50 mg IV daily; OR **Mica** 100 mg IV daily; OR **Anidula** 200 mg IV loading dose then 100 mg IV daily. Note: Reduce **Caspo** dose for renal impairment **Funduscopic examination** within first week of therapy to exclude ophthalmic involvement. Ocular disease present in ~15% of patients with candidemia, but endophthalmitis is uncommon (~2%) *(CID 53:262, 2011)*. Intraocular injections of Ampho B required for endophthalmitis as echinocandins have poor penetration into the eye. For **septic thrombophlebitis,** catheter removal and incision and drainage and resection of the vein, as needed, are recommended; duration of therapy at least 2 weeks after last positive blood culture.	**Flu** 800 mg (12 mg/kg) loading dose, then 400 mg daily IV OR **Lipid-based Ampho B** 3-5 mg/kg IV daily; OR **Ampho B** 0.7 mg/kg IV daily; OR **Vori** 400 mg (6 mg/kg) IV twice daily for 2 doses then 200 mg q12h.	**Echinocandin** is recommended for empiric therapy, particularly for patients with recent azole exposure or with moderately severe or severe illness, hemodynamic instability. **An echinocandin should be used for treatment of *Candida glabrata* unless susceptibility to fluconazole or voriconazole has been confirmed.** Echinocandin preferred empiric therapy in centers with high prevalence of non-albicans candida species. Echinocandin vs. polyenes or azole associated with better survival *(Clin Infect Dis 54:1110, 2012)*. A double-blind randomized trial of anidulafungin (n=127) and fluconazole (n=118) showed an 88% microbiologic response rate (119/135 candida species) with anidulafungin vs a 76% (99/130 candida species) with fluconazole (p=0.02) *(NEJM 356: 2472, 2007)*. **Fluconazole** is not recommended for empiric therapy but could be considered recommended for patients with mild-to-moderate illness, hemodynamically stable, with no recent azole exposure. **Fluconazole not recommended for treatment of documented *C. krusei*: use an echinocandin or voriconazole or posaconazole (note: echinocandins have better in vitro activity than either Vori or Posa against *C. glabrata*).** **Fluconazole recommended for treatment of *Candida parapsilosis*** because of reduced susceptibility of this species to echinocandins. Transition from echinocandin to fluconazole for stable patients with *Candida albicans* or other azole-susceptible species. **Voriconazole** with little advantage over fluconazole (more drug-drug interactions) except for oral step-down therapy of *Candida krusei* or voriconazole-susceptible *Candida glabrata*. Recommended **duration of therapy** is 14 days after last positive blood culture. Duration of systemic therapy should be extended to 4-6 weeks for eye involvement.

TABLE 11A (3)

TYPE OF INFECTION/ORGANISM/ SITE OF INFECTION	ANTIMICROBIAL AGENTS OF CHOICE		COMMENTS
	PRIMARY	ALTERNATIVE	
Candidiasis: Bloodstream infection *(continued)*			
Bloodstream: neutropenic patient Remove all intravascular catheters if possible; replace catheters at a new site (not over a wire).	**Capso** 70 mg IV loading dose, then 50 mg IV daily, 35 mg for moderate hepatic insufficiency; OR **Mica** 100 mg IV daily; OR **Anidula** 200 mg IV loading dose then 100 mg IV daily; OR **Lipid-based Ampho B** 3-5 mg/kg IV daily.	**Flu** 800 mg (12 mg/kg) loading dose, then 400 mg daily IV or po; OR **Vori** 400 mg (6 mg/kg) IV twice daily for 2 doses then 200 mg (3 mg/kg) IV q12h.	**Duration of therapy** in absence of metastatic complications is for 2 weeks after last positive blood culture, resolution of signs, and resolution of neutropenia. Perform funduscopic examination after recovery of white count as signs of ophthalmic involvement may not be seen during neutropenia. *See comments above for recommendations concerning choice of specific agents.*
Candidiasis: Bone and joint infections			
Osteomyelitis	**Flu** 400 mg (6 mg/kg) daily IV or po; OR **Lipid-based Ampho B** 3–5 mg/kg daily x several weeks, then oral fluconazole.	**Caspo**, **Mica** or **Anidula** or **Ampho B** 0.5–1 mg/kg IV daily x several weeks then oral **Flu**.	Treat for a total of 6-12 months. **Surgical debridement** often necessary; **remove hardware** whenever possible.
Septic arthritis	**Flu** 400 mg (6 mg/kg) daily IV or po; OR **Lipid-based Ampho B** 3–5 mg/kg IV daily x several weeks, then oral fluconazole.	**Caspo**, **Mica** or **Anidula** or **Ampho B** 0.5–1 mg/kg IV daily for several weeks then oral **Flu**.	**Surgical debridement** in all cases; removal of prosthetic joints whenever possible. Treat for at least 6 weeks and indefinitely if retained hardware.
Candidiasis: Cardiovascular infections			
Endocarditis, Myocarditis, Pericarditis *(See Eur J Clin Microbiol Infect Dis 27:519, 2008)*	**Caspo** 50–150 mg/day IV; OR **Mica** 100–150 mg/day IV; OR **Anidula** 100–200 mg/day IV; OR **Lipid-based Ampho B** 3–5 mg/kg IV daily + **Flucytosine** 25 mg/kg po qid.	**Ampho B** 0.6–1 mg/kg IV daily + **Flucytosine** 25 mg/kg po qid	Consider use of higher doses of echinocandins for endocarditis or other endovascular infections. Can switch to **Fluconazole 400-800 mg orally in stable patients** with negative blood cultures and fluconazole susceptible organism. *See Med 90:237, 2011.* Valve replacement strongly recommended, particularly if prosthetic valve endocarditis. Duration of therapy not well defined, but treat for at least 6 weeks after valve replacement and longer in those with complications (e.g., perivalvular or myocardial abscess, extensive disease, delayed resolution of candidemia). Pericarditis: Pericardial window or pericardiectomy also is recommended. Long-term (life-long?) suppression with Fluconazole 400-800 mg daily for native valve endocarditis and no valve replacement; life-long suppression for prosthetic valve endocarditis if no valve replacement.
Candidiasis: Mucosal, esophageal, and oropharyngeal			
Candida esophagitis Primarily encountered in HIV-positive patients Dysphagia or odynophagia predictive of esophageal candidiasis.	**Flu** 200-400 (3-6 mg/kg) mg IV/po daily; OR (**Caspo** 50 mg IV daily; OR **Mica** 150 mg IV daily; OR **Anidula** 200 mg IV loading dose then 100 mg IV daily); OR **Ampho B** 0.5 mg/kg IV daily.	An azole (**Itra** solution 200 mg daily; or **Posa** suspension 400 mg bid for 3 days then 400 mg daily or **Vori** IV/po 200 mg q12h.	**Duration of therapy** 14-21 days. IV Echinocandin or Ampho B for patients unable to tolerate oral therapy. For Fluconazole refractory disease, Itra (80% will respond), Posa, Vori, an Echinocandin, or Ampho B. Echinocandins associated with higher relapse rate than fluconazole. ART recommended. Suppressive therapy with fluconazole 200 mg po 3x/wk until CD4 >200/mm^3.

See page 2 for abbreviations. All dosage recommendations are for adults (unless otherwise indicated) and assume normal renal function.

TABLE 11A (4)

TYPE OF INFECTION/ORGANISM/ SITE OF INFECTION	ANTIMICROBIAL AGENTS OF CHOICE		COMMENTS
	PRIMARY	ALTERNATIVE	
Candidiasis: Mucosal, esophageal, and oropharyngeal *(continued)*			
Oropharyngeal candidiasis			
Non-AIDS patient	**Clotrimazole troches** 10 mg 5 x daily; OR **Nystatin suspension** or pastilles po qid; OR **Flu** 100-200 mg daily.	**Itra** solution 200 mg daily; OR **Posa** suspension 400 mg bid for 3 days then 400 mg daily; or **Vori** 200 mg q12h; OR (**Capso** 70 mg loading dose then 50 mg IV daily; or **Mica** 100 mg IV daily; or **Anidula** 200 mg IV loading dose then 100 mg IV daily); OR **Ampho B** 0.3 mg/kg daily.	**Duration of therapy** 7-14 days. Clotrimazole or nystatin recommended for mild disease; Fluconazole preferred for moderate-to-severe disease. Alternative agents reserved for refractory disease.
AIDS patient	**Flu** 100-200 mg po daily x 7-14 days.	Same as for non-AIDS patient x 7-14 days.	ART in HIV-positive patients. Suppressive therapy until CD4 >200/mm³, but if required fluconazole 100 mg po thrice weekly. Oral Itra, Posa, or Vori for 28 days for Fluconazole-refractory disease. IV echinocardin also an option. Dysphagia or odynophagia predictive of esophageal candidiasis.
Vulvovaginitis			
Non-AIDS Patient	**Topical azole therapy: Butoconazole 2% cream** (5 gm) q24h at bedtime x 3 days or 2% cream SR 5 gm x 1; OR **Clotrimazole 100 mg vaginal tabs** (2 at bedtime x 3 days) or 1% cream (5 gm) at bedtime times 7 days (14 days may ↑ cure rate) or 100 mg vaginal tab x 7 days or 500 mg vaginal tab x 1; OR **Miconazole 200 mg vaginal suppos** (1 at bedtime x 3 days) or 100 mg vaginal suppos. q24h x 7 days or 2% cream (5 gm) at bedtime x 7 days; OR **Terconazole 80 mg vaginal tab** (1 at bedtime x 3 days) or 0.4% cream (5 gm) at bedtime x 7 days or 0.8% cream 5 gm intravaginal q24h x 3 days; or **Tioconazole** 6.5% vag. ointment x 1 dose. **Oral therapy:** **Flu** 150 mg po x 1; OR If severe, **Flu** 150 mg q72h x 3 OR **Itra** 200 mg po bid x 1 day.		**Recurrent vulvovaginal candidiasis: Fluconazole** 150 mg weekly for 6 months. If severe can induce with Flu 150 mg q10-14 days, then weekly.
AIDS Patient	Topical **azoles** (clotrimazole, buto, mico, tico, or tercon) x3–7d; OR Topical **Nystatin** 100,000 units/day as vaginal tablet x14d; OR **Flu** 150 mg po x1 dose.		For recurrent disease 10-14 days of topical azole or oral Flu 150 mg, then **Flu** 150 mg po weekly for 6 mos.
Candidiasis: Other infections			
CNS Infection	**Lipid-based Ampho B** 3–5 mg/kg IV daily + 5-FC 25 mg/kg po qid.	**Flu** 400–800 mg (6-12 mg/kg) IV or po.	Removal of **intraventricular devices** recommended. Flu 400-800 mg as step-down therapy in the stable patient and in patient intolerant of Ampho B. Experience too limited to recommend echinocandins at this time. **Treatment duration** for several weeks until resolution of CSF, radiographic, and clinical abnormalities.
Cutaneous *(including paronychia, Table 1, page 29)*	Apply topical **Ampho B, Clotrimazole, Econazole, Miconazole, or Nystatin** 3-4 x daily for 7–14 days or ketoconazole 400 mg po once daily x 14 days. Ciclopirox olamine 1% cream/lotion; apply topically bid x 7–14 days.		

TABLE 11A (5)

TYPE OF INFECTION/ORGANISM/ SITE OF INFECTION	ANTIMICROBIAL AGENTS OF CHOICE		COMMENTS
	PRIMARY	ALTERNATIVE	
Candidiasis: Other infections *(continued)*			
Endophthalmitis /Chorioretinitis • Occurs in 10% of candidemia, thus ophthalmological consult for all pts • Diagnosis: typical white exudates on retinal exam and/or positive vitrectomy culture • Chorioretinitis accounts for 85% of ocular disease while endophthalmitis occurs in only 15% *(Clin Infect Dis 53:262, 2011)*.	Chorioretinitis or Endophthalmitis: Lipid-based **Ampho B** 3-5 mg/kg daily + **Flucytosine** 25 mg/kg qid OR **Vori** 6 mg/kg po/IV q12 x 2 doses and then 4 mg/kg po/IV q12. Consider intravitreal **Ampho B** 5–10 mcg in 0.1 mL or intravitreal **Vori** 100 mcg in 0.1 mL for sight threatening disease.	Chorioretinitis or Endophthalmitis: **Flu** 6-12 mg/kg IV daily (poor activity against C. glabrata or C. krusei) and consider intravitreal **Ampho B** 5-10 mcg in 0.1 mL for sight-threatening disease. Consider vitrectomy in advanced disease. *Clin Infect Dis. 52:648, 2011.*	**Duration of therapy:** 4-6 weeks or longer, based on resolution determined by repeated examinations. Vitrectomy may be necessary for those with vitritis or endophthalmitis *(Br J Ophthalmol 92:466, 2008; Pharmacotherapy 27:1711, 2007)*.
Neonatal candidiasis	**Ampho B** 1 mg/kg IV daily; OR **Flu** 12 mg/kg IV daily.	**Lipid-based Ampho B** 3-5 mg/kg IV daily.	**Lumbar puncture** to rule out CNS disease, **dilated retinal examination,** abdominal ultrasound and **intravascular catheter removal** strongly recommended. Lipid-based Ampho B used only if there is no renal involvement. Echinocandins considered 3rd line therapy. **Duration of therapy is at least 3 weeks.**
Peritonitis (Chronic Ambulatory Peritoneal Dialysis) *See Table 19, page 255.*	**Flu** 400 mg po q24h x 2–3 wks; or **Caspo** 70 mg IV on day 1 followed by 50 mg IV q24h x 14 days; or **Mica** 100 mg IV q24h x 14 days.	**Ampho B,** continuous intraperitoneal dosing at 1.5 mg/L of dialysis fluid x 4–6 wks.	Remove cath immediately or if no clinical improvement in 4–7 days.
Candidiasis: Urinary tract infections			
Cystitis **Asymptomatic** *See CID 52:s427, 2011; CID 52:s452, 2011.*	**If possible, remove catheter or stent.** No therapy indicated except in patients at high risk for dissemination or undergoing a urologic procedure.		**High risk patients** (neonates and neutropenic patients) should be managed as outlined for treatment of bloodstream infection. For patients undergoing urologic procedures, Flu 200 mg (3 mg/kg) IV/po daily or Ampho B 0.5 mg/kg IV daily (for flu-resistant organisms) for several days pre- and post-procedure.
Symptomatic	**Flu** 200 mg (3 mg/kg) IV/po daily x 14 days.	**Ampho B** 0.5 mg/kg IV daily (for fluconazole resistant organisms) x 7-10 days.	Concentration of echinocandins is low; case reports of efficacy versus azole resistant organisms *(Can J Infect Dis Med Microbiol 18:149, 2007; CID 44:e46, 2007)*. Persistent candiduria in immunocompromised pt warrants ultrasound or CT of kidneys to rule out fungus ball.
Pyelonephritis	**Flu** 200–400 mg (3–6 mg/kg) po once daily.	**Ampho B** 0.5 mg/kg daily IV + 5-FC 25 mg/kg po qid.	**Treat for 2 weeks.** For suspected disseminated disease treat as if bloodstream infection is present.
Chromoblastomycosis *(Clin Exp Dermatol, 34:849, 2009)*. (Cladophialophora, Phialophora, or Fonsecaea); Cutaneous (usually feet, legs): raised scaly lesions, most common in tropical areas	If lesions small & few, **surgical excision or cryosurgery with liquid nitrogen.** If lesions chronic, extensive, burrowing: **Itraconazole.**	**Itra:** 200-400 mg oral sol'n q24h or 400 mg pulse therapy once daily for 1 week of each month x 6-12 months (or until response)[NAI].	**Terbinafine**[NAI] 500-1000 mg once daily alone or in combination with **Itra** 200-400 oral sol'n mg; or **Posa** (800 mg/d) po may be effective. Anecdotal report of efficacy of topical imiquimod 5%: 5x/wk *(CID 58:1734, 2014)*.

TABLE 11A (6)

TYPE OF INFECTION/ORGANISM/ SITE OF INFECTION	ANTIMICROBIAL AGENTS OF CHOICE		COMMENTS
	PRIMARY	ALTERNATIVE	
Coccidioidomycosis *(Coccidioides immitis) (IDSA Guidelines: CID 63: e112, 2016; see also Mayo Clin Proc 83:343, 2008)*			
Primary pulmonary (San Joaquin or Valley Fever): **For pts at low risk of persistence/complication**	**Antifungal rx not generally recommended.** Treat if fever, wt loss and/or fatigue that does not resolve within 4-8 wks		Uncomplicated pulmonary in normal host common in endemic areas *(Emerg Infect Dis 12:958, 2006)* Influenza-like illness of 1–2 wks duration.
Primary pulmonary in pts with ↑ risk for complications or dissemination. Rx indicated: • Immunosuppressive disease, post-transplantation, hematological malignancies or therapies (steroids, TNF-α antagonists) • Pregnancy in 3rd trimester. • Diabetes • CF antibody >1:16 • Pulmonary Infiltrates • Dissemination (identification of spherules or culture of organism from ulcer, joint effusion, pus from subcutaneous abscess or bone biopsy, etc.)	**Mild to moderate severity** *(EID 20:983, 2014)*: **Itra** solution 200 mg po or IV bid; OR **Flu** 400 mg po q24h x 3–12 mos **Locally severe or disseminated disease** **Ampho B** 0.6–1 mg/kg per day x 7 days then 0.8 mg/kg every other day or **liposomal Ampho B** 3-5 mg/kg/d IV or **ABLC** 5 mg/kg/d IV, until clinical improvement (usually several wks or longer in disseminated disease), followed by **Itra** or **Flu** for at least 1 year. Some use combination of Ampho B & Flu for progressive severe disease; controlled series lacking. **Consultation with specialist recommended:** surgery may be required. Suppression in HIV+ patients until CD4 >250 & infection controlled: **Flu** 200 mg po q24h or Itra oral sol'n 200 mg po bid *(Mycosis 46:42, 2003)*.		**Ampho B cure rate 50–70%. Responses to azoles are similar. Itra** may have slight advantage esp. in soft tissue infection. Relapse rates after rx 40%: Relapse rate ↑ if ↑ CF titer ≥1:256. Following CF titers after completion of rx important; rising titers warrant retreatment. **Posaconazole** reported successful in 73% of pts with refractory non-meningeal cocci *(Chest 132:952, 2007)*. Not frontline therapy. Treatment of pediatric cocci to include salvage therapy with Vori & Caspo *(CID 56:1573, 1579 & 1587, 2013)*. Can detect delayed hypersensitivity with skin test antigen called Spherusol; helpful if history of Valley Fever.
Meningitis: occurs in 1/3 to 1/2 of pts with disseminated coccidioidomycosis			
Adult *(CID 42:103, 2006)*	**Flu** 400–1,000 mg po q24h indefinitely	**Ampho B** IV as for pulmonary *(above)* + 0.1–0.3 mg daily intra-thecal (intraventricular) via reservoir device. **OR Itra** oral sol'n 400–800 mg q24h **OR Vori** *(See Comment)*	**80% relapse rate, continue flucon indefinitely,** **Voriconazole** successful in high doses (6 mg/kg IV q12h) followed by oral suppression (200 mg po q12h). For practical spects of intrathecal ampho B, see *CID 2017,64:519*. Small retrospective study suggests benefit from adjunctive corticosteroids *(CID 2017,65:338)*.
Child *(Cryptococcus neoformans, C. gattii)*	**Flu** (Pediatric dose not established, 6 mg per kg po q24h used)		
Cryptococcosis *IDSA Guideline: CID 50:291, 2010.*			
Non-meningeal (non-AIDS) Risk 57% in organ transplant & those receiving other forms of immunosuppressive agents *(EID 13:953, 2007)*.	**Flu** 400 mg/day IV or po x 8 wks to 6 mos **For more severe disease:** **Ampho B** 0.5–0.8 mg/kg per day IV till response then change to **Flu** 400 mg po q24h x 8–10 wks course	**Itra** 200-400 mg solution q24h x 6-12 mos OR (**Ampho B** 0.3 mg/kg per day IV + **Flucytosine** 37.5 mg/kg po qid) x 6 wks (use ideal body wt)	**Flu alone 90% effective for meningeal and non-meningeal forms.** Fluconazole as effective as Ampho B. Addition of **interferon-g** (IFN-γ-Ib 50 mcg per M² subcut. 3x per wk x 9 wks) to liposomal Ampho B assoc. with response in pt failing antifungal rx *(CID 38: 910, 2004)*. Posaconazole 400-800 mg also effective in a small series of patients *(CID 45:562, 2007; Chest 132:952, 2007)*

Meningitis (non-AIDS) IDSA Guidelines: *CID 50:291, 2010.*	• Induction phase: (**Liposomal Ampho B** 3-4 mg/kg IV q24h or **Ampho B lipid complex** 5 mg/kg IV q24h) + **Flucytosine** 25 mg/kg po q6h
	  ○ Duration: Minimum 2 weeks for transplant recipients and minimum 4 weeks in non-immunocompromised patients. Treat until patient is afebrile and cultures are negative.
	  ○ Need to monitor intracranial pressure; If over 25 cm, need to remove CSF. *See comment.*
	• Consolidation phase: **Flu** 400-800 mg po daily x 8 weeks
	• Maintenance phase: **Flu** 200 mg po daily x 6-12 months
			If CSF opening pressure >25 cm H_2O, repeat LP to drain fluid to control pressure.
			C. gattii meningitis reported in the Pacific Northwest *(EID 13:42, 2007)*; severity of disease and prognosis appear to be worse than with C. neoformans; initial therapy with **Ampho B + Flucytosine** recommended.
			C. gattii less susceptible to flucon than C. neoformans *(Clin Microbiol Inf 14:727, 2008)*.
			Outcomes in both AIDS and non-AIDS cryptococcal meningitis improved with Ampho B + 5-FC induction therapy for 14 days in those with neurological abnormalities or high organism burden *(PLoS ONE 3:e2870, 2008)*.

TABLE 11A (7)

TYPE OF INFECTION/ORGANISM/ SITE OF INFECTION	ANTIMICROBIAL AGENTS OF CHOICE: PRIMARY	ANTIMICROBIAL AGENTS OF CHOICE: ALTERNATIVE	COMMENTS
Cryptococcosis *(continued)*			
HIV+/AIDS: Cryptococcemia and/or Meningitis			
Treatment *See Clin Infect Dis 50:291, 2010 (IDSA Guidelines).* ↓ with ARV but still common presenting OI in newly diagnosed AIDS pts. Cryptococcal infection may be manifested by positive blood culture or positive serum cryptococcal antigen (CRAG: >95% sens). CRAG no help in monitoring response to therapy. With ARV, symptoms of acute meningitis may return: immune reconstitution inflammatory syndrome (IRIS). ↑ CSF pressure **(>250 mm H2O)** associated with high mortality: lower with CSF removal. If frequent LPs not possible, ventriculoperitoneal shunts an option *(Surg Neurol 63:529 & 531, 2005).*	**Ampho B** 0.7 mg/kg IV q24H or Liposomal **Ampho B** 3-4 mg/kg IV q24 or **Ampho B** lipid complex 5 mg/kg IV q24 + **Flucytosine** 25 mg/kg po q6h for at least two weeks or longer until CSF is sterilized. *See Comment.* **Then** **Consolidation therapy: Flu** 400-800 mg po q24h to complete a 10-wks course then suppression *(see below).* Deferring ART for 5 wks after initiation cryptococcal meningitis therapy significantly improved survival as compared to starting ART during the first 2 wks *(NEJM 370:2487, 2014).*	**If 5-FC not possible**: Ampho B product + Fluc 800-1200 mg/day IV/po x 2 weeks **If Ampho B product not possible**: Fluc 800-1200 mg/day IV/po + 5-FC 25 mg/kg po q6h x 4-6 weeks **If Ampho B nor 5-FC possible**: Fluc 1200-2000 mg po daily x 10-12 weeks	• Outcome of treatment: treatment failure associated with dissemination of infection & high serum antigen titer, indicative of high burden of organisms and lack of 5FC use during inductive Rx, abnormal neurological evaluation & underlying hematological malignancy. Mortality rates still high, particularly in those with concomitant pneumonia *(Postgrad Med 121:107, 2009).* Early Dx essential for improved outcome *(PLOS Medicine 4:e47, 2007).* • Ampho B + 5FC treatment ↓ crypto CFUs more rapidly than ampho + Flu or Ampho + 5FC + Flu. Ampho B 1 mg/kg/d alone much more rapidly fungicidal in vivo than Flu 400 mg/d *(CID 45:76&81, 2007).* Use of lipid-based Ampho B associated with lower mortality compared to Ampho B deoxycholate in solid organ transplant recipients *(CID 48:1566, 2009).* • Monitor 5-FC levels: peak 70-80 mg/L, trough 30-40 mg/L. Higher levels assoc. with bone marrow toxicity. No difference in outcome if given IV or po *(AAC 51:1038, 2007).* • 5-FC is renally cleared therefore if renal failure occurs during treatment with Ampho B, 5-FC dose needs adjustment. • Trend toward improved outcomes with fluconazole 400-800 mg combined with Ampho B versus Ampho B alone in AIDS patients *(CID 48:1775, 2009).* Role of other azoles uncertain: successful outcomes were observed in 14/29 (48%) subjects with cryptococcal meningitis treated with posaconazole *(JAC 56:745, 2005).* Voriconazole also may be effective. • **When to initiate antiretroviral therapy (ART)?** Defer ART to allow for 5 weeks of anti-fungal treatment. When ART was started 1-2 weeks after diagnosis of cryptococcal meningitis mortality was increased when compared to initiation of ART >5 weeks after diagnosis *(NEJM 370:2487, 2014).*
Suppression (chronic maintenance therapy) Discontinuation of antifungal rx can be considered among pts who remain asymptomatic, with CD4 >100–200/mm³ for ≥6 months. Some perform a lumbar puncture before discontinuation of maintenance rx. Reappearance of pos. serum CRAG may predict relapse	**Flu** 200 mg/day po [If CD4 count rises to >100/mm³ with effective antiretroviral rx, some authorities recommend dc suppressive rx. *See www.hivatis.org.* Authors would only dc if CSF culture negative.]	**Itra** 200 mg po q12h if Flu intolerant or failure. No data on Vori for maintenance.	Itraconazole less effective than fluconazole & not recommended because of higher relapse rate (23% vs 4%). Recurrence rate of 0.4 to 3.9 per 100 patient-years with discontinuation of suppressive therapy in 100 patients on ARV with CD4 >100 cells/mm³.

TABLE 11A (8)

TYPE OF INFECTION/ORGANISM/ SITE OF INFECTION	ANTIMICROBIAL AGENTS OF CHOICE		COMMENTS
	PRIMARY	ALTERNATIVE	
Dermatophytosis			
Onychomycosis *(Tinea unguium)* (primarily cosmetic) **Laser rx FDA approved:** modestly effective, expensive *(Med Lett 55:15, 2013)*. Review: *JAMA 2018,319:397.*	**Fingernail Rx Options:** **Terbinafine**[1] 250 mg po q24h [children <20 kg: 62.5 mg/day, 20–40 kg: 125 mg/day, >40 kg: 250 mg/day] x 6 wks (79% effective) OR **Itra**[2] 200 mg po q24h x 3 mos.^{NAI} OR **Itra** 200 mg po bid x 1 wk/mo x 2 mos OR **Flu** 150–300 mg po q wk x 3–6 mos.^{NAI} Note: Cure rates for all options are low.		**Toenail Rx Options:** **Terbinafine**[1] 250 mg po q24h [children <20 kg: 62.5 mg/day, 20–40 kg: 125 mg/day, >40 kg: 250 mg/day] x 12 wks (76% effective) OR **Itra** 200 mg po q24h x 3 mos (59% effective) OR **Efinaconazole** 10% solution applied to nail once daily for 48 wks OR **Itra** 200 mg bid x 1 wk/mo. x 3–4 mos (63% effective)^{NAI} OR **Flu** 150–300 mg po q wk x 6–12 mos (48% effective)^{NAI} OR topical **Tavaborole** (Kerydin) or topical **Efinaconazole** (Jublia)
Tinea capitis ("ringworm") *(Trichophyton tonsurans, Microsporum canis*, N. America; other sp. elsewhere) *(PIDJ 18:191, 1999)*	**Terbinafine**[1] 250 mg po q 24h x 2-4 wks (adults); 4-6 mg/kg/day (children) 10-20 kg: 62.5 mg q24h x2 weeks 20-40 kg: 125 mg q24h x2 weeks >40 kg: 250 mg q24h x2 weeks	**Itra**[2] 5 mg/kg per day x 4 wks^{NFDA}. **Flu** 6 mg/kg q wk x 8-12 wks.^{NAI} Cap at 150 mg po q wk for adults **Griseo:** adults 500 mg po q24h x 6-8 wks; children age >2 years: Micro susp: 20-25 mg/kg/day; Ultramicro tabs: 10-15 mg/kg/day Dur: at least 6 wks, continue until clear	Durations of therapy are for T. tonsurans; treat for approx. twice as long for M. canis. All agents with similar cure rates (60-100%) in clinical studies. Addition of topical ketoconazole or selenium sulfate shampoo reduces transmissibility *(Int J Dermatol 39:261, 2000)*
Tinea corporis, cruris, or pedis *(Trichophyton rubrum, T. mentagrophytes, Epidermophyton floccosum)* "Athlete's foot, jock itch", and ringworm	**Topical rx:** Generally applied 2x/day. Available as creams, ointments, sprays, by prescription & "over the counter". Apply 2x/day for 2–3 wks. Recommend: Lotrimin Ultra or Lamisil AT; contain butenafine & terbinafine—both are fungicidal	**Terbinafine** 250 mg po q24h x 2 wks^{NAI} OR **Keto** 200 mg po q24h x 4 wks OR **Flu** 150 mg po 1x/wk for 2–4 wks^{NAI} **Griseo:** adults 500 mg po q24h times 4–6 wks, children 10–20 mg/kg per day. Duration: 2-4 wks for corporis, 4-8 wks for pedis.	**Keto** po often effective in severe recalcitrant infection. Follow for hepatotoxicity; many drug-drug interactions.
Tinea versicolor *(Malassezia furfur or Pityrosporum orbiculare)* Rule out erythrasma—*see Table 1, page 58*	**Keto** (400 mg po single dose)^{NAI} or (200 mg q24h x 7 days) or (2% cream 1x q24h x 2 wks)	**Flu** 400 mg po single dose or **Itra** 400 mg po q24h x 3–7 days	**Keto** (po) times 1 dose was 97% effective in 1 study. Another alternative: **Selenium sulfide** (Selsun), 2.5% lotion, apply as lather, leave on 10 min then wash off, 1/day x 7 day or 3–5/wk times 2–4 wks
Fusariosis			
Third most common cause of invasive mold infections, after *Aspergillus* and *Mucorales* and related molds, in patients with hematologic malignancies *(Mycoses 52:197, 2009)*. Pneumonia, skin infections, bone and joint infections, and disseminated disease occur in severely immunocompromised patients. In contrast to other molds, blood cultures are frequently positive. *Fusarium solani, F. oxysporum, F. verticillioides* and *F. moniliforme* account for approx. 90% of isolates *(Clin Micro Rev 20: 695, 2007)* Frequently fatal, outcome depends on decreasing the level of immunosuppression.	**Lipid-based Ampho B** 5-10 mg/kg/d IV; OR **Ampho B** 1-1.5 mg/kg/d IV.	**Posa** 400 mg po bid with meals (if not meals, 200 mg qid); OR **Vori** IV: 6 mg per kg q12h times 1 day, then 4 mg per kg q12h; po: 400 mg q12h, then 200 mg q12h. *See comments.*	**Surgical debridement** for localized disease. *Fusarium* spp. resistance to most antifungal agents, including echinocandins. *F. solani* and *F. verticillioides* typically are resistant to azoles. *F. oxysporum* and *F. moniliforme* may be susceptible to voriconazole and posaconazole. Role of combination therapy not well defined but case reports of response *(Mycoses 50: 227, 2007)*. Given variability in susceptibilities can consider combination therapy with Vori and Ampho B awaiting speciation. Outcome dependent on reduction or discontinuation of immuno-suppression. Duration of therapy depends on response; long-term suppressive therapy for patients remaining on immunosuppressive therapy.

[1] **Serious but rare cases of hepatic failure** have been reported in pts receiving Terbinafine & should not be used in those with chronic or active liver disease *(see Table 11B, page 145)*.
[2] Use of Itraconazole has been associated with myocardial dysfunction and with onset of congestive heart failure.

See page 2 for abbreviations. All dosage recommendations are for adults (unless otherwise indicated) and assume normal renal function.

TABLE 11A (9)

TYPE OF INFECTION/ORGANISM/ SITE OF INFECTION	ANTIMICROBIAL AGENTS OF CHOICE: PRIMARY	ANTIMICROBIAL AGENTS OF CHOICE: ALTERNATIVE	COMMENTS
Histoplasmosis *(Histoplasma capsulatum): See IDSA Guideline: CID 45:807, 2007.* Best diagnostic test is urinary, serum, or CSF histoplasma antigen: MiraVista Diagnostics (1-866-647-2847)			
Acute pulmonary histoplasmosis	**Mild to moderate disease, symptoms <4 wks:** No rx; If symptoms last over one month: **Itra** oral sol'n 200 mg po tid for 3 days then once or twice daily for 6-12 wks. **Moderately severe or severe: Liposomal Ampho B,** 3-5 mg/kg/d IV or **ABLC** 5 mg/kg/d IV or Ampho B 0.7-1.0 mg/kg/d for 1-2 wks, then Itra 200 mg tid for 3 days, then bid for 12 wks. + **methylprednisolone** 0.5-1 mg/kg/d for 1-2 wks.		Ampho B for patients at low risk of nephrotoxicity. Check for Itra drug-drug interactions.
Chronic cavitary pulmonary histoplasmosis	**Itra** oral sol'n 200 mg po tid for 3 days then once or twice daily for at least 12 mos (some prefer 18-24 mos).		Document therapeutic itraconazole blood levels at 2 wks. Relapses occur in 9-15% of patients.
Mediastinal lymphadenitis, mediastinal granuloma, pericarditis; and rheumatologic syndromes	**Mild cases:** Antifungal therapy not indicated. Nonsteroidal anti-inflammatory drug for pericarditis or rheumatologic syndromes. If no response to non-steroidals, **Prednisone** 0.5-1 mg/kg/d tapered over 1-2 weeks for 1) pericarditis with hemodynamic compromise, 2) lymphadenitis with obstruction or compression syndromes, or 3) severe rheumatologic syndromes. **Itra** 200 oral sol'n mg po once or twice daily for 6-12 wks for moderately severe to severe cases, or if prednisone is administered.		Check Itra blood levels to document therapeutic concentrations. Check for Itra drug-drug interactions.
Progressive disseminated histoplasmosis	**Mild to moderate disease: Itra** 200 mg po tid for 3 days then bid for at least 12 mos. **Moderately severe to severe disease: Liposomal Ampho B,** 3 mg/kg/d or **ABLC** 5 mg/kg/d for 1-2 weeks then **Itra** 200 mg tid for 3 days, then bid for at least 12 mos.		**Ampho B** 0.7-1.0 mg/kg/d may be used for patients at low risk of nephrotoxicity. Confirm therapeutic Itra blood levels. Azoles are teratogenic; Itra should be avoided in pregnancy; use a lipid ampho formulation. Urinary antigen levels useful for monitoring response to therapy and relapse.
CNS histoplasmosis	**Liposomal Ampho B,** 5 mg/kg/d, for a total of 175 mg/kg over 4-6 wks, then **Itra** 200 mg 2-3x a day for at least 12 mos. Vori likely effective for CNS disease or Itra failures. *(Arch Neurology 65: 666, 2008; J Antimicro Chemo 57:1235, 2006).*		Monitor CNS histo antigen, monitor Itra blood levels. PCR may be better for Dx than histo antigen. Absorption of Itra (check levels) and CNS penetration may be an issue; case reports of success with Fluconazole *(Braz J Infect Dis 12:555, 2008)* and Posaconazole *(Drugs 65:1553, 2005)* following Ampho B therapy.
Prophylaxis (immunocompromised patients)	**Itra** 200 mg po daily. Check for Itra drug-drug interactions *(Table 22A).*		Consider primary **prophylaxis in HIV-infected** patients with <150 CD4 cells/mm^3 in high prevalence areas. Secondary prophylaxis (i.e., suppressive therapy) indicated in HIV-infected patients with <150 CD4 cells/mm^3 and other immunocompromised patients in who immunosuppression cannot be reversed

TABLE 11A (10)

TYPE OF INFECTION/ORGANISM/ SITE OF INFECTION	ANTIMICROBIAL AGENTS OF CHOICE		COMMENTS
	PRIMARY	ALTERNATIVE	
Madura foot *(See Nocardia & Scedosporium)*			
Mucormycosis & other related species—*Rhizopus, Rhizomucor, Lichtheimia (CID 54:1629, 2012).* Rhinocerebral, pulmonary due to angioinvasion with tissue necrosis. Key to successful rx: early dx with symptoms suggestive of sinusitis (or lateral facial pain or numbness): think mucor with palatal ulcers, &/or black eschars, onset unilateral blindness in immunocompromised or diabetic pt. Rapidly fatal without rx. Dx by culture of tissue or stain: wide ribbon-like, non-septated with variation in diameter & right angle branching. Diabetics are predisposed to mucormycosis due to microangiopathy & ketoacidosis. Iron overload also predisposes: iron stimulates fungal growth.	**Liposomal Ampho B** 5-10 mg/kg/day; OR **Ampho B** 1-1.5 mg/kg/day.	**Isavuconazonium sulfate** loading dose of 372 mg (equivalent to isavuconazole 200 mg) IV/po q8 x 6 doses then 372 mg IV/po daily OR **Posaconazole** delayed-release tabs/IV loading dose of 300 mg q12 x 2 doses then 300 mg daily (posaconazole oral suspension 200 mg po QID)	**Ampho B** (ABLC) monotherapy relatively ineffective with 20% success rate vs 69% for other polyenes *(CID 47:364, 2008).* Complete or partial response rates of 60-80% in **Posa** salvage protocols *(JAC 61, Suppl 1, i35, 2008).* **Isavuconazole:** Approved for treatment of invasive mucor infection based on historical controls *(Ln 2016;387:760)* **Combination therapy:** Adjunctive echinocandin to liposomal Amphotericin B is promising given safety profile, synergy in murine models, and observational clinical data *(Clin Infect Dis 54(S1):S73, 2012).* Adjunctive Deferasirox therapy to liposomal Amphotericin B failed to demonstrate benefit *(J Antimicrob Chemother. 67:715, 2012).* Resistant to **Vori:** prolonged use of voriconazole prophylaxis predisposes to mucormycosis infections. Total duration of therapy based on response: continue therapy until 1) resolution of clinical signs and symptoms of infection, 2) resolution or stabilization of radiographic abnormalities; and 3) resolution of underlying immunosuppression. Posaconazole for secondary prophylaxis for those on immunosuppressive therapy *(CID 48:1743, 2009).*
Paracoccidioidomycosis (South American blastomycosis) *P. brasiliensis (Dermatol Clin 26:257, 2008; Expert Rev Anti Infect Ther 6:251, 2008).* Important cause of death from fungal infection in HIV-infected patients in Brazil *(Mem Inst Oswaldo Cruz 104:513, 2009).*	Mild-moderate disease: **Itra** 200 mg po daily for 6-9 months for mild and x 12-18 months for moderate disease. Severe disease: **Ampho B** 0.7-1 mg/kg IV daily to a cumulative total of 30 mg/kg followed by **Itra** 200 mg po daily for at least 12 months	**Keto** 200-400 mg daily x 6-18 months; OR **Ampho B** total dose >30 mg/kg OR **TMP/SMX** 800/160 mg bid-tid x 30 days, then 400/80 mg/day indefinitely (up to 3-5 years)	Improvement in >90% pts on Itra or Keto.[NAI] **Ampho B** reserved for severe cases and for those intolerant to other agents. TMP-SMX suppression life-long in HIV+. Check for Itra or Keto drug-drug interactions.
Lobomycosis (keloidal blastomycosis)/ P. loboi	**Surgical excision**, **clofazimine** or **itra**.		
Penicilliosis *(Talaromyces marneffei, formerly Penicillium marneffei)*: Common disseminated fungal infection in AIDS pts in SE Asia (esp. Thailand & Vietnam).	**Ampho B** 0.5–1 mg/kg per day times 2 wks followed by **Itra** 400 mg/day x 10 wks followed by 200 mg/day po **indefinitely for HIV-infected pts.**	For less sick patients **Itra** oral sol'n 200 mg po tid x 3 days, then 200 mg po bid x 12 wks, then 200 mg po q24h. (IV if unable to take po) (Oral sol'n better absorbed)	3rd most common OI in AIDS pts in SE Asia following TBc and cryptococcal meningitis. Prolonged fever, lymphadenopathy, hepatomegaly. Skin nodules are umbilicated (mimic cryptococcal infection or molluscum contagiosum). Preliminary data suggests Vori effective: *CID 43:1060, 2006.*
Phaeohyphomycosis, Black molds, Dematiaceous fungi *(See Clin Microbiol Rev 27:527, 2014.)* Opportunistic infection in immunocompromised hosts (e.g., HIV/AIDS, transplants). Most often presents with skin and soft tissue infection or mycetoma but can cause disease in bone and joint, brain abscess, endocarditis, and disseminated disease. Most clinically relevant species are within the genera of *Exophiala, Cladophialophora, Coniosporium, Cyphellophora, Fonsecaea, Phialophora,* and *Rhinocladiella.*	**Surgery** + **Itra** oral sol'n 400 mg/day po, duration not defined, probably 6 mo[NAI]	Voriconazole 6 mg/kg po bid x 1 day and then 4 mg/kg po bid or Posaconazole (suspension) 400 mg po bid	Both Vori and Posa have demonstrated efficacy *(Med Mycol 48:769, 2010; Med Mycol 43:91, 2005)* often in addition to surgical therapy. Consider obtaining anti-fungal susceptibility testing.

See page 2 for abbreviations. All dosage recommendations are for adults (unless otherwise indicated) and assume normal renal function.

TABLE 11A (11)

TYPE OF INFECTION/ORGANISM/ SITE OF INFECTION	ANTIMICROBIAL AGENTS OF CHOICE		COMMENTS
	PRIMARY	ALTERNATIVE	
Pneumocystis pneumonia (PJP) caused by ***Pneumocystis jirovecii***. Ref: *JAMA 301:2578, 2009.*			
Not acutely ill, able to take po meds. PaO_2 >70 mmHg Diagnosis: sputum PCR. Serum Beta-D Glucan may help; reasonable sensitivity & specificity, but also many false positives *(JCM 51:3478, 2013).*	(**TMP-SMX-DS**, 2 tabs po q8h x 21 days) OR (**Dapsone** 100 mg po q24h + **TMP** 5 mg/kg po tid x 21 days)	[**Clinda** 300–450 mg po q6h + **Primaquine** 15 mg base po q24h] x 21 days OR **Atovaquone** suspension 750 mg po bid with food x 21 days	Mutations in gene of the enzyme target (dihydropteroate synthetase) of sulfamethoxazole identified. Unclear whether mutations result in resist to TMP-SMX or dapsone + TMP *(EID 10:1721, 2004)*. Dapsone ref.: *CID 27:191, 1998.* **After 21 days, chronic suppression in AIDS pts *(see below—post-treatment suppression).***
	NOTE: Concomitant use of corticosteroids usually reserved for sicker pts with PaO_2 <70 *(see below)*		
Acutely ill, po rx not possible. PaO_2 <70 mmHg. Still unclear whether antiretroviral therapy (ART) should be started during treatment of PCP *(CID 46: 634, 2008).*	[**Prednisone** (15–30 min. before **TMP-SMX**): 40 mg po bid times 5 days, then 40 mg q24h times 5 days, then 20 mg po q24h times 11 days] + [**TMP-SMX** (15 mg of TMP component per kg per day) IV div. q6–8h times 21 days]	**Prednisone** as in primary rx + [(**Clinda** 600 mg IV q8h) + (**Primaquine** 30 mg base po q24h)] times 21 days OR **Pentamidine** 4 mg per kg per day IV times 21 days. **Caspo** active in animal models: *CID 36:1445, 2003*	**After 21 days, chronic suppression in AIDS pts** *(see post-treatment suppression).* **PJP can occur in absence of HIV infection & steroids** *(CID 25:215 & 219, 1997).* Wait 4–8 days before declaring treatment failure& switching to clinda + primaquine or pentamidine *(JAIDS 48:63, 2008)*, or adding caspofungin *(Transplant 84:685, 2007).*
	Can substitute IV prednisolone (reduce dose 25%) for po prednisone		
Primary prophylaxis and post-treatment suppression	(**TMP-SMX-DS or -SS**, 1 tab po q24h or 1 DS 3x/wk) OR (**Dapsone** 100 mg po q24h). DC when CD4 >200 x/3 mos *(NEJM 344:159, 2001).*	(**Pentamidine** 300 mg in 6 mL sterile water by aerosol q4 wks) OR (**Dapsone** 200 mg po + **Pyrimethamine** 75 mg po + **folinic acid** 25 mg po —**all once a week**) or **Atovaquone** 1500 mg po q24h with food.	TMP-SMX-DS regimen provides cross-protection vs Toxo and other bacterial infections. Dapsone + pyrimethamine protects vs Toxo. Atovaquone suspension 1500 mg once daily as effective as daily dapsone *(NEJM 339:1889, 1998)* or inhaled pentamidine *(JID 180:369, 1999).*
Scedosporium species *(Scedosporium apiospermum [Pseudallescheria boydii] and Scedosporium prolificans [now Lomentospora prolificans])* Infection occurs via inhalation or inoculation of skin. Normal hosts often have cutaneous disease. Immunocompromised hosts can have pulmonary colonization -> invasive disease in lung or skin -> disseminated disease.	*Scedosporium apiospermum:* **Vori** 6 mg/kg IV/po q12h on day 1, then 4 mg/kg IV/po q12h. *Scedosporium prolificans:* Surgical debridement and reduction of immuno-suppression, consider addition of Vori as above although usually resistant.	**Posa** 400 mg po bid with meals (may be less active)	Surgical debridement should be considered in most cases. S. apiospermum is resistant Amphotericin B and Scedosporium prolificans is resistant to all antifungal agents. Synergy with Terbinafine and echinocandins has been reported in vitro although clinical data is limited *(AAC 56:2635, 2012)*. S. prolificans osteomyelitis responded to miltefosine *(CID 48:1257, 2009)* in a case report. Consider susceptibility testing. Treatment guidelines/review: *Clin Microbiol Infect 3:27, 2014. Clin Microbiol Rev 21:157, 2008.*

See page 2 for abbreviations. All dosage recommendations are for adults (unless otherwise indicated) and assume normal renal function.

TABLE 11A (12)

TYPE OF INFECTION/ORGANISM/ SITE OF INFECTION	ANTIMICROBIAL AGENTS OF CHOICE		COMMENTS
	PRIMARY	ALTERNATIVE	
Sporotrichosis *IDSA Guideline: CID 45:1255, 2007.*			
Cutaneous/Lymphocutaneous	**Itra** oral sol'n po 200 mg/day for 2-4 wks after all lesions resolved, usually 3-6 mos.	If no response, **Itra** 200 mg po bid or **Terbinafine** 500 mg po bid or **SSKI** 5 drops (eye drops) tid & increase to 40-50 drops tid	**Flu** 400-800 mg daily only if no response to primary or alternative suggestions. Pregnancy or nursing: local hyperthermia *(see below)*.
Osteoarticular	**Itra** oral sol'n 200 mg po bid x 12 mos.	**Liposomal Ampho B** 3-5 mg/kg/d IV or **ABLC** 5 mg/kg/d IV or **Ampho B Deoxycholate** 0.7-1 mg/kg IV daily; if response, change to **Itra** oral sol'n 200 mg po bid x total 12 mos.	After 2 wks of therapy, document adequate serum levels of itraconazole.
Pulmonary	If severe, **Lipid Ampho B** 3-5 mg/kg IV or **standard Ampho B** 0.7-1 mg/kg IV once daily until response, then **Itra** 200 mg po bid. Total of 12 mos.	Less severe: **Itra** 200 mg po bid x 12 mos.	After 2 weeks of therapy document adequate serum levels of Itra. Surgical resection plus Ampho B for localized pulmonary disease.
Meningeal or Disseminated	**Lipid Ampho B** 5 mg/kg IV once daily x 4-6 wks, then—if better—**Itra** 200 mg po bid for total of 12 mos.	AIDS/Other immunosuppressed pts: chronic therapy with **Itra** oral sol'n 200 mg po once daily.	After 2 weeks, document adequate serum levels of Itra.
Pregnancy and children	**Pregnancy:** Cutaneous—local hyperthermia. Severe: **Lipid Ampho B** 3-5 mg/kg IV once daily. **Avoid Itra.**	**Children:** Cutaneous: **Itra** 6-10 mg/kg (max of 400 mg) daily. Alternative is **SSKI** 1 drop tid increasing to max of 1 drop/kg or 40-50 drops tid/day, whichever is lowest.	For children with disseminated sporotrichosis: Standard **Ampho B** 0.7 mg/kg IV once daily & after response, Itra 6-10 mg/kg (max 400 mg) once daily.

TABLE 11B – ANTIFUNGAL DRUGS: DOSAGE, ADVERSE EFFECTS, COMMENTS

DRUG NAME, GENERIC (TRADE)/ USUAL DOSAGE	ADVERSE EFFECTS/COMMENTS
Non-lipid Amphotericin B deoxycholate (Fungizone): 0.5-0.7 mg/kg IV per day as single infusion **Ampho B predictably not active vs. Scedosporium, Candida lusitaniae & Aspergillus terreus**	**Admin:** Ampho B is a colloidal suspension that must be prepared in electrolyte-free D5W at 0.1 mg/mL to avoid precipitation. No need to protect suspensions from light. Infusions cause chills/fever, myalgia, anorexia, nausea, rarely hemodynamic collapse/hypotension. Postulated due to proinflammatory cytokines, doesn't appear to be histamine release *(Pharmacol 23:966, 2003)*. **Infusion duration usu. 4+ hrs.** No difference found in 1 vs 4 hr infus. except chills/fever occurred sooner with 1 hr infus. Febrile reactions ↓ with repeat doses. Rare pulmonary reactions (severe dyspnea & focal infiltrates suggest pulmonary edema) assoc with rapid infus. **Severe rigors respond to meperidine (25–50 mg IV).** Premedication with acetaminophen, diphenhydramine, hydrocortisone (25–50 mg) and heparin (1000 units) had no influence on rigors/fever. If cytokine postulate correct, NSAIDs or high-dose steroids may prove efficacious but their use may risk worsening infection under rx or increased risk of **nephrotoxicity** (i.e., NSAIDs). Clinical side effects ↓ with ↑ age. **Toxicity:** Major concern is nephrotoxicity. Manifest initially by kaliuresis and **hypokalemia**, then fall in serum bicarbonate (may proceed to renal tubular acidosis), ↓ in renal erythropoietin and anemia, and rising BUN/serum creatinine. Hypomagnesemia may occur. Can reduce risk of renal injury by **(a) pre- & post-infusion hydration with 500 mL saline (if clinical status allows salt load), (b)** avoidance of other nephrotoxins, eg, radiocontrast, aminoglycosides, cis-platinum, **(c)** use of lipid prep of Ampho B.
Lipid-based Ampho B products[1]: Amphotericin B lipid complex (ABLC) (Abelcet): 5 mg/kg per day as single infusion	**Admin:** Consists of Ampho B complexed with 2 lipid bilayer ribbons. Compared to standard Ampho B, larger volume of distribution, rapid blood clearance and high tissue concentrations (liver, spleen, lung). Dosage: **5 mg/kg once daily;** infuse at 2.5 mg/kg per hr; adult and ped. dose the same. Saline pre- and post-dose lessens toxicity. Do NOT use an in-line filter. Do not dilute with saline or mix with other drugs or electrolytes.[2] **Toxicity:** Fever and chills 14–18%; nausea 9%, vomiting 8%; serum creatinine ↑ in 11%; renal failure 5%; anemia 4%; ↓ K 5%; rash 4%. A fatal fat embolism following ABLC infusion *(Exp Mol Path 177:246, 2004)*. Majority of pts intolerant of liposomal Ampho B can tolerate ABLC *(CID 56:701, 2013)*.
Liposomal Amphotericin B (LAB, AmBisome): 3–5 mg/kg IV per day as single infusion. If intolerant, majority OK with lipid form *(CID 56:701, 2013)*.	**Admin:** Consists of vesicular bilayer liposome with Ampho B intercalated within the membrane. Dosage: **3–5 mg/kg per day** IV as single dose infused over a period of approx. 120 min. If tolerated, infusion time reduced to 60 min. *(See footnote[2])*. Saline pre- and post-dose lessens toxicity. **Major toxicity:** Gen less than Ampho B. Nephrotoxicity 18.7% vs 33.7% for Ampho B, chills 47% vs 75%, nausea 39.7% vs 38.7%, vomiting 31.8% vs 43.9%, rash 24% for both, ↓ Ca 18.4% vs 20.9%, ↓ K 20.4% vs 25.6%, ↓ mg 20.4% vs 25.6%. Acute reactions common with liposomal Ampho B, 20– 40%. 86% occur within 5 min of infusion, incl chest pain, dyspnea, hypoxia or severe abdom, flank or leg pain; 14% dev flushing & urticaria near end of 4 hr infusion. All responded to diphenhydramine (1 mg/kg) & interruption of infusion. Reactions may be due to complement activation by liposome *(CID 36:1213, 2003)*.
Caspofungin (Cancidas) 70 mg IV on day 1 followed by 50 mg IV q24h (reduce to 35 mg IV q24h with moderate hepatic insufficiency)	An echinocandin which inhibits synthesis of β-(1,3)-D-glucan. Fungicidal against candida (MIC <2 mcg/mL) including those resistant to other antifungals & active against aspergillus (MIC 0.4–2.7 mcg/mL). Approved indications: empirical rx for febrile, neutropenic pts; rx of candidemia, candida intraabdominal abscesses, peritonitis, & pleural space infections; esophageal candidiasis; & invasive aspergillosis in pts refractory to or intolerant of other therapies. Serum levels on rec. dosages = peak 12, trough 1.3 (24 hrs) mcg/mL. **Toxicity:** remarkably non-toxic. Most common adverse effect: pruritus at infusion site & headache, fever, chills, vomiting, & diarrhea assoc with infusion. ↑ serum creatinine in 8% on caspo vs 21% short-course Ampho B in 422 pts with candidemia *(Ln, Oct. 12, 2005, online)*. Drug metab in liver & dosage ↓ to 35 mg in moderate to severe hepatic failure. Class C for preg (embryotoxic in rats & rabbits). *See Table 22A, page 259 for drug-drug interactions, esp. cyclosporine (hepatic toxicity) & tacrolimus (drug level monitoring recommended)*. Reversible thrombocytopenia reported *(Pharmacother 24:1408, 2004)*. **No drug in CSF, urine or vitreous humor of the eye.**
Micafungin (Mycamine) 50 mg IV q24h for prophylaxis post-bone marrow stem cell trans; 100 mg IV q24h candidemia, 150 mg IV q24h candida esophagitis.	Approved for rx of esophageal candidiasis & prophylaxis against candida infections in HSCT[3] recipients. Active against most strains of candida sp. & aspergillus sp. incl those resist to fluconazole such as C. glabrata & C. krusei. No antagonism seen when combo with other antifungal drugs. No dosage adjust for severe renal failure or moderate hepatic impairment. Watch for drug-drug interactions with sirolimus or nifedipine. Micafungin well tolerated & common adverse events incl nausea 2.8%, vomiting 2.4%, & headache 2.4%. Transient ↑ LFTs, BUN, creatinine reported; rare cases of significant hepatitis & renal insufficiency. *See CID 42:1171, 2006.* **No drug in CSF or urine**. ECMO: 200 mg IV qd *(Crit Care 22:289, 2018)*.

[1] Published data from patients intolerant of or refractory to conventional Ampho B deoxycholate. **None of the lipid Ampho B preps has shown superior efficacy compared to Ampho B in prospective trials (except liposomal Ampho B was more effective vs Ampho B in rx of disseminated histoplasmosis at 2 wks). Dosage equivalency has not been established** *(CID 36:1500, 2003)*. Nephrotoxicity ↓ with all lipid Ampho B preps.

[2] Comparisons between Abelcet & AmBisome suggest higher infusion-assoc. toxicity (rigors) & febrile episodes with Abelcet (70% vs 36%) but higher frequency of mild hepatic toxicity with AmBisome (59% vs 38%, p=0.05). Mild elevations in serum creatinine were observed in 1/3 of both *(BJ Hemat 103:198, 1998; Focus on Fungal Inf #9, 1999; Bone Marrow Tx 20:39, 1997; CID 26:1383, 1998)*.

[3] HSCT = hematopoietic stem cell transplant.

See page 2 for abbreviations. All dosage recommendations are for adults (unless otherwise indicated) and assume normal renal function.

TABLE 11B (2)

DRUG NAME, GENERIC (TRADE)/ USUAL DOSAGE	ADVERSE EFFECTS/COMMENTS
Anidulafungin (Eraxis) For Candidemia; 200 mg IV on day 1 followed by 100 mg/day IV). Esophageal candida: 100 mg IV x 1, then 50 mg IV once/d.	An echinocandin with antifungal activity (cidal) against candida sp. & aspergillus sp. including Ampho B- & triazole-resistant strains. FDA approved for treatment of esophageal candidiasis (EC), candidemia, and other complicated Candida infections. Effective in clinical trials of esophageal candidiasis & in 1 trial was superior to fluconazole in rx of invasive candidiasis/candidemia in 245 pts (75.6% vs 60.2%). Like other echinocandins, remarkably non-toxic; most common side-effects: nausea, vomiting, ↓ mg, ↓ K & headache in 11–13% of pts. No dose adjustments for renal or hepatic insufficiency. *See CID 43:215, 2006.* **No drug in CSF or urine**.
Fluconazole (Diflucan) 100 mg tabs 150 mg tabs 200 mg tabs 400 mg IV Oral suspension: 50 mg per 5 mL.	IV=oral dose because of excellent bioavailability. **Pharmacology:** absorbed po, water solubility enables IV. For peak serum levels *(see Table 9A, page 103)*. T½ 30hr (range 20–50 hr). 12% protein bound. **CSF levels 50–90% of serum in normals,** ↑ in meningitis. No effect on mammalian steroid metabolism. **Drug-drug interactions common,** *see Table 22A.* Side-effects overall 16% [more common in HIV+ pts (21%)]. Nausea 3.7%, headache 1.9%, skin rash 1.8%, abdominal pain 1.7%, vomiting 1.7%, diarrhea 1.5%, ↑ SGOT 20%. Alopecia (scalp, pubic crest) in 12–20% pts on ≥400 mg po q24h after median of 3 mos (reversible in approx. 6mo). Rare: severe hepatotoxicity *(CID 41:301, 2005)*, exfoliative dermatitis. **Note: Candida krusei and Candida glabrata resistant to Flu.**
Flucytosine (Ancobon, 5-FC) 500 mg cap **Expensive:** $11,000 for 100 capsules (Sep 2015 US price)	AEs: Overall 30%. GI 6% (diarrhea, anorexia, nausea, vomiting); hematologic 22% [leukopenia, thrombocytopenia, when serum level >100 mcg/mL (esp. in azotemic pts)]; hepatotoxicity (asymptomatic ↑ SGOT, reversible); skin rash 7%; aplastic anemia (rare—2 or 3 cases). False ↑ in serum creatinine on EKTACHEM analyzer. Bioavailability 100%. Good levels in CSF, eye & urine.
Griseofulvin (Fulvicin, Grifulvin, Grisactin) 500 mg, susp 125 mg/mL.	Photosensitivity, urticaria, GI upset, fatigue, leukopenia (rare). Interferes with warfarin drugs. Increases blood and urine porphyrins, should not be used in patients with porphyria. Minor disulfiram-like reactions. Exacerbation of systemic lupus erythematosus.
Imidazoles, topical For vaginal and/or skin use	Not recommended in 1st trimester of pregnancy. Local reactions: 0.5-1.5%: dyspareunia, mild vaginal or vulvar erythema, burning, pruritus, urticaria, rash. Rarely similar symptoms in sexual partner.
Isavuconazonium sulfate (prodrug Isavuconazole) (Cresemba) po: 186 mg caps IV: 372 mg vials No drug in CSF. Ref: *Med Lett 2016,58:33*	An azole antifungal agent for treatment of invasive aspergillosis and invasive mucormycosis in adults. **Contraindications:** Coadministration with strong CYP3A4 inhibitors, e.g., Ketoconazole or high-dose Ritonavir, or strong CYP3A4 inducers, e.g., Rifampin, carbamazepine, St. John's wort, or long-acting barbiturates is contraindicated. Do not use in patients with shortened QT interval. **Dosing: Isavuconazonium sulfate** loading dose of 372 mg (equivalent to isavuconazole 200 mg) IV/po q8 x 6 doses then 372 mg IV/po daily. **AEs:** Most common: nausea, vomiting, diarrhea, headache, elevated liver chemistry tests, hypokalemia, constipation, dyspnea, cough, peripheral edema, and back pain. Hepatic: increased ALT, AST. **Teratogenic.**
Itraconazole (Sporanox) 100 mg cap 10 mg/mL oral solution IV usual dose 200 mg bid x 4 doses followed by 200 mg q24h for a max of 14 days	**Itraconazole tablet & solution forms not interchangeable, solution preferred.** Many authorities recommend measuring drug serum concentration after 2 wks to ensure satisfactory absorption. To obtain highest plasma concentration, tablet is given with food & acidic drinks (e.g., cola) while solution is taken in fasted state; under these conditions, the peak conc. of capsule is approx. 3 mcg/mL & of solution 5.4 mcg/mL. Peak levels reached faster (2.2 vs 5 hrs) with solution. **Peak plasma concentrations after IV injection (200 mg) compared to oral capsule (200 mg): 2.8 mcg/mL (on day 7 of rx) vs 2 mcg/mL (on day 36 of rx).** Protein-binding for both preparations is over 99%, which explains virtual absence of penetration into CSF **(do not use to treat meningitis).** Adverse effects: dose-related nausea 10%, diarrhea 8%, vomiting 6%, & abdominal discomfort 5.7%. Allergic rash 8.6%, ↑ bilirubin 6%, edema 3.5%, & hepatitis 2.7% reported. ↑ doses may produce hypokalemia 8% & ↑ blood pressure 3.2%. Delirium, peripheral neuropathy & tremor reported *(J Neur Neurosurg Psych 81:327, 2010)*. **Reported to produce impairment in cardiac function.** Severe liver failure req transplant in pts receiving pulse rx for onychomycosis: FDA reports 24 cases with 11 deaths out of 50 mill people who received the drug prior to 2001. Other concern, as with fluconazole and ketoconazole, is **drug-drug interactions;** *see Table 22A.* Some can be life-threatening.
Ketoconazole (Nizoral) 200 mg tab	**Gastric acid required for absorption**—cimetidine, omeprazole, antacids block absorption. In achlorhydria, dissolve tablet in 4 mL 0.2N HCl, drink with a straw. Coca-Cola ↑ absorption by 65%. CSF levels "none". **Drug-drug interactions important,** *see Table 22A.* **Some interactions can be life-threatening.** **Dose- dependent nausea and vomiting.** Liver toxicity of hepatocellular type reported in about 1:10,000 exposed pts—usually after several days to weeks of exposure. At doses of ≥800 mg per day serum testosterone and plasma cortisol levels fall. With high doses, adrenal (Addisonian) crisis reported.
Miconazole (Monistat IV) 200 mg—*not available in U.S.*	IV miconazole indicated in patient critically ill with Scedosporium (Pseudallescheria boydii) infection. Very toxic due to vehicle needed to get drug into solution.

TABLE 11B (3)

DRUG NAME, GENERIC (TRADE)/ USUAL DOSAGE	ADVERSE EFFECTS/COMMENTS
Nystatin (Mycostatin) 30 gm cream 500,000 units oral tab	Topical: virtually no adverse effects. Less effective than imidazoles and triazoles. po: large doses give occasional GI distress and diarrhea.
Posaconazole (Noxafil) **Suspension** (40 mg/mL): 400 mg po bid with meals (if not taking meals, 200 mg qid). 200 mg po tid (with food) for prophylaxis. **Delayed-release tabs** (100 mg): 300 mg bid x 1 day and then 300 mg daily for prophylaxis. **Intravenous formulation:** 300 mg IV bid x 1 day the 300 mg daily (prophylaxis). Takes 7-10 days to achieve steady state. **Takes 7-10 days to achieve steady state. No IV formulation.**	**Suspension is dosed differently than delayed-release tablets (not interchangeable) – check dose carefully.** An oral triazole with activity against a wide range of fungi refractory to other antifungal rx including: aspergillosis, mucormycosis (variability by species), fusariosis, Scedosporium (Pseudallescheria), phaeohyphomycosis, histoplasmosis, refractory candidiasis, refractory coccidioidomycosis, refractory cryptococcosis, & refractory chromoblastomycosis. **Should be taken with high fat meal for maximum absorption.** Approved for prophylaxis of invasive aspergillus and candidiasis. Clinical response in 75% of 176 AIDS pts with azole-refractory oral/esophageal candidiasis. Posaconazole has similar toxicities as other triazoles: nausea 9%, vomiting 6%, abd. pain 5%, headache 5%, diarrhea, ↑ ALT, AST, & rash (3% each). In pts rx for >6 mos., serious side-effects have included adrenal insufficiency, nephrotoxicity, & QTc interval prolongation. Significant drug-drug interactions; inhibits CYP3A4 *(see Table 22A)*. Consider monitoring serum concentrations *(AAC 53:24, 2009)*. **100 mg delayed-release tablets:** loading dose of 300 mg (three 100 mg delayed-release tablets) twice daily on the first day, followed by a once-daily maintenance dose of 300 mg (three 100 mg delayed-release tablets) starting on the second day of therapy. Approved for prophylaxis only and not treatment. Tablets allow patients to achieve better levels than the suspension. Treatment dose unknown but prophylactic dose often achieves therapeutic levels. **The tablet and solution are not interchangeable.** Intravenous formulation approved for prophylaxis at 300 mg IV daily after a loading dose of 300 mg bid x 1 day. Consider therapeutic drug monitoring with a goal trough of >0.7 for prophylaxis and >1.0 *for treatment.* *JAC 69:1162, 2014.*
Terbinafine (Lamisil) 250 mg tab Discontinued in U.S. in May 2017.	In pts given terbinafine for onychomycosis, rare cases (8) of idiosyncratic & symptomatic hepatic injury & more rarely liver failure leading to death or liver transplant. The drug is **not recommended** for pts with **chronic or active liver disease;** hepatotoxicity may occur in pts with or without pre-existing disease. Pretreatment serum transaminases (ALT & AST) advised & alternate rx used for those with abnormal levels. Pts started on terbinafine should be warned about symptoms suggesting liver dysfunction (persistent nausea, anorexia, fatigue, vomiting, RUQ pain, jaundice, dark urine or pale stools). If symptoms develop, drug should be discontinued & liver function immediately evaluated. In controlled trials, changes in ocular lens and retina reported—clinical significance unknown. Major drug-drug interaction is 100% ↑ in rate of clearance by rifampin. **AEs:** usually mild, transient and rarely caused discontinuation of rx. % with AE, terbinafine vs placebo: nausea/diarrhea 2.6–5.6 vs 2.9; rash 5.6 vs 2.2; taste abnormality 2.8 vs 0.7. Inhibits CYP2D6 enzymes *(see Table 22A)*. An acute generalized exanthematous pustulosis and subacute cutaneous lupus erythematosus reported.
Voriconazole (Vfend) **IV: Loading dose 6 mg per kg q12h times 1 day, then 4 mg per kg q12h IV** for invasive aspergillus & serious mold infections; **3 mg per kg IV q12h** for serious candida infections. **Oral: >40 kg body weight:** 400 mg po q12h, then 200 mg po q12h. **<40 kg body weight:** 200 mg po q12h, then 100 mg po q12h **Take oral dose 1 hour before or 1 hour after eating.** Oral suspension (40 mg per mL). Oral suspension dosing: Same as for oral tabs. Reduce to ½ maintenance dose for moderate hepatic insufficiency	A triazole with activity against Aspergillus sp., **including Ampho resistant strains of A. terreus.** Active vs Candida sp. (including krusei), Fusarium sp., & various molds. Steady state serum levels reach 2.5–4 mcg per mL. Up to 20% of patients with subtherapeutic levels with oral administration: check levels for suspected treatment failure, life threatening infections. 300 mg bid oral dose or 8 mg/kg/d IV dose may be required to achieve target steady-state drug concentrations of 1-6 mcg/mL. **Toxicity** similar to other azoles/triazoles including uncommon serious hepatic toxicity (hepatitis, cholestasis & fulminant hepatic failure. Liver function tests should be monitored during rx & drug dc'd if abnormalities develop. **Photosensitivity is common and can be severe.** Many reports of associated skin cancers. Strongly recommend sun protective measures. *CID 58:997, 2014* & hallucinations & anaphylactoid infusion reactions with fever and hypertension. 1 case of QT prolongation with ventricular tachycardia in a 15 y/o pt with ALL reported. **Approx. 21% experience a transient visual disturbance** following IV or po ("altered/enhanced visual perception", blurred or colored visual change or photophobia) within 30–60 minutes. Visual changes resolve within 30–60 min. after administration & are attenuated with repeated doses **(do not drive at night for outpatient rx)**. Persistent visual changes occur rarely. Cause unknown. In patients with ClCr <50 mL per min., the intravenous vehicle (SBECD-sulfobutylether-B cyclodextrin) may accumulate but not obviously toxic *(CID 54:913, 2012)*. Hallucinations, hypoglycemia, electrolyte disturbance & pneumonitis attributed to ↑ drug concentrations. Potential for drug-drug interactions high—*see Table 22A.* **With prolonged use, fluoride in drug can cause a painful periostitis.** *(CID 59:1237, 2014)* **NOTE: Not in urine in active form. No activity vs. mucormycosis.**

See page 2 for abbreviations. All dosage recommendations are for adults (unless otherwise indicated) and assume normal renal function.

TABLE 12A – TREATMENT OF MYCOBACTERIAL INFECTIONS*

Diagnosis of M. tuberculosis, Updated Guidelines *(IDSA, ATS, CDC): CID 64:e1, 2017.*

Tuberculin skin test (TST). Same as PPD *[Chest 138:1456, 2010].* Criteria for positive TST after 5 tuberculin units (intermediate PPD) read at 48–72 hours:

- ≥5 mm induration: + HIV, immunosuppressed, ≥15 mg prednisone per day, healed TBc on chest x-ray, recent close contact
- ≥10 mm induration: foreign-born, countries with high prevalence; IVD Users; low income; NH residents; chronic illness; silicosis
- ≥15 mm induration: otherwise healthy

Two-stage to detect sluggish positivity: If 1st PPD + but <10 mm, repeat intermediate PPD in 1 wk. Response to 2nd PPD can also happen if pt received BCG in childhood.

BCG vaccine as child: If ≥10 mm induration and from country with TB, should be attributed to MTB. Prior BCG may result in booster effect in 2-stage TST. Routine anergy testing not recommended.

Interferon Gamma Release Assays (IGRAs): IGRAs detect sensitivities to MTB by measuring IFN-γ release in response to MTB antigens (for review see *JAMA 308:241, 2012* and *MMWR 59 (RR-5):1, 2010)*:

- Approved tests: T-SPOT.TB (Oxford Immunotec) and QuantiFERON-TB Gold and QuantiFERON-TB Gold Plus (Quaigen).
- May be used in place of TST in all situations in which TST is indicated.
- CDC recommends IGRA over TST in most circumstances the exception being children age < 5 years (although some experts recommend an age < 3 years.

IGRAs are relatively specific for MTB and do not cross-react with BCG or most nontuberculous mycobacteria. CDC recommends IGRA over TST for persons unlikely to return for reading TST & for persons who have received BCG. IGRA or TST may be used without preference for recent contacts of TB with special utility for follow-up testing since IGRAs do not produce "booster effect".

- May also be used without preference over TBc for occupational exposures.
- As with TST, testing with IGRAs in low prevalence populations will result in false-positive results *(CID 53:234, 2011).*
- Manufacturer's IFN-gamma cutoff ≥0.35 IU/mL for QFT-GIT may be too low for low prevalence settings, inflating positivity and conversion rates, and a higher cut-off may be more appropriate *(Am J Respir Crit Care Med 188:1005, 2013).* For detailed discussion of IGRAs, *see MMWR 59 (RR-5), 2010 and JAMA 308:241, 2012.* False positive IGRA *(JCM 54:845, 2016).*

Rapid (24-hr or less) diagnostic tests for MTB: (1) the Amplified Mycobacterium tuberculosis Direct Test amplifies and detects MTB ribosomal RNA; (2) the AMPLICOR Mycobacterium tuberculosis Test amplifies and detects MTB DNA. Both tests have sensitivities & specificities >95% in sputum samples that are AFB-positive. In negative smears, specificity remains >95% but sensitivity is 40–77% *(MMWR 58:7, 2009; CID 49:46, 2009)* to 60-90% *(see: http://www.cdc.gov/tb/publications/guidelines/amplification_tests/default.htm (3)* COBAS TaqMan MTB Test: real-time PCR test for detection of M. tuberculosis in respiratory specimens (not available in the U.S.) with performance characteristics similar to other rapid tests *(J Clin Microbiol 51:3225, 2013).*

Xpert MTB/RIF is a rapid test (2 hrs) for MTB in sputum samples which also detects RIF resistance with specificity of 99.2% and sensitivity of 72.5% in smear negative patients *(NEJM 363:1005, 2010).* Current antibody-based and ELISA-based rapid tests for TBc not recommended by WHO because they are less accurate than microscopy ± culture *(Lancet ID 11:736, 2011).*

Xpert MTB/RIF Ultra (Xpert Ultra) (not yet available in the US) *(Lancet Infect Dis 018 Jan;18(1):76-84)*: Higher sensitivity than Xpert MTB/RIF for detection of M. tuberculosis in smear-negative specimens, pediatric patients, HIV-infected patients, and in extra-pulmonary disease; slightly lower specificity than Xpert MTB/RIF. Recommended by WHO as initial diagnostic test for suspected tuberculous meningitis *(Lancet Infect Dis. 2018 Jan;18(1):68-75.)*

CAUSATIVE AGENT/ DISEASE	MODIFYING CIRCUMSTANCES	SUGGESTED REGIMENS	
		INITIAL THERAPY	CONTINUATION PHASE OF THERAPY
I. **Mycobacterium tuberculosis exposure baseline TST/IGRA negative** (household members & other close contacts of potentially infectious cases)	Neonate- Rx essential NOTE: If fever, abnormal CXR (pleural effusion, hilar adenopathy, infiltrate) at baseline, treat for active TBc and not with INH alone.	**INH** (10 mg/kg/ day for 8-10 wks) **RIF** 10-20 mg/kg/d also an option *(NEJM 379:454, 2018)*	Repeat tuberculin skin test (TST) in 8-12 wks: if TST neg & CXR normal & infant age at exposure >6 mos., stop INH, if TST (≥5 mm) or age ≤ 6 mos, treat with INH for total of 9 mos (4 mos if RIF used). If follow-up CXR abnormal, treat for active TB.
	Children <5 years of age—Rx indicated	As for neonate for 1st 8-10 wks.	If repeat TST at 8-10 wks is negative, stop. If repeat TST ≥5 mm, continue INH for total of 9 mos. If INH not given initially, repeat TST at 3 mos, if TST is positive, treat with INH for 9 mos. *(see Category II below).*
	Older children & adults— Risk 2–4% 1st yr		Pts at high risk of progression (e.g., HIV+, immunosuppressed or on immunosuppressive therapy) and no evidence of active infection should be treated for LTBI *(see below).* For others repeat TST/IGRA at 8-10 wks: no rx if repeat TST/IGRA neg.

See page 2 for abbreviations

* Dosages are for adults (unless otherwise indicated) and assume normal renal function

† **DOT** = directly observed therapy; **SAT** = self-administered therapy

TABLE 12A (2)

CAUSATIVE AGENT/ DISEASE	MODIFYING CIRCUMSTANCES	SUGGESTED REGIMENS	
		INITIAL THERAPY	**ALTERNATIVE**
II. Tuberculosis (LTBI, positive TST or IGRA as above, active TB ruled out) *See FIGURE 1 for treatment algorithm for pt with abnormal baseline CXR (e.g., upper lobe fibronodular disease) suspected active TBc.)* *Review: NEJM 372:2127, 2015* Estimating risk of active TB in pts with positive TST or IGRA (www.tst3d.com)	Age no longer an exclusion, all persons with LTBI should be offered therapy. If pre-anti-TNF therapy, recommend at least one month of treatment for LBTI prior to start of anti-TNF therapy *(Arth Care & Res 64:625, 2012)*. Overall, regimens containing a rifamycin (RIF, RFB or RFP) are most effective at preventing active tuberculosis *(AnUM 161:419 & 449, 2014)*. For patients on **Isoniazid (INH)** educate and monitor clinically for signs and symptoms of hepatitis. Baseline lab testing of liver function at start of therapy not routinely indicated but is indicated for patients with HIV infection, pregnant women, and women within 3 mo of delivery, persons with a history of chronic liver disease, persons who use alcohol regularly, and persons at risk for chronic liver disease. Lab monitoring of liver function during therapy is indicated if baseline liver function tests are abnormal, if risk factors for hepatic disease are present, or to evaluate for possible adverse effects.	**INH** po once daily (adult: 5 mg/kg/day, max 300 mg/day; child: 10-15 mg/kg/day not to exceed 300 mg/day) x 9 mos. For current recommendations for monitoring hepatotoxicity on INH see *MMWR 59:227, 2010*. Supplemental pyridoxine 50 mg/day for HIV+ patients. - - - - - **3HP**: a 12 dose once weekly 3-month regimen of **INH + Rifapentine (RFP)**: INH po 15 mg/kg (max dose 900 mg); RFP po (wt-based dose): 10-14 kg: 300 mg; 14.1-25 kg: 450 mg; 25.1-32 kg: 600 mg; 32.1-49.9 kg: 750 mg; 50 kg: 900 mg. Recommended for treatment of LTBI 1) in adults; 2) in persons with LTBI aged 2–17 years; 3) in persons with LTBI who have HIV infection, including AIDS, and are taking antiretroviral medications with acceptable drug-drug interactions with rifapentine; and 4) by DOT† or SAT† in persons aged ≥2 years *(MMWR 67:723, 2018)*. Not recommended for children age <2 yrs. HIV Note: Increase in flu-like sx when INH/RFP combined with dolutegravir *(CID 2018;67:193)*.	**INH** 300 mg once daily for 6 mo (but slightly less effective than 9 mos.; not recommended in children, HIV+ persons, or those with fibrotic lesions on chest film). **INH** 2x/wk (adult: 15 mg/kg, max 900 mg; child: 20-30 mg/kg, max dose 900 mg) x 9 mo. **RIF** once daily po (adult: 10 mg/kg/day, max dose 600 mg/day; child: 10-20 mg/kg/day, max dose 600 mg/day) for 4 mos *(NEJM 379:440, 454, 2018)*. **INH** + **RIF** once daily x 3 mos *(AnIM 2017;167:248)*. Rates of flu-like symptoms, cutaneous reactions, and severe drug reactions (rare, 0.3%) higher with 3 mo INH+RFP than with 9 mo INH *(CID 61:527, 2015)*, but hepatotoxicity higher with INH (1.8% vs. 0.4%) *(Int J Tuberc Lung Dis 19:1039, 2015)*. Randomized trial of HIV-infected patients in Africa living in areas of high tuberculosis prevalence found that once daily RFP 600 mg (weight of >45 kg) plus INH 300 mg once daily administered for 1 month was non-inferior to a 9-month regimen of INH in preventing active tuberculosis *(NEJM. 2019; 380:1001)*; completion rate was significantly higher in the 1 month group.
	Pregnancy	Regimens as above. Once active disease is excluded may delay initiation of therapy until after delivery unless patient is recent contact to an active case, HIV+. Supplemental pyridoxine 10-25 mg/d recommended	
LTBI, suspected INH-resistant organism		**RIF** once daily po (adult: 10 mg/kg/day, max dose 600 mg/day; child: 10-20 mg/kg/day, max dose 600 mg/day) for 4 mos.	**RFB** 300 mg once daily po may be substituted for RIF (in HIV+ patient on anti-retrovirals, dose may need to be adjusted for drug interactions).
LTBI, suspected INH and RIF resistant organism		**Moxi** 400 mg ± **EMB** 15 mg/kg once daily x 12 months	**Levo** 500 mg once daily + (**EMB** 15 mg/kg or **PZA** 25 mg/kg) once daily x 12 months. **NOTE:** PZA combo regimen, although perhaps most efficacious, poorly tolerated and may be overall less effective than FQ + EMB *(CID 64:1670, 2017)*

See page 2 for abbreviations

* Dosages are for adults (unless otherwise indicated) and assume normal renal function

† **DOT** = directly observed therapy; **SAT** = self-administered therapy

TABLE 12A (3)

CAUSATIVE AGENT/ DISEASE	MODIFYING CIRCUM-STANCES	SUGGESTED REGIMENS							COMMENTS
		INITIAL THERAPY			CONTINUATION PHASE OF THERAPY (in vitro susceptibility known)				
		SEE COMMENTS FOR DOSAGE AND DIRECTLY OBSERVED THERAPY (DOT) REGIMENS							
		Regimen: in order of preference	Drugs	Interval/Doses (min. duration)	Regimen	Drugs	Interval/Doses (min. duration)	Range of Total Doses (min. duration)	
III. Mycobacterium tuberculosis **A. Pulmonary TB** General reference on rx in adults & children: *MMWR 52 (RR-11):1, 2003.* In pts with newly diagnosed HIV and TB, Rx for both should be started as soon as possible *(NEJM 362:697, 2010).*	**Rate of INH resistance known to be <4%** (drug-susceptible organisms)	1 *(See Figure 2 page 152)*	**INH RIF PZA EMB**	7 days per wk times 56 doses (8 wks) or 5 days per wk (DOT) times 40 doses (8 wks) If cavitary disease, treat for 9 mos. Fixed dose combination of INH, RIF, PZA & EMB currently being evaluated *(JAMA 305:1415, 2011)*.	1a	**INH/ RIF**[9]	7 days per wk times 126 doses (18 wks) or 5 days per wk (DOT) times 90 doses (18 wks). If cavitary disease, treat for 9 mos.	182–130 (26 wks)	See dose chart below
					1b	**INH/ RIF**	2 times per wk times 36 doses (18 wks)	92–76 (26 wks) (Not AIDS pts)	
Isolation essential! Hospitalized pts with suspected or documented active TB should be isolated in single rooms using airborne precautions until deemed non-infectious. DC isolation if 3 negative AFB smears or 1-2 neg NAAT (Xpert MTB/ RIF) *(CID 59:1353 & 1361, 2014).*					1c	**INH/ RFP**	1 time per wk times 18 doses (18 wks) (only if HIV-neg)	74–58 (26 wks)	
		2 *(See Figure 2 page 152)*	**INH RIF PZA EMB**	7 days per wk times 14 doses (2 wks), then 2 times per wk times 12 doses (6 wks) or 5 days per wk (DOT) times 10 doses (2 wks) then 2 times per wk times 12 doses (6 wks)	2a	**INH/ RIF**	2 times per wk times 36 doses (18 wks)	62–58 (26 wks) (Not AIDS pts)	
					2b[5]	**INH/ RFP**	1 time per wk times 18 doses (18 wks) (only if HIV-neg)	44–40 (26 wks)	
		3 *(See Figure 2 page 152)*	**INH RIF PZA EMB**	3 times per wk times 24 doses (8 wks)	3a	**INH/ RIF**	3 times per wk times 54 doses (18 wks)	78 (26 wks)	
USE DOT REGIMENS IF POSSIBLE		4 *(See Figure 2 page 152)*	**INH RIF EMB**	7 days per wk times 56 doses (8 wks) or 5 days per wk (DOT) times 40 doses (8 wks)	4a	**INH/ RIF**	7 days per wk times 217 doses (31 wks) or 5 days per wk (DOT) times 155 doses (31 wks)	273–195 (39 wks)	
					4b	**INH/ RIF**	2 times per wk times 62 doses (31 wks)	118–102 (39 wks)	

(continued on next page)

COMMENTS

Regimen*	Dose in mg per kg (max. q24h dose) INH	RIF	PZA	EMB	SM	RFB
Q24h:						
Child	10-20 (300)	10-20 (600)	15-30 (2000)	15-25	20-40 (1000)	10-20 (300)
Adult	5 (300)	10 (600)	15-30 (2000)	15-25	15 (1000)	5 (300)
2 times per wk (DOT):						
Child	20-40 (900)	10-20 (600)	50-70 (4000)	50	25-30 (1500)	10-20 (300)
Adult	15 (900)	10 (600)	50-70 (3000)	50	25-30 (1500)	5 (300)
3 times per wk (DOT):						
Child	20-40 (900)	10-20 (600)	50-70 (3000)	25-30	25-30 (1500)	NA
Adult	15 (900)	10 (600)	50-70 (3000)	25-30	25-30 (1500)	NA

Second-line anti-TB agents can be dosed as follows to facilitate DOT: Cycloserine 500–750 mg po q24h (5 times per wk)
Ethionamide 500–750 mg po q24h (5 times per wk)
Kanamycin or capreomycin 15 mg per kg IM/IV q24h (3–5 times per wk)
Ciprofloxacin 750 mg po q24h (5 times per wk)
Ofloxacin 600–800 mg po q24h (5 times per wk)
Levofloxacin 750 mg po q24h (5 times per wk)
(CID 21:1245, 1995)

Risk factors for drug-resistant (MDR) TB: Recent immigration from Latin America or Asia or living in area of ↑ resistance (≥4%) or previous rx without RIF; exposure to known MDR TB. Incidence of MDR TB in **US steady** at 0.7%. Incidence of primary drug resistance is particularly high (>25%) in parts of China, Thailand, Russia, Estonia & Latvia; ~80% of US MDR cases in foreign born.

NOTE: Thrice weekly therapy for both the initial and continuation phase and twice weekly therapy in the continuation phase have higher rates of relapse and microbiological failure, acquired drug resistance compared to daily therapy *(CID 64:1211, 2017).*

(continued on next page)

* Dosages are for adults (unless otherwise indicated) and assume normal renal function

† **DOT** = directly observed therapy; **SAT** = self-administered therapy

TABLE 12A (4)

CAUSATIVE AGENT/ DISEASE	MODIFYING CIRCUM-STANCES	SUGGESTED REGIMEN[8]	DURATION OF TREATMENT (mos.)[8]	SPECIFIC COMMENTS[8]	COMMENTS
III. Mycobacterium tuberculosis **A. Pulmonary TB** *(continued from previous page)*	**INH resistance**	**RIF, PZA, EMB** (a **FQ** may strengthen the regimen for pts with extensive disease).	6	INH should be stopped in cases of INH resistance. Outcome similar for drug susceptible and INH-mono-resistant strains *(CID 48:179, 2009)*.	*(continued from previous page)* Mono-rifampin resistance is rare; resistance to rifampin is a marker for MDR, which should be assumed pending documentation of susceptibility to INH. Expert consultation recommended for MDR and XDR cases. Pretomanid FDA-approved for use in combination with bedaquiline and linezolid for treatment of MDR or XDR TB based on 89% success rate in an open-label trial of 107 patients, 56 of whom were HIV-infected. This 3-drug oral regimen is a major advance over WHO recommended multi-drug regimen (5 preferred, but at least 4 active agents) of levofloxacin (or moxifloxacin) + bedaquiline + linezolid + clofazimine + cycloserine + other agents (e.g., amikacin, ethionamide, delamanid) as needed to construct an active multi-drug regimen administered for 18-24 months. **See ATS/CDC/ ERSIDSA Guidelines for most up-to-date recommendations** ***(Am J. Respir Crit Care Med 200:e93, 2019)***
Multidrug-Resistant Tuberculosis (MDR TB): Defined as resistant to at least 2 drugs including INH & RIF. Pt clusters with high mortality *(NEJM 363:1050, 2010)*. **Extensively Drug-Resistant TB** (XDR-TB): Defined as resistant to INH & RIF plus any FQ and at least 1 of the 3 second-line drugs: capreomycin, kanamycin or amikacin *(MMWR 56:250, 2007; CID 51:379, 2010)*.	**Resistance to RIF**	**INH, EMB, FQ,** supplemented with **PZA** for the first 2 mos (an IA may be included for the first 2-3 mos. for pts with extensive disease)	12–18	Extended use of an IA may not be feasible. An all-oral regimen times 12-18 mos. should be effective but for more extensive disease &/or to shorten duration (e.g., to 12 mos.), an IA may be added in the initial 2 mos. of rx.	
	Resistance to INH & RIF	**Bedaquiline** 400 mg po once daily x 2 wks, then 200 mg 3 times per week, for 24 wks for a total of 26 weeks + **Pretomanid** 200 mg po once daily for 26 weeks + **Linezolid** 1200 mg po once daily for up to 26 weeks. Administer with food.	6	Recently FDA-approved all oral treatment for MDR TB *(see Comments)*	
	XDR-TB	Expert consultation strongly advised. *See comments*	18-24	Therapy requires administration of 4-6 drugs to which infecting organism is susceptible, including multiple second-line drugs *(MMWR 56:250, 2007)*. Increased mortality seen primarily in HIV+ patients. Cure with outpatient therapy likely in non-HIV+ patients when regimens of 4 or 5 or more drugs to which organism is susceptible are employed *(NEJM 359:563, 2008; CID 47:496, 2008)*. Successful sputum culture conversion correlates to initial susceptibility to FQs and kanamycin *(CID 46:42, 2008)*. Bedaquiline *(CID 60:188, 2015)* and Linezolid are options.	

See page 2 for abbreviations

* Dosages are for adults (unless otherwise indicated) and assume normal renal function

† **DOT** = directly observed therapy; **SAT** = self-administered therapy

TABLE 12A (5)

CAUSATIVE AGENT/DISEASE; MODIFYING CIRCUMSTANCES	SUGGESTED REGIMENS: INITIAL THERAPY	SUGGESTED REGIMENS: CONTINUATION PHASE OF THERAPY (in vitro susceptibility known)	COMMENTS
III. Mycobacterium tuberculosis *(continued)*			
B. Extrapulmonary TB Steroids: *see Comment*	**INH** + **RIF** (or **RFB**) + **PZA** + **EMB** q24h x 2 months	**INH** + **RIF** (or **RFB**)	IDSA recommends 6 mos for lymph node, pleural, pericarditis, disseminated disease, genitourinary & peritoneal TBc; 6–9 mos for bone & joint; 9-12 mos for CNS (including meningeal) TBc. **Corticosteroids** "strongly rec" only for meningeal TBc *[MMWR 52(RR-11):1, 2003]*. Steroids not recommended for pericarditis *(NEJM 371:1121 & 1155, 2014)*.
	Some add **pyridoxine** 25–50 mg po q24h to regimens that include INH.		
C. Tuberculous meningitis Excellent summary of clinical aspects and therapy *(IDSA guidelines: Clin Infect Dis, Aug 10. pii: ciw376. [Epub ahead of print], 2016)*	**(INH** + **RIF** + **EMB** + **PZA)** + prednisone 60 mg/day x 4 wks, then 30 mg/day x 4 wks, then 15 mg/day x 2 wks, then 5 mg/day x 1 wk	May omit **EMB** when susceptibility to **INH** and **RIF** established. Can D/C PZA after 2 months. Treat for total of 12 months. *See Table 9, page 103,* for CSF drug penetration. Initial reg of **INH + RIF + SM + PZA** also effective, even in patients with INH resistant organisms.	**3 drugs often rec for initial rx; we prefer 4** *(J Infect 59:167, 2009)*. Infection with MDR TB ↑ mortality & morbidity. Adjunctive corticosteroids improve survival *(Cochrane Database Syst Rev, Apr 28;4:CD002244, 2016)* and strongly recommended; Adult - dexamethasone 0.4 mg/kg/day week 1, 0.3 mg/kg/day week 2, 0.2 mg/kg/day week 3, 0.1 mg/kg/day week 4, then tapered to stop over 3-4 weeks; Child - dexamethasone 0.6 mg/kg/day or prednisolone 4 mg/kg/day for 4 weeks then tapered to stop over 4 weeks.
D. Tuberculosis during pregnancy	**INH** + **RIF** + **EMB** x 9 mos	SM should not be substituted for EMB due to toxicity. AMK, capreomycin, kanamycin, FQs also contraindicated. PZA is recommended for routine use in pregnant women by the WHO but has not been recommended for general use in U.S. due to lack of safety data, although PZA has been used in some US health jurisdictions without reported adverse events. Breast-feeding should not be discouraged. If PZA is not included in the initial treatment regimen, the minimum duration of therapy is 9 months. Pyridoxine, 25 mg/ day, should be administered.	
E. Treatment failure or relapse Usually due to poor compliance or resistant organisms, or subtherapeutic drug levels *(CID 55:169, 2012)*.	Directly observed therapy (DOT). Check susceptibilities. *(See section III. A, page 148 & above)*	Pts whose sputum is culture-positive after 5–6 mos. = treatment failures. Failures may be due to non-compliance or resistant organisms. Confirm susceptibilities of original isolates and obtain susceptibility to first and second line agents on current isolates. Non-compliance common, therefore institute DOT. If isolates show resistance, modify regimen to include at least 2 (preferably 3) new active agents, ones that the patient has not previously received if at all possible. Patients with MDR-TB usually convert sputum within 12 weeks of successful therapy.	
F. HIV infection or AIDS—pulmonary or extrapulmonary All HIV infected patients with TB should be treated with ARVs. If CD4 <50, initiation of ARVs within 2 weeks of starting TB meds associated with improved survival (Ann Intern Med 163:32, 2015). If CD4 >50 no proven survival benefit with early ARVs: initiate ARVs at 2-4 weeks of TB meds for moderately severe or severe TB, 8-12 weeks for less severe TB.	**INH** + **RIF** (or **RFB**) + **PZA** q24h x 2 mos.	**INH** + **RIF** (or **RFB**) q24h x 4 months (total 6 mos.). Treat up to 9 mos. in pts with delayed response, cavitary disease.	1. Co-administration of RIF not recommended for these anti-retroviral drugs: nevirapine, etravirine, rilpivirine; maraviroc, elvitegravir (integrase inhibitor in four drug combination Stribild), all HIV protease inhibitors. Use RFB instead). 2. RIF may be coadministered with efavirenz; nucleoside reverse transcriptase inhibitors. Coadministration of RIF with raltegravir best avoided (use RFB instead) but if necessary increase raltegravir dose to 800 mg q12h: RIF + dolutegravir OK at 50 mg bid of latter. 3. Because of possibility of developing resistance to RIF or RFB in pts with low CD4 cell counts who receive wkly or biwkly (2x/wk) therapy, daily dosing (preferred), or at a min 3x/wk dosing (failure rate likely higher) recommended for initial or continuation phase of rx. 4. Clinical & microbiologic response similar to that of HIV-neg patient. 5. Post-treatment suppression not necessary for drug-susceptible strains. 6. In RBPCT, prednisone reduced IRIS from 47% to 33% *(NEJM 2018,379:1915)*.
	Add pyridoxine 50 mg po q24h to regimens that include INH		
Concomitant protease inhibitor (PI) therapy	**INH** 300 mg q24h + **RFB** (150 mg q24h or 300 mg tiw) + **EMB** 15 mg/kg q24h + **PZA** 25 mg/kg q24h x 2 mos.; then INH + RFB x 4 mos. (up to 7 mos.)	**INH** + **RFB** x 4 mos. (7 mos. in slow responders, cavitary disease)	Rifamycins induce cytochrome CYP450 enzymes (RIF > RFP > RFB) & reduce serum levels of concomitantly administered PIs. Conversely, PIs inhibit CYP450 & cause ↑ serum levels of RFP & RFB. If dose of RFB is not reduced, toxicity ↑.

* Dosages are for adults (unless otherwise indicated) and assume normal renal function

† **DOT** = directly observed therapy; **SAT** = self-administered therapy

TABLE 12A (6)

FIGURE 1: TREATMENT ALGORITHM FOR ACTIVE, CULTURE-NEGATIVE PULMONARY TUBERCULOSIS AND INACTIVE TUBERCULOSIS *(modified from MMWR 52(RR-11):1, 2003).*

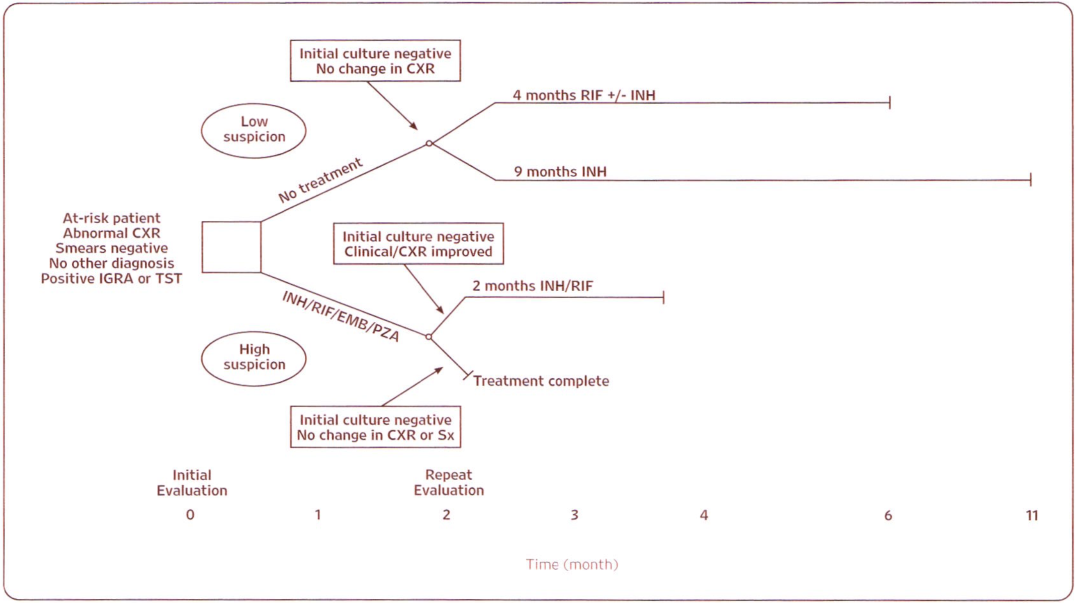

Patients at high clinical suspicion of active TB should be started on 4-drug therapy, pending results of cultures. If cultures are negative and there is no change in symptoms or CXR, the 4-drug regimen can be stopped and no further therapy is required. If cultures are negative and there is clinical or CXR improvement, continue INH/RIF for 2 additional months. For patients at low suspicion for active TB, treat for LTBI once cultures are negative.

 * Dosages are for adults (unless otherwise indicated) and assume normal renal function † **DOT** = directly observed therapy; **SAT** = self-administered therapy

TABLE 12A (7)

FIGURE 2: TREATMENT ALGORITHM FOR CULTURE-POSITIVE PULMONARY TUBERCULOSIS *[Modified from MMWR 52(RR-11):1, 2003]*

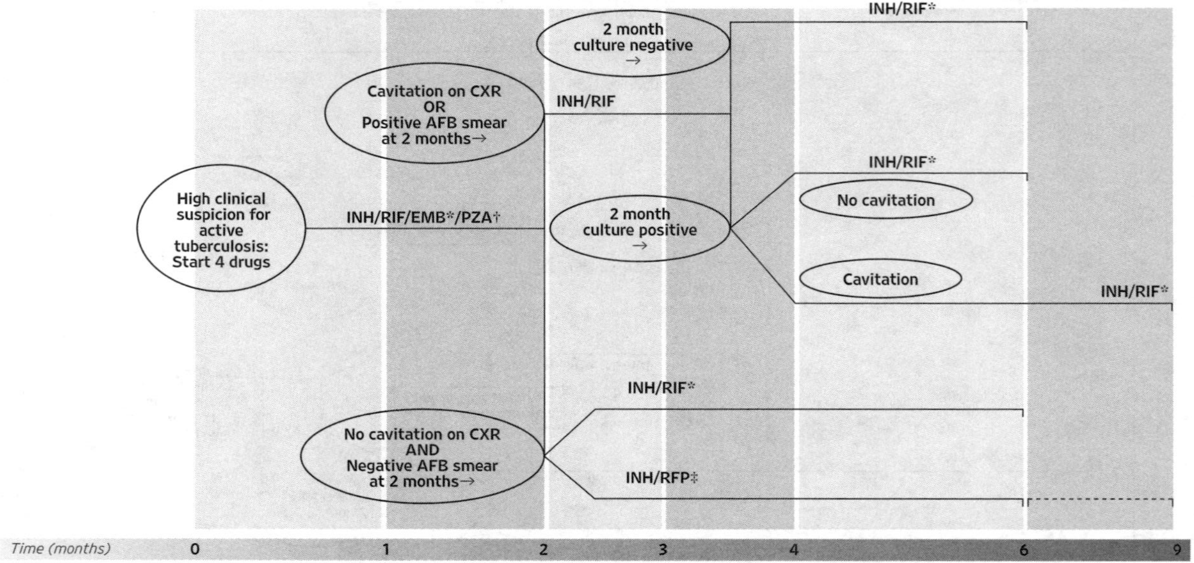

If the pt has HIV infection & the CD4 cell count is < 100 per mcL, the continuation phase should consist of daily or 3x weekly Isoniazid (INH) + Rifampin (RIF) for 4--7 mo. If pt HIV-neg. administered INH/RIF daily, thrice, or twice weekly.

* EMB may be discontinued in <2 months if drug susceptibility testing indicates no drug resistance.

† PZA may be discontinued after 2 months (56 doses).

‡ Once weekly INH/RFP, do not use in HIV-infected patients with tuberculosis or in patients with extrapulmonary tuberculosis. Therapy should be extended to 9 months if 2 mo. culture is positive.

TABLE 12A (8)

CAUSATIVE AGENT/DISEASE	MODIFYING CIRCUMSTANCES	SUGGESTED REGIMENS PRIMARY	SUGGESTED REGIMENS ALTERNATIVE	COMMENTS
IV. Nontuberculous Mycobacteria (NTM) *(See ATS Consensus: AJRCCM 175:367, 2007; EID 17:506, 2011)*				
A. Mycobacterium bovis		**INH + RIF + EMB** x 2 months then INH + RIF x 7 months		The M. tuberculosis complex includes M. bovis and regimens effective for MTB (except PZA based) also likely to be effective for M. bovis. **All isolates resistant to PZA**. Isolation not required. Increased prevalence of extrapulmonary disease in U.S. born Hispanic populations and elsewhere *(CID 47:168, 2008; EID 14:909, 2008; EID 17:457, 2011)*.
B. Bacillus Calmette-Guerin (BCG) (derived from M. bovis)	Only fever (>38.5°C) for 12–24 hrs	**INH** 300 mg q24h times 3 months		Intravesical BCG effective in superficial bladder tumors and carcinoma in situ. With sepsis, consider initial adjunctive prednisolone. Also susceptible to RFB, CIP, oflox, levo, moxi, streptomycin, amikacin, capreomycin. BCG may cause regional adenitis or pulmonary disease in HIV-infected children. **Resistant to PZA**.
	Systemic illness or sepsis	Same as for M. bovis.		
C. Mycobacterium avium-intracellulare complex (MAC, MAI, or Battey bacillus) *ATS/IDSA Consensus Statement: AJRCCM 175:367, 2007; See http://aidsinfo.nih.gov/guidelines/html/4/adult-and-adolescent-oi-prevention-and-treatment-guidelines/0 for updated CDC recommendations for AIDS patients.*	**Immunocompetent patients**			Intermittent (tiw) therapy not recommended for patients with cavitary disease, patients who have been previously treated or patients with moderate of severe disease. Intermittent therapy may be an option in nodular bronchiectatic form of the disease *(Am J Respir Crit Care Med 191:96, 2015)*. The primary microbiologic goal of therapy is 12 months of negative sputum cultures on therapy. **"Classic" pulmonary MAC:** Men 50–75, smokers, COPD. May be associated with hot tub use *(Clin Chest Med 23:675, 2002)*. **"New" pulmonary MAC:** Women 30–70, scoliosis, mitral valve prolapse, (bronchiectasis), pectus excavatum ("Lady Windermere syndrome") and fibronodular disease in elderly women *(EID 16:1576, 2010)*. May also be associated with interferon gamma deficiency *(AJM 113:756, 2002)*. For cervicofacial lymphadenitis (localized) in immunocompetent children, surgical excision is as effective as chemotherapy *(CID 44:1057, 2007)*. Moxifloxacin and gatifloxacin, active in vitro & in *vivo (AAC 51:4071, 2007)*.
	Nodular/Bronchiectatic disease	[**Clarithro** 1000 mg or **Azithro** 500 mg] tiw + **EMB** 25 mg/kg tiw + [**RIF** 600 mg or **RFB** 300 mg] tiw		
	Cavitary disease or severe nodular/bronchiectatic disease	[**Clarithro** 500-1000 mg/day (lower dose for wt <50 kg) or **Azithro** 250 mg/day] + **EMB** 15 mg/kg/day + [RIF 600 mg/day or **RFB** 150-300 mg/day] ± [**Strep** or **AMK**] If sputum remains MAC+, can add FDA-approved inhalations of liposomal AMK per day		
	HIV infection: **Primary prophylaxis**—Pt's CD4 count <50–100 per mm³ Discontinue when CD4 count >100 per mm³ in response to ART	**Azithro** 1200 mg po weekly OR **Clarithro** 500 mg po bid	**RFB** 300 mg po q24h OR **Azithro** 1200 mg po weekly + **RIF** 300 mg po q24h	**Many drug-drug interactions,** *see Table 22A, page 259*. Drug-resistant MAI disease seen in 29-58% of pts in whom disease develops while taking clarithro prophylaxis & in 11% of those on azithro but has not been observed with RFB prophylaxis. Clarithro resistance more likely in pts with extremely low CD4 counts at initiation. Need to be sure no active MTB; RFB used for prophylaxis may promote selection of rifamycin-resistant MTB.
	Treatment Either presumptive dx or after + culture of blood, bone marrow, or usually, sterile body fluids, eg liver	(**Clarithro** 500 mg po bid + **EMB** 15 mg/kg/day ± **RFB** 300 mg po q24h (adjust dose)	**Azithro** 500 mg po/day + **EMB** 15 mg/kg/day +/- **RFB** 300-450 mg po/day	Adjust RFB dose as needed for drug-drug interactions. Addition of a third or fourth drug should be considered for patients with advanced immunosuppression (CD4+ count <50 cells/µL), high mycobacterial loads (>2 log CFU/mL of blood), or in the absence of effective ART: AMK 10–15 mg/kg IV daily; Strep 1 gm IV or IM daily; CIP 500-750 mg PO bid; Levo 500 mg PO daily; Moxi 400 mg PO daily. Testing of susceptibility to clarithromycin and azithromycin is recommended. Short term (4–8 weeks) of systemic corticosteroid (equivalent to 20–40 mg of prednisone) can be used for IRIS.

* Dosages are for adults (unless otherwise indicated) and assume normal renal function

† **DOT** = directly observed therapy; **SAT** = self-administered therapy

TABLE 12A (9)

CAUSATIVE AGENT/DISEASE	MODIFYING CIRCUMSTANCES	SUGGESTED REGIMENS PRIMARY/ALTERNATIVE		COMMENTS
IV. Nontuberculous Mycobacteria (NTM) *(continued)*				
C. Mycobacterium avium-intracellulare complex *(continued)*	**Chronic post-treatment suppression—secondary prophylaxis**	**Always necessary.** [**Clarithro** or azithro] + **EMB** 15 mg/kg/day *(dosage above)*	**Clarithro** or **Azithro** or **RFB** *(dosage above)*	Recurrences almost universal without chronic suppression. Can discontinue if no signs and symptoms of MAC disease and sustained (>6 months) CD4 count >100 cells/μL in response to ART.
D. Mycobacterium celatum	Treatment; optimal regimen not defined	May be susceptible to **clarithro**, **FQ** Treat as if MAC.		Isolated from pulmonary lesions and blood in AIDS patients. Easily confused with M. xenopi (and MAC).
E. Mycobacterium abscessus	Treatment; Surgical excision may facilitate clarithro rx in subcutaneous abscess and is important adjunct to rx. For role of surgery in M. abscessus pulmonary disease, *see CID 52:565, 2011.*	**Cutaneous infection:** Surgical debridement + **Azithro** 500 mg once daily x 4-6 months OR **Azithro** 500 mg once daily + **Moxi** 400 mg po once daily x 4-6 months **Pulmonary or disseminated disease:** **Intensive phase:** (**Imipenem** 1000 mg IV q12h or **Cefoxitin** 8-12 gm/day IV in 2-3 divided doses) + **Azithro** 250-500 mg po once daily + **Amikacin** 15 mg/kg once daily IV (adjust dose to obtain a peak serum concentration of 20-30 μg/mL and a trough of < 5-10 μg/mL) + **Tigecycline** 100 mg loading dose then 50 mg q12h IV; treat for 2-3 months depending on severity of infection, clinical response, tolerability, and toxicity, ideally with the goal of converting sputum cultures to negative. **Continuation phase: Azithro** 250-500 mg + one or two other oral agents depending on tolerability and disease severity; optimal duration of therapy is unknown but target is 12 months after sputum cultures convert to negative.		**M. abscesses** is a complex of 3 species: *M. abscessus, M. massiliense, M. bolletii*. Treatment outcomes poor with half or more of patients remaining culture-positive or relapsing with infection due to strains with inducible macrolide resistance, i.e., M. abscessus subspecies abscessus *(CID 64:301, 309, 2017)*. Inducible resistance to macrolides not seen in M. abscessus subspecies massiliense due to non-functional macrolide resistance gene; Outcomes better with infection from *M. massiliense* compared to other members of the complex *(Int J Tuberc Lung Dis 18:1141, 2014)*. 2-4 week regimen of IV **amikacin** + IV **cefoxitin** (or **IMP**) + an oral macrolide (**clarithro** 1000 mg/d or **azithro** 250 mg/d) followed by oral macrolide administered for 12-15 months after culture conversion for M. massiliense pulmonary infection highly effective (98% culture conversion at end of treatment) in one study *(Chest 150:1211, 2016)*. M. abscessus susceptibilities: Amikacin (70%), Clarithromycin (95%) (however, M. abscessus subspecies abscessus often has inducible resistance requiring prolonged incubation for detection), Cefoxitin (70%), Rifabutin, Ciprofloxacin, Doxycycline *(EID 21:doi: 10.3201/2109.141634, 2015)* Linezolid, Clofazimine. Omadacycline has in vitro activity similar to tigecycline *(AAC 63:e00470, 2019)*. Pulmonary and disseminated disease notoriously refractory to therapy and outcomes are poor with half or more of patients remaining culture-positive or relapsing, particularly with infection due to strains with inducible macrolide resistance such as M. abscessus subspecies abscessus; long-term suppressive therapy often needed to control symptoms or disease progression *(Int J Tuberc Lung Dis 18:1141, 2014)*. Significant toxicity *(Int J Tuberc Lung Dis. 2017; 21:818)* and uncertain efficacy of Amikacin *(AAC 2016;60(10):6374-6 and AAC 2017;61(11). pii: e01206-17)*. Inhalation therapy with nebulised Amikacin may be an option for refractory cases or as an adjunct during the continuation phase, although lack of a commercially available product and lack of quality data on efficacy, tolerability, and duration of treatment are limitations.
Mycobacterium chelonae	Rapid grower assoc. with skin, wound, soft tissue infection; rarely disseminated/pulmonary	Skin: **Clarithro** 500 mg po bid + one other active agent x 4-6 months; More serious infection: **Clarithro** 500 mg po bid + **Tobra** 5 mg/kg IV once daily + one additional active agent x 2-8 wk then **Clarithro** 500 mg po bid plus one additional active agent for up to 12 mo.		*M. chelonae* susceptible to AMK (80%), clarithro (92-100%), azithro, tobramycin (100%), IMP (8-50%), moxifloxacin (0-50%), Doxy (25%), linezolid (50-100%), omadacycline (MIC90 = 0.25 μg/mL), tigecycline (MIC90 = 0.125 μg/mL). Resistant to cefoxitin. Tigecycline successfully used as salvage in combination regimens *(J Antimicrob Chemother 69:1945, 2014)*.
F. Mycobacterium fortuitum	Treatment; optimal regimen not defined. Surgical excision of infected areas.	**AMK** + **Cefoxitin** + **Probenecid** 2–6 wks, then po **TMP- SMX**, or **doxy** 2–6 mos. Usually responds to 6–12 mos of oral rx with 2 drugs to which it is susceptible.		**Resistant to all standard anti-TBc drugs.** Sensitive in vitro to doxycycline, minocycline, cefoxitin, IMP, AMK, TMP-SMX, CIP, oflox, azithro, clarithro, linezolid, tigecycline, but some strains resistant to azithromycin, rifabutin. For M. fortuitum pulmonary disease treat with at least 2 agents active in vitro until sputum cultures negative for 12 months *(AJRCCM 175:367, 2007)*. Disseminated disease associated with auto-antibodies to *interferon-γ (Intern Med 53:1361, 2014)*.

TABLE 12A (10)

CAUSATIVE AGENT/DISEASE	MODIFYING CIRCUMSTANCES	SUGGESTED REGIMENS PRIMARY/ALTERNATIVE	COMMENTS
IV. Nontuberculous Mycobacteria (NTM) *(continued)*			
G. Mycobacterium haemophilum	Combination of **CIP** + **RFB** + **Clarithro** *(EID 2019, 25:1648)*. Surgical debridement may be necessary.		Ulcerative skin lesions, tenosynovitis, osteomyelitis, lymphadenitis, pulmonary infection, disseminated infection usually in immunocompromised host. Lab: Requires supplemented media to isolate.
H. Mycobacterium genavense	2 or more drugs: **Clarithro**, **EMB**, **RFB**; **CLO**, **Amikacin**, Moxifloxacin as alternatives.		Seen in AIDS patients with CD4 <50 and in non-HIV severely immunocompromised hosts. *For review see Clin Microbiol Infect 19:432, 2013.*
I. Mycobacterium gordonae	Rarely a true pathogen.		Frequent colonizer, not associated with disease. In vitro: sensitive to EMB, RIF, AMK, CIP, clarithro, linezolid. Resistant to INH. Surgical excision.
J. Mycobacterium kansasii	[(**Azithro** 500 mg or **Clarithro** 1000 mg) + **RIF** 600 mg + **EMB** 15 mg/kg] po q24h	**INH** 300 mg + **Pyridoxine** 50 mg + **RIF** 600 mg + EMB 15 mg/kg) po q24h **For Rifampin resistant organism:** [**INH** 900 mg + **Pyridoxine** 50 mg + **EMB** 15 mg/kg + (**Moxi** 400 mg or **Azithro** 500 mg or **Clarithro** 1000 mg)] po q24h	**All isolates are resistant to PZA.** Treat until sputum cultures have been negative for 12 mo. For HIV+ patients on a protease inhibitor, substitute Rifabutin (150 mg/day) for Rifampin
K. Mycobacterium marinum	Two active agents for 1-2 months after surgical incision: **Clarithro** 500 mg bid + **EMB** 25 mg/kg q24h or **RIF** 600 mg q24h + **EMB** 25 mg/kg q24h Surgical excision.		For deep tissue involvement a three drug combination therapy with Rifampin 600 mg q24h + [Minocycline 100–200 mg q24h or Doxycycline 100–200 mg q24h] + Clarithromycin 500 mg bid. Monotherapy may be considered for minimal disease: Minocycline 100–200 mg q24h or Doxycycline 100–200 mg q24h or TMP-SMX 160/800 mg po bid.
L. Mycobacterium scrofulaceum	Surgical excision. Chemotherapy seldom indicated. Although regimens not defined, **Clarithro** + **CLO** with or **without EMB**. **INH**, **RIF**, **strep** + **cycloserine** have also been used.		In vitro resistant to INH, RIF, EMB, PZA, AMK, CIP. Susceptible to clarithro, strep, erythromycin.
M. Mycobacterium simiae	Regimen(s) not defined. Start 4 drugs as for disseminated MAC		Most isolates resistant to all 1st-line anti-TBc drugs. Isolates often not clinically significant.
N. Mycobacterium ulcerans (Buruli ulcer)	WHO recommends **RIF** + **SM** for 8 weeks. **RIF**+ **CIP** recommended as alternatives by WHO *(CMN 31:119, 2009)*.		Susceptible in vitro to RIF, strep, CLO, clarithro, CIP, oflox, amikacin, moxi, linezolid. Australian guidelines *(MJA 200:267, 2014)* recommend oral combination of RIF + Clarithro or RIF + a FQ (moxifloxacin or CIP). Surgery not required for cure and reserved for those declining or intolerant of antibiotic, debridement of necrotic tissue, large defects.
O. Mycobacterium xenopi	Regimen(s) not defined. **Clarithro** 500 mg bid + **RIF** 600 mg or **Rifabutin** 300 mg + **EMB** 15 mg/kg once daily + **INH** 300 mg once daily.		In vitro: sensitive to clarithro and many standard antimycobacterial drugs. MOXI active in vitro and may be an alternative.

TABLE 12A (11)

CAUSATIVE AGENT/DISEASE	MODIFYING CIRCUMSTANCES	SUGGESTED REGIMENS PRIMARY/ALTERNATIVE	COMMENTS
IV. Nontuberculous Mycobacteria (NTM) *(continued)*			
P. Mycobacterium leprae (leprosy) Classification: *CID 44:1096, 2007.* Overview: *Lancet ID 11:464, 2011.*	There are 2 sets of therapeutic recommendations here: one from USA (National Hansen's Disease Program [NHDP], Baton Rouge, LA) and one from WHO. Both are based on expert recommendations and neither has been subjected to controlled clinical trial.		
Paucibacillary Forms: (Intermediate, Tuberculoid, Borderline tuberculoid)	(**Dapsone** 100 mg/day + **RIF** 600 mg po/day) for 12 months	(**Dapsone** 100 mg/day (unsupervised) + **RIF** 600 mg 1x/mo (supervised)) for 6 mos	Side effects overall 0.4%
Single lesion paucibacillary	**Treat as paucibacillary leprosy for 12 months.**	Single dose ROM therapy: (**RIF** 600 mg + **Oflox** 400 mg + **Mino** 100 mg) *(Ln 353:655, 1999).*	
Multibacillary forms: Borderline Borderline-lepromatous Lepromatous *See Comment for erythema nodosum leprosum (ENL)* Rev.: *Lancet 363:1209, 2004*	(**Dapsone** 100 mg/day + **CLO** 50 mg/day + **RIF** 600 mg/day) for 24 mos **Alternative regimen:** (**Dapsone** 100 mg/day + **RIF** 600 mg/day + **Minocycline** 100 mg/day) for 24 mos if **CLO** is refused or unavailable.	(**Dapsone** 100 mg/day + **CLO** 50 mg/day (both unsupervised) + **RIF** 600 mg + **CLO** 300 mg once monthly (supervised)). Continue regimen for 12 months.	Side-effects overall 5.1%. For **erythema nodosum leprosum:** prednisone 60–80 mg/day or thalidomide 100-400 mg/day. Thalidomide available in US at 1-800-4-CELGENE. Altho thalidomide effective, WHO no longer rec because of potential toxicity however the majority of leprosy experts feel thalidomide remains drug of choice for ENL under strict supervision. **CLO (Clofazimine)** available from NHDP under IND protocol; contact at 1-800-642-2477. **Ethionamide** (250 mg q24h) or prothionamide (375 mg q24h) may be subbed for CLO. Etanercept effective in one case refractory to above standard therapy *(CID 52:e133, 2011).* Regimens incorporating clarithro, minocycline, dapsone monotherapy have been abandoned due to emergence of resistance *(CID 52:e127, 2011),* but older patients previously treated with dapsone monotherapy may remain on lifelong maintenance therapy. Moxi highly active in vitro and produces rapid clinical response *(AAC 52:3113, 2008).*

 * Dosages are for adults (unless otherwise indicated) and assume normal renal function † **DOT** = directly observed therapy; **SAT** = self-administered therapy

TABLE 12B – DOSAGE AND ADVERSE EFFECTS OF ANTIMYCOBACTERIAL DRUGS

AGENT (TRADE NAME)[1]	USUAL DOSAGE*	ROUTE/1º DRUG RESISTANCE (RES) US[2,§]	SIDE-EFFECTS, TOXICITY AND PRECAUTIONS	SURVEILLANCE
FIRST LINE DRUGS				
Ethambutol (Myambutol) (100, 400 mg tab)	25 mg/kg/day for 2 mos then 15 mg/ kg/day q24h as 1 dose (<10% protein binding) [Bacteriostatic to both extra-cellular & intracellular organisms]	RES: 0.3% (0–0.7%) po 400 mg tab	**Optic neuritis** with decreased visual acuity, central scotomata, and loss of green and red perception; peripheral neuropathy and headache (~1%), rashes (rare), arthralgia (rare), hyperuricemia (rare). Anaphylactoid reaction (rare). *Comment:* Primarily used to inhibit resistance. Disrupts outer cell membrane in M. avium with ↑ activity to other drugs.	Monthly visual acuity & red/ green with dose >15 mg/kg/ day. ≥10% loss considered significant. Usually reversible if drug discontinued.
Isoniazid (INH) (Nydrazid, Laniazid, Teebaconin) (50, 100, 300 mg tab)	Q24h dose: 5–10 mg/kg/day up to 300 mg/day as 1 dose. 2x/wk dose: 15 mg/kg (900 mg max dose) (<10% protein binding) [Bactericidal to both extracellular and intracellular organisms] Add pyridoxine in alcoholic, pregnant, or malnourished pts.	RES: 4.1% (2.6–8.5%) po 300 mg tab IM 100 mg/mL in 10 mL (IV route not FDA-approved but has been used, esp. in AIDS)	Overall ~1%. Liver: **Hep** (children 10% mild ↑ SGOT, normalizes with continued rx, age <20 yrs rare, 20–34 yrs 1.2%, ≥50 yrs 2.3%) [also ↑ with q24h alcohol & previous exposure to Hep C (usually asymptomatic—*CID 36:293, 2003*)]. May be fatal. With prodromal sx, dark urine do LFTs; discontinue if SGOT >3–5x normal. **Peripheral neuropathy** (17% on 6 mg/kg per day, less on 300 mg, incidence ↑ in slow acetylators); **pyridoxine 10 mg q24h will decrease incidence;** other neurologic sequelae, convulsions, optic neuritis, toxic encephalopathy, psychosis, muscle twitching, dizziness, coma (all rare); allergic skin rashes, fever, minor disulfiram-like reaction, flushing after Swiss cheese; blood dyscrasias (rare); + antinuclear (20%). **Drug-drug interactions** common, *see Table 22A*.	Pre-rx liver functions. Repeat if symptoms (fatigue, weakness, malaise, anorexia, nausea or vomiting) >3 days *(AJRCCM 152: 1705, 1995)*. Some recommend SGOT at 2, 4, 6 mos esp. if age >50 yrs. Clinical evaluation every mo.
Pyrazinamide (500 mg tab)	25 mg per kg per day (maximum 2.5 gm per day) q24h as 1 dose [Bactericidal for intracellular organisms]	po 500 mg tab	**Arthralgia; hyperuricemia** (with or without symptoms); hepatitis (not over 2% if recom-mended dose not exceeded); gastric irritation; photosensitivity (rare).	Pre-rx liver functions. Monthly SGOT, uric acid. Measure serum uric acid if symptomatic gouty attack occurs.
Rifamate®— combination tablet	2 tablets single dose q24h	po (1 hr before meal)	1 tablet contains 150 mg INH, 300 mg RIF	As with individual drugs
Rifampin (Rifadin, Rimactane, Rifocin) (100, 300, 450, 600 mg cap)	10.0 mg per kg per day up to 600 mg per day q24h as 1 dose (60–90% protein binding) [Bactericidal to all populations of organisms]	RES: 0.2% (0–0.3%) po 300 mg cap (IV available, Merrell-Dow)	INH/RIF dc'd in ~3% for toxicity; gastrointestinal irritation, antibiotic-associated colitis, drug fever (1%), pruritus with or without skin rash (1%), anaphylactoid reactions in HIV+ pts, mental confusion, thrombocytopenia (1%), leukopenia (1%), hemolytic anemia, transient **abnormalities in liver function. "Flu syndrome"** (fever, chills, headache, bone pain, shortness of breath) seen if RIF taken irregularly or if q24h dose restarted after an interval of no rx. **Discolors urine, tears, sweat, contact lens an orange-brownish color.** May cause drug-induced lupus erythematosus *(Ln 349: 1521, 1977)*.	Pre-rx liver function. Repeat if symptoms. **Multiple significant drug-drug interactions,** *see Table 22A*.
Rifater®— combination tablet *(See Side-Effects)*	Wt ≥55 kg, 6 tablets single dose q24h	po (1 hr before meal)	1 tablet contains 50 mg INH, 120 mg RIF, 300 mg PZA. Used in 1st 2 months of rx (PZA 25 mg per kg). Purpose is convenience in dosing, ↑ compliance *(AnIM 122: 951, 1995)* but cost 1.58 more. Side-effects = individual drugs.	As with individual drugs, PZA 25 mg per kg
Streptomycin (IV/IM sol'n)	15 mg per kg IM q24h, 0.75–1.0 gm per day initially for 60–90 days, then 1.0 gm 2–3 times per week (15 mg per kg per day) q24h as 1 dose	RES: 3.9% (2.7–7.6%) IM (or IV)	Overall 8%. **Ototoxicity:** vestibular dysfunction (vertigo); paresthesias; dizziness & nausea (all less in pts receiving 2–3 doses per week); tinnitus and high frequency loss (1%); nephrotoxicity (rare); peripheral neuropathy (rare); allergic skin rashes (4–5%); drug fever. Available from X-Gen Pharmaceuticals, 607-732-4411. Ref. re: IV—*CID 19:1150, 1994*. Toxicity similar with qd vs tid dosing *(CID 38:1538, 2004)*.	Monthly audiogram. In older pts, serum creatinine or BUN at start of rx and weekly if pt stable

[1] Note: Malabsorption of antimycobacterial drugs may occur in patients with AIDS enteropathy. For review of adverse effects, see *AJRCCM 167:1472, 2003*.

[2] **RES** = % resistance of M. tuberculosis

See page 2 for abbreviations

* Dosages are for adults (unless otherwise indicated) and assume normal renal function

† **DOT** = directly observed therapy; **SAT** = self-administered therapy

§ Mean (range) (higher in Hispanics, Asians, and patients <10 years old)

TABLE 12B (2)

AGENT (TRADE NAME)[1]	USUAL DOSAGE*	ROUTE/1º DRUG RESISTANCE (RES) US[2,§]	SIDE-EFFECTS, TOXICITY AND PRECAUTIONS	SURVEILLANCE
SECOND LINE DRUGS (more difficult to use and/or less effective than first line drugs)				
Amikacin (Amikin) (IV sol'n)	7.5–10.0 mg per kg q24h [Bactericidal for extracellular organisms]	RES: (est. 0.1%) IM/IV 500 mg vial	*See Table 10C, page 128* Toxicity similar with qd vs tid dosing *(CID 38:1538, 2004)*.	Monthly audiogram. Serum creatinine or BUN weekly if pt stable
Amikacin liposomal suspension (for inhalation)	One daily oral inhalation	Via inhalation	Risk of respiratory AEs: hypersensitivity, pneumonitis, hemoptysis, bronchospasm.	
Bedaquiline (Sirturo) (100 mg tab) Ref: *JAC 69:2310, 2014; NEJM 371:723, 2014; CID 60:188, 2015.*	Directly observed therapy (DOT): 400 mg once daily for 2 weeks, then 200 mg 3 times weekly for 22 weeks, taken with food and always used in combination with other anti-TB medications.	Does not exhibit cross-resistance to other TB drugs; always use in combination with other TB drugs to prevent selection of resistant mutants	Most common: nausea, vomiting, arthralgia, headache, hyperuricemia. Elevated transaminases. Bedaquiline in clinical trials was administered as one component of a multiple drug regimen, so side-effects were common, yet difficult to assign to a particular drug. Resistance reported: *CID 2018,66:1625.*	Moderate QTc increases (average of 10-16 ms over the 24 weeks of therapy. Potential risks of pancreatitis, myopathy, myocardial injury, severe hepatotoxicity.
Capreomycin sulfate (Capastat sulfate)	1 gm per day (15 mg per kg per day) q24h as 1 dose	RES: 0.1% (0–0.9%) IM/IV	Nephrotoxicity (36%), ototoxicity (auditory 11%), eosinophilia, leukopenia, skin rash, fever, hypokalemia, neuromuscular blockade.	Monthly audiogram, biweekly serum creatinine or BUN
Ciprofloxacin (Cipro) (250, 500, 750 mg tab)	750 mg bid	500 mg or 750 mg po IV 200-400 mg vial	TB not an FDA-approved indication for CIP. Desired CIP serum levels 4–6 mcg per mL. *See Table 10A, page 122 for adverse effects.*	None
Clofazimine (Lamprene) (50, 100 mg cap)	50 mg per day (unsupervised) + 300 mg 1 time per month supervised or 100 mg per day	50 mg (with meals)	Skin: **pigmentation (pink-brownish black)** 75–100%, dryness 20%, pruritus 5%. GI: abdominal pain 50% (rarely severe leading to exploratory laparoscopy), splenic infarction (VR), bowel obstruction (VR), GI bleeding (VR). Eye: conjunctival irritation, retinal crystal deposits.	None
Cycloserine (Seromycin) (250 mg tab)	750–1000 mg per day (15 mg per kg per day) 2–4 doses per day [Bacteriostatic for both extra-cellular & intracellular organisms]	RES: 0.1% (0–0.3%) 250 mg cap	Convulsions, **psychoses** (5–10% of those receiving 1.0 gm per day); headache; somnolence; hyperreflexia; increased CSF protein and pressure, **peripheral neuropathy.** 100 mg pyridoxine (or more) q24h should be given concomitantly. Contraindicated in epileptics.	None
Dapsone (25, 100 mg tab)	100 mg per day	100 mg tab	Blood: ↓ hemoglobin (1–2 gm) & ↑ retics (2–12%), in most pts. Hemolysis in G6PD deficiency. ↑ hemolysis due to concomitant atazanavir *(AAC 56:1081, 2012).* **Methemoglobinemia.** CNS: peripheral neuropathy (rare). GI: nausea, vomiting. Renal: albuminuria, nephrotic syndrome. Erythema nodosum leprosum in pts rx for leprosy (½ pts 1st year). Hypersensitivity syndrome in 0.5-3.6% *(See Surveillance)*.	Hypersensitivity syndrome: fever, rash, eosinophilia, lymphadenopathy, hepatitis, pneumonitis. Genetic marker identified *(NEJM 369:1620, 2013).*
Ethionamide (Trecator-SC) (120, 250 mg tab)	500–1000 mg per day (15–20 mg per kg per day) divided 1–3 doses per day [Bacteriostatic for extracellular organisms only]	RES: 0.8% (0–1.5%) 250 mg tab	**Gastrointestinal irritation** (up to 50% on large dose); goiter; peripheral neuropathy (rare); convulsions (rare); changes in affect (rare); difficulty in diabetes control; rashes; hepatitis; purpura; stomatitis; gynecomastia; menstrual irregularity. Give drug with meals or antacids; 50–100 mg pyridoxine per day concomitantly; SGOT monthly. Possibly teratogenic.	

See page 2 for abbreviations

* Dosages are for adults (unless otherwise indicated) and assume normal renal function

§ Mean (range) (higher in Hispanics, Asians, and patients <10 years old)

† **DOT** = directly observed therapy; **SAT** = self-administered therapy

TABLE 12B (3)

AGENT (TRADE NAME)[1]	USUAL DOSAGE*	ROUTE/1º DRUG RESISTANCE (RES) US[2,§]	SIDE-EFFECTS, TOXICITY AND PRECAUTIONS	SURVEILLANCE
SECOND LINE DRUGS *(continued)*				
Linezolid (Zyvox) (600 mg tab, oral suspension 100 mg/mL)	600 mg once daily	PO or IV	Not FDA-approved indication. High rate of adverse events (>80% with 4 months or longer of therapy: myelosuppression, peripheral neuropathy, optic neuropathy. Avoid tyramine-containing foods, soy products, adrenergic agents (e.g., pseudoephedrine, phenylpropanol-amine) MOA inhibitors, SSRIs. 600 mg >300 mg dose for toxicity; consider reducing dose to 300 mg for toxicity or after 4 mos of therapy or culture-conversion to reduce toxicity.	Baseline and monthly complete blood count, visual acuity checks, screen for symptoms of peripheral neuropathy, neurologic examination.
Moxifloxacin (Avelox) (400 mg tab)	400 mg qd	400 mg cap	Not FDA-approved indication. Concomitant administration of rifampin reduces serum levels of moxi *(CID 45:1001, 2007)*.	None
Ofloxacin (Floxin) (200, 300, 400 mg tab)	400 mg bid	400 mg cap	Not FDA-approved indication. Overall adverse effects 11%, 4% discontinued due to side-effects. GI: nausea 3%, diarrhea 1%. **CNS:** insomnia 3%, headache 1%, dizziness 1%.	
Para-aminosalicylic acid (PAS, Paser) (Na^+ or K^+ salt) (4 gm cap)	4–6 gm bid (200 mg per kg per day) [Bacteriostatic for extracellular organisms only]	RES: 0.8% (0–1.5%) 450 mg tab *(see Comment)*	**Gastrointestinal irritation** (10–15%); goitrogenic action (rare); depressed prothrombin activity (rare); G6PD-mediated hemolytic anemia (rare), drug fever, rashes, hepatitis, myalgia, arthralgia. Retards hepatic enzyme induction, may ↓ INH hepatotoxicity. Available from CDC, (404) 639-3670, Jacobus Pharm. Co. (609) 921-7447.	None
Rifabutin (Mycobutin) (150 mg cap)	300 mg per day (prophylaxis or treatment)	150 mg tab	Polymyalgia, polyarthralgia, granulocytopenia. Uveitis rare with 300 mg/day but increases to 8-38% if higher dose or combined with clarithro, PI or azole antifungal. Reddish urine, orange skin (pseudojaundice).	None
Rifapentine (Priftin) (150 mg tab)	600 mg twice weekly for 1st 2 mos., then 600 mg q week	150 mg tab	Similar to other rifabutins. *(See RIF, RFB)*. Hyperuricemia seen in 21%. Causes red-orange discoloration of body fluids. Flu-like illness in pts given weekly Rifapentine + INH for latent MTB *(CID 61:527, 2015)*.	None
Thalidomide (Thalomid) (50, 100, 200 mg cap)	100–300 mg po q24h (may use up to 400 mg po q24h for severe erythema nodosum leprosum)	50 mg tab	**Contraindicated in pregnancy. Causes severe life-threatening birth defects. Both male and female patients must use barrier contraceptive methods (Pregnancy Category X).** Frequently causes drowsiness or somnolence. May cause peripheral neuropathy. *(AJM 108:487, 2000)* For review, *see Ln 363:1803, 2004*.	In US: contact Celgene (800-4-CELGENE)

See page 2 for abbreviations

* Dosages are for adults (unless otherwise indicated) and assume normal renal function

§ Mean (range) (higher in Hispanics, Asians, and patients <10 years old)

† **DOT** = directly observed therapy; **SAT** = self-administered therapy

TABLE 13A – TREATMENT OF PARASITIC INFECTIONS

- ***See Table 13D* for sources for antiparasitic drugs not otherwise commercially available.**
- The following resources are available through the Centers for Disease Control and Prevention (CDC) in Atlanta. Website is www.cdc.gov. General advice for parasitic diseases other than malaria: (+1) (404) 718-4745 (day), (+1) (770) 488-7100 (after hours). For CDC Drug Service 8:00 a.m. – 4:30 p.m. EST: (+1) (404) 639-3670; fax: (+1) (404) 639-3717. *See www.cdc.gov/laboratory/drugservice/index.html* For malaria: Prophylaxis advice (+1) (770) 488-7788; treatment (+1) (770) 488-7788; or after hours (+1) (770) 488-7100; toll-free (US) 1-855-856-4713; website: *www.cdc.gov/malaria*
- **NOTE: All dosage regimens are for adults with normal renal function unless otherwise stated.** Many of the suggested regimens are not FDA approved.
- For licensed drugs, suggest checking package inserts to verify dosage and side-effects. Occasionally, post-licensure data may alter dosage as compared to package inserts.

INFECTING ORGANISM	SUGGESTED REGIMENS		COMMENTS
	PRIMARY	ALTERNATIVE	
PROTOZOA—INTESTINAL (non-pathogenic: E. hartmanni, E. dispar, E. moshkovskii, E. coli, Iodamoeba bütschlii, Endolimax nana, Chilomastix mesnili)			
Balantidium coli	**Tetracycline** 500 mg po qid x 10 days	**Metronidazole** 750 mg po tid x 5 days	Another alternative: Iodoquinol 650 mg po tid x 20 days.
Blastocystis hominis Ref: *Trends Parasitol 28:305, 2012; Trends Parasitol. 2018; 34:369*	**Metronidazole** 1.5 gm po 1x/day x 10 days or 750 mg po tid x 10 days (need to treat is dubious).	**Alternatives: Iodoquinol*** 650 mg po tid x 20 days or **TMP-SMX-DS,** one bid x 7 days or **Nitazoxanide** 500 mg po bid x 3 days	Role as pathogen unclear; may serve as marker of exposure to contaminated food/water. Some genotypes may be more virulent.
Cryptosporidium parvum & hominis Treatment is unsatisfactory Ref.: *Ln ID 15:85, 2015*	**Immunocompetent—No HIV: Nitazoxanide** 500 mg po bid x 3 days (expensive)	**HIV with immunodeficiency:** Effective antiretroviral therapy best therapy. **Nitazoxanide** no clinical or parasite response compared to placebo.	**Nitazoxanide:** Approved in liquid formulation for rx of children & 500 mg tabs for adults who are immunocompetent. Ref.: *CID 40:1173, 2005*. **C. hominis** assoc. with ↑ in post-infection eye & joint pain, recurrent headache, & dizzy spells *(CID 39:504, 2004)*.
Cyclospora cayetanensis; cyclosporiasis Ref: *Ln ID 19:e226, 2019*	**Immunocompetent pts: TMP-SMX-DS** tab 1 po bid x 7–10 days. Other options: *see Comments.*	**AIDS pts: TMP-SMX-DS** tab 1 po qid for up to 3-4 wks. Immunocompromised pts: may require suppressive rx with **TMP-SMX** DS 1 tab 3x/wk	If sulfa-allergic: **CIP** 500 mg po bid x 7 days but results inconsistent. Biliary disease described in HIV pts.
Dientamoeba fragilis Ref: *Clin Micro Rev 54:2243, 2017; J Clin Microbiol pii: JCM.00400-16, 2016*	**Iodoquinol*** 650 mg po tid x 20 days or **Paromomycin*** 25-35 mg/kg/day po in 3 div doses x 7 days or **Metronidazole** 750 mg tid x 10 days.	For treatment failures: **Tetracycline** 500 mg po qid x 10 days + **Iodoquinol*** 650 mg po tid x 10 days OR (**Iodoquinol*** + **Paromomycin***) May try second course of Iodoquinol	**Metronidazole** failed in prospective random placebo-control DB study *(CID 58:1692, 2014). In vitro tinidazole, metronidazole most active. AAC 56:487, 2012*
Entamoeba histolytica; amebiasis. If available, use stool PCR for diagnosis. E. histolytica, E. dispar, E. moshkovskii, are microscopically identical; antigen testing needed to distinguish.			
Asymptomatic cyst passer	**Paromomycin*** 25-35 mg/kg/day po in 3 divided doses x 7 days OR **Iodoquinol*** 650 mg po tid x 20 days	**Diloxanide furoate*** (Furamide) 500 mg po tid x 10 days.	
Patient with diarrhea/dysentery; mild/moderate disease. Oral therapy possible	**Metronidazole** 500–750 mg po tid x 7-10 days or **Tinidazole** 2 gm po daily x 3 days, followed by: Either [**Paromomycin*** 25-35 mg/kg/day po divided in 3 doses x 7 days] or [**Iodoquinol*** 650 mg po tid x 20 days] to clear intestinal cysts. *See comment.*		General review: *Open Forum Infect Dise 2018, 5:ofy161*. Colitis can mimic ulcerative colitis; ameboma can mimic adenocarcinoma of colon. **Nitazoxanide** 500 mg po bid x 3 days may be effective *(JID 184:381, 2001 & Tran R Soc Trop Med & Hyg 101:1025, 2007)*
Severe or extraintestinal infection, e.g., hepatic abscess	(**Metronidazole** 750 mg **IV to po** tid x 10 days or **Tinidazole** 2 gm 1x/day x 5 days) followed by **Paromomycin*** 25-35 mg/kg/day po divided in 3 doses x 7 days or **Iodoquinol*** 650 mg po tid x 20 days.		Serology positive (antibody present) with extraintestinal disease.

* For source of drug, see *Table 13D, page 177*.

TABLE 13A (2)

INFECTING ORGANISM	SUGGESTED REGIMENS		COMMENTS
	PRIMARY	ALTERNATIVE	
PROTOZOA—INTESTINAL *(continued)*			
Giardia duodenalis also known as **Giardia lamblia, Giardia intestinalis.**	**Tinidazole** 2 gm po x 1	**Metronidazole** 250 mg po tid x 5 days; Nitazoxanide 500 mg po bid x 3 days; Albendazole 400 mg po once daily with food x 5 days. Cochrane Database Syst *Rev.2012 Dec 12; 12:CD007787.*	**Refractory pts: Quinacrine** 100 mg po tid x 5 days or **(metro 750 mg po + quinacrine 100 mg po)** or (**Paromomycin** 10 mg/kg po) 3x/day x 3 wks *(CID 33:22, 2001)* giardia genetically heterogeneous *(J Clin Invest 123:2346, 2013)*. **Pregnancy: Paromomycin*** 25-35 mg/kg/day po in 3 divided doses x 5-10 days.
Cystoisospora belli (formerly Isospora belli) Diagnosis requires special order: AFB stain of stool	**Immunocompetent: TMP-SMX-DS** tab 1 po bid x 7-10 days; **Immunocompromised: TMP-SMX-DS** qid for up to 4 wks. If CD4<200 may not respond; need ART.	**CIP** 500 mg po bid x 7 days is second-line alternative *(AnIM 132:885, 2000)* OR **Pyrimethamine** 50-75 mg/day + **Folinic acid** 10-25 mg/day (po).	**Chronic suppression in AIDS pts:** either **TMP-SMX-DS** 1 tab po 3x/wk OR tab 1 po daily OR (**Pyrimethamine** 25 mg/day po + **Folinic acid** 10 mg/day po) OR as 2nd-line alternative: **CIP** 500 mg po 3x/wk.
Microsporidiosis	For HIV pts: antiretroviral therapy key. *See guidelines aidsinfo.nih.gov updated 2019 for microsporidia.* Rec to treat until CD4 >200		
Ocular: Encephalitozoon hellum or cuniculi, Vittaforma (Nosema) corneae, Nosema ocularum	**Albendazole** 400 mg po bid x 3 wks plus fumagillin eye drops *(see Comment)*.	In HIV+ pts, reports of response of E. hellum to **Fumagillin*** eyedrops *(see Comment)*. For V. corneae, may need keratoplasty.	To obtain fumagillin: 800-292-6773 or *www.leiterrx.com*. Neutropenia & thrombocytopenia serious adverse events. Dx: Most labs use modified trichrome stain. Need electron micrographs for species identification. FA and PCR methods in development. Peds dose ref.: *PIDJ 23:915, 2004*
Intestinal (diarrhea): Enterocytozoon bieneusi (HIV), Encephalitozoon (Septata) intestinalis	**Albendazole** 400 mg po bid x 3 wks; peds dose: 15 mg/kg per day div. into 2 daily doses x 7 days for **E. intestinalis.** Fumagillin equally effective. For HIV-associated, treat until CD4 >200 for 6 mos.	Oral **Fumagillin*** 20 mg po tid reported effective for **E. bieneusi** *(NEJM 346:1963, 2002)* (where available). For HIV-associated, treat until CD4 >200. *(see Comment)*. Albendazole not effective.	
Disseminated: E. hellum, cuniculi or intestinalis; Pleistophora sp., *others in Comment. Ref: JCM 52:3839, 2014.*	**Albendazole** 400 mg po bid x 3 wks. Fumagillin 20 mg po tid (where available). For HIV-associated, treat until CD4 >200.	No established rx for Pleistophora sp.	For Trachipleistophora sp., try itraconazole + albendazole *(NEJM 351:42, 2004)*. Other pathogens: Brachiola vesicularum & algerae *(NEJM 351:42, 2004)*.
PROTOZOA—EXTRAINTESTINAL			
Amebic meningoencephalitis Review of US experience *(CID 68:1815, 2019)*. CDC no longer provides miltefosine. *See www.impavido.com*			
Acanthamoeba sp.— no proven rx Rev.: *FEMS Immunol Med Micro 50:1, 2007*	Adult IV therapy: [**Pentamidine + Fluconazole**] + **Miltefosine*** 50 mg po tid. May add **TMP-SMX**, **Metronidazole**, and **Azithromycin**		For Acanthamoeba keratitis: miltefosine or voriconazole. Need brain tissue for dx.
Balamuthia mandrillaris	**Albendazole** + (**Fluconazole** or **Itraconazole**) + **Miltefosine*** 50 mg po tid ± **pentamidine** (poorly tolerated)		Need brain tissue for dx.
Naegleria fowleri. >95% mortality. Ref. *MMWR 57:573, 2008.*	**Amphotericin** B 1.5 mg/kg/day ± intrathecal + **Rifampin** 10 mg/kg/day + **Fluconazole** 10 mg/kg/day IV/po + **Miltefosine*** 50 mg po tid + **Azithromycin** 500 mg IV/po. Duration of therapy is empiric as there are few survivors		
Babesia microti (US), **Babesia duncani** (US West Coast), and **Babesia divergens** (EU) *(NEJM 366:366:2397, 2012)*	**For mild/moderate disease: Atovaquone** 750 mg po bid + **Azithro** 500 mg po on day 1, then 250-1000 mg po daily for total of 7-10 days. If relapse, treat x 6 wks & until blood smear neg x 2 wks.	**For severe babesiosis:** (**Clindamycin** 600 mg po tid) + (**Quinine** 650 mg po tid) x 7–10 days For adults, can give **Clinda** IV as 1.2 gm bid. Compelling in vivo data for tafenoquine *(JID 220:442, 2019)*.	Overwhelming infection in asplenic patients. In immunocompromised patients, treat for 6 or more weeks *(CID 46:370, 2008)*. Transfusion related cases occur.

* For source of drug, see *Table 13D, page 177.*

TABLE 13A (3)

INFECTING ORGANISM	SUGGESTED REGIMENS		COMMENTS
	PRIMARY	ALTERNATIVE	
PROTOZOA—EXTRAINTESTINAL *(continued)*			
Leishmaniasis *(Suggest consultation – CDC (+1) 404-718-4745).* Therapy needs individualization according to species and many options for each manifestation. **Note: Miltefosine available directly from Profounda, Inc. (+1 407-270-7790), www.impavido.com.** Definitive guidelines from IDSA/ASTMH *academic.oup.com/cid/article/63/12/e202/2645609* and include geographic distribution maps for each species. Diagnosis of cutaneous disease: Sample full depth punch biopsy from raised edge of ulcer. PCR mandatory to speciate; culture and histology also available. Rapid diagnosis often possible using needle aspirate, slit skin smear, brushings, or scraping of lesion edge with giemsa staining. Serology not useful. Available from CDC Drug Service, *see Table 13D.*			
Cutaneous: Mild Disease 4 or less lesions (1 cm or more), none > or = to 5 cm in diameter; no lesions in cosmetically sensitive areas, no lesions over joints or genitalia; may observe. Otherwise, consider Complex Disease which includes failure of previous treatment, or substantial local or lymphatic nodules, or large regional lymphadenopathy.	**Mild Disease** in travelers frequently responds to observation or local therapy and is preferred approach if patient agrees **Paromomycin*** 15% paromomycin and 12% MBCL ointment bid x 10 days rest for 10 days and then 10 more days; cryotherapy (freeze up to 3 x with liquid nitrogen); intralesional Antimony up to 5 mL into lesions weekly x 8-10 wks with cryotherapy at end of each treatment. CDC antimony IND does not cover intralesional use, common outside US. **Alternative: Miltefosine** (w/food) 50 mg po bid (wt 30-44 kg); 50 mg tid (wt ≥45 kg). Treat for 28 days. Response in about 70% of pts.	**Moderate Disease:** **Sodium stibogluconate*** (Pentostam) or **Meglumine antimoniate** (Glucantime) 20 mg/kg/day Sb IV x 20 days. Dilute in 120 mL of D5W and infuse over 1-2 hrs OR Liposomal **Amphotericin B** (3 mg/kg IV once daily days 1-5 and 10. Alternatives: **Fluconazole** 200 mg po daily x 6 weeks (for *L. mexicana, L. panamensis, L. major*) or **Ketoconazole** 600 mg po daily x 30 days *(L. mexicana)* or **Miltefosine** (dose as for mild disease). Some experts use **Ampho B** 0.5-1 mg/kg IV daily or qod to total dose of 15-30 mg/kg	Observation, oral therapy, topical paromomycin* only when low potential for mucosal spread; never use for lesions of any severity which are or may be *L. brasiliensis, L. panamensis* or *L. guyanensis* which always require therapy as per mucosal leishmaniasis below. Generic pentavalent antimony varies in quality and safety. Mild disease in travelers frequently responds to observation *(CID 57:370, 2013)* and is acceptable per IDSA/ASTMH guidelines. Monitor for gradual healing. Miltefosine is preg cat D (do not use in pregnancy).
Leishmaniasis, Mucosal (Espundia) All cutaneous lesions due to *L. brasiliensis, L. guyanensis*, or *L. panamensis* is proven or possible.	• **Cutaneous *L. braziliensis* of any severity:** ○ [**Sodium Stibogluconate** (Pentostam) or **Meglumine antimoniate** (Glucantime)] 20 mg/kg/day IV/IM x 20 days ○ **Liposomal Ampho B** (3 mg/kg IV once daily days 1-5 and days 14, 21 or days 1-5 and 10. • **Mucosal: Pentavalent antimony (Sb)*** 20 mg/kg/day Sb IV x 28 days for mucosal disease, or **Liposomal Amphotericin B** (regimens vary) with total cumulative dose of 20-60 mg/kg or **Amphotericin B** 0.5-1 mg/kg IV daily or qod to total dose of 20 45 mg/kg.	**Miltefosine*** (w/food) 50 mg po bid (wt 30-44 kg); 50 mg tid (wt ≥45 kg). Treat for 28 days. Complete resolution in 62% of pts.	Antimony available from CDC drug service. *See Table 13D for contact information.* Miltefosine has variable activity against mucosal disease according to geographic location. Expert consultation needed.
Visceral leishmaniasis (Kala-Azar) *New World & Old World* *L. donovani: India, Africa* *L. infantum: Mediterranean* *L. chagasi: New World (identical to L. infantum)*	*Immunocompetent:* **Liposomal Ampho B** 3 mg/kg once daily days 1-5 & days 14, 21 (increase to 40 mg/kg total dose for East African VL) HIV/AIDS: **Liposomal Ampho B** 4 mg/kg qd on days 1-5, 10, 17, 24, 31, 38 *(Curr Opin Infect Dis 26:1, 2013).*	**Standard Ampho B** 1 mg/kg IV daily x 15-20 days or qod x 8 wks (to total of 15-20 mg/kg) OR **pentavalent antimony*** 20 mg/kg/day IV x 28 days OR **Miltefosine*** (w/food) 50 mg po bid (wt 30-44 kg); 50 mg tid (wt ≥45 kg).	In HIV patients, need suppression with Amphotericin B q 2-4 wks. While CD4 remains <200. VL from South Asia is resistant to antimony. Miltefosine may be less effective against *L. infantum-chagasi* and less efficacy data for *L. donovani* in Africa.
Malaria (Plasmodia species) —NOTE: *CDC Malaria info— prophylaxis/treatment (770) 488-7788. After hours: 770-488-7100. US toll-free 1-855-856-4713. CDC offers species confirmation and drug resistance testing. Refs: JAMA 297:2251, 2264 & 2285, 2007.* See: *www.cdc.gov/malaria* Review of rapid diagnostic tests: *CID 54:1637, 2012.*			
Prophylaxis—Drugs plus personal protection: screens, nets, 30–35% DEET skin repellent (avoid >50% DEET) *(JAMA 2016,316:766)*, permethrin spray on clothing and mosquito nets. Country risk from CDC *(https://www.cdc.gov/malaria/travelers/country_table/a.html)* or WHO *(http://www.who.int/ith/ith-country-list.pdf?ua=1)*			

* For source of drug, see *Table 13D, page 177.*

TABLE 13A (4)

INFECTING ORGANISM	SUGGESTED REGIMENS		COMMENTS
	PRIMARY	ALTERNATIVE	
PROTOZOA—EXTRAINTESTINAL/Malaria (Plasmodia species) *(continued)*			
For areas free of chloroquine (CQ)-resistant P. falciparum: Central America (west of Panama Canal), Caribbean, Korea, Middle East (most)	**CQ** phosphate 500 mg (300 mg base) po per wk starting 1–2 wks before travel, during travel, & 4 wks post-travel **or Atovaquone-Proguanil (AP)** 1 adult tab per day (1 day prior to, during, & 7 days post-travel) or **Tafenoquine** 200 mg once daily x3 days (starting 3 days before travel) then 200 mg once weekly (starting 7 days after last loading regimen dose) then a 200 mg one-time dose (7 days after last dose in malaria area in non-pregnant G6PD-normal travelers. Note: **CQ** may exacerbate psoriasis.	**CQ Peds dose:** 8.3 mg/kg (5 mg/kg of base) po 1x/wk up to 300 mg (base) max. dose **or AP** by weight (peds tabs): 5-8 kg 1/2 tab, 9-10 kg 3/4 tab, 11–20 kg, 1 tab; 21–30 kg, 2 tabs; 31–40 kg, 3 tabs; >40 kg, 1 adult tab per day. **Adults: Doxy** or **MQ** as below.	AP must be taken with food for adequate absorption. CQ safe during pregnancy. **The areas free of CQ-resistant falciparum malaria continue to shrink:** *See CDC or WHO maps for most current information on CQ resistance.* **Doxy AEs:** photosensitivity, candida vaginitis, gastritis. For Tafenoquine must document on at least 1 occasion during life a quantitative level of >70% normal level of G6PD activity before use. Do not use screening or qualitative G6PD tests.
For areas with CQ-resistant P. falciparum Details on considerations for malaria prophylaxis: *N Engl J Med. 2016; 375:247.*	**Atovaquone** 250 mg—**Proguanil** 100 mg **(Malarone)** comb. tablet, 1 per day with food 1–2 days prior to, during, & 7 days post-travel. **Not in pregnancy.** Malarone preferred for trips of a week or less; expense may preclude use for longer trips. Native population: intermittent pregnancy prophylaxis/treatment programs in a few countries. Fansidar 1 tab po 3 times during pregnancy *(Expert Rev Anti Infect Ther 8:589, 2010).*	**Doxycycline** 100 mg po daily for adults & children >8 yrs of age. Take 1-2 days before, during & for 4 wks after travel **OR TQ** 200 mg once daily x3 days (starting 3 days before travel) then 200 mg once weekly (starting 7 days after last loading regimen dose) then a 200 mg one-time dose (7 days after last dose in malaria area) **OR Mefloquine (MQ)** 250 mg (228 mg base) po once per wk, 1-2 wks before, during, & for 4 wks after travel *(see Comment).* **Doxy**: 2.2 mg/kg po per day,(max 100 mg/day) **MFQ**: ≤ 9 kg: 5 mg/kg weekly (4.6 mg/kg base) 10-19 kg: ¼ adult tab weekly 20-30 kg: ½ tab weekly 31-45 kg: ¾ tab weekly > 45 kg: 1 tab weekly **Doxy AEs:** photosensitivity, candida vaginitis, gastritis.	**Pregnancy: MQ current best option.** Insufficient but reassuring data with **Malarone** *(Trav Med ID 27:20, 2019)*. **Avoid doxycycline and tafenoquine.** **Tafenoquine** (TQ), **Primaquine: Can cause hemolytic anemia if G6PD deficiency present. For TQ must test for G6PD (as above). TQ causes benign vortex keratopathy in 21% after 6 months use.** **MQ not recommended** if cardiac conduction abnormalities, seizures, or psychiatric disorders, e.g., depression, psychosis. If used, can start 3 wks before travel to assure tolerability. Children: Weekly dosing may make MFQ preferable; TQ not licensed in children. If 8 yr or older doxycycline liquid is available. For children under 10 kg. MFQ needs to be compounded but AP pediatric tablets can be cut. TQ good option when weekly dosing preferable such as for long-stay trips. TQ not approved for use for >6 months consecutively; use 3-month washout.
Treatment of Malaria. *Diagnosis is by microscopy. Alternative: rapid antigen detection test (Binax NOW): detects 96-100% of P. falciparum and 50% of other plasmodia (CID 49:908, 2009; CID 54:1637, 2012). Need microscopy to speciate. Can stay positive for over a month after successful treatment.*			
Uncomplicated P. falciparum (or species unidentified). 2015 WHO Guidelines suggest artemisinin combination therapy for adults (except in pregnancy) for all malaria species. E.g., Artemether-Lumefantrine.			
Acquired in Cen. Amer., west of Panama Canal; Haiti, Dom. Repub., & most of Mid-East **CQ sensitive**	**Adults: CQ phosphate** 1 gm salt (600 mg base) po, then 0.5 gm in 6 hrs, then 0.5 gm daily x 2 days. Total: 2500 mg salt	**Peds: CQ** 10 mg/kg of base po; then 5 mg/kg of base at 6, 24, & 48 hrs. Total: 25 mg/kg base	Other chloroquine salts available in some countries, total dose may differ **Peds dose should never exceed adult dose. CQ + MQ prolong QTc. Doses >2x recommended may be fatal.**

* For source of drug, see *Table 13D, page 177.*

TABLE 13A (5)

INFECTING ORGANISM	SUGGESTED REGIMENS		COMMENTS
	PRIMARY	ALTERNATIVE	
PROTOZOA—EXTRAINTESTINAL/Malaria (Plasmodia species)/Treatment of Malaria *(continued)*			
CQ-resistant or unknown resistance. Note: If >2% parasitemia or Hb <7, treat as severe malaria regardless of clinical findings or lack thereof. CDC IND for IV artesunate requires >5% parasitemia if no other severe malaria criteria met. Note to reader re dosing: For Peds, developing world drugs are listed under Primary; drugs of choice are listed under Alternative; Pregnancy alternatives are listed under Comments.	**Adults: Atovaquone-Proguanil** 1 gm–400 mg (4 adult tabs) po 1x/day x 3 days w/ food OR [**QS** 650 mg po tid x 3 days (7 days if SE Asia)] + [(**Doxy** 100 mg po bid) or (**Tetra** 250 mg po qid) or **Clinda** 20 mg/kg/d divided tid) x 7 days] OR **Artemether-Lumefantrine*** tabs 20/120 mg: 4 tabs po (at 0, 8 hrs) then bid x 2 days (total 6 doses); take with food OR a less desirable adult alternative, **Mefloquine** 750 mg po x 1 dose, then 500 mg po x 1 dose 6-12 hr later. **MQ** is 2nd line alternative due to neuropsychiatric reaction and cannot use in SE Asia due to resistance. Clinda or Tetra only if doxy not available. Other options: Available in Europe and endemic countries, WHO pre-qualified and EMA approved is **Dihydroartemisinin-piperaquine**. Available as PPQ 320 mg/DHA 40 mg (adult tabs) and PPQ 160 mg/DHA 20 mg (pediatric tabs). 5 to <7 kg PPQ 80 mg/DHA 10 mg po q24h x3 days 7 to <13 kg PPQ 160 mg/DHA 20 mg po q24h x3 days 13 to <24 kg PPQ 320 mg/DHA 40 mg po q24h x3 days 24 to <36 kg PPQ 640 mg/DHA 80 mg po q24h x3 days 36 to <75 kg PPQ 960 mg/DHA 120 mg po q24h x3 days 75 to 100 kg PPQ 1280 mg/DHA 160 mg po q24h x3 days >100 kg no data Available in many endemic countries and WHO pre-qualified and EMA approved ACT is **Pyronaridine/ Artesunate** 2 tablets (180 mg/60 mg) as a single dose each day for 3 days for 24 to >45 kg or 1 tablet if 20 to <24 kg. Pediatric granule formulation for oral suspension (60 mg/20 mg) • 5 - <8 kg 1 sachet Daily for 3 days • 8 - <15 kg 2 sachets Daily for 3 days • 15 - <20 kg 3 sachets Daily for 3 days	**Peds (drugs of choice): QS** 10 mg/kg po tid x 3 days + **Doxy** 2.2 mg/kg/ bid up to 100 mg per dose both x 7 days. AAP now recommends that doxy can safely be administered for durations ≤21 days regardless of age. OR **Atovaquone-Proguanil** (all once daily x 3 d) by weight: • 5-8 kg: 2 peds tabs; • 9-10 kg: 3 peds tabs; • 11-20 kg: 1 adult tab; • 21-30 kg: 2 adult tabs; • 31-40 kg: 3 adult tabs; • >40 kg: 4 adult tabs. OR **MQ Salt:** 15 mg/kg x 1, then 6-12 hrs later, 10 mg/kg ALL po. OR **Artemether-Lumefantrine*** • 5 kg to <15 kg: 1 tablet (20 mg/ 120 mg) as a single dose, then 1 tablet again after 8 hours, then 1 tablet every 12 hours for 2 days • 15 kg to <25 kg: 2 tablets (40 mg/ 240 mg) as a single dose, then 2 tablets again after 8 hours, then 2 tablets every 12 hours for 2 days • 25 kg to <35 kg: 3 tablets (60 mg/ 360 mg) as a single dose, then 3 tablets again after 8 hours, then 3 tablets every 12 hours for 2 days • ≥35 kg: as per adult dose	**Pregnancy:** • **Artemether-Lumefantrine** 4 tablets (80 mg/ 480 mg) as a single dose, then 4 tablets again after 8 hours, then 4 tablets every 12 hours for 2 days (take with food)). Drug of choice in 2nd/3rd trimester. Artemether-Lumefantrine is safer than quinine in the first trimester of pregnancy *(Malar J. 13:197, 2014)*. Lumefantrine appears safe *(Malar J 14:77, 2015)* and is safer than quinine in the first trimester of pregnancy *(Malaria J 13:197, 2014)* and *PLoS Med. 2017;14(5):e1002290* and is recommended by experts in the 1st trimester but not yet in official guidelines OR • **Quinine sulfate** 10 mg/kg po tid x 3 days (7 days if SE Asia)) + Clindamycin 20 mg/kg/day divided tid x 7 days • Do not delay therapy if quinine available and Artemether-Lumefantrine is not In U.S., QS is only available as quinine 324 mg capsule, thus hard to use to treat children. **Note: Oral Artemether-Lumefantrine tabs FDA-approved but not widely stocked.** Call 1-800-COARTEM to obtain.
Uncomplicated/P. malariae or P. knowlesi *(JID 199: 1107 & 1143, 2009)*. All regions **– always CQ-sensitive**	**CQ** as above: adults & peds. In South Pacific, beware of P. knowlesi: looks like P. malariae, but behaves like P. falciparum *(CID 46:165, 2007)*.	**Artemether-Lumefantrine*** (20/120 mg tab) 4 tabs po x 1 dose, repeat in 8 hrs, then repeat q12h x 2 days (take with food) OR **Atovaquone-Proguanil** (250/100 mg tab) 4 adult tabs po daily x 3 days or **DHA-PPQ** or **Pyronaridine-artesunate**	

* For source of drug, see *Table 13D, page 177*.

TABLE 13A (6)

INFECTING ORGANISM	SUGGESTED REGIMENS: PRIMARY	SUGGESTED REGIMENS: ALTERNATIVE	COMMENTS
PROTOZOA—EXTRAINTESTINAL/Malaria (Plasmodia species)/Treatment of Malaria *(continued)*			
Uncomplicated/P. vivax or P. ovale **CQ-sensitive** (except Papua New Guinea, Indonesia which are CQ-resistant-*see below)*	**Adults: CQ** as above + **PQ/TQ** base. PQ/TQ to start or be given on day 1 or 2 of appropriate blood-stage therapy with CQ (or alternative drug). For PQ 30 mg po once daily x 14 days Each primaquine phosphate tab is 26.3 mg of salt and 15 mg of base. 30 mg of base = 2 x 26.3 mg tabs prim. phos. Where available Tafenoquine (TQ) 300 mg single dose preferable to PQ. **Peds:** CQ as above + PQ base 0.5 mg po once daily x 14 days.	**Artemether-Lumefantrine** or **DHA-PPQ** or **Pyronaridine-artesunate** as above + **PQ base** 0.5 mg po once daily x 14 days. Where available TQ 300 mg single dose preferable to PQ; not approved for age ≤ 16 yrs	TQ/PQ added to eradicate latent parasites in liver. **Screen for G6PD def.** (must have 70% normal G6PD activity to use TQ) **before starting PQ or TQ;** if mildly G6PD deficient dose PQ as 45 mg po once weekly x 8 wks (cannot use TQ). **Note: rare severe reactions.** CQ safe in pregnancy. Avoid PQ in pregnancy. If P. vivax or P. ovale during pregnancy, after pregnancy check for G6PD deficiency & give PQ 30 mg po daily x 14 days or TQ x 300 mg.
Uncomplicated/P. vivax **CQ-resistant:** Papua, New Guinea & Indonesia	**Adults/Peds:** [**QS** + (**doxy** or **tetra**) + **PQ/TQ**] as above or **Artemether-Lumefantrine** or DHA-PPQ (same dose as for P. falciparum) + **PQ/TQ**	**Adults: MQ** + **PQ/TQ** as above.	Rarely acute. Lung injury and other serious complications: *LnID 8:449, 2008*. If pregnant treat as for uncomplicated P. falciparum in pregnancy. AAP now recommends that doxy can safely be administered for ≤21 days regardless of age.
Severe malaria, i.e., impaired consciousness, severe anemia, renal failure, pulmonary edema, ARDS, DIC, jaundice, acidosis, seizures, parasitemia >5%. One or more of latter. **Almost always P. falciparum.** *Ref: NEJM 358:1829, 2008; Science 320:30, 2008.* All regions Note: • IV Artesunate is drug of choice but not FDA-approved. Available from CDC Drug Service, see Antiparasitic Drugs, Sources, *see Table 13D.*	**Artesunate*** 2.4 mg/kg IV at 0, 12, 24, 48 hrs. Continue q24h if unable to take oral medication. Follow IV Artesunate with a complete oral course of one of: **Atovaquone/Proguanil, Artemether/Lumefantrine or Dihydroartemisinin/piperaquine** (not available in US). **Doxy** 100 mg po/IV q12h is less preferred alternative. Pregnancy (all trimesters): IV **artesunate** as above followed by **Clinda** 10 mg/kg po/IV loading dose, then 5 mg/kg po/IV(as tolerated) q8h x 7 days.	**Peds: Artesunate*** 2.4 mg/kg IV (3.0 mg/kg if wt less than 20 kg) at 0, 12, 24, 48 hrs. Continue q24h if unable to take oral medication. Follow IV Artesunate with a complete oral course of one of: **Atovaquone/Proguanil, Artemether/Lumefantrine or Dihydroartemisinin/Piperaquine** (not available in US). **Doxy** 2.2 mg/kg po/iv q12h x 7 days (less preferred regimen) if wt <45 kg. Adult dose for wt >45 kg. American Academy of Pediatrics now permits <21 days of doxy for any acute infection for children of all ages. IV **quinine dihydrochloride** still available in many endemic countries but second line only to be used if no IV **artemisinin** derivative is available.	Exchange transfusion no longer recommended. Switch to QS po + Doxy when patient able to take oral drugs. AAP now recommends that doxy can be used for ≤21 days regardless of age. **Steroids not recommended for cerebral malaria.** IV Artesunate from CDC (8 hr transport time post-approval), *see Table 13D (Ref: CID 44:1067 & 1075, 2007)*. Can cause non-life threatening, but transfusion requiring, hemolytic anemia up to 15 days post-therapy *(AnIM 163:498, 2015)*. If needed, give interim po treatment until IV artesunate arrives (if oral medications are not tolerated, consider administration via nasogastric tube or after an antiemetic): Artemether-lumefantrine, Atovaquone proguanil, Quinine sulfate Dosing as above.
Malaria—self-initiated treatment: Only for people at high risk. Carry a reliable supply of recommended treatment (to avoid counterfeit meds). Use only if malaria is lab-diagnosed and no available reliable meds.	**Artemether-Lumefantrine** (20/120 mg tab) 4 tabs po x 1 dose, repeat in 8 hrs, then repeat q12h x 2 days (take with food) OR **Atovaquone-Proguanil (AP)** 4 adult tabs (1 gm/400 mg) po daily x 3 days	**Peds:** Using adult **AP** tabs for 3 consecutive days: 11-20 kg, 1 tab; 21–30 kg, 2 tabs; 31–40 kg, 3 tabs; >41 kg, 4 tabs. For Peds dosing of Artemether-Lumefantrine, *see Uncomplicated/P. falciparum, page 163.*	Do not use for renal insufficiency pts. Do not use if weight <11 kg, pregnant, or breast-feeding. **Artemether-Lumefantrine:** sold as Riamet (EU) and Coartem (US & elsewhere).

* For source of drug, see *Table 13D, page 177.*

TABLE 13A (7)

INFECTING ORGANISM	SUGGESTED REGIMENS		COMMENTS
	PRIMARY	ALTERNATIVE	
PROTOZOA—EXTRAINTESTINAL *(continued)*			
Toxoplasma gondii (Toxoplasmosis) (Reference: *Ln 363:1965, 2004)*			
Immunologically normal patients *(For pediatric doses, see reference)*			
Acute illness w/ lymphadenopathy	No specific rx unless severe/persistent symptoms or evidence of vital organ damage		
Acq. via transfusion (lab accident)	Treat as for active chorioretinitis.		
Active chorioretinitis; meningitis; lowered resistance due to steroids or cytotoxic drugs	[**Pyrimethamine** (pyri) 200 mg po once on 1st day, then 50–75 mg q24h] + [**Sulfadiazine** *(see footnote[1])* S 1–1.5 gm po qid] + [**Leucovorin (folinic acid)** 5–20 mg 3x/wk]—*see Comment.* Treat 1–2 wks beyond resolution of signs/symptoms; continue leucovorin 1 wk after stopping pyri.		For congenital Toxo, Toxo meningitis in adults, & chorioretinitis, **add prednisone 1 mg/kg/day in 2 div. doses** until CSF protein conc. falls or vision-threatening inflammation subsides. Adjust folinic acid dose by following CBC results.
Acute in pregnant women. Ref*: CID 47:554, 2008*.	**If <18 wks gestation at diagnosis: Spiramycin*** 1 gm po q8h until 16-18 wks; dc if amniotic fluid PCR is negative. Positive PCR: treat as below. **If >18 wks gestation & documented fetal infection by positive amniotic fluid PCR: (Pyrimethamine** 50 mg po q12h x 2 days, then 50 mg/day + **Sulfadiazine** 75 mg/kg po x 1 dose, then 50 mg/kg q12h (max 4 gm/day) + **Folinic acid** 10-20 mg po daily) for minimum of 4 wks or for duration of pregnancy.		Screen patients with IgG/IgM serology at commercial lab. IgG+ /IgM neg = remote past infection; IgG+/IgM+ = seroconversion. For Spiramycin, consult with Palo Alto Medical Foundation Toxoplasma Serology Lab: 650-853-4828 or toxlab@pamf.org
Fetal/congenital	Mgmt complex. Combo rx with pyrimethamine + sulfadiazine + leucovorin—*see Comment*		Details in *Ln 363:1965, 2004*. **Consultation advisable.**
AIDS			
Cerebral toxoplasmosis Ref: *MMWR 58(RR-4) 1, 2009.*	[**Pyrimethamine** (pyri) 200 mg x 1 po, then 75 mg/day po] + (**Sulfadiazine** [Wt based dose: 1 gm if <60 kg, 1.5 gm if ≥60 kg] po q6h) + (**Folinic acid** 10–25 mg/day po) for minimum of 6 wks after resolution of signs/ symptoms, and then suppressive rx *(see below)* OR **TMP-SMX** 10/50 mg/kg per day po or IV div. q12h x 30 days *(AAC 42:1346, 1998)*	[**Pyri** + **Folinic acid** (as in primary regimen)] + 1 of the following: (1) **Clinda** 600 mg po/IV q6h or (2) **TMP-SMX** 5/25 mg/kg/day po or IV bid or (3) **Atovaquone** 750 mg po q6h. Treat 4–6 wks after resolution of signs/symptoms, then suppression.	Use alternative regimen for pts with severe sulfa allergy. If multiple ring-enhancing brain lesions (CT or MRI), >85% of pts respond to 7–10 days of empiric rx; if no response, suggest brain biopsy. Pyri penetrates brain even if no inflammation; folinic acid prevents pyrimethamine hematologic toxicity.
Primary prophylaxis, AIDS pts—IgG Toxo antibody + CD4 count <100 per mcL	(**TMP-SMX-DS**, 1 tab po q24h or 3x/wk) or (**TMP-SMX-SS**, 1 tab po q24h)	[(**Dapsone** 50 mg po q24h) + (**Pyri** 50 mg po q wk) + (**Folinic acid** 25 mg po q wk)] OR **Atovaquone** 1500 mg po q24h	Prophylaxis for pneumocystis also effective vs Toxo. Ref: *MMWR 58(RR-4):1, 2009.* **Another alternative:** (Dapsone 200 mg po + pyrimethamine 75 mg po + folinic acid 25 mg po) once weekly.
Suppression after rx of cerebral Toxo	(**Sulfadiazine** 2-4 gm po divided in 2-4 doses/day) + (**Pyri** 25–50 mg po q24h) + (**Folinic acid** 10–25 mg po q24h). DC if CD4 count >200 x 3 mos	[(**Clinda** 600 mg po q8h) + (**Pyri** 25–50 mg po q24h) + (**Folinic acid** 10–25 mg po q24h)] OR **Atovaquone** 750 mg po q6–12h. **TMP-SMX** 1DS bid or qd becoming standard due to difficulty obtaining Pyri.	(Pyri + sulfa or TMP-SMX) prevents PCP and Toxo; (clinda + pyri) prevents Toxo only. Additional drug needed to prevent PCP.
Trichomonas vaginalis	*See Vaginitis, Table 1, page 28.*		

[1] Sulfonamides for Toxo. Sulfadiazine now commercially available. Sulfisoxazole much less effective.

* For source of drug, see *Table 13D, page 177.*

TABLE 13A (8)

INFECTING ORGANISM	SUGGESTED REGIMENS		COMMENTS
	PRIMARY	ALTERNATIVE	
PROTOZOA—EXTRAINTESTINAL *(continued)*			
Trypanosomiasis. Ref.: *Ln 362:1469, 2003.* **Note: Drugs for African trypanosomiasis may be obtained free from WHO or CDC.** See *Table 13D, page 177,* **for source information**. Fexinidazole, a completely oral regimen effective against both stages of disease in both species of African trypanosomiasis is approved by EMA and declared drug of choice for most g-HAT cases but not yet available. *Lancet 201W8,e 3s9t 1A:1f4ri4c.*			
West African sleeping sickness (T. brucei gambiense)			
Early: Blood/lymphatic—CNS OK	**Pentamidine** 4 mg/kg IV/IM daily x 7-10 days	In US, free from CDC drug service: **Suramin*** 100 mg IV (test dose), then 1 gm IV on days 1, 3, 7, 14, & 21. Peds dose is 20 mg/kg.	Suramin effective but avoid if possible due to possible co-infection with O. volvulus in W. Africa.
Late: Encephalitis	Combination of IV **Eflornithine***, 400 mg/kg/day divided q12h x 7 days, plus **Nifurtimox***, 15 mg/kg/day po, divided q8h x 10 days (abbreviated NECT) now WHO standard of care *(Lancet 374:56, 2009; CID 56:195 2013)*	**Melarsoprol*** 2.2 mg/kg/day IV x 10 days; toxic arsenical now superseded by NECT	
East African sleeping sickness (T. brucei rhodesiense)			
Early: Blood/lymphatic. Clinical series in travelers *Int J Infect Dis (2018); https://doi.org/10.1016/j.ijid.2018.08.012*	**Suramin*** 100 mg IV (test dose), then 1 gm IV on days 1 3, 7, 14, & 21	Peds: **Suramin*** 2 mg/kg test dose, then 20 mg/kg IV on days 1, 3, 7, 14 & 21	Suramin & Melarsoprol: CDC Drug Service or WHO (at no charge) *(see Table 13D)*
Late: Encephalitis (prednisolone may prevent encephalitis) Pre-treatment with Suramin advised by some.	**Melarsoprol*** 2.2 mg/kg/day IV x 10 days *(PLoS NTD 6:e1695, 2012)*		Early illness: patient waiting for Suramin, use pentamidine 4 mg/kg/day IV/IM x 1-2 doses. Does not enter CSF.
T. cruzi—**Chagas disease** or acute American trypanosomiasis *Ref: NEJM 373:456, 2015.* For chronic disease: no benefit in established cardiomyopathy *(NEJM 373:1295, 2015)* US burden reviewed *PLoS Negl Trop Dis 2016;10:e0005033.*	*Adult (Age ≥12 years):* **Benznidazole*** 5-7 mg kg/day po in 2 doses (q12h) x 60 days *Pediatric (Age <12 years):* **Benznidazole*** 7.5 mg/kg/day po in 2 doses (q12h) x 60 days. South American pediatric tablet formulation (LAFEPE and ELEA) not widely available. U.S.: available from Exeltis, Inc., Tel: +1 877-303-7181; www.benznidazoletablets.com. **Benznidazole** 12.5 & 100 mg approved tabs for 2-12 yr olds. CDC advocates off-label use in adults.	**Nifurtimox*** 8–10 mg/kg per day po div. 4x/day after meals x 120 days; Ages 11–16 yrs: 12.5–15 mg/kg per day div. qid po x 90 days; Children <11yrs: 15–20 mg/kg per day div. qid po x 90 days. **For AEs:** *Table 13B.* Ref: *CID 2016;63:1056* **Diagnosis:** Two separate confirmatory serological tests based on different antigens and/or techniques (EIA and immunoblot (TESA)) needed to make diagnosis in those who screen positive in blood bank testing (Ortho EIA kit). **Non-blood bank screening:** EIA (Wiener kit) plus confirmatory TESA/IFA; all available via CDC Many US commercial labs use Hemagen or Inbios EIA kits which appear to have high false-positive rates in Central American populations. Positive commercial EIA tests should be confirmed at CDC before any treatment.	Due to adverse effects may give Benznidazole 300 mg per day for 60 days, regardless of body weight OR give 300 mg per day but prolong treatment to complete the total dose corres-ponding to 5 mg/kg per day for 60 days. *N Engl J Med 373:456, 2015.* Immunosuppression for heart transplant can reactivate chronic Chagas disease. Can transmit by organ/transfusions. Do not use benznidazole in pregnancy.
NEMATODES—INTESTINAL (Roundworms). Eosinophilia? Think Strongyloides, toxocariasis and filariasis: *CID 34:407, 2005; 42:1781 & 1655, 2006-- See Table 13C.*			
Anisakis simplex (**anisakiasis**) Anisakiasis differentiated from Anisakidosis *(CID 51:806, 2010).* Other: A. pegreffii, A. physeteris, Pseudoterranova decipiens.	Physical removal: endoscope or surgery. IgE antibody test vs *A. simplex* may help diagnosis. No antimicrobial therapy.	Anecdotal reports of possible treatment benefit from albendazole *(Ln 360:54, 2002; CID 41:1825, 2005)*	Anisakiasis acquired by eating raw fish: herring, salmon, mackerel, cod, squid. Similar illness due to Pseudoterranova species acquired from cod, halibut, red snapper.
Ascaris lumbricoides (**ascariasis**) *Ln 367:1521, 2006*	**Albendazole** 400 mg po x 1 dose OR **Mebendazole** 100 mg po bid X 3 days or 500 mg po x 1 dose	**Ivermectin** 150–200 mcg/kg po x 1 dose	Review of efficacy of single dose: *JAMA 299:1937, 2008.* Mebendazole 500 mg tabs not widely available.
Capillaria philippinensis (**capillariasis**)	**Albendazole** 400 mg po bid x 10 days	**Mebendazole** 500 mg po daily x 20 days	Albendazole preferred.

* For source of drug, see *Table 13D, page 177.*

TABLE 13A (9)

INFECTING ORGANISM	SUGGESTED REGIMENS		COMMENTS
	PRIMARY	ALTERNATIVE	
NEMATODES—INTESTINAL (Roundworms) *(continued)*			
Enterobius vermicularis (**pinworm**)	**Mebendazole** 500 mg po x 1 dose, repeat in 2 weeks OR **Pyrantel pamoate** 11 mg/kg base (to max. dose of 1 gm) po x 1 dose; repeat in 2 wks	**Albendazole** 400 mg po x 1 dose, repeat in 2 wks.	*Side-effects in Table 13B, page 175.* Treat whole household.
Gongylonemiasis (adult worms in oral mucosa)	Surgical removal	**Albendazole** 400 mg/day po x 3 days	Ref: *CID 32:1378, 2001; J Helminth 80:425, 2006.*
Hookworm (Necator americanus and Ancylostoma duodenale)	**Albendazole** 400 mg po daily x 3 days	**Mebendazole** 500 mg po daily x 3 days OR **Pyrantel pamoate** 11 mg/kg (to max. dose of 1 gm) po daily x 3 days	**NOTE:** Ivermectin not effective. Single dose therapy as used in public health programs has lower cure rates and 3-day albendazole superior to 3-day mebendazole, *PLoS One 6:e25003, 2011.*
Strongyloides stercoralis (**strongyloidiasis**) *(Hyperinfection, See Comment)*	**Ivermectin** 200 mcg/kg per day po x 2 days	**Albendazole** 400 mg po bid x 7 days ; less effective	For disseminated disease with larvae in stool and sputum, repeat treatment every 15 days while stools positive and then 1 more treatment cycle. For hyperinfection with sepsis, treat daily for at least 10 days or until larvae undetectable. For hyperinfection: veterinary ivermectin given subcutaneously or rectally *(CID 49:1411, 2009).*
Trichostrongylus orientalis, T. colubriformis	**Pyrantel pamoate** 11 mg/kg (maximum 1 gm) po x 1 dose OR **Albendazole** 400 mg po daily x 10 doses OR **Mebendazole** 500 mg po qd x 10 days	**Albendazole** 400 mg po x 1 dose	
Trichuris trichiura (**whipworm**) *NEJM 370:610, 2014; PLoS One 6:e25003, 2011*	**Mebendazole** 100 mg po twice daily x 3 days. Low cure rates with either mebendazole or albendazole	**Albendazole** 400 mg po qd x 3 days or **Ivermectin** 200 mcg/kg po qd x 3 days	Mebendazole clearly superior for trichuris *(PLoS One.6:e25003, 2011; N Engl J Med 370:610, 2014).* Single dose Mebendazole 500 mg tab significantly less effective than 3 days (the references quoted currently support this).
NEMATODES—EXTRAINTESTINAL (Roundworms)			
Ancylostoma braziliense & caninum: causes **cutaneous larva migrans**	**Albendazole** 400 mg po bid x 3-7 days *(Ln ID 8:302, 2008).*	**Ivermectin** 200 mcg/kg po x 1 dose/day x 1–2 days (not in children wt <15 kg)	Also called "creeping eruption", dog and cat hookworm. Ivermectin cure rate 81-100% (1 dose) to 97% (2–3 doses) *(CID 31:493, 2000).*
Angiostrongylus cantonensis (Angiostrongyliasis); causes eosinophilic meningitis *(Hawaii J Med PH 72:35, 2013)*	Mild/moderate disease: Analgesics, serial LPs (if necessary). Prednisone 60 mg/day x 14 days reduces headache & need for LPs.	Adding **Albendazole** 15 mg/kg/day to prednisone 60 mg/day both for 14 days may reduce duration of headaches and need for repeat LPs.	**Do not use Albendazole without prednisone,** *see TRSMH 102:990, 2008.* Gnathostoma and Baylisascaris also cause eosinophilic meningitis.
Baylisascariasis (Raccoon roundworm); eosinophilic meningitis	No drug proven efficacious. Try po **Albendazole,** Peds: 25–50 mg/kg/day po; Adults: 400 mg po bid with corticosteroids. Treat for one month.		*Clin Microbiol Rev. 29:375, 2016.* Other causes of eosinophilic meningitis: Gnathostoma & Angiostrongylus.
Dracunculus medinensis: **Guinea worm** Dog reservoir found in 3 countries hampering eradication. *Am J Trop Med Hyg. 2018, 99:388*	Slow extraction of pre-emergent worm over several days	No drugs effective. Oral analgesics, anti-inflammatory drugs, topical antiseptics/antibiotic ointments to alleviate symptoms and facilitate worm removal by gentle manual traction over several days.	

* For source of drug, see *Table 13D, page 177.*

TABLE 13A (10)

INFECTING ORGANISM	SUGGESTED REGIMENS		COMMENTS
	PRIMARY	ALTERNATIVE	
NEMATODES—EXTRAINTESTINAL (Roundworms) *(continued)*			
Filariasis: Determine if co-infection with either Loa loa or Onchocerca			
Lymphatic filariasis (**Elephantiasis**): Etiologies: Wuchereria bancrofti Brugia malayi, Brugia timori	*Mono-infection:* **Diethylcarbamazine[2] (DEC)*** 6 mg/kg/day po in 3 divided doses x 12 days + **Doxy** 200 mg/day po x 6 wks	*Dual infection with Onchocerciasis:* Treat Onchocerciasis first: **Ivermectin** 150 mcg/kg po x 1 dose, wait 1 month, then start **DEC** as for mono-infection *Dual infection with Loa Loa:* DEC drug of choice for both but can cause severe encephalopathy if >2500 Loa Loa microfilaria/mL in blood. Refer to expert center for apheresis pre-DEC or prednisone + small doses of DEC. If <2500 microfilaria/mL, start regular dose of **DEC**	Doxy x 6 wks may improve mild/moderate lymphedema independent of parasite infection *(CID 55:621, 2012)*. **Note: DEC can cause irreversible eye damage if concomitant Onchocerciasis.**
Loiasis, Loa loa, eye worm disease: **Look for dual infection with either Onchocerciasis or Lymphatic filariasis.** Moxidectin pivotal study *Lancet. 2018 Jan 17. pii: S0140-6736(17)32844-1*			
	Mono-infection with <2500 L. loa microfilaria/mL: **DEC** 8-10 mg/kg/day po in 3 divided doses x 21 days *Mono-infection with >2500 L. loa microfilaria/mL:* Refer to expert center for apheresis prior to **DEC** therapy; alternatively: **Albendazole** 200 mg po bid x 21 days	*Dual infection with Lymphatic filariasis:* See Lymphatic filariasis, above *Dual infection with Onchocerciasis:* Treat Onchocerciasis first with **Ivermectin**, then treat L. loa with **DEC**	If >5000 L. loa microfilaria/mL in blood & given Ivermectin for Onchocerciasis, can facilitate entry of L. loa into CNS with severe encephalopathy. May require multiple 21 day courses of DEC to clear mono-infection
Onchocerca volvulus (Onchocerciasis), river blindness: **Look for dual infection with either Loa loa or Lymphatic filariasis**			
	Mono-infection: **Ivermectin** 150 mcg/kg x 1 dose, then repeat every 3-6 months until asymptomatic + **Doxy** 200 mg/day x 6 wks. No accepted alternative therapy. **Moxidectin** 8 mg po (age 12 or over) to be used instead of Ivermectin but not widely available	*Dual infection with Lymphatic filariasis:* See Lymphatic filariasis, above *Dual infection with L. loa:* Treat Onchocerciasis first with **Ivermectin**, then treat L. loa with **DEC**. If >5000 L. Loa microfilaria/mL in blood. Refer to expert center for apheresis before starting DEC	Onchocerciasis and Loa loa are mildly co-endemic in West and Central Africa.
Body cavity			
Mansonella perstans	In randomized trial, **Doxy** 200 mg po once daily x 6 weeks cleared microfilaria from blood in 67 of 69 patients *(NEJM 361:1448, 2009)*. Doxy may not work outside Mali and Cameroon due to strain variation.	**Albendazole** in high dose x 3 weeks. Doxy may not work outside Mali and Cameroon due to strain variation.	Efficacy of doxy believed to be due to inhibition of endosymbiont wolbachia; Ivermectin has no activity. Ref: *Trans R Soc Trop Med Hyg 100:458, 2006*.
Mansonella streptocerca	**Ivermectin** 150 µg/kg x 1 dose.	**Diethylcarbamazine** 6 mg/kg x 12 days kills microfilaria in adults but causes transient exacerbation of clinical symptoms and may cause vision loss and hypotension if co-infected with O. volvulus.	May need antihistamine or corticosteroid for allergic reaction from disintegrating organisms. Chronic pruritic hypopigmented lesions that may be confused with leprosy. Can be asymptomatic.
Mansonella ozzardi	**Ivermectin** 200 µ/kg x 1 dose likely effective. *Am J Trop Med Hyg 90:1170, 2014; Am J Trop Med Hyg. 2018, 98: 786*	Usually asymptomatic. Articular pain, pruritus, lymphadenopathy reported. May have allergic reaction from dying organisms.	
Dirofilariasis: **Heartworms**			
D. immitis, dog heartworm	No effective drugs; surgical removal only option		Can lodge in pulmonary artery → coin lesion. Eosinophilia rare.

[2] May need antihistamine or corticosteroid for allergic reaction from disintegrating organisms.

* For source of drug, see *Table 13D, page 177*.

TABLE 13A (11)

INFECTING ORGANISM	SUGGESTED REGIMENS		COMMENTS
	PRIMARY	ALTERNATIVE	
NEMATODES—EXTRAINTESTINAL (Roundworms)/Filariasis/Dirofilariasis: Heartworms *(continued)*			
D. tenuis (raccoon), D. ursi (bear), D. repens (dogs, cats)	No effective drugs	Worms migrate to conjunctivae, subcutaneous tissue including face, scrotum, breasts, extremities. D. repens emerging throughout Europe *Clin Microbiol Rev 25:507, 2012*	
Gnathostoma spinigerum			
Cutaneous larva migrans	**Albendazole** 400 mg po q24h or bid times 21 days	**Ivermectin** 200 μg/kg/day po x 2 days.	*Other etiology of larva migrans: Ancylostoma sp., see page 168*
Eosinophilic meningitis	Supportive care; monitor for cerebral hemorrhage	Case reports of steroid use: both benefit and harm from Albendazole or ivermectin *(EIN 17:1174, 2011).*	Other causes of eosinophilic meningitis: **Angiostrongylus** *(see page 168)* & **Baylisascaris** *(see page 168)*
Toxocariasis *(Lancet Infect Dis. 2018, ;18:e14)*	**Rx directed at relief of symptoms as infection self-limited, e.g., steroids & antihistamines; use of anthelmintics controversial.**		
Visceral larval migrans	**Albendazole** 400 mg po bid x 5 days ± **Prednisone** 60 mg/day	**Mebendazole** 100–200 mg po bid times 5 days	Severe lung, heart or CNS disease may warrant steroids *(Clin Micro Rev 16:265, 2003).* Differential dx of larval migrans syndromes: Toxocara canis & catis, Ancylostoma spp., Gnathostoma spp., Spirometra spp.
Ocular larval migrans	First 4 wks of illness: (Oral **Prednisone** 30–60 mg po q24h + subtenon **Triamcinolone** 40 mg/wk) x 2 wks (Surgery is sometimes necessary)		No added benefit of anthelmintic drugs. Rx of little effect after 4 wks. Some use steroids *(Clin Micro Rev 16:265, 2003).*
Trichinella spiralis (**Trichinellosis**) — muscle infection *(Review: Clin Micro Rev 22:127, 2009).*	**Albendazole** 400 mg po bid x 8–14 days	**Mebendazole** 500 mg po tid x 10 days (still with concomitant prednisone)	Use albendazole/mebendazole with caution during pregnancy. ↑ IgE, ↑ CPK, ESR 0, massive eosinophilia: >5000/μL.
	Concomitant **prednisone** 40–60 mg po q24h		
TREMATODES (Flukes) – Liver, Lung, Intestinal. All flukes have snail intermediate hosts; transmitted by ingestion of metacercariae on plants, fish or crustaceans.			
Liver flukes: Clonorchis sinensis, Metorchis conjunctus, Opisthorchis viverrini	**Praziquantel** 25 mg/kg po tid x 2 days	**Albendazole** 10 mg/kg per day po x 7 days	Same dose in children
Fasciola hepatica (sheep liver fluke), Fasciola gigantica	**Triclabendazole*** once, may repeat after 12-24 hrs. 10 mg/kg po x 1 dose. Single 20 mg/kg po dose effective in treatment failures.		
Intestinal flukes: Fasciola buski Heterophyes heterophyes; Metagonimus yokogawai. Nanophyetus salmincola	**Praziquantel** 25 mg/kg po tid x 1 days		Same dose in children
Lung fluke: Paragonimus sp.	**Praziquantel** 25 mg/kg po tid x 2 days	**Triclabendazole*** 10 mg/kg po x 2 doses over 12-24 hrs.	Same dose in children
Schistosoma sp.	• Travelers and temporary residents lightly infected with no chronic disease. o Light infection detected by serology, eggs not usually present in stool or urine. o Uncommon CNS involvement including spinal cord. o Almost all travel related cases are from Africa.		
Schistosoma haematobium; GU bilharziasis.	**Praziquantel** 40 mg/kg po on the same day (one dose of 40 mg/kg or two doses of 20 mg/kg)		Same dose in children. (this applies to all schisto species) Some clinicians use 60 mg/kg praziquantel for all species for travelers and temporary residents not expecting re-exposure.
Schistosoma intercalatum	**Praziquantel** 20 mg/kg po on the same day in 1 or 2 doses		Same dose in children
Schistosoma japonicum; Oriental schisto.	**Praziquantel** 60 mg/kg po on the same day (3 doses of 20 mg/kg)		Same dose in children. Cures 60–90% pts.

* For source of drug, see *Table 13D, page 177.*

TABLE 13A (12)

INFECTING ORGANISM	SUGGESTED REGIMENS		COMMENTS
	PRIMARY	ALTERNATIVE	
TREMATODES (Flukes) *(continued)*			
Schistosoma mansoni (intestinal bilharziasis)	**Praziquantel** 40 mg/kg po on the same day in (one dose of 40 mg/kg or two doses of 20 mg/kg)		Praziquantel: Same dose for children and adults. Cures 60–90% pts. No advantage to splitting dose in 2 Cochrane Database Syst Rev. *8:CD000053, 2014*
Schistosoma mekongi	**Praziquantel** 60 mg per kg po on the same day (3 doses of 20 mg/kg)		Same dose for children
Toxemic schisto; Katayama fever	**Praziquantel** 20 mg per kg po bid with short course of high dose prednisone. Repeat Praziquantel in 4-6 wks *(Clin Micro Rev 16:225, 2010).*		Reaction to onset of egg laying 4-6 wks after infection exposure in fresh water.
CESTODES (Tapeworms)			
Echinococcus granulosus (hydatid disease) *(Curr Opin Infect Dis 31:383,2018; LnID 12:871, 2012; BMC Infect Dis 2018, 18:306).* Dead or calcified cysts as determined by experienced radiologist require no therapy. Watch and wait for asymptomatic or non-compromising cysts.	**Liver cysts:** Image-based (U/S not CT/MRI) staging first. <5 cm CE1, CE3a cysts and possibly <5 cm CE2, CE3b cysts consider trial of albendazole 400 mg po bid for 3-6 months and assess response; 30-50% response rate. Uncomplicated 5-10 cm CE1 and CE3a cysts: Percutaneous aspiration-injection-reaspiration (PAIR) + Albendazole. Before & after drainage: **Albendazole** ≥60 kg, 400 mg po bid or <60 kg, 15 mg/kg/day divided bid, for a total of at least 30 days. Multivesicular or relapsing cysts may require longer therapy. Inject contrast after aspiration and before instilling scolocidal agent to ensure no biliary communication. Surgical resection (experienced surgeon only) with Albendazole starting 1 week pre-operatively and for 4 weeks post-operatively for CE2 and CE3b 5-10 cm and all viable cysts large than 10 cm. Complicated, multi vesicular, or infected cysts almost always require surgical intervention. Large hepatic cysts >7.5 cm likely to have biliary communication and require surgery. Laparoscopic and large bore non-surgical approaches being developed in endemic areas. Lung cysts Surgical resection. Avoid pre-operative Albendazole. May give Albendazole 400 mg po.		
Lung cysts	Surgical resection. Avoid pre-operative Albendazole. May give Albendazole 400 mg po bid x at least 28 days post-operatively. Ruptured or complicated cysts may require longer therapy. **Note:** Brain, cardiac, splenic, renal, bone locations uncommonly occur requiring surgical intervention. Metastatic spread into body cavities with spontaneous or iatrogenic (during surgery) cyst rupture require Albendazole 400 mg po bid indefinitely until clinical response with periodic surgical debulking if feasible.		
Echinococcus multilocularis (alveolar cyst disease) *(COID 16:437, 2003)*	**Albendazole** efficacy not clearly demonstrated, can try in dosages used for hydatid disease. Wide surgical resection only reliable rx; technique evolving. Post-surgical resection or if inoperable: Albendazole for several years *(Acta Tropic 114:1, 2010).*		
Intestinal tapeworms			
Diphyllobothrium latum (fish), Dipylidium caninum (dog), Taenia saginata (beef), & Taenia solium (pork)	**Praziquantel** 5–10 mg/kg po x 1 dose for children and adults.	**Niclosamide*** 2 gm po x 1 dose	Niclosamide from Expert Compounding Pharm, *see Table 13D.*
Hymenolepis diminuta (rats) and H. nana (humans)	**Praziquantel** 25 mg/kg po x 1 dose for children and adults.	**Niclosamide*** 2 gm po daily x 7 days	
Neurocysticercosis (NCC) New review: *Curr Opin Infect Dis. 2018, 31:377* Larval form of T. solium IDSA treatment guidelines. *CID 2018,66:1159*	**NOTE: Treat concomitant T. solium intestinal tapeworms,** if present, with **praziquantel** 5-10 mg/kg po x 1 dose after starting steroid. Both CT and MRI should be performed. Immunoblot preferred; ELISA lacks specificity. Serology insensitive for single lesions, calcified lesions. For multiple parenchymal lesions, subarachnoid NCC, intraventricular NCC, serology almost 100% sensitive; CSF testing no advantage over serum testing. Parenchymal scolex on imaging is diagnostic, serology not necessary. In non-endemic areas, check stools of household contacts of confirmed cases for tapeworm eggs.		
Parenchymal NCC			
1-20 "Viable" or degenerating cysts by CT/MRI. Meta-analysis: Treatment assoc with cyst resolution, ↓ seizures, and ↓ seizure recurrence.	**Albendazole** 15 mg/kg/d po (max 800 mg/d) + **Praziquantel** 50 mg/kg/d po + **Dexamethasone** 0.1 mg/kg/d po. Start steroid 1 day before anti-parasitics. Treat for 10 days. Continue seizure meds for 1 yr. Slow steroid taper after 10 days increasing back if seizures develop. Albendazole alone adequate if only 1-2 cysts on an MRI.	**Albendazole** alone 800 mg per day plus **Dexamethasone** 0.1 mg/kg per day ± Anti-seizure medication). *See Comment.* Limited data indicates that increasing dexamethasone to 8 mg/day X 28 days with 2-week taper decreases seizures but prolongs steroid exposure. *Epilepsia 55:1452, 2014*	Retreat after 6 months if any viable cysts remain. Methotrexate at ≤20 mg/wk allows a reduction in steroid use *(CID 44:449, 2007).* Some recommend longer courses of albendazole (even >30 days) if large number of parenchymal cysticerci.
Dead calcified cysts	**No treatment indicated**		

* For source of drug, see *Table 13D, page 177.*

TABLE 13A (13)

INFECTING ORGANISM		SUGGESTED REGIMENS		COMMENTS
		PRIMARY	ALTERNATIVE	
CESTODES (Tapeworms)/Neurocysticercosis *(continued)*				
Subarachnoid NCC		Albendazole 15 mg/kg per day (max. 1200 mg/day) + Dexamethasone (doses as above with very slow taper) + v-p shunt prior to therapy. 30 day course, may need to repeat multiple times or give continuously for months according to clinical and MRI evolution *(Expert Rev Anti Infect Ther 9:123, 2011)*; continue until radiologic resolution. Intracranial pressure must be monitored and managed by an experienced clinician. If diffuse cerebral edema or raised ICP, control with steroids or shunting prior to any anti-parasitic therapy.	Long courses of combination therapy with Albendazole/praziquantel combination therapy for refractory disease.	
Intraventricular NCC		Neuroendoscopic removal is treatment of choice with or without obstruction. If surgery not possible, **Albendazole + Dexamethasone; observe closely for evidence of obstruction of flow of CSF.**	**Albendazole** + **Dexamethasone** (as above); place v-p shunt prior to therapy when no access to neuroendoscopy.	
Sparganosis (Spirometra mansonoides) Larval cysts; source—frogs/snakes		Surgical resection. No antiparasitic therapy. Can inject alcohol into subcutaneous masses.		
ECTOPARASITES. Ref.: *CID 36:1355, 2003; Ln 363:889, 2004.* **NOTE: Due to potential neurotoxicity and risk of aplastic anemia, lindane not recommended.**				
DISEASE	**INFECTING ORGANISM**			
Head lice *Med Lett 54:61, 2012.*	Pediculus humanus, var. capitis. Re-treatment often necessary as current drugs do not kill eggs.	**Permethrin** 1% lotion: Apply to shampooed dried hair for 10 min.; repeat in 9-10 days. **OR** **Malathion** 0.5% lotion (Ovide): Apply to dry hair for 8–12 hrs, then shampoo. 2 doses 7-9 days apart. **OR** **Spinosad** 0.9% suspension; wash off after 10 min (85% effective). Repeat in 7 days, if needed. Use nit comb initially & repeat in 7-10 days	**Ivermectin** 200-400 µg/kg po once; 3 doses at 7 day intervals effective in 95% *(JID 193:474, 2006)*. Topical ivermectin 0.5% lotion, 75% effective. **Malathion:** Report that 1–2 20-min. applications 98% effective *(Ped Derm 21:670, 2004)*. In alcohol—potentially flammable. **Benzyl alcohol:** 76% effective.	**Permethrin:** success in 78%. Resistance increasing. No advantage to 5% permethrin. **Spinosad** is effective, but expensive. Wash hats, scarves, coats & bedding in hot water, then dry in hot dryer for 20+ minutes.
Pubic lice (crabs)	Phthirus pubis	**Pubic hair: Permethrin** OR **Malathion** as for head lice. Shave pubic hair.	**Eyelids: Petroleum jelly** applied qid x 10 days OR **yellow oxide of mercury** 1% qid x 14 days	**Do not use lindane.** Treat sex partners of the last 30 days.
Body lice	Pediculus humanus, var. corporis	No drugs for the patient. Organism lives in & deposits eggs in seams of clothing. Discard clothing; if not possible, treat clothing with 1% malathion powder or 0.5% permethrin powder. Success with ivermectin in homeless shelter: 12 mg po on days 0, 7, & 14 *(JID 193:474, 2006)*		
Myiasis Due to larvae of flies		Usually cutaneous/subcutaneous nodule with central punctum. Treatment: Occlude punctum to prevent gas exchange with petrolatum, fingernail polish, makeup cream or bacon. When larva migrates, manually remove. Ref: *Clin Microbiol Rev 25:79, 2012.*		
Scabies	Sarcoptes scabiei			
Immunocompetent patients Refs: *MMWR 64(RR-3):1, 2015; NEJM 362:717, 2010.*		**Permethrin** 5% cream (ELIMITE) under nails (finger and toe). Apply entire skin from chin down to and including under fingernails and toenails. Leave on 8–14 hrs. Repeat in 1-2 wks. Safe for children age >2 mos.	**Ivermectin** 200 µg/kg po with food x 1, then second dose in 2 wks. **Less effective: Crotamiton** 10% cream, apply x 24 hr, rinse off, then reapply x 24 hr.	Trim fingernails. Reapply cream to hands after handwashing. Treat close contacts; wash and heat dry linens. Pruritus may persist times 2 wks after mites gone.
AIDS and HTLV-infected patients (CD4 <150 per mm^3), debilitated or developmentally disabled patients (**Norwegian scabies**—*see Comments)*		For Norwegian crusted scabies: **Permethrin** 5% cream daily x 7 days, then twice weekly until cured. Add **Ivermectin** po (dose in Alternative)	**Ivermectin** 200 mcg/kg po on days 1, 2, 8, 9 & 15+ **Permethrin** cream. May need addt'l doses of Ivermectin on days 22 & 29.	**Norwegian scabies** in AIDS pts: Extensive, crusted. Can mimic psoriasis. Not pruritic. Highly contagious—isolate!

* For source of drug, see *Table 13D, page 177.*

TABLE 13B – DOSAGE AND SELECTED ADVERSE EFFECTS OF ANTIPARASITIC DRUGS

Doses vary with indication. For convenience, drugs divided by type of parasite; some drugs used for multiple types of parasites, e.g., albendazole.

CLASS, AGENT, GENERIC NAME (TRADE NAME)	USUAL ADULT DOSAGE	ADVERSE REACTIONS/COMMENTS
Antiprotozoan Drugs		
Intestinal Parasites		
Diloxanide furoate[NUS] (Furamide)	500 mg po tid x 10 days	Source: *See Table 13D, page 177.* Flatulence, N/V, diarrhea.
Iodoquinol (Yodoxin)	Adults: 650 mg po tid (or 30-40 mg/kg/day div. tid); children: 40 mg/kg per day div. tid.	Rarely causes nausea, abdominal cramps, rash, acne. **Contraindicated if iodine intolerance** (contains 64% bound iodine). Can cause iododerma (papular or pustular rash) and/or thyroid enlargement.
Metronidazole	Side-effects similar for all. *See metronidazole in Table 10A, page 125*	
Nitazoxanide (Alinia)	Adults: 500 mg po q12h. Children 4–11: 200 mg susp. po q12h. Take with food. Expensive.	Abdominal pain 7.8%, diarrhea 2.1%. Rev.: *CID 40:1173, 2005; Expert Opin Pharmacother 7:953, 2006.* Headaches; rarely yellow sclera (resolves after treatment).
Paromomycin (Humatin)	15-35 mg/kg/day po in 3 divided doses x 5-10 days (250 mg tabs). Source: *See Table 13D.*	**Aminoglycoside similar to neomycin;** if absorbed due to concomitant inflammatory bowel disease can result in oto/nephrotoxicity. Doses >3 gm daily are associated with nausea, abdominal cramps, diarrhea.
Quinacrine	100 mg po tid x 5 days. *See Table 13D.*	**Contraindicated for pts with history of psychosis or psoriasis. Yellow staining of skin.** Dizziness, headache, vomiting, toxic psychosis (1.5%), hemolytic anemia, leukopenia, thrombocytopenia, urticaria, rash, fever, minor disulfiram-like reactions.
Tinidazole (Tindamax)	250-500 mg tabs, with food. Regimen varies with indication.	**Chemical structure similar to metronidazole but better tolerated.** Seizures/peripheral neuropathy reported. **Adverse effects:** Metallic taste 4–6%, nausea 3–5%, anorexia 2–3%.
Antiprotozoan Drugs: Non-Intestinal Protozoa		
Extraintestinal Parasites		
Antimony compounds[NUS] Stibogluconate sodium (Pentostam) from CDC or Meglumine antimonate (Glucantime)—French trade name	For IV use: vials with 100 mg antimony/mL. Dilute selected dose in 50 mL of D5W shortly before use. Infuse over at least 10 minutes. Intralesional injection used in many countries; 20 mg/kg qwk X 5-10 weeks.	**AEs in 1st 10 days:** headache, fatigue, elevated lipase/amylase, clinical pancreatitis. After 10 days: elevated AST/ALT/ALK/PHOS. CBC, biochemistry weekly, EKG q2 weeks if prolonged therapy. **NOTE: Reversible T wave changes in 30-60%. Risk of QTc prolongation. Renal excretion; modify dose if renal insufficiency. Metabolized in liver; lower dose if hepatic insufficiency. Generic drug may have increased toxicity due to antimony complex formation.**
Artemether-Lumefantrine, po (Coartem, FDA-approved)	4 (20 mg Artemether and 120 mg Lumefantrine) combination tablets X 6 doses over 3 days for adults. Take with food. Can be crushed and mixed with a few teaspoons of water	**Can prolong QT_c:** avoid in patients with congenital long QT_c, family history of sudden death or long QT_c, or need for drugs known to prolong QT_c *(see list under fluoroquinolones, Table 10A, page 122).* Artemether induces CYP3A4 and both Artemether & Lumefantrine are metabolized by CYP3A4 *(see drug-drug interactions, Table 22A, page 259).* Adverse effects experienced by >30% of adults: headache, anorexia, dizziness, arthralgia and myalgia. Non-life threatening, but transfusion requiring, hemolytic anemia can occur up to 15 days post-therapy *(AnIM 163:498, 2015).*
Artesunate, IV Ref: *NEJM 358:1829, 2008*	Available from CDC Malaria Branch. 2.4 mg/kg IV at 0, 12, 24, & 48 hrs for adults. Follow with 2nd drug po.	**More effective than quinine & safer than quinidine.** Contact CDC at 770-488-7758 or 770-488-7100 after hours. No dosage adjustment for hepatic or renal insufficiency. No known drug interactions.
Atovaquone (Mepron) Ref.: *AAC 46:1163, 2002*	Suspension: 1 tsp (750 mg) po bid 750 mg/5 mL.	No. pts stopping rx due to side-effects was 9%; rash 22%, GI 20%, headache 16%, insomnia 10%, fever 14%
Atovaquone and Proguanil (Malarone) For prophylaxis of P. falciparum; little data on P. vivax. Generic available in US.	**Prophylaxis:** 1 tab po (250 mg + 100 mg) q24h with food **Treatment:** 4 tabs po (1000 mg + 400 mg) once daily with food x 3 days. Adult tab: 250/100 mg; Peds tab 62.5/25 mg. *Treatment see comment, page 164.*	Adverse effects in rx trials: Adults—abd. pain 17%, N/V 12%, headache 10%, dizziness 5%. Rx stopped in 1%. Asymptomatic mild ↑ in ALT/AST. Children—cough, headache, anorexia, vomiting, abd. pain. *See drug interactions, Table 22A.* Safe in G6PD-deficient pts. Can crush tabs for children and give with milk or other liquid nutrients. Renal insufficiency: contraindicated if CrCl <30 mL per min.

* For source of drug, see *Table 13D, page 177.*

TABLE 13B (2)

CLASS, AGENT, GENERIC NAME (TRADE NAME)	USUAL ADULT DOSAGE	ADVERSE REACTIONS/COMMENTS
Antiprotozoan Drugs: Non-Intestinal Protozoa/Extraintestinal Parasites *(continued)*		
Benznidazole* Benznidazole 12.5 & 100 mg approved tabs for 2-12 yr olds. CDC advocates off-label use in adults *(www.benznidazoletablets.com)*	5 mg/kg per day po. 100 mg tabs. May use 300 mg per day for 60 days, regardless of body weight OR give 300 mg per day but prolong treatment to complete the total dose corresponding to 5 mg/kg per day for 60 days.	**Photosensitivity in 50% of pts.** GI: abdominal pain, nausea/vomiting/anorexia. Dermatitis including Stevens-Johnson. CNS: disorientation, insomnia, twitching/seizures, paresthesias, polyneuritis. Discontinue if leucopenia or thrombocytopenia. **Contraindicated in pregnancy**. Recommended dose range 5-7.5 mg/kg/day but more than 5 mg/kg has unacceptable side effects in adults, higher doses better tolerated in children.
Chloroquine phosphate (Aralen)	Dose varies—*see Malaria Prophylaxis and rx, pages 162-163.*	Minor: anorexia/nausea/vomiting, headache, dizziness, blurred vision, pruritus in dark-skinned pts. Major: protracted rx in rheumatoid arthritis can lead to retinopathy. Can exacerbate psoriasis. Can block response to intradermally administered rabies vaccine. **Contraindicated in pts with epilepsy.**
Dapsone *See Comment re methemoglobinemia*	100 mg po q24h	Usually tolerated by pts with rash after TMP-SMX. **Dapsone is common etiology of acquired methemoglobinemia** *(NEJM 364:957, 2011)*. Metabolite of dapsone converts heme iron to + 3 charge (no O2 transport) from normal +2. Normal blood level 1%; cyanosis at 10%; headache, fatigue, tachycardia, dizziness at 30-40%, acidosis & coma at 60%, death at 70-80%. Low G6PD is a risk factor. Treatment: methylene blue 1-2 mg/kg IV over 5 min x 1 dose.
Eflornithine (Ornidyl) (WHO or CDC drug service)	400 mg/kg/day IV divided q12h x 7 days in combination with Nifurtimox for West African Trypanosomiasis	Diarrhea in ½ pts, vomiting, abdominal pain, anemia/leukopenia in ½ pts, seizures, alopecia, jaundice, ↓ hearing. Contraindicated in pregnancy.
Fumagillin	Eyedrops + po. 20 mg po tid. Leiter's: 800-292-6772.	Adverse events: Neutropenia & thrombocytopenia
Mefloquine	One 250 mg tab/wk for **malaria prophylaxis**; for rx, 1250 mg x 1 or 750 mg & then 500 mg in 6–8 hrs. In U.S.: 250 mg tab = 228 mg base; outside U.S.: 275 mg tab = 250 mg base	Side-effects in roughly 3%. Minor: headache, irritability, insomnia, weakness, diarrhea. **Toxic psychosis, seizures can occur.** Do not use with quinine, quinidine, or halofantrine. Rare: Prolonged QT interval and toxic epidermal necrolysis *(Ln 349:101, 1997)*. **Not used for self-rx due to neuropsychiatric side-effects.** FDA black box for possible prolonged effects. Avoid if pre-existing overlay of depression or other psychiatric disorders.
Melarsoprol (Mel B, Arsobal) (CDC)	2.2 mg/kg/day IV x 10 days	**Post-rx encephalopathy (2-10%) with 50% mortality overall, risk of death 2° to rx 8-14%.** Prednisolone 1 mg per kg per day po may ↓ encephalopathy. Other: Heart damage, albuminuria, abdominal pain, vomiting, peripheral neuropathy, Herxheimer-like reaction, pruritus. o Prednisone may prevent/attenuate encephalopathy. o Pretreatment with Suramin (dose as above) is often used in late-stage East African trypanosomiasis to clear the hemolymphatic system of trypanosomes before administration of melarsoprol.
Miltefosine (Impavido) No longer available from CDC, purchase from www.impavido.com	50 mg po bid (wt 33-44 kg); 50 mg po tid (wt ≥45 kg) (max 150 mg/d). Treat for 28 days	**Pregnancy—No;** teratogenic. Side-effects vary: kala-azar pts, vomiting in up to 40%, diarrhea in 17%; "motion sickness", headache & increased creatinine. Metabolized by liver; virtually no urinary excretion.
Nifurtimox (Lampit) *(CDC)* (Manufactured in Germany by Bayer)	8–10 mg/kg per day po div. 4 x per day for 90-120 days for Chaga's. 15 mg/kg/day po, divided q8h x 10 days for West African trypanosomiasis	**Side-effects in 40–70% of pts.** GI: abdominal pain, nausea/vomiting. CNS: polyneuritis (1/3), disorientation, insomnia, twitching, seizures. Skin rash. Hemolysis with G6PD deficiency. Monitor CBC, biochemistry after 4-6 weeks. Monitor frequently for neuropathy. Ref: *CID 2016;63:1056.*
Pentamidine	4 mg/kg IV or IM daily x 7-10 days for African Trypanosomiasis. 300 mg via aerosol q month.	Hypotension, hypocalcemia, hypoglycemia followed by hyperglycemia, pancreatitis. Neutropenia (15%), thrombocytopenia. Nephrotoxicity. Others: nausea/vomiting, ↑ liver tests, rash.
Primaquine phosphate	26.3 mg (=15 mg base). Adult dose is 30 mg of base po daily.	**In G6PD def. pts, can cause hemolytic anemia with hemoglobinuria, esp. African, Asian peoples.** Methemoglobinemia. Rapid G6PD screening tests now readily available. Nausea/abdominal pain if pt. fasting. *(CID 39:1336, 2004)*. **Pregnancy: No.**

* For source of drug, see *Table 13D, page 177.*

TABLE 13B (3)

CLASS, AGENT, GENERIC NAME (TRADE NAME)	USUAL ADULT DOSAGE	ADVERSE REACTIONS/COMMENTS
Antiprotozoan Drugs: Non-Intestinal Protozoa/Extraintestinal Parasites *(continued)*		
Pyrimethamine (Daraprim, Malocide) Also combined with Sulfadoxine as **Fansidar** (25–500 mg)	100 mg po, then 25 mg/day. **Very expensive:** $75,000 for 100 tabs (25 mg). Financial assistance may be available by calling 1-877-258-8033. Consider compounding pharmacy (imprimusrx.com).	**Major problem is hematologic:** megaloblastic anemia, ↓ WBC, ↓ platelets. Can give 5 mg folinic acid per day to ↓ bone marrow depression and not interfere with antitoxoplasmosis effect. If high-dose pyrimethamine, ↑ folinic acid to 10–50 mg/day. Pyrimethamine + sulfadiazine can cause mental changes due to carnitine deficiency *(AJM 95:112, 1993)*. Other: Rash, vomiting, diarrhea, xerostomia.
Quinine sulfate (Qualaquin)	324 mg tabs. No IV prep. in US. Oral rx of chloroquine-resistant falciparum malaria: 624 mg po tid x 3 days, then (tetracycline 250 mg po qid or doxy 100 mg bid) x 7 days	Cinchonism; tinnitus, headache, nausea, abdominal pain, blurred vision. Rarely: blood dyscrasias, drug fever, asthma, hypoglycemia. Transient blindness in <1% of 500 pts *(AnIM 136:339, 2002)*. **Contraindicated if prolonged QTc, myasthenia gravis, optic neuritis or G6PD deficiency.**
Spiramycin (Rovamycin)	1 gm po q8h *(see Comment)*.	GI and allergic reactions have occurred. Available at no cost after consultation with Palo Alto Medical Foundation Toxoplasma Serology Lab: 650-853-4828 or from U.S. FDA 301-796-1600.
Sulfadiazine	1–1.5 gm po q6h.	*See Table 10A, page 126, for sulfonamide side-effects*
Sulfadoxine & Pyrimethamine combination (Fansidar)	Contains 500 mg Sulfadoxine & 25 mg Pyrimethamine	Long half-life of both drugs: Sulfadoxine 169 hrs, pyrimethamine 111 hrs allows weekly dosage. In African, used empirically in pregnancy for intermittent preventative treatment (ITPp) against malaria: dosing at 3 set times during pregnancy. Reduces material and fetal mortality if HIV+. *See Expert Rev Anti Infect Ther 8:589, 2010.* **Fatalities reported due to Stevens-Johnson syndrome and toxic epidermal necrolysis.** Renal excretion—caution if renal impairment.
Tafenoquine (Arakoda, Krintafel) (for P. vivax malaria, age ≥ 16 yrs, ≥ 18 yrs for prophylaxis) Arakoda: 100 mg tab Krintafel: 150 mg tab	Radical cure (prevention of relapse): 300 mg single dose on day 1 or 2 of appropriate blood-stage therapy. Prophylaxis: 200 mg qd x 3 days (starting 3 days before travel), then 200 mg qwk maintenance starting 7 days after last loading dose, then after leaving endemic area, 200 mg once, 7 days after last maintenance dose	Test for G6PD deficiency before use. **Must have 70% normal G6PD activity on quantitative testing to use TQ;** do not use screening tests or qualitative tests. AEs: hemolytic anemia (G6PD deficiency), methemoglobinemia, psychiatric effects only if previous psychosis, hypersensitivity.
DRUGS USED TO TREAT NEMATODES, TREMATODES, AND CESTODES		
Albendazole (Albenza)	Doses vary with indication. Take with food; fatty meal increases absorption. See *Table 13D* for US availability	FDA Pregnancy Category C due to lack of data but available evidence suggests no difference in congenital abnormalities. WHO allows use of albendazole in 2nd and 3rd trimesters. CDC suggests consideration in 3rd trimester if infection is compromising the pregnancy. Abdominal pain (with prolonged courses), nausea/vomiting, alopecia, ↑ serum transaminase. Rare leukopenia.
Diethylcarbamazine *(CDC)*	Dose varies with species of filaria.	Headache, dizziness, nausea, fever. In Onchocerciasis, host may experience inflammatory reaction to death of microfilariae: fever, urticaria, asthma, GI upset **(Mazzotti reaction). Pregnancy—No.**
Ivermectin (Stromectol, Mectizan) (3 mg tab & topical 0.5% lotion for head lice). Take on empty stomach.	Strongyloidiasis dose: 200 µg/kg/day po x 2 days Onchocerciasis: 150 µg/kg x 1 po Scabies: 200 µg/kg po x 1; if AIDS, wait 14 days & repeat	Mild side-effects: fever, pruritus, rash. In rx of onchocerciasis, can *see tender lymphadenopathy,* headache, bone/joint pain.
Mebendazole (Vermox)	In developing world chewable tablet, 500 mg po once in public health campaigns. 100 mg po twice/day for 3 days is optimal for most intestinal nematodes. 100 mg single dose adequate for pinworm. See Table 13D for US availability	Rarely causes abdominal pain, nausea, diarrhea. FDA Pregnancy Category C due to lack of data but available evidence suggests no difference in congenital abnormalities. WHO allows use of mebendazole in 2nd and 3rd trimesters. CDC suggests consideration in 3rd trimester if infection is compromising the pregnancy.

* For source of drug, see *Table 13D, page 177.*

TABLE 13B (4)

CLASS, AGENT, GENERIC NAME (TRADE NAME)	USUAL ADULT DOSAGE	ADVERSE REACTIONS/COMMENTS
DRUGS USED TO TREAT NEMATODES, TREMATODES, AND CESTODES *(continued)*		
Praziquantel (Biltricide)	Doses vary with parasite; *see Table 13A*.	Mild: dizziness/drowsiness, N/V, rash, fever. **Only contraindication is ocular cysticercosis**. Potential exacerbation of neurocysticercosis. Metab.-induced by anticonvulsants and steroids; can negate effect with cimetidine 400 mg po tid. Reduce dose if advanced liver disease. Praziquantel is pregnancy category B. Available evidence suggests no difference in adverse birth outcomes. WHO encourages the use of praziquantel in any stage of pregnancy. CDC advises individual risk-benefit assessment according to clinical disease in the mother.
Pyrantel pamoate (over-the-counter)	Oral suspension. Dose for all ages: 11 mg/kg (to max. of 1 gm) x 1 dose	Rare GI upset, headache, dizziness, rash
Suramin (Germanin) *(CDC)*	Drug powder mixed to 10% solution with 5 mL water and used within 30 min. First give test dose of 0.1 gm IV. Try to avoid during pregnancy.	Does not cross blood-brain barrier; no effect on CNS infection. Side-effects: vomiting, pruritus, urticaria, fever, paresthesias, albuminuria (discontinue drug if casts appear). Do not use if renal/liver disease present. Deaths from vascular collapse reported.
Triclabendazole (Egaten) *(CDC)* Available at no charge from Novartis. *See Table 13D*	Used for fasciola hepatica liver fluke infection: 10 mg/kg po x 1 dose. May repeat in 12-24 hrs. 250 mg tabs	AEs ≥10%: sweating and abdominal pain. AEs 1-10%: weakness, chest pain, fever, anorexia, nausea, vomiting. **Note: use with caution if G6PD def. or impaired liver function.**

TABLE 13C – PARASITES THAT CAUSE EOSINOPHILIA (EOSINOPHILIA IN TRAVELERS)

Frequent and Intense (>5000 eos/mcL)	Moderate to Marked Early Infections	During Larval Migration; Absent or Mild During Chronic Infections	Other	
Strongyloides (absent in compromised hosts); Lymphatic Filariasis; Toxocara (cutaneous larva migrans); Trichinella; Angiostrongylus; Opisthorchis	Ascaris; Hookworm; Clonorchis; Paragonimus; Fasciola; Schistosomiasis	Opisthorchis; Baylisascaris	Schistosomiasis; Cysticercosis; Trichuris; Angiostrongylus; Onchocerciasis; echinococcus	Non-lymphatic filariasis; Gnathostoma; Capillaria; Trichostrongylus

* For source of drug, see *Table 13D, page 177*.

TABLE 13D – SOURCES FOR HARD-TO-FIND ANTIPARASITIC DRUGS

Source	Drugs Available	Contact Information
CDC Drug Service	Artesunate, Diethylcarbamazine (DEC), Eflornithine, Melarsoprol, Nifurtimox, Sodium stibogluconate, Suramin, Triclabendazole	www.cdc.gov/laboratory/drugservice/index.html (+1) 404-639-3670 or drugservice@cdc.gov
CDC Malaria Branch	Contact for the availability of: Artesunate (IV) for severe malaria, any case of malaria where the person is not tolerating oral medications, or any highly suspected cases of severe malaria. Criteria for release broadened in April 2019 and additional supply of imported artesunate was obtained. Artesunate now pre-positioned at 18 locations nationally.	CDC Malaria Hotline (770-488-7788) from 9:00 am to 5:00 pm Eastern Time. After hours or on weekends and holidays, call the CDC Emergency Operation Center at 770-488-7100 and ask to page the person on call for the Malaria Branch
WHO	Drugs for treatment of African trypanosomiasis	priottog@who.int; (+41) 794-682-726; (+41) 227-911-345 francoj@who.int; (+41) 796-198-535; (+41) 227-913-313
Compounding Pharmacies, Specialty Distributors, Direct from Mfgr		
Expert Compounding Pharmacy	Albendazole, Furazolidone, Iodoquinol, Mebendazole (100 mg tabs), Niclosamide, Paromomycin (oral), Praziquantel, Pyrantel pamoate, Quinacrine, Thiabendazole, Tinidazole	www.expertpharmacy.org 1-800-247-9767; (+1) 818-988-7979
Exeltis, Inc. / Benznidazole	Commercial FDA approved tab for child age 2-12 yrs, may use off-label in adults (www.benznidazoletablets.com)	+1 800-964-9650
Leiter's Pharmacy	Fumagillin	www.leiterrx.com 1-800-292-6772; +1-408-292-6772
Novartis, Inc.	Triclabendazole. Available and shipped for free to any pharmacy having a valid prescription on hand. Novartis will request patient name, DOB, and pharmacy address/phone.	Tel: +1 888-669-6682.
Profounda, Inc.	Miltefosine (leishmaniasis or free-living ameba)	www.impavido.com; +1 407-270-7790
Victoria Apotheke Zurich will ship worldwide if sent physicians prescription.	Paromomycin (oral and topical), Triclabendazole. Other hard to find anti-parasitic drugs	www.pharmaworld.com (+41) 43-344-6060
Palo Alto Medical Foundation, Toxoplasma Serology Lab	Spiramycin (consultation required for release)	(+1) 650-853-4828; toxlab@pamf.org
Imprimis (compounding pharmacy)	Pyrimethamine	+1 844-446-6979; www.imprimisrx.com

Note: In the U.S. FDA-approved branded Albendazole (Albenza) and Mebendazole marketed by Amedra is very costly and is difficult for retail pharmacies to access. Vermox brand mebendazole 500 mg tablets is FDA-approved but for donation only and not sold in the U.S.

TABLE 14A – ANTIVIRAL THERAPY*

For HIV, *see Table 14C*; for Hepatitis, *see Table 14E* and *Table 14F*. For Antiviral Activity Spectra, *see Table 4C, page 87*

VIRUS/DISEASE	DRUG/DOSAGE	SIDE EFFECTS/COMMENTS
Adenovirus: Cause of RTIs including fatal pneumonia in children & young adults and 60% mortality in transplant pts. Frequent cause of cystitis in transplant patients. Adenovirus 14 associated with severe pneumonia in otherwise healthy young adults. **Findings include:** fever, ↑ liver enzymes, leukopenia, thrombocytopenia, diarrhea, pneumonia, or hemorrhagic cystitis. Encephalitis: *NEJM 381:1459, 2019.* Treatment Guidelines: https://doi.org/10.1111/ctr.13527	In severe cases of pneumonia or post HSCT[1]: **Cidofovir** • 5 mg/kg/wk x 2 wks, then q 2 wks + **Probenecid** 1.25 gm/M^2 given 3 hrs before cidofovir and 3 & 9 hrs after each infusion • Or 1 mg/kg IV 3x/wk. For adenovirus hemorrhagic cystitis *(CID 40:199, 2005; Transplantation. 2006; 81:1398):* Intravesical **Cidofovir** (5 mg/kg in 100 mL saline instilled into bladder).	Routine monitoring with HAdV viral load recommended 1- 2 times/wk in high-risk patients: Allo-HSCT with haploidentical donor or unrelated cord blood graft; Severe GVHD; Severe lymphopenia; and/or Rx with alemtuzumab. Monitoring should continue until immune reconstitution. Those with at least 1 risk factor and viremia should be Rx'd with cidofovir. Ribavirin not recommended. Vidarabine and Ganciclovir have in vitro activity against adenovirus; little to no clinical data. Donor specific T-cells should be reserved for those who have failed antiviral therapy and administered as part of a clinical trial.
Bunyaviridae: Severe fever with thrombocytopenia syndrome virus (SFTSV) Possibly transmitted by *Haemaphysalis longicomis* and *Amblyomma americanum (lone star)* ticks.	No therapy recommended. Ribavirin ineffective. Clinical symptoms: Fever, weakness, myalgias, GI symptoms	Lab: Elevated LDH (>1200) and CPK (>800) associated with higher mortality rates. Initially thought to be an anaplasma infection, but serology showed a new virus. Epi update: *Clim Exp Vacc Res 7:43-50, 2018*. Reservoir in animals (goats/cattle/dogs/cats)
Coronavirus— **SARS-CoV:** Severe acute respiratory syndrome *(NEJM 348:1953 & 1967, 2003)* **MERS-CoV:** Middle East respiratory syndrome *(NEJM 2017,376:584)* **2019-nCoV.** Novel respiratory CoV emerged in Wuhan, China in late 2019. See *https://www.cdc.gov/coronavirus/2019-nCoV/summary.html* for criteria for testing of suspected cases and most current information. Cases reported from multiple countries as of early 2020.	**SARS:** • Ribavirin—ineffective. • Interferon alfa ± steroids—small case series. • Pegylated IFN-α effective in monkeys. • Low dose steroids alone successful in one Beijing hospital. High dose steroids ↑ serious fungal infections. • Inhaled nitric oxide improved oxygenation & improved chest x-ray *(CID 39:1531, 2004)*. **MERS:** Increased 14 day survival with **Ribavirin** po + **PEG-IFN** 180 mcg/kg sc x 2 wks *(LnID 14:1090, 2014)*. Other therapies: *LnID 14:1136, 2014.*	**SARS: Transmission by close contact:** effective infection control practices (**mask [changed frequently]**, eye protection, gown, gloves) key to stopping transmission. **MERS:** Suspected reservoirs are camels and perhaps other animals. *Review: Clin Micro Rev. 28:465, 2015*. Korean guidelines recommend IFN-1+ lopinavir/ritonavir + ribavirin (though no clinical trials) *(Korean J Intern Med. 2018 Mar; 33(2): 233–246)*.
Enterovirus—Meningitis: most common cause of aseptic meningitis. Rapid CSF PCR test is accurate; reduces costs and hospital stay for infants *(Peds 120:489, 2007)*	**No rx currently recommended.**	No clinical benefit from Pleconaril. Up to 1/3rd of adults have neutrophilic pleocytosis in CSF. Reviewed *(J Clin Virology, 104, 56-60, 2018)*.
Hemorrhagic Fever Virus Infections: *Review: LnID 6:203, 2006.*		
Congo-Crimean Hemorrhagic Fever (HF) Tick-borne; symptoms include N/V, fever, headache, myalgias, & stupor (1/3). Signs: *conjunctival* injection, hepatomegaly, petechiae (1/3). Lab: ↓ platelets, ↓ WBC, ↑ ALT, AST, LDH & CPK (100%).	**RBV** 30 mg/kg/day po loading dose, then 15 mg/kg q6h x 4 days, then 7.5 mg/kg q8h x 6 days (WHO recommendation) *(see Comment)*. Reviewed *Antiviral Res 78:125, 2008.*	3/3 healthcare workers in Pakistan had complete recovery *(Ln 346:472, 1995)* & 61/69 (89%) with confirmed CCHF rx with ribavirin survived in Iran *(CID 36:1613, 2003)*. Shorter time of hospitalization among ribavirin treated pts (7.7 vs. 10.3 days), but no difference in mortality or transfusion needs in study done in Turkey *(J Infection 52: 207-215, 2006)*. Suggested benefit from ribavirin & dexamethasone *(281 pts) (CID 57:1270, 2013)*.

[1] HSCT = Hematopoietic stem cell transplant

* *See page 2 for abbreviations.* *NOTE: All dosage recommendations are for adults (unless otherwise indicated) and assume normal renal function.*

TABLE 14A (2)

VIRUS/DISEASE	DRUG/DOSAGE	SIDE EFFECTS/COMMENTS
Hemorrhagic Fever Virus Infections *(continued)*		
Ebola/Marburg HF (Central Africa) Largest ever documented outbreak of Ebola virus (EVD), West Africa, 2014. Diagnostic testing at U.S. CDC. Within a few days of symptom onset, diagnosis is most commonly made by antigen-capture enzyme linked immunosorbent assay (ELISA), IgM antibody ELISA, NAAT or viral culture. Updated in: *http://emergency.cdc.gov/han/han00365.asp* See also: *https://www.cdc.gov/vhf/ebola/outbreaks/index-2018.html* Review: *PLOS Neglect Trop Dis 2017 https://doi.org/10.1371/journal.pntd.0005700*	(PALM [together save lives]) study is a randomized, controlled trial of four investigational agents (ZMapp, remdesivir, Monoclonal antibodies mAb114 and REGN-EB3 are the treatment of choice. Randomized PALM study showed these two Rx's superior to ZMapp and remdesivir for the treatment Ebola virus disease. Rx works better in those with lower viral load *(https://www.niaid.nih.gov/news-events/independent-monitoring-board-recommends-early-termination-ebola-therapeutics-trial-drc)*	**Abrupt onset of symptoms typically 8-10 days after exposure (range 2-21 days).** Nonspecific symptoms, which may include fever, chills, myalgias, and malaise. Fever, anorexia, asthenia / weakness are the most common signs and symptoms. Patients may develop a diffuse erythematous maculopapular rash (days 5-7) (usually involving the face, neck, trunk, and arms) that can desquamate. EVD can **often be confused with** other more common infectious diseases such as malaria, typhoid fever, meningococcemia, and other bacterial infections (e.g., pneumonia). **Gastrointestinal symptoms:** severe watery diarrhea, nausea, vomiting and abdominal pain. **Other:** chest pain, shortness of breath, headache or confusion, may also develop. Patients often have conjunctival injection. Hiccups reported. Seizures may occur, and cerebral edema reported. Bleeding is not universally present but can manifest later in the course as petechiae, ecchymosis/bruising, or oozing from venipuncture sites and mucosal hemorrhage. Frank hemorrhage is less common. Pregnant women may experience spontaneous miscarriages.
With pulmonary syndrome: Hantavirus pulmonary syndrome, "sin nombre virus"	**No benefit from RBV demonstrated** *(CID 39:1307, 2004)*. Early recognition of disease and supportive (usually ICU) care is key to successful outcome.	Acute onset of fever, headache, myalgias, non-productive cough, thrombocytopenia, increased PT and non-cardiogenic pulmonary edema with respiratory insufficiency following exposure to droppings of infected rodents.
With renal syndrome: Lassa, Venezuelan, Korean, HF, Sabia, Argentinian HF, Bolivian HF, Junin, Machupo (>90% occur in China *CID 59:1040, 2014*)	**RBV** 30 mg/kg/day po loading dose, then 15 mg/kg q6h x 4 days, then 7.5 mg/kg x 6 days (WHO recommendation) *(see Comment)*.	Toxicity low, hemolysis reported but recovery when treatment stopped. No significant changes in WBC, platelets, hepatic or renal function. *See CID 36:1254, 2003,* for management of contacts. ARF in Lassa associated with 15-fold higher mortality *(Lancet ID 18, (6): 684-695, 2018)*. Favipiravir effective in Macaques *(https://www.ncbi.nlm.nih.gov/pubmed/29882740)*.
Dengue and dengue hemorrhagic fever (DHF) *www.cdc.gov/ncidod/dvbid/dengue/dengue-hcp.htm* Think dengue in traveler to tropics or subtropics (incubation period usually 4-7 days) with fever, bleeding, thrombocytopenia, or hemoconcentration with shock. Dx by viral isolation or serology; serum to CDC (telephone 787-706-2399).	**No data on antiviral rx.** Fluid replacement with careful hemodynamic monitoring critical. Review of treatment: *Current Treatment Opinion ID 9:185-93, 2017.*	Diagnosis: ELISA detects IgM antibody. Has some cross-reactivity with West Nile Virus infection. Should only be used in pts with symptoms c/w Dengue Fever. Many candidate antiviral drugs in development; non effective yet. Rupatadine shortened symptoms and modestly reduced severity of illness in small clinical trial *(Scientific Reports 8: 3857, 2018)*.
West Nile virus *(JAMA 310:308, 2013)* A flavivirus transmitted by mosquitoes, blood transfusions, transplanted organs & breast-feeding. Birds (>200 species) are main host with humans & horses incidental hosts.	**No proven rx**. Supportive care (See www.cdc.gov/westnile/healthcareproviders). RCT of IVIG of no benefit *(BMC Infect Dis 2014;14:248)*.	Usually nonspecific febrile disease but 1/150 cases develops meningoencephalitis, aseptic meningitis or polio-like paralysis *(NEJM 2017;377:1878)*. Long-term sequelae (neuromuscular weakness & psychiatric) common. Diagnosis: increased IgM antibody in serum & CSF or CSF PCR (contact State Health Dept./CDC). Blood supply now tested in U.S.
Yellow fever	**No data on antiviral rx** **Guidelines for use of preventative vaccine:** *(http://www.cdc.gov/mmwr/preview/mmwrhtml/mm6423a5.htm?s_cid=mm6423a5_w)* Sofosbuvir being evaluated as potential treatment.	Reemergence in Africa & S. Amer. due to urbanization of susceptible population *(https://www.nejm.org/doi/full/10.1056/NEJMp1702172)*. Vaccination Diagnosis: increased IgM antibody safe and effective in HIV patients, especially in those with suppressed VL and higher CD4 counts *(CID 48:659, 2009)*. A purified whole-virus, inactivated, cell-culture-derived vaccine (XRX-001) using the 17D strain proven safe and resulted in neutralizing antibodies after 2 doses in a de-escalation, phase I study. *(N Engl J Med 2011 Apr 7; 364:1326)*
Chikungunya fever: brake bone fever A self-limited arbovirus illness spread by Aedes mosquito. High epidemic potential (Caribbean).	**No antiviral therapy.** Fluids, analgesics, anti-pyretics *(NEJM 371:885, 2014; Ann Rev Med 69: 395, 2018)*.	Clinical presentation: high fever, severe myalgias & headache, morbilliform rash with occ. thrombocytopenia. Rarely hemorrhagic complications. Dx mostly clinical; definitive diagnosis by PCR *(NEJM 372:1231, 2015; JCI 27: 737, 2017)*.

** See page 2 for abbreviations.   NOTE: All dosage recommendations are for adults (unless otherwise indicated) and assume normal renal function.*

TABLE 14A (3)

VIRUS/DISEASE	DRUG/DOSAGE	SIDE EFFECTS/COMMENTS
Hemorrhagic Fever Virus Infections *(continued)*		
SFTSV (Severe fever with thrombocytopenia syndrome virus)	*See Bunyaviridae, page 178*	
Hepatitis Viral Infections	*See Table 14E (Hepatitis A & B), Table 14F (Hepatitis C)*	
Herpesvirus Infections		
Cytomegalovirus (CMV) At risk pts: HIV/AIDS, cancer chemotherapy, post-transplant Solid Organ Treatment Guidelines *(Transplantation 102:900-31, 2018)* Review of anti-CMV drugs *(Curr Opin Organ Transplant 2019, 24:469)*	**Primary prophylaxis** not generally recommended except in certain transplant populations *(see Table 15E)*. Preemptive therapy in pts with ↑ CMV DNA plasma VL & CD4 <100/mm³. If used: **valganciclovir** 900 mg po q12h *(CID 32: 783, 2001)*. Primary prophylaxis may be dc if response to ART with ↑ CD4 >100 for 6 mos.	Risk for developing CMV disease correlates with quantity of CMV DNA in plasma: each $\log_{10}$ ↑ associated with 3.1-fold ↑ in disease *(CID 28:758, 1999)*. Resistance demonstrated in 5% of transplant recipients receiving primary prophylaxis *(J Antimicrob Chemother 65:2628. 2010)*. Brincidofovir not effective against CMV in transplant patients. Letermovir effective as primary preventative therapy.
CMV: Colitis, Esophagitis, Gastritis Symptoms relate to site of disease	*Mild:* **Valganciclovir** 900 mg po bod with food x 14-21 days *Severe:* **Ganciclovir** 5 mg/kg IV q12h x 14-21 days OR **Foscarnet** (60 mg/kg IV q8h or 90 mg/kg q12h) x 14-21 days *Post-treatment suppression:* **Valganciclovir** 900 mg po once daily until CD4 >100 x 6 mos	Diagnosis: Elevated whole blood quantitative PCR & histopathology. Severe bouts of Inflammatory Bowel Disease (IBD) colitis may be complicated by CMV; Rx of CMV in this setting is recommended *(European J Clin Micro & Inf Dis 34:13, 2015)*. Rx of CMV in less severe bouts of IBD colitis is unclear.
CMV: Neurologic disease, Encephalitis Myelitis, polyradiculopathy, peripheral neuropathy Symptoms relate to site of disease	Treat as for colitis, esophagitis, gastritis above	Diagnosis: Elevated whole blood and/or CSF quantitative PCR. NOTE: **Severe or fatal IRIS** has occurred in AIDS pts; suggest delay starting ART for 2 wks after initiation of CMV therapy.
CMV: Pneumonia At risk: 1st 6 months post-transplant & 3 months post-stopping prophylaxis Require evidence of invasive disease. Diagnosis: prefer whole blood quantitative PCR and/or positive lung biopsy histopathology Ref: *Transplantation 96:333, 2013; Am J Transplant 13(Suppl 4):93, 2013*	*Viremic but no/mild symptoms:* **Valganciclovir** 900 mg po bid *(Am J Transplant 7:2106, 2007)*. *Severe in lung transplant or AIDS pts:* **Ganciclovir** 5 mg/kg IV q12h (adjust for renal insufficiency). Treat until clinical resolution & neg blood PCR; min duration: 2 wks *If Ganciclovir-resistant:* **Foscarnet** (60 mg/kg q8h or 90 mg/kg q12h) IV (adjust for renal insufficiency). Try to reduce immunosuppression.	*Post-treatment suppression:* Valganciclovir 900 mg po once daily x 1-3 months if high risk of relapse. Suspect resistant CMV if treatment failure or relapse. Do genotype resistance testing *(CID 56:1018, 2013)*. NOTE: IVIG or CMV specific immunoglobulin did not improve overall or attributable mortality in retrospective study of 421 bone marrow transplant pts *(CID 61:31, 2015)*.
CMV: Retinitis Most common ocular complication of HIV/AIDS. Rare in pts on ART with CD4 >200. If not on ART, wait to start until after 2 wks of CMV therapy. Ref: aidsinfo.nih.gov/guidelines **CMV immune recovery retinitis:** new retinitis after starting ART. Do not stop ART or Valganciclovir. No steroids.	*Not sight-threatening:* **Valganciclovir** 900 mg po bid with food x 14-21 days, then 900 mg po once daily until CD4 >100 x 6 months. Sight-threatening *(see Comment)*: **Valganciclovir** + intravitreal **Ganciclovir** 2 mg (1-4 doses over 7-10 days).	Sight-threatening: <1500 microns from fovea or next to head of optic nerve. If can't use Valganciclovir, Ganciclovir 5 mg/kg IV q12h x 14-21 days, then 5 mg/kg IV once daily. If suspect Ganciclovir resistance: Foscarnet (60 gm/kg q8h or 90 mg/kg q12h) x 14-21 days. Ganciclovir ocular implants no longer available.
CMV in Transplant patients: *See Table 15E for CMV prophylaxis.* CMV disease can manifest as CMV syndrome with or without end-organ disease. **Guidelines for CMV therapy** *(Transplantation 102:900-31, 2018)*. **Ganciclovir** 5 mg/kg IV q12h OR **Valganciclovir** 900 mg po q12h *(Am J Transplant 7:2106, 2007)* are effective treatment options. Treatment duration should be individualized. Continue treatment until (1) CMV PCR or antigenemia has become undetectable, (2) clinical evidence of disease has resolved, and (3) at least 2-3 weeks of treatment *(Am J Transplant 13(Suppl 4):93, 2013; Blood 113:5711, 2009)*. Secondary prophylaxis (**Valganciclovir** 900 mg daily) should be considered for 1-3 month course in patients recently treated with high-dose immunosuppression such as lymphocyte depleting antibodies, those with severe CMV disease, or those with >1 episode of CMV disease. In HSCT recipients, secondary prophylaxis should be considered in similar cases balancing the risk of recurrent infection with drug toxicity. Brincidofovir not effective against CMV in transplant patients.		
CMV in pregnancy: Hyperimmune globulin 200 IU/kg maternal weight as single dose during pregnancy (early), administered IV reduced complications of CMV in infant at one year of life. *(CID 55: 497, 2012)*.		

** See page 2 for abbreviations. NOTE: All dosage recommendations are for adults (unless otherwise indicated) and assume normal renal function.*

TABLE 14A (4)

VIRUS/DISEASE	DRUG/DOSAGE	SIDE EFFECTS/COMMENTS
Herpesvirus Infections *(continued)*		
CMV: Congenital/Neonatal Symptomatic	**Valganciclovir** 16 mg/kg po bid x 6 mos	Better outcome after 6 mos compared to 6 wks with no difference in AEs *(NEJM 372:933, 2015)*. Monitor for neutropenia.
Epstein Barr Virus (EBV) — Mononucleosis	**No treatment.** Corticosteroids for tonsillar obstruction, CNS complications, or threat of splenic rupture.	Potential therapies reviewed *(Cancers 10: 197, 2018)*. **Diff dx of atypical lymphocytes:** EBV, CMV, Hep A, Hep B, Toxo, measles, mumps, drugs, HHV6, HHV7, HIV & others.
EBV, chronic active disease	Bone Marrow Transplant is most commonly used Rx (Allo-HSCT	Newly appreciated disorder: Dx base on > 3 months mononucleosis like symptoms; Elevated EBV genomic DNA in peripheral blood; EBV infection of T-cells or NK cells in tissue or peripheral blood; Exclusion of other causes of chronic disease. Most cases in Asia; more cases now identified world-wide. Review: *Front. Pediatr., 05 February 2019 (https://doi.org/10.3389/fped.2019.00014)*
HHV-6—Cause of roseola (exanthem subitum) & other febrile diseases of childhood *(NEJM 352:768, 2005)*. Fever & rash in transplant pts *(JID 179:311, 1999)*. Reactivation in 47% of 110 U.S. hematopoietic stem cell transplant pts *(CID 40:932, 2005)*. Associated with meningoencephalitis, infectious mono & DRESS syndrome in immunocompetent adults *(NEJM 2018;379:775)*. Diagnosis made by pos. PCR in CSF & compatible clinical syndrome. CSF film array PCR, 15 pos. for HHV-5, only 1 of 15 with compatible clin. illness *(CID 67:1125, 2018)*. RX; **Ganciclovir** is primary regimen.		
HHV-7—Ubiquitous virus (>90% of the population is infected by age 3 yrs). No relationship to human disease. Infects CD4 lymphocytes via CD4 receptor; transmitted via saliva.		
HHV-8—The agent of Kaposi's sarcoma, Castleman's disease, & body cavity lymphoma. Associated with diabetes in sub-Saharan Africa *(JAMA 299:2770, 2008)*.	**No antiviral treatment.** Effective anti-HIV therapy may help.	Localized lesions: radiotherapy, laser surgery or intralesional chemotherapy. Systemic: chemotherapy. Castleman's disease responded to ganciclovir *(Blood 103:1632, 2004)* & valganciclovir *(JID 2006)*.
Herpes simplex virus (HSV Types 1 & 2)		
Bell's palsy H. simplex most implicated etiology. Other etiologic considerations: VZV, HHV-6, Lyme disease.	As soon as possible after onset of palsy: **Valacyclovir** 500 mg bid x first 5 days + **Prednisone** 1 mg/kg po divided bid x 5 days then taper to 5 mg bid over the next 5 days (total of 10 days Prednisone).	Cochrane Review *(2015)(JAMA 2016,316:874)* "compared with oral corticosteroids alone, addition of valacyclovir or famciclovir associated with greater number of recoveries at 3-12 mos".
Encephalitis Review: *Clin ID Reports 19:13, 2017* HSV-1 is most common cause of sporadic encephalitis. Survival & recovery from neurological sequelae are related to mental status at time of initiation of rx. **Early dx and rx imperative**. *N Engl J Med 2018; 379:557.*	**Acyclovir** 10-12.5 mg/kg IV (infuse over 1 hr) q8h x 14-21 days. 20 mg/kg q8h in children <12 yrs. Dose calculation in obese patients uncertain. To lessen risk of nephrotoxicity with larger doses seems reasonable to infuse each dose over more than 1 hour. In morbid obesity, use actual body weight. In morbid obesity, use "adjusted" body weight. Adjusted BW = ideal BW + 0.4 (actual BW- ideal BW).	Mortality rate reduced from >70% to 19% with acyclovir rx. PCR analysis of CSF for HSV-1 DNA is 100% specific & 75–98% sensitive. 8/33 (25%) CSF samples drawn before day 3 were neg. by PCR; neg. PCR assoc. with ↓ protein & <10 WBC per mm^3 in CSF *(CID 36:1335, 2003)*. All were + after 3 days. Relapse after successful rx reported in 7/27 (27%) children. Relapse was associated with a lower total dose of initial acyclovir rx (285 ± 82 mg per kg in relapse group vs. 462 ± 149 mg per kg, p <0.03). *(CID 30:185, 2000; Neuropediatrics 35:371, 2004)*. Series in 106 adults *J Clin Virol 60:112, 2014*
Genital Herpes: *Sexually Transmitted Treatment Guidelines MMWR 64(RR-3):1, 2015; NEJM 2016,375:666.*		
Primary (initial episode)	**Acyclovir** (Zovirax or generic) 400 mg po tid x 7–10 days	↓ by 2 days time to resolution of signs & symptoms, ↓ by 4 days time to healing of lesions, ↓ by 7 days duration of viral shedding. Does not prevent recurrences. For severe cases only: 5 mg per kg IV q8h times 5–7 days.
	Valacyclovir (Valtrex) 1000 mg po bid x 7-10 days	An ester of acyclovir, which is well absorbed, bioavailability 3–5 times greater than acyclovir.
	Famciclovir (Famvir) 250 mg po bid or tid x 7–10 days	Metabolized to penciclovir, which is active component. Side effects and activity similar to acyclovir. **Famciclovir** 250 mg po tid **equal to acyclovir** 200 mg 5 times per day.

* See page 2 for abbreviations. *NOTE: All dosage recommendations are for adults (unless otherwise indicated) and assume normal renal function.*

TABLE 14A (5)

VIRUS/DISEASE	DRUG/DOSAGE	SIDE EFFECTS/COMMENTS
Herpesvirus Infections/Herpes simplex virus (HSV Types 1 & 2)/Genital Herpes *(continued)*		
Episodic recurrences	**Acyclovir** 800 mg po tid **x 2 days** or 400 mg po tid **x 5 days** or **Famciclovir** 1000 mg bid **x 1 day**, 250 mg bid x 2 days or 125 mg po bid x 5 days or **Valacyclovir** 500 mg po bid **x 3 days** or 1 gm po once daily **x 5 days** Valacyclovir more effective overall *(Meta-analysis in J Oral Path Med 46:561, 2017).* For HIV patients, *see Comment*	For episodic recurrences in **HIV patients:** **Acyclovir** 400 mg po tid x 5-10 days or **Famciclovir** 500 mg po bid x 5-10 days or **Valacyclovir** 1 gm po bid x 5-10 days
Chronic daily suppression	Suppressive therapy reduces the frequency of genital herpes recurrences by 70–80% among pts who have frequent recurrences (i.e., >6 recurrences per yr) & many report no symptomatic outbreaks. **Acyclovir** 400 mg po bid , **or Famciclovir** 250 mg po bid, **or Valacyclovir** 1 gm po q24h; pts with <9 recurrences per yr could use 500 mg po q24h and then use **Valacyclovir** 1 gm po q24h if breakthrough at 500 mg. For HIV patients, *see Comment.*	For chronic suppression in HIV patients: (all regimens equally efficacious: *Cochrane Database System Rev 8:CD009036, 2014)* (Often not needed with current era ART) **Acyclovir** 400-800 mg po bid or tid or **Famciclovir** 500 mg po bid or **Valacyclovir** 500 mg po bid
Genital, immunocompetent		
Gingivostomatitis, primary (children)	**Acyclovir** 15 mg/kg po 5x/day x 7 days	Efficacy in randomized double-blind placebo-controlled trial *(BMJ 314:1800, 1997).*
Keratoconjunctivitis and recurrent epithelial keratitis	**Trifluridine** (Viroptic), 1 drop 1% solution q2h (max. 9 drops per day) for max. of 21 days *(see Table 1, page 15)*	In controlled trials, response % > idoxuridine. Suppressive rx with acyclovir (400 mg bid) reduced recurrences of ocular HSV from 32% to 19% *(NEJM 339:300, 1998).*
Mollaret's recurrent "aseptic" meningitis (usually HSV-2) *(Ln 363:1772, 2004)*	No controlled trials of antiviral rx & resolves spontaneously. If therapy is to be given, **Acyclovir** (15–30 mg/kg/day IV) or **Valacyclovir** 1-2 gm po qid should be used.	Pos. PCR for HSV in CSF confirms dx *(EJCMID 23:560, 2004).* In randomized controlled trial, no benefit from valacyclovir suppressive rx *(CID 2012,54:1304).*
Mucocutaneous *(for Genital see page 181)*		
Oral labial, "fever blisters":		
Normal host *See Ann Pharmacotherapy 38:705, 2004; JAC 53:703, 2004*	Start rx with prodrome symptoms (tingling/burning) before lesions show. **Drug** / **Dose** / **Sx Decrease** **Oral: Valacyclovir** — 2 gm po q12h x 1 day — ↓ 1 day **Famciclovir**[2] — 500 mg po bid x 7 days — ↓ 2 days **Acyclovir**[NFDA] — 400 mg po 5 x per day (q4h while awake) x 5 days) — ↓ ½ day **Topical:** **Penciclovir** 1% cream — q2h during day x 4 days — ↓ 1 day **Acyclovir** 5% cream[3] — 6x/day (q3h) x 7 days — ↓ ½ day	Penciclovir *(AAC 46: 2848, 2002).* Oral acyclovir 5% cream *(AAC 46:2238, 2002).* Oral famciclovir *(JID 179:303, 1999).* Topical fluocinonide (0.05% Lidex gel) q8h times 5 days in combination with famciclovir ↓ lesion size and pain when compared to famciclovir alone *(JID 181:1906, 2000).* Acyclovir 5% cream + 1% hydrocortisone (Xerese) superior to acyclovir alone *(AAC 58:1273, 2014).*
Herpes Whitlow	*See Table 1, page 29*	

[2] FDA approved only for HIV pts

[3] Approved for immunocompromised pts

** See page 2 for abbreviations. NOTE: All dosage recommendations are for adults (unless otherwise indicated) and assume normal renal function.*

TABLE 14A (6)

VIRUS/DISEASE	DRUG/DOSAGE	SIDE EFFECTS/COMMENTS
Herpesvirus Infections/Herpes simplex virus (HSV Types 1 & 2)/Mucocutaneous *(continued)*		
Oral labial or genital: Immunocompromised		
(includes pts with AIDS) and critically ill pts in ICU setting/large necrotic ulcers in perineum or face. *(See Comment)* Primary HSV in pregnancy: increased risk of dissemination, including severe hepatitis, Risk greatest in 3rd trimester *(NEJM 370:2211, 2014)*.	**Acyclovir** 5 mg per kg IV (infused over 1 hr) q8h times 7 days (250 mg per M^2) or 400 mg po 5 times per day times 14-21 days *(see Comment if suspect acyclovir-resistant)* **OR** **Famciclovir:** In HIV infected, 500 mg po bid for 7 days for recurrent episodes of genital herpes **OR** **Valacyclovir**[NAI]**:** In HIV-infected, 500 mg po bid for 5–10 days for recurrent episodes of genital herpes or 500 mg po bid for chronic suppressive rx.	**Acyclovir-resistant HSV: IV foscarnet** 90 mg/kg IV q12h x 7 days. Suppressive therapy with famciclovir (500 mg po bid), valacyclovir (500 mg po bid) or acyclovir (400-800 mg po bid) reduces viral shedding and clinical recurrences.
Neonatal herpes. 3 distinct syndromes: **Skin, eye and mouth** (SEM): typically presents 9-11 days of life (range 4-14 days). **Disseminated**: presents with septic appearance, LFT abnormalities 9-11 days of life (range 4-14 days). **Central nervous system** (CNS): presents 16-17 days of life (range 10-21 days)	**Acyclovir** 60mg/kg/d div q 8h. Duration 14 days for SEM, 21 days for disseminated or CNS. For CNS, repeat HSV PCR of CSF before stopping. Continue 7 more days if PCR still positive.	Infants can progress from one syndrome to another. After treatment, suppressive therapy reduces recurrence, improves outcome. Acyclovir 900 mg/m2/day po divided 3 times daily x 6 months. For management of asymptomatic infant born to mother with active lesions see *Pediatrics. 2013 Feb;131(2):e635-4.*
Pregnancy and genital H. simplex	Acyclovir safe even in first trimester. No proof that acyclovir at delivery reduces risk/severity of neonatal Herpes. In contrast, C-section in women with active lesions reduces risk of transmission. Ref. *Obstet Gyn 106:845, 2006.*	
Herpes simiae (Herpes B virus): **Monkey bite** *CID 35:1191, 2002* Decision whether to initiate prophylaxis after exposure based on an algorithm: McGill Criteria. Algorithm and approach to assessment/wound management in this article *(Emerg Infect Dis. 2019 Sep; 25(9): e190045)*	**Postexposure prophylaxis: Valacyclovir** 1 gm po q8h times 14 days or acyclovir 800 mg po 5 times per day times 14 days. **Treatment of disease:** (1) CNS symptoms absent: **Acyclovir** 12.5–15 mg per kg IV q8h or ganciclovir 5 mg per kg IV q12h. (2) CNS symptoms present: **Ganciclovir** 5 mg per kg IV q12h.	Fatal human cases of myelitis and hemorrhagic encephalitis have been reported following bites, scratches, or eye inoculation of saliva from monkeys. Initial sx include fever, headache, myalgias and diffuse adenopathy, incubation period of 2–14 days *(EID 9:246, 2003)*. In vitro ACV and ganciclovir less active than other nucleosides (penciclovir or 5-ethyldeoxyuridine may be more active; clinical data needed) *(AAC 51:2028, 2007)*.
Varicella-Zoster Virus (VZV)		
Varicella: Diagnosis *(JEADV 31:9, 2017)* and treatment *(JEADV 31:20, 2017)*. Immunization: *www.cdc.gov/vaccines/schedules/hcp/imz/child-adolescent* or *Med Lett 2018;60:73.*		
Normal host (chickenpox)		
Child (2–12 years)	**In general, treatment not recommended.** Might use oral **acyclovir** for healthy persons at ↑ risk for moderate to severe varicella, i.e., >12 yrs of age; chronic cutaneous or pulmonary diseases; chronic salicylate rx (↑ risk of Reye syndrome), **Acyclovir** dose: 20 mg/kg po qid x 5 days (start within 24 hrs of rash) or **Valacyclovir** 20 mg/kg tid x 5 days.	Acyclovir slowed development and ↓ number of new lesions and ↓ duration of disease in children: 9 to 7.6 days *(PIDJ 21:739, 2002)*. Oral dose of acyclovir in children should not exceed 80 mg per kg per day or 3200 mg per day.
Adolescents, young adults	Start within 24 hrs of rash: **Valacyclovir** 1000 mg po tid x 7 days or **Famciclovir** 500 mg po tid x 7 days (probably effective, but data lacking)	↓ duration of fever, time to healing, and symptoms.
Pneumonia or chickenpox in 3rd trimester of pregnancy	**Acyclovir** 800 mg po 5 times per day or 10 mg per kg IV q8h times 5 days. Risks and benefits to fetus and mother still unknown. Many experts recommend rx, especially in 3rd trimester. Some would add VZIG (varicella-zoster immune globulin).	Varicella pneumonia associated with 41% mortality in pregnancy Acyclovir ↓ incidence and severity *(JID 185:422, 2002)*. If varicella-susceptible mother exposed and respiratory symptoms develop within 10 days after exposure, start acyclovir

* *See page 2 for abbreviations.* *NOTE: All dosage recommendations are for adults (unless otherwise indicated) and assume normal renal function.*

TABLE 14A (7)

VIRUS/DISEASE	DRUG/DOSAGE	SIDE EFFECTS/COMMENTS
Herpesvirus Infections/Varicella-Zoster Virus (VZV)/Varicella *(continued)*		
Immunocompromised host	**Acyclovir** 10–12 mg per kg (500 mg per M^2) IV (infused over 1 hr) q8h times 7 days	Disseminated 1º varicella infection reported during infliximab rx of rheumatoid arthritis *(J Rheum 31:2517, 2004)*. Continuous infusion of high-dose acyclovir (2 mg per kg per hr) successful in 1 pt with severe hemorrhagic varicella *(NEJM 336:732, 1997)*.
Prevention—Postexposure prophylaxis Varicella deaths still occur in unvaccinated persons *(MMWR 56 (RR-4) 1-40, 2007)*	**CDC Recommendations for Prevention:** Since <5% of cases of varicella but >50% of varicella-related deaths occur in adults >20 yrs of age, the CDC recommends a more aggressive approach in this age group: **1st, varicella-zoster immune globulin** (VZIG) (125 units/10 kg (22 lbs) body weight IM up to a max. of 625 units; minimum dose is 125 units) is recommended for postexposure prophylaxis in susceptible persons at greater risk for complications (immunocompromised such as HIV, malignancies, pregnancy, and steroid therapy) as soon as possible after exposure (<96 hrs). If varicella develops, initiate treatment quickly (<24 hrs of rash) with **Acyclovir** as below. Some would rx presumptively with acyclovir in high-risk pts. **2nd,** susceptible adults should be vaccinated. Check antibody in adults with negative or uncertain history of varicella (10–30% will be AB-neg.) and vaccinate those who are Ab-neg. **3rd,** susceptible children should receive vaccination. Recommended routinely before age 12–18 mos. but OK at any age.	
Herpes zoster (shingles) *(See NEJM 369:255, 2013)*		
Normal host ▪ Effective therapy most evident in pts age >50 yrs. ▪ *(For treatment of post-herpetic neuralgia, see CID 36: 877, 2003; Ln 374:1252, 2009)* ▪ Herpes zoster subunit vaccine (Shingrix) preferred for immunocompetent adults age 50 yrs or older *(NEJM 2016;375:1019)* ▪ Analgesics for acute pain associated with Herpes zoster *(NEJM 369:255, 2013)*	**[NOTE: Trials showing benefit of therapy: only in pts treated within 3 days of onset of rash]** **Valacyclovir** 1000 mg po tid times 7 days (adjust dose for renal failure) *(See Table 17A)* **OR**	Increasing recognition of ↑risk of stroke during 6 mos after episode of Shingles. Oral antivirals during clinical H. zoster infection may have protective effect *(CID 58:1497, 1504, 2014)*. VZV found in wall of cerebral and temporal arteries of pts with giant cell arteritis *(Neurology 84:1948, 2015; JID 51:537, 2015)*.
	Famciclovir 500 mg tid x 7 days. Adjust for renal failure *(see Table 17A)* **OR**	Time to healing more rapid. Reduced incidence of post-herpetic neuralgia (PHN) vs placebo in pts >50 yrs of age. Famciclovir similar to acyclovir in reduction of acute pain and incidence of PHN *(J Micro Immunol Inf 37:75, 2004)*.
	Acyclovir 800 mg po 5 times per day times 7 days Add **Prednisone** in pts over 50 yrs old to decrease discomfort during acute phase of zoster. Does not decrease incidence of post-herpetic neuralgia. Dose: 30 mg po bid days 1–7, 15 mg bid days 8–14 and 7.5 mg bid days 15–21.	A meta-analysis of 4 placebo-controlled trials (691 pts): acyclovir accelerated by approx. 2-fold pain resolution and reduced incidence of post-herpetic neuralgia at 3 & 6 mos *(CID 22:341, 1996)*; med. time to resolution of pain 41 days vs 101 days in those >50 yrs. In post-herpetic neuralgia, controlled trials demonstrated effectiveness of **gabapentin**, the **lidocaine patch** (5%) & **opioid analgesic** in controlling pain *(Drugs 64:937, 2004; J Clin Virol 29:248, 2004)*. **Nortriptyline** & **amitriptyline** are equally effective but nortriptyline is better tolerated *(CID 36:877, 2003)*. Role of antiviral drugs in rx of PHN unproven *(Neurol 64:21, 2005)* but 8 of 15 pt improved with IV acyclovir 10 mg/kg q 8 hrs x 14 days followed by oral valacyclovir 1 gm 3x a day for 1 month *(Arch Neur 63:940, 2006)*. Review: *NEJM 371:1526, 2014; Expert Opin Pharmacotherapy 15:61, 2014*
Immunocompromised host		
Not severe Guidelines: *Clinical Transplantation (June 2019) https://doi.org/10.1111/ctr.13622*	**Acyclovir** 800 mg po 5 times per day times 7 days. (**Options: Famciclovir** 750 mg po q24h or 500 mg bid or 250 mg 3 times per day times 7 days **OR Valacyclovir** 1000 mg po tid times 7 days, though both are not FDA-approved for this indication)	If progression, switch to IV. RA pts on TNF-alpha inhibitors at high risk for VZV. Zoster more severe, but less post-herpetic neuralgia *(JAMA 301:737, 2009)*.
Severe: >1 dermatome, trigeminal nerve or disseminated	**Acyclovir** 10-12.5 mg per kg IV (infusion over 1 hr) q8h times 7 days. In older pts, ↓ to 7.5 mg per kg. If nephrotoxicity and pt improving, ↓ to 5 mg per kg q8h.	A common manifestation of immune reconstitution following HAART in HIV-infected children *(J All Clin Immun 113:742, 2004)*. Rx must be begun within 72 hrs. For Acyclovir-resistant VZV in HIV+ pts previously treated with acyclovir: **Foscarnet** (40 mg per kg IV q8h for 14–26 days).

TABLE 14A (8)

VIRUS/DISEASE	DRUG/DOSAGE	SIDE EFFECTS/COMMENTS
Herpesvirus Infections/Varicella-Zoster Virus (VZV)/Herpes zoster (shingles)/Immunocompromised host *(continued)*		
Progressive Outer Retinal Necrosis (PORN) Reviewed *(Ophthalmology 24(3): 382-392, 2017)*	**Ganciclovir** 5 mg/kg and/or **Foscarnet** 90 mg/kg IV q12h + **Ganciclovir** 2 mg/0.05 mL and/or **Foscarnet** 1.2 mg/0.05 mL intravitreal twice weekly.	Expert consultation with an ophthalmologist. NB: **Ganciclovir** ocular implants no longer manufactured. If HIV pt, optimize ARV therapy.
Human T-cell Leukotrophic Virus-1 (HTLV-1) Causes illness in only 5% of infected persons. Two are associated with HTLV-1: Adult T-cell leukemia/ lymphoma *(NEJM 367:552, 2012)* and HTLV-1-associated myelopathy (HAM), also known as tropical spastic paraparesis (TSP).	No proven therapy. Some nucleoside antiretroviral therapies used with limited success. Mogamulizumab (anti-CCR4) antibody being evaluated for refractory T-cell cutaneous lymphoma (Blood: *https://doi.org/10.1182/blood-2018-02-835991).*	Laboratory diagnosis is by blood and CSF. Anti-HTLV-1 antibodies are detected by ELISA antibody testing; Western Blot is used for confirmation (Focus Diagnostics or Quest Diagnostics). HTLV DNA can be detected by PCR in circulating CD4 cells. One tube multiplex qPCR highly specific / sensitive *(Retrovirology 11(Suppl): P105, 2014).*

TABLE 14A (9)

Influenza A & B and novel influenza viruses. IDSA Influenza Guideline: *CID 68:895, 2019.*
Vaccine info *(http://www.cdc.gov/flu/professionals/acip/index.htm); Med Lett 56:97, 2014; MMWR 63:691, 2014.*

- **Oseltamivir and zanamivir are recommended drugs.** Amantadine and rimantidine should not be used because of widespread resistance.
- Novel H1N1 (referred to as pandemic H1N1, pH1N1, H1N1pdm and formerly swine flu) emerged in 2009 and now is the dominant H1N1 strain worldwide. Old distinction from seasonal H1N1 is still sometimes used but not relevant
- Rapid influenza tests are can be falsely negative in 20-50%. PCR is gold standard test.
- Initiate therapy as close to the onset of symptoms as possible, and certainly within 48 hrs of onset of symptoms. Starting therapy after 48 hours of onset of symptoms is associated with reduced therapeutic benefit. However, starting therapy up to 5 days after onset in patients who are hospitalized is associated with improved survival *(Clin Infect Dis 55:1198, 2012).*
- Empiric therapy should be started for all patients who are hospitalized, have severe or progressive influenza or are at higher risk of complications due to age or underlying medical conditions.
- Look for concomitant bacterial pneumonia.
- Other important influenza viruses causing human disease
  - **H3N2v influenza:** 159 cases of influenza A/H3N2v reported over the summer of 2012. Most of the cases of influenza A/H3N2v occurred in children under the age of 10 with direct contact with pigs. This variant is susceptible to the neuraminidase inhibitors, oseltamivir and zanamivir. *See MMWR 61:619, 2012.*
  - **Avian influenza H5N1:** Re-emerged in Asia in 2003 and human cases detected in 15 countries mostly in Asia as well as Egypt, Nigeria and Djibouti. Circulation associated with massive poultry die off. Imported cases rare – one in Canada. As of January 2014, 648 confirmed cases and 384 deaths (59%). Human infection associated with close contact with poultry; very limited human to human transmission. Mortality associated with high viral load, disseminated virus and high cytokine activity *(Nature Medicine 12:1203-1207 2006).* Sensitive to oseltamivir but oseltamivir resistance has emerged on therapy *(NEJM 353:267-272 2005).* Use oseltamivir and consider IV zanamivir
  - **Avian influenza H7N9:** Emerged in Eastern China in March 2013 and 132 cases documented during Spring 2013 with 44 deaths (33%). Cases appeared again in early winter 2013-2014 and continue to increase. Infection associated with close contact with live bird markets; extremely limited human to human transmission to date. Mortality highest among older persons and those with medical conditions. Oseltamivir active against most but not all strains. No zanamivir resistance documented to date.

Virus/Disease	Susceptible to (Recommended Drug/Dosage):	Resistant to:	Alternatives/Side Effects/Comments
• **A/H1N1 (current seasonal resembles pandemic H1N1)** • Influenza B • Influenza A (A/H3N2, A/H3N2v*, A/H5N1, A/H7N9**)	**Oseltamivir** Adult: Oseltamivir 75 mg po bid x 5 days Pediatric (child age 1-12 years): Infant 2 wks-11 months: 3 mg/kg bid x 5 days ≤15 kg: 30 mg bid x 5 days >15 kg to 23 kg: 45 mg bid x 5 days >23 kg to 40 kg: 60 mg bid x 5 days >40 kg: 75 mg bid x 5 days or **Zanamivir** 2 inhalations (5 mg each) bid x 5 days or **Baloxavir** 40 mg po single dose if >12 years (80 mg if > 80 kg) or **Peramivir** 600 mg IV once daily x 5-10 days For IV Zanamivir, *see Comment* **Laninamivir** (approved in Japan): Age < 10 yrs: 20 mg once daily by inhalation Age > 10 yrs: 40 mg once daily by inhalation	Amantadine and rimantidine (100%) * A/H3N2v strain are susceptible ** A/H7N9 resistant to oseltamivir (rarely)	• **A/H1N1:** Higher dose (150 mg bid) **not** more effective for H1N1 • **Zanamivir** not recommended for children <7 years or those with reactive airway disease • **IV zanamivir** is available under compassionate use IND and clinical trials for hospitalized influenza patients with suspected or known gastric stasis, gastric malabsorption, gastrointestinal bleeding, or for patients suspected or confirmed with oseltamivir-resistant influenza virus infection. For compassionate use, contact GlaxoSmithKline at (+1) 919-315-5215 or email: gskclinicalsupportHD@GSK.com. • **Influenza B:** Baloxavir was more effective than oseltamivir in one trial *(IDWeek 20018 LB)*. One study suggested virologic benefit to higher dose oseltamivir for critically ill patients with influenza B. • **A/H5N1:** Given high mortality, consider obtaining investigational drug. Zanamivir retains activity against most oseltamivir resistant H5N1 • Association between corticosteroid rx & increased mortality *(JID 212:183, 2015).* For now, avoid steroids unless indicated for another reason.

** See page 2 for abbreviations.   NOTE: All dosage recommendations are for adults (unless otherwise indicated) and assume normal renal function.*

TABLE 14A (10)

VIRUS/DISEASE	DRUG/DOSAGE	SIDE EFFECTS/COMMENTS
Measles Increasing reports of measles in unvaccinated children and adults *(NEJM 391:349, 2019)*.		
Children	**Vitamin A:** 50,000 IU (age < 6 mos); 100,000 IU (age 6-11 mos); 200,000 IU (age > 12 mos)	Vitamin A may ↓ severity of measles.
Children & Adults	Post-exposure prophylaxis: Vaccine within 72 hrs of exposure or IVIG within 6 days of exposure (0.5 mL/kg up to wt 30 kg; wt > 30 kg: 400 mg). Need MMR vaccine within 6 mos of IVIG.	↓ severity of illness in adults.
Metapneumovirus (HMPV)		
A paramyxovirus isolated from pts of all ages, with mild bronchiolitis/bronchospasm to pneumonia. Review: *Infect Dis Clin N Amer 2017;31:455.*	**No proven antiviral therapy** (intravenous ribavirin used anecdotally with variable results) Investigational Agents Reviewed *(Clin Vaccine Immunol 22:8 & 858, 2015)*	Human metapneumovirus isolated from 6-21% of children with RTIs *(NEJM 350:443, 2004)*. Dual infection with RSV assoc. with severe bronchiolitis *(JID 191:382, 2005)*. Clinical picture in elderly *(JID 2018;218:868)*. Aerosolized ribavirin not recommended.
Monkeypox (orthopox virus) *(see LnID 4:17, 2004)*		
Outbreak from contact with ill prairie dogs. Source likely imported Gambian giant rats *(CID 58:260, 2014)*	**No proven antiviral therapy. Tecovirimat** (Tpoxx) 600 mg (three 200 mg capsules) twice daily x 14 days (active in monkey models; likely effective in humans. Not an FDA approved indication) Cidofovir is active in vitro & in mouse model.	Incubation period of 12 days, then fever, headache, cough, adenopathy, & a vesicular papular rash that pustulates, umbilicates, & crusts on the head, trunk, & extremities. Transmission in healthcare setting rare.
Norovirus (Norwalk-like virus, or NLV)		
Vast majority of outbreaks of non-bacterial gastroenteritis *(JID 213(Suppl 1):1, 2016)*.	**No antiviral therapy.** Replete volume. Transmission by contaminated food, fecal-oral contact with contaminated surfaces, or fomites.	Sudden onset of nausea, vomiting, and/or watery diarrhea lasting 12-60 hours. Ethanol-based hand rubs effective *(J Hosp Inf 60:144, 2005)*.
Papillomaviruses: Warts		
External Genital Warts Also look for warts in anal canal *(MMWR 64(3):1, 2015)*	**Patient applied:** **Podofilox** (0.5% solution or gel): apply 2x/day x 3 days, 4th day no therapy, repeat cycle 4x; OR **Imiquimod** 5% cream: apply once daily hs 3x/wk for up to 16 wks. **Sinecatechins**: Apply to external genital warts only 3x/day until effect or adverse effect **Provider administered:** Cryotherapy with liquid nitrogen; repeat q1-2 wks; OR **Trichloroacetic acid** (TCA): repeat weekly as needed; OR surgical removal.	**Podofilox:** Inexpensive and safe (pregnancy safety not established). Mild irritation after treatment. **Imiquimod:** Mild to moderate redness & irritation. Topical imiquimod effective for treatment of vulvar intraepithelial neoplasms *(NEJM 358:1465, 2008)*. Safety in pregnancy not established. **Sinecatechins**: Local irritation, redness, pain, and itching **Cryotherapy:** Blistering and skin necrosis common. **Podophyllin resin:** No longer recommended as other less toxic regimens available. **TCA:** Caustic. Can cause severe pain on adjacent normal skin. Neutralize with soap or sodium bicarbonate.
Warts on cervix	Need evaluation for evolving neoplasia	Gynecological consult advised.
Vaginal warts	Cryotherapy with liquid nitrogen or **TCA**	
Urethral warts	Cryotherapy with liquid nitrogen	
Anal warts	Cryotherapy with liquid nitrogen or **TCA** or surgical removal	Advise anoscopy to look for rectal warts.
Skin papillomas	**Topical α-lactalbumin. Oleic acid** (from human milk) applied 1x/day for 3 wks	↓ lesion size & recurrence vs placebo ($p < 0.001$) *(NEJM 350:2663, 2004)*. Further studies warranted.

TABLE 14A (11)

VIRUS/DISEASE	DRUG/DOSAGE	SIDE EFFECTS/COMMENTS
Parvo B19 Virus (Erythrovirus B19). *Review: NEJM 350:586, 2004. Wide range of manifestation.* **Treatment options for common symptomatic infections:**		
Erythema infectiosum	Symptomatic treatment only	Diagnostic tools: IgM and Igb antibody titers. Perhaps better: blood parvovirus PCR. Dose of IVIG not standardized; suggest 400 mg/kg IV of commercial IVIG for 5 or 10 days or 1000 mg/kg IV for 3 days. Most dramatic anemias in pts with pre-existing hemolytic anemia. Bone marrow shows erythrocyte maturation arrest with giant pronormoblasts *(Rev Med Virol 25:224, 2015).*
Arthritis/arthralgia	Nonsteroidal anti-inflammatory drugs (NSAID)	
Transient aplastic crisis	Transfusions and oxygen	
Fetal hydrops	Intrauterine blood transfusion	
Chronic infection with anemia	**IVIG** and transfusion *(CID 56:968, 2013)* For dose, *see Comment*	
Chronic infection without anemia	Perhaps **IVIG**	
Papovavirus/Polyomavirus		
Progressive multifocal leukoencephalopathy (PML) Serious demyelinating disease due to JC virus in immunocompromised pts.	No specific therapy for JC virus. Two general approaches: 1. In HIV pts: HAART. Cidofovir may be effective. 2. Stop or decrease immunosuppressive therapy.	Failure of treatment with interferon alfa-2b, cytarabine and topotecan. Immunosuppressive **Natalizumab** temporarily removed from market due to reported associations with PML. Mixed reports on **cidofovir.** Most likely effective in ART-experienced pts. **Watch for IRIS when starting ARV Rx.**
BK virus induced nephropathy in immunocompromised pts and hemorrhagic cystitis	Decrease immunosuppression if possible. Suggested antiviral therapy based on anecdotal data. If progressive renal dysfunction: 1. **Fluoroquinolone** first; 2. **IVIG** 500 mg/kg IV; 3. **Leflunomide** 100 mg po daily x 3 days, then 10-20 mg po daily; 4. **Cidofovir** only if refractory to all of the above *(see Table 14B for dose).*	Use PCR to monitor viral "load" in urine and/or plasma. Report of cidofovir as potentially effective for BK hemorrhagic cystitis *(CID 49:233, 2009).* Adoptive immunotransfer of BKV specific T-cell being explored to treat hemorrhagic cystitis *(E J Haematology 98:632, 2017).*
Rabies *(see Table 20B, page 257; diagnosis and management: www.cdc.gov/rabies)*		
Rabid dogs account for 50,000 cases per yr worldwide. Most cases in the U.S. are cryptic, 70% assoc. with 2 rare bat species *(EID 9:151, 2003).* An organ donor with early rabies infected 4 recipients (2 kidneys, liver & artery) all died avg. 13 days after transplant *(NEJM 352:1103, 2005).*	**Mortality 100% with only survivors those who receive rabies vaccine before the onset of illness/symptoms** *(CID 36:61, 2003).*	Corticosteroids ↑ mortality rate and ↓ incubation time in mice. Therapies that have failed after symptoms develop include rabies vaccine, rabies immunoglobulin, rabies virus neutralizing antibody, ribavirin, alfa interferon, induced coma & ketamine. For post-exposure prophylaxis, *see Table 20B, page 257.*
Respiratory Syncytial Virus (RSV) Major cause of morbidity in neonates/infants. Diagnosis: airway swab for RSV PCR Review: *Infect Dis Clin N Amer 2017;31:455.*	*All ages:* Hydration, O2 as needed. If wheezing, trial of beta-agonist. *Corticosteroids:* children-no; adults-maybe *Nebulized Ribavirin:* for severe RSV in children, adults *(CID 57:1731, 2013).* *Nebulized Ribavirin + RSV immune globulin:* immunocompromised adults (HSCT) *(CID 56:258, 2013).* Oral ribavirin may be as effective as aerosolized, and much less expensive, in immunocompromized patients *(Transplant ID 20:e12844, 2018).*	In adults, RSV accounted for 10.6% of hospitalizations for pneumonia, 11.4% of AECB, 7.2% for asthma & 5.4% for CHF in pts >65 yrs of age *(NEJM 352:1749, 2005).* RSV caused 11% of clinically important respiratory illnesses in military recruits *(CID 41:311, 2005).*
Prevention of RSV in: (1) Children <24 mos. old with chronic lung disease of prematurity (formerly broncho-pulmonary dysplasia) requiring supplemental O_2 or (2) Premature infants (<32 wks gestation) and <6 mos. old at start of RSV season or (3) Children with selected congenital heart diseases	**Palivizumab** (Synagis) 15 mg per kg IM q month Nov-Apr. *See Pediatrics 126:e16, 2010.*	Expense argues against its use, Guidance from the Academy of Pediatrics recommends use of Palivizumab only in newborn infants born at 29 weeks gestation (or earlier) and in special populations (e.g., those infants with significant heart disease) *(Pediatrics 2014;134:415–420).*

** See page 2 for abbreviations. NOTE: All dosage recommendations are for adults (unless otherwise indicated) and assume normal renal function.*

TABLE 14A (12)

VIRUS/DISEASE	DRUG/DOSAGE	SIDE EFFECTS/COMMENTS
Respiratory Syncytial Virus (RSV) *(continued)*		
Rhinovirus (Colds) *See Infect Dis Clin N Amer 2017;31:455; Chest 2017;152:1021.* Found in 1/2 of children with community-acquired pneumonia; role in pathogenesis unclear *(CID 39:681, 2004).* High rate of rhinovirus identified in children with significant lower resp tract infections *(Ped Inf Dis 28:337, 2009)*	No antiviral rx indicated *(Ped Ann 34:53, 2005).* Symptomatic rx: • **Ipratropium bromide** nasal (2 sprays per nostril tid) • **Clemastine** 1.34 mg 1–2 tab po bid–tid (OTC). • Oral zinc preparations reduce duration of symptoms by ~ 1 day; does not reduce severity of symptoms *(JAMA 311:1440, 2014)* Avoid intranasal zinc products *(see Comment).*	Sx relief: ipratropium nasal spray ↓ rhinorrhea and sneezing vs placebo *(AnIM 125:89, 1996).* Clemastine (an antihistamine) ↓ sneezing, rhinorrhea but associated with dry nose, mouth & throat in 6–19% *(CID 22:656, 1996).* **Echinacea** didn't work *(CID 38:1367, 2004 & 40:807, 2005)* —put it to rest! Public health advisory advising that three over-the-counter cold remedy products containing **zinc** (e.g., Zicam) should not be used because of multiple reports of permanent anosmia *(www.fda.gov/Safety/MedWatch/SafetyInformation/SafetyAlertsforHumanMedicalProducts/ucm166996.htm).*
Rotavirus: Leading recognized cause of diarrhea-related illness among infants and children world-wide and kills ½ million children annually.	**No antiviral rx available;** oral hydration life-saving.	**Two live-attenuated vaccines highly effective (85 and 98%)** and safe in preventing rotavirus diarrhea and hospitalization *(NEJM 354; 1 & 23, 2006).* ACIP recommends either of the two vaccines, RV1 or RV5, for infants *(MMWR 58(RR02): 1, 2009).*
Smallpox *(NEJM 346:1300, 2002)*	Smallpox vaccine (if within 4 days of exposure) + **Tecovirimat** (Tpoxx) 600 mg (three 200 mg capsules) po bid x 14 days OR **cidofovir** (dosage uncertain but likely similar to CMV) 5 mg/kg IV once weekly for 2 weeks followed by once weekly dosing. Must be used with hydration and Probenecid; *contact CDC: 770-488-7100).*	
Contact vaccinia *(JAMA 288:1901, 2002)*	From vaccination: Progressive vaccinia—vaccinia immune globulin may be of benefit. To obtain immune globulin, contact CDC: 770-488-7100. *(CID 39:759, 776 & 819, 2004)*	
West Nile virus: *See page 179*		
Zika Virus: Mosquito (Aedes sp.) transmitted flavivirus CDC updates at: *http://www.cdc.gov/zika/index.html* *NEJM 381:1444, 2019*	No treatment available. Symptomatic support (avoid aspirin, NSAIDs until Dengue ruled out. Most serious manifestation of infection is **congenital birth defect(s)**: microcephaly and fetal demise. Sexual transmission occurs. For preconception counseling and prevention, *see MMWR 65(39):1077, 2016.*	3-7 day incubation. Asymptomatic infection most often; when symptoms occur, usually consists of low grade fever, arthralgias, morbiliform rash, and / or conjunctival redness (non-purulent conjunctivitis). Duration of symptoms ranges from a few days to one week. Rare Guillain-Barré syndrome. Hospitalization very infrequent, fatalities are very rare.

TABLE 14B – ANTIVIRAL DRUGS (NON-HIV)

DRUG NAME(S) GENERIC (TRADE)	DOSAGE/ROUTE IN ADULTS*	COMMENTS/ADVERSE EFFECTS
CMV		
Cidofovir (Vistide)	5 mg per kg IV once weekly for 2 weeks, then once every other week. **Properly timed IV prehydration with normal saline & Probenecid must be used with each cidofovir infusion:** 2 gm po 3 hrs before each dose and further 1 gm doses 2 & 8 hrs after completion of the cidofovir infusion. Renal function (serum creatinine and urine protein) must be monitored prior to each dose *(see pkg insert for details)*. Contraindicated if creatinine >1.5 mg/dL, CrCl ≤55 mL/min or urine protein ≥100 mg/dL.	**Adverse effects: Nephrotoxicity;** dose-dependent proximal tubular injury (Fanconi-like syndrome): proteinuria, glycosuria, bicarbonaturia, phosphaturia, polyuria (nephrogenic diabetic insipidus, ↑ creatinine. Concomitant saline prehydration, probenecid, extended dosing intervals allow use but still highly nephrotoxic. Other major toxicities: neutropenia (give G-CSF as needed); eye: monthly intra-ocular pressure. Dc cidofovir if pressure decreases 50% or uveitis occurs. **Black Box warning.** Renal impairment can occur after ≤2 doses. Contraindicated in pts receiving concomitant nephrotoxic agents. Monitor for ↓ WBC. In animals, carcinogenic, teratogenic, causes ↓ sperm and ↓ fertility. FDA indication only CMV retinitis in HIV pts. **Comment:** Dose must be reduced or discontinued if changes in renal function occur during rx. For ↑ of 0.3-0.4 mg per dL in serum creatinine, cidofovir dose must be ↓ from 5 to 3 mg per kg; discontinue cidofovir if ↑ of 0.5 mg per dL above baseline or 3+ proteinuria develops (for 2+ proteinuria, observe pts carefully and consider discontinuation).
Foscarnet (Foscavir)	Induction: 90 mg per kg IV, over 1.5-2 hours, q12h **OR** 60 mg per kg, over 1 hour, q8h Maintenance: 90 –120 mg per kg IV, over 2 hours, q24h Dosage adjustment with renal dysfunction *(see Table 17A)*.	Use infusion pump to control rate of administration. **Adverse effects: Major toxicity is renal impairment (1/3 of patients).** Can cause infusion-related ionized hypocalcemia: manifests as arrhythmia, tetany, paresthesia, changes in mental status. Slow infusion rate and avoid drugs that lower Ca++, e.g., pentamidine. --↑ creatinine, proteinuria, nephrogenic diabetes insipidus, ↓K+, ↓Ca++, ↓ Mg++. Adequate hydration may ↓ toxicity. Other: headache, mild (100%); fatigue (100%), nausea (80%), fever (25%). CNS: seizures. Hematol: ↓ WBC, ↓ Hgb. Hepatic: liver function tests ↑. Neuropathy. Penile and oral ulcers.
Ganciclovir (Cytovene)	IV: 5 mg per kg q12h times 14 days (induction) 5 mg per kg IV q24h or 6 mg per kg 5 times per wk (maintenance) Dosage adjust. with renal dysfunction *(see Table 17A)*	**Adverse effects: Black Box warnings:** cytopenias, carcinogenicity/teratogenicity & aspermia in animals. Absolute neutrophil count dropped below 500 per mm³ in 15%, thrombocytopenia 21%, anemia 6%. Fever 48%. GI 50%: nausea, vomiting, diarrhea, abdominal pain 19%, rash 10%. Confusion, headache, psychiatric disturbances and seizures. Neutropenia may respond to granulocyte colony stimulating factor (G-CSF or GM-CSF). Severe myelosuppression may be ↑ with coadministration of zidovudine or azathioprine. 32% dc/interrupted rx, principally for neutropenia. Avoid extravasation.
Letermovir (Prevymis)	480 mg po/IV once daily starting between days 0-28 post-transplant & continuing to day 100	**Adverse effects:** N/V, diarrhea, peripheral edema, cough, headache, abdominal pain **Drug interactions:** if concomitant cyclosporine, reduce dose to 240 mg once daily. Avoid if severe hepatic impairment.
Valganciclovir (Valcyte)	450 mg tablets; take with food. Oral solution: 50 mg/mL. Adult does 900 mg. Treatment (induction): 900 mg po q12h with food; Prophylaxis (maintenance): 900 mg po q24h. Dosage adjustment for renal dysfunction *(See Table 17A)*.	A prodrug of ganciclovir with better bioavailability than oral ganciclovir: 60% with food. Preg cat: C (may be teratogenic, contraceptive precaution for females). **Adverse effects:** Similar to ganciclovir. May cause dose limiting neutropenia, anemia, thrombocytopenia. Acute renal failure may occur. Diarrhea (16-41%), nausea (8-30%), vomiting (3-21%). **CMV retinitis** (sight-threatening lesions): 900 mg po q12h + intravitreal Ganciclovir: 900 mg po q12h x 14-21 days, then 900 mg po q24h for maintenance.
Herpesvirus		
Acyclovir (Zovirax or generic)	Doses: *see Table 14A for various indications* 400 mg or 800 mg tab 200 mg cap Suspension 200 mg per 5 mL Ointment or cream 5% IV injection Dosage adjustment for renal dysfunction *(See Table 17A)*.	**po:** Generally well-tolerated with occ. diarrhea, vertigo, arthralgia. Less frequent rash, fatigue, insomnia, fever, menstrual abnormalities, acne, sore throat, muscle cramps, lymphadenopathy. **IV:** Phlebitis, caustic with vesicular lesions with IV infiltration. **IV or po:** Renal (5%): ↑ creatinine, hematuria. With high doses may crystallize in renal tubules → obstructive uropathy (rapid infusion, dehydration, renal insufficiency and ↑ dose ↑ risk). Adequate pre-hydration may prevent such nephrotoxicity. Hepatic: ↑ ALT, AST. Uncommon: neutropenia, rash, diaphoresis, hypotension, headache, nausea. **Neurotoxicity:** hallucination, death delusions, involuntary movements. To avoid, lower dose if renal impairment *(AJM 128:692, 2015)*.

* *See page 2 for abbreviations.* *NOTE: All dosage recommendations are for adults (unless otherwise indicated) and assume normal renal function.*

TABLE 14B (2)

DRUG NAME(S) GENERIC (TRADE)	DOSAGE/ROUTE IN ADULTS*	COMMENTS/ADVERSE EFFECTS
Herpesvirus *(continued)*		
Famciclovir (Famvir)	125 mg, 250 mg, 500 mg tabs Dosage depends on indication: *(see label and Table 14A).*	Metabolized to penciclovir. **Adverse effects:** similar to acyclovir, included headache, nausea, diarrhea, and dizziness but incidence does not differ from placebo. May be taken without regard to meals. Dose should be reduced if CrCl <60 mL per min *(see package insert & Table 14A, page 181 & Table 17A, page 248)*. May be taken with or without food.
Penciclovir (Denavir)	Topical 1% cream	Apply to area of recurrence of herpes labialis with start of sx, then q2h while awake times 4 days. Well tolerated.
Trifluridine (Viroptic)	Topical 1% solution: 1 drop q2h (max. 9 drops/day) until corneal re-epithelialization, then dose is ↓ for 7 more days (one drop q4h for at least 5 drops/day), not to exceed 21 days total rx.	Mild burning (5%), palpebral edema (3%), punctate keratopathy, stromal edema. For HSV keratoconjunctivitis or recurrent epithelial keratitis.
Valacyclovir (Valtrex)	500 mg, 1 gm tabs Dosage depends on indication and renal function *(see label, Table 14A & Table 17A)*	An ester pro-drug of acyclovir that is well-absorbed, bioavailability 3–5 times greater than acyclovir. **Adverse effects** similar to acyclovir. Thrombotic thrombocytopenic purpura/hemolytic uremic syndrome reported in pts with advanced HIV disease and transplant recipients participating in clinical trials at doses of 8 gm per day. Death delusion with high serum levels.
Valganciclovir (Valcyte)	450 mg tablets; take with food. Oral solution: 50 mg/mL. Adult does 900 mg. Treatment (induction): 900 mg po q12h with food; Prophylaxis (maintenance): 900 mg po q24h. Dosage adjustment for renal dysfunction *(See Table 17A).*	A prodrug of ganciclovir with better bioavailability than oral ganciclovir: 60% with food. Preg cat: C (may be teratogenic, contraceptive precaution for females). **Adverse effects:** Similar to ganciclovir. May cause dose limiting neutropenia, anemia, thrombocytopenia. Acute renal failure may occur. Diarrhea (16-41%), nausea (8-30%), vomiting (3-21%). **CMV retinitis** (sight-threatening lesions): 900 mg po q12h + intravitreal Ganciclovir: 900 mg po q12h x 14-21 days, then 900 mg po q24h for maintenance.
Hepatitis B		
Adefovir dipivoxil (Hepsera)	10 mg po q24h (with normal CrCl) 10 mg tab	It is an acyclic nucleotide analog with activity against hepatitis B (HBV) at 0.2-2.5 mM (IC_{50}). *See Table 9* for Cmax & T½. Active against lamivudine-resistant HBV strains and in vitro vs. entecavir- resistant strains. To minimize resistance, use in combination with lamivudine for lamivudine-resistant virus; consider alternative therapy if viral load remains >1,000 copies/mL with treatment. Primarily renal excretion—adjust dose. No food interactions. Generally few side effects, but **Black Box warning** regarding lactic acidosis/hepatic steatosis with nucleoside analogs. At 10 mg per day potential for delayed nephrotoxicity. Monitor renal function, esp. with pts with pre-existing or other risks for renal impairment. Pregnancy Category C. **Hepatitis may exacerbate when treatment discontinued;** Up to 25% of pts developed ALT ↑ 10 times normal within 12 wks; usually responds to re-treatment or self-limited, but hepatic decompensation has occurred. **Do not use adefovir in HIV infected patients.**
Entecavir (Baraclude)	0.5 mg q24h. If refractory or resistant to lamivudine or telbivudine: 1 mg per day Tabs: 0.5 mg & 1 mg. Oral solution: 0.05 mg/mL. Administer on an empty stomach.	A nucleoside analog active against HBV including lamivudine-resistant mutants. Minimal adverse effects reported: headache, fatigue, dizziness, & nausea reported in 22% of pts. Alopecia, anaphylactoid reactions reported. Potential for lactic acidosis and exacerbation of hepB at discontinuation (**Black Box warning**). Do not use as single anti-retroviral agent in HIV co-infected pts; M134 mutation can emerge *(NEJM 356:2614, 2007)*. Adjust dosage in renal impairment *(see Table 17A, page 247)*.
Lamivudine (3TC) (Epivir-HBV)	**HBV** dose: 100 mg po q24h Dosage adjustment with renal dysfunction *(see label)*. Tabs 100 mg and oral solution 5 mg/mL.	**Black Box warnings:** caution, dose is lower than HIV dose, so must exclude co-infection with HIV before using this formulation; lactic acidosis/hepatic steatosis; severe exacerbation of liver disease can occur on dc. YMDD-mutants resistant to lamivudine may emerge on treatment. **Adverse effects:** *See Table 14D.*

* *See page 2 for abbreviations. NOTE: All dosage recommendations are for adults (unless otherwise indicated) and assume normal renal function.*

TABLE 14B (3)

DRUG NAME(S) GENERIC (TRADE)	DOSAGE/ROUTE IN ADULTS*	COMMENTS/ADVERSE EFFECTS
Hepatitis B *(continued)*		
Telbivudine (Tyzeka)	**HBV:** 600 mg orally q24h, without regard to food. Dosage adjustment with renal dysfunction, Ccr <50 mL/min *(see label)*. 600 mg tabs; 100 mg per 5 mL solution.	An oral nucleoside analog approved for Rx of Hep B. It has ↑ rates of response and superior viral suppression than lamivudine *(NEJM 357:2576, 2007)*. **Black Box warnings** regarding lactic acidosis/hepatic steatosis with nucleosides and potential for severe exacerbation of HepB on dc. Generally well-tolerated with ↓ mitochondrial toxicity vs other nucleosides and no dose limiting toxicity observed *(Medical Letter 49:11, 2007)*. Myalgias, myopathy and rhabdomyolysis reported. Peripheral neuropathy. Genotypic resistance rate was 4.4% by one yr, ↑ to 21.5% by 2 yrs of rx of eAg+ pts. Selects for YMDD mutation like lamivudine. Combination with lamivudine was inferior to monotherapy *(Hepatology 45:507, 2007)*.
Tenofovir (TDF/TAF)	*See page 209*	
Hepatitis C - (For all HCV direct acting agents (DAA) a **Black Box warning** exists regarding potential flare of HBV when HCV is cured among those coinfected with HBV and HCV)		
Direct Acting Agents:		
Daclatasvir (Daklinza)	60 mg 1 tab po once daily (dose adjustment when used with CYP 3A4 inhibitors / inducers)	Contraindicated with strong CYP3A inducers, e.g., phenytoin, carbamazepine, Rifampin, St. John's wort. Most common AE: headache and fatigue. Bradycardia when administered in combination with Sofosbuvir and Amiodarone. **Co-administration with Amiodarone not recommended**. If used, cardiac monitoring advised.
Elbasvir + Grazoprevir (Zepatier)	Combination formulation (Elbasvir 50 mg + Grazoprevir 100 mg) 1 tab po once daily	NS5A and NS3-4a PI inhibitors with activity against genotypes 1 and 4. Contraindicated in patients with moderate or severe hepatic impairment (Child-Pugh Class B or C). Also contraindicated with concomitant use of organic ion transporter polypeptide 1B (OATP1B) inhibitors, strong inducers of cytochrome P450 3A (CYP3A), and efavirenz.
Glecaprevir + Pibrentasvir (Mavyret)	Combination formulation (Glecaprevir 100 mg + Pibrentasvir 40 mg) 3 tabs po once daily with food	Contraindicated if severe hepatic impairment (Child-Pugh C). **Do not co-administer with Atazanavir or Rifampin.** Most common AEs: headache and fatigue.
Ledipasvir + Sofosbuvir (Harvoni); **Velpatasvir + Sofosbuvir** (Epclusa); **Voxilaprevir + Velpatasvir + Sofosbuvir** (Vosevi)	Combination formulations: (Ledipasvir 90 mg + Sofosbuvir 400 mg) 1 tab po once daily; (Velpatasvir 100 mg + Sofosbuvir 400 mg) 1 tab po daily; Voxilaprevir 100 mg + Velpatasvir 100 mg + Sofosbuvir 400 mg) 1 tab po once daily with food	NS5A/NS5B inhibitor combination for Genotype 1 HCV. First agent for HCV treatment without Ribavirin or Interferon. No adjustment for mile/moderate renal or hepatic impairment. Most common AEs: fatigue (16%), headache (14%), nausea (7%), diarrhea (3%), insomnia (5%). Antacids and H2 blockers interfere with absorption of ledipasvir. The drug solubility decreases as pH increases. Recommended to separate administration of ledipasvir and antacid Rx by at least 4 hours.
Paritaprevir + Ritonavir + Ombitasvir + Dasabuvir (PrOD) (Viekira Pak); **Paritaprevir + Ritonavir + Ombitasvir** (Technivie)	Ombitasvir 12.5 mg, Paritaprevir 75 mg, and Ritonavir 50 mg co-packaged with tablets of Dasabuvir 250 mg (Viekira Pak); or without Dasabuvir (Technivie)	Do not co-administer with drugs that are highly dependent on CYP3A for clearance; strong inducers of CYP3A and CYP2C8; and strong inhibitors of CYP2C8. Do not use if known hypersensitivity to Ritonavir (e.g., toxic epidermal necrolysis, Stevens-Johnson syndrome). If used with Ribavirin: fatigue, nausea, pruritus, other skin reactions, insomnia and asthenia. When used without Ribavirin: nausea, pruritus and insomnia. **Warning: Hepatic decompensation and hepatic failure, including liver transplantation or fatal outcomes, have been reported mostly in patients with** advanced cirrhosis.
Simeprevir (Olysio)	150 mg 1 cap po once daily with food + both Ribavirin and Interferon	NS3/4A inhibitor. Need to screen patients with HCV genotype 1a for the Q80K polymorphism; if present consider alternative therapy. Contraindicated in pregnancy and in men whose female partners are pregnant (risk category C); concern is combination with ribavirin (risk category X). No dose adjustment required in patients with mild, moderate or severe renal impairment; no dose adjustment for mild hepatic impairment. Most common AEs (in combination with Ribavirin, Interferon): rash, pruritus, nausea. CYP3A inhibitors affect plasma concentration of Simeprevir.
Sofosbuvir (Sovaldi)	400 mg 1 tab po once daily with food + both Pegylated Interferon and Ribavirin. For combination formulation, *see Ledipasvir.*	NS5B inhibitor for Genotypes 1, 2, 3, 4 HCV. Efficacy established in patients awaiting liver transplant and in patients with HIV-1/HCV co-infection. No adjustment needed for mild to moderate renal impairment. No dose adjustment for mild, moderate, or severe hepatic impairment. Most common AEs (in combination with interferon and ribavirin): fatigue, headache, nausea, insomnia, anemia. Rifampin and St. John's wort may alter concentrations of Sofosbuvir.

** See page 2 for abbreviations.*   *NOTE: All dosage recommendations are for adults (unless otherwise indicated) and assume normal renal function.*

TABLE 14B (4)

DRUG NAME(S) GENERIC (TRADE)	DOSAGE/ROUTE IN ADULTS*	COMMENTS/ADVERSE EFFECTS
Hepatitis C *(continued)*		
Other:		
Interferon alfa is available as alfa-2a (Roferon-A), **alfa-2b** (Intron-A)	For HCV combination therapy, usual Roferon-A and Intron-A doses are 3 million international units 3x weekly subQ.	Depending on agent, available in pre-filled syringes, vials of solution, or powder. **Black Box warnings:** can cause/aggravate psychiatric illness, autoimmune disorders, ischemic events, infection. Withdraw therapy if any of these suspected. **Adverse effects: Flu-like syndrome** is common, esp. during 1st wk of rx: fever 98%, fatigue 89%, myalgia 73%, headache 71%. **GI:** anorexia 46%, diarrhea 29%. CNS: dizziness 21%. Hemorrhagic or ischemic stroke. Rash 18%, may progress to Stevens Johnson or exfoliative dermatitis. Alopecia. ↑ TSH, autoimmune thyroid disorders with ↓- or ↑- thyroidism. **Hematol:** ↓ WBC 49%, ↓ Hgb 27%, ↓ platelets 35%. Post-marketing reports of antibody-mediated pure red cell aplasia in patients receiving interferon/ribavirin with erythropoiesis-stimulating agents. Acute reversible hearing loss &/or tinnitus in up to 1/3 *(Ln 343:1134, 1994)*. Optic neuropathy (retinal hemorrhage, cotton wool spots, ↓ in color vision) reported *(AIDS 18:1805, 2004)*. Doses may require adjustment (or dc) based on individual response or adverse events, and can vary by product, indication (eg, HCV or HBV) and mode of use (mono- or combination-rx). (Refer to labels of individual products and to ribavirin if used in combination for details of use.)
PEG interferon alfa-2b (PEG-Intron)	0.5–1.5 mcg/kg subQ q wk	
Pegylated-40k interferon alfa-2a (Pegasys)	180 mcg subQ q wk	
Ribavirin (Rebetol, Copegus)	For use with an interferon for hepatitis C. Available as 200 mg caps and 40 mg/mL oral solution (Rebetol) or 200 mg and 400 mg tabs (Copegus) *(See Comments regarding dosage).*	**Black Box warnings:** ribavirin monotherapy of HCV is ineffective; hemolytic anemia may precipitate cardiac events; teratogenic/ embryocidal (**Preg Category X**). Drug may persist for 6 mos, avoid pregnancy for at least 6 mos after end of rx of women *or their partners.* Only approved for pts with Ccr >50 mL/min. Do not use in pts with severe heart disease or hemoglobinopathies. ARDS reported *(Chest 124:406, 2003)*. **Adverse effects:** hemolytic anemia (may require dose reduction or dc), dental/periodontal disorders, and all adverse effects of concomitant interferon used *(see above)*. Postmarketing: retinal detachment, ↓ hearing, hypersensitivity reactions. See *Table 14A* for specific regimens, but dosing depends on: interferon used, weight, HCV genotype, and is modified (or dc) based on side effects (especially degree of hemolysis, with different criteria in those with/without cardiac disease). **Initial Rebetrol dose with Intron A (interferon alfa-2b) is wt-based:** 400 mg am & 600 mg pm for ≤75 kg, and 600 mg am & 600 mg pm for wt >75 kg, but with Pegintron approved dose is 400 mg am & 400 mg pm with meals. Doses and duration of Copegus with peg-interferon alfa-2a are less in pts with genotype 2 or 3 (800 mg per day divided into 2 doses, for 24 wks) than with genotypes 1 or 4 (1000 mg per day divided into 2 doses for wt <75 kg and 1200 mg per day divided into 2 doses for ≥75 kg for 48 wks); in HIV/HCV co-infected pts, dose is 800 mg per day regardless of genotype. *(See individual labels for details, including initial dosing and criteria for dose modification in those with/without cardiac disease.)*
Influenza A		
Amantadine (Symmetrel) or **Rimantadine** (Flumadine) Influenza B intrinsically resistant and most circulating Influenza A is resistant.	**Amantadine** 100 mg caps, tabs; 50 mg/mL oral solution & syrup. Treatment or prophylaxis: 100 mg bid; or 100 mg daily if age ≥65 y; dose reductions with CrCl starting at ≤50 mL/min. **Rimantadine** 100 mg tabs, 50 mg/5 mL syrup. Treatment or prophylaxis: 100 mg bid, or 100 mg daily in elderly nursing home pts, or severe hepatic disease, or CrCl ≤10 mL/min. For children, rimantadine only approved for prophylaxis.	**Side-effects/toxicity: CNS** (can be mild: nervousness, anxiety, difficulty concentrating, and lightheadedness). Serious: delirium, hallucinations, and seizures—are associated with high plasma drug levels resulting from renal insufficiency, esp. in older pts, those with prior seizure disorders, or psychiatric disorders.

* *See page 2 for abbreviations.* *NOTE: All dosage recommendations are for adults (unless otherwise indicated) and assume normal renal function.*

TABLE 14B (5)

DRUG NAME(S) GENERIC (TRADE)	DOSAGE/ROUTE IN ADULTS*	COMMENTS/ADVERSE EFFECTS
Influenza A and B—For both drugs, initiate within 48 hrs of symptom onset		
Baloxavir marboxil (Xofluza)	For age ≥12 yrs & within 48 hr of symptoms onset. Wt 40-80 kg: 40 mg po x 1 dose Wt ≥80 kg: 80 mg po x 1 dose	FDA indicated for uncomplicated influenza. One trial demonstrated efficacy in high risk patients with similar efficacy against flu A and superior activity against flu B. Active against oseltamivir-resistant influenza. Compared to oseltamivir, faster decrease in viral load in airway and, if Influenza B, faster clinical recovery. **AEs:** diarrhea (3%) headache (1%), nausea (1%) Distinct mechanism of action: inhibits viral endonuclease. Cost: $150 per dose compared to $50 for 5 days of oseltamivir.
Zanamivir (Relenza) For pts ≥ 7 yrs of age (treatment) or ≥5 yrs (prophylaxis)	Powder is inhaled by specially designed inhalation device. Each blister contains 5 mg zanamivir. **Treatment:** oral inhalation of 2 blisters (10 mg) bid for 5 days. **Prophylaxis:** oral inhalation of 2 blisters (10 mg) once daily for 10 days (household outbreak) to 28 days (community outbreak).	Active by inhalation against neuraminidase of both influenza A and B and inhibits release of virus from epithelial cells of respiratory tract. Approx. 4–17% of inhaled dose absorbed into plasma. Excreted by kidney but with low absorption, dose reduction not necessary in renal impairment. Minimal side-effects: <3% cough, sinusitis, diarrhea, nausea and vomiting. **Reports of respiratory adverse events in pts with or without h/o airways disease, should be avoided in pts with underlying respiratory disease.** Allergic reactions and neuropsychiatric events have been reported. **Caution: do not reconstitute zanamivir powder for use in nebulizers or mechanical ventilators** (MedWatch report of death). **Zanamivir for IV** administration is available for compassionate use through an emergency IND application. Contact GSK *(919-315-5215)* for forms, then contact FDA *(301-796-1500 or 301-796-9900).*
Oseltamivir (Tamiflu) For pts ≥1 yr (treatment or prophylaxis)	For adults: **Treatment,** 75 mg po bid for 5 days; 150 mg po bid has been used for morbidly obese patients but this dose is not FDA-approved. **Prophylaxis,** 75 mg po once daily for 10 days to 6 wks. *(See label for pediatric weight-based dosing.)* Adjust doses for CrCl ≤30 mL/min. 30 mg, 45 mg, 75 mg caps; powder for oral suspension.	Well absorbed (80% bioavailable) from GI tract as ethyl ester of active compound GS 4071. T½ 6–10 hrs; excreted unchanged by kidney. Adverse effects include diarrhea, nausea, vomiting, headache. Nausea ↓ with food. Rarely, severe skin reactions (toxic epidermal necrolysis, Stevens-Johnson syndrome, erythema multiforme). **Delirium** & abnormal behavior reported *(CID 48:1003, 2009).* No benefit from higher dose in non- critically ill; not recommended *(CID 57:1511, 2013).*
Peramivir (Rapivab)	600 mg IV single dose (acute uncomplicated influenza)	FDA indication is for single dose use in acute uncomplicated influenza. No approved dose for hospitalized patients but 200-400 mg IV daily for 5 days used in trial. Flu with H275Y oseltamivir resistance has moderate resistance to peramivir.
Pox viruses (Smallpox, Monkeypox)		
Tecovirimat (Tpoxx)	600 mg (three 200 mg caps) po bid x 14 days	Inhibitor of the orthopoxvirus VP37 envelope wrapping protein. **No Clinical Trial data in humans** (approval by FDA for smallpox based on animal treatment studies).
Respiratory Syncytial Virus (RSV) monoclonal antibody		
Palivizumab (Synagis) Used for prevention of RSV infection in high-risk children	15 mg per kg IM q month throughout RSV season Single dose 100 mg vial	A monoclonal antibody directed against the surface F glycoprotein; **AEs:** uncommon, occ. ↑ ALT. Anaphylaxis <1/10⁵ pts; acute hypersensitivity reaction <1/1000. Postmarketing reports: URI, otitis media, fever, ↓ plts, injection site reactions. Preferred over polyclonal immune globulin in high risk infants & children.
Warts Regimens are from drug labels specific for external genital and/or perianal condylomata acuminata only *(see specific labels for indications, regimens, age limits).*		
Interferon alfa-2b (IntronA)	Injection of 1 million international units into base of lesion, thrice weekly on alternate days for up to 3 wks. Maximum 5 lesions per course.	Interferons may cause "flu-like" illness and other systemic effects. 88% had at least one adverse effect. **Black box warning:** alpha interferons may cause or aggravate neuropsychiatric, autoimmune, ischemic or infectious disorders.
Interferon alfa-N3 (Alferon N)	Injection of 0.05 mL into base of each wart, up to 0.5 mL total per session, twice weekly for up to 8 weeks.	Flu-like syndrome and hypersensitivity reactions. Contraindicated with allergy to mouse IgG, egg proteins, or neomycin.
Imiquimod (Aldara)	5% cream. Thin layer applied at bedtime, washing off after 6-10 hr, thrice weekly to maximum of 16 wks; 3.75% cream apply qd.	Erythema, itching & burning, erosions. Flu-like syndrome, increased susceptibility to sunburn (avoid UV).

* *See page 2 for abbreviations.* *NOTE: All dosage recommendations are for adults (unless otherwise indicated) and assume normal renal function.*

TABLE 14B (6)

DRUG NAME(S) GENERIC (TRADE)	DOSAGE/ROUTE IN ADULTS*	COMMENTS/ADVERSE EFFECTS
Warts *continued)*		
Podofilox (Condylox)	0.5% gel or solution twice daily for 3 days, no therapy for 4 days; can use up to 4 such cycles.	Local reactions—pain, burning, inflammation in 50%. Can ulcerate. Limit surface area treated as per label.
Sinecatechins (Veregen)	15% ointment. Apply 0.5 cm strand to each wart three times per day until healing but not more than 16 weeks.	Application site reactions, which may result in ulcerations, phimosis, meatal stenosis, superinfection.

See page 2 for abbreviations. *NOTE: All dosage recommendations are for adults (unless otherwise indicated) and assume normal renal function.*

TABLE 14C – ANTIRETROVIRAL THERAPY (ART) IN TREATMENT-NAÏVE ADULTS (HIV/AIDS)

Overview

- Human immunodeficiency virus (HIV)
- Antiretroviral therapy (ART) in **treatment-naïve adults** *(aidsinfo.nih.gov/guidelines/html/1/adult-and-adolescent-treatment-guidelines/0)*
- Guidelines: *www.aidsinfo.nih.gov; iasusa.org; JAMA 2018; 320:379*

When to Start ART

- **All patients with HIV regardless of CD4 count** *(NEJM 373:795, 2015; NEJM 373:808, 2015)*
- Only exceptions are:
    - Patient is not ready to start (for personal reasons or lack of commitment to take medications)
    - Patient is an "Elite Controller", i.e., HIV RNA undetectable for extended period without ART. Controversy exists about treating such patients, though many experts suggest ART owing to inflammation resulting from ongoing de novo HIV replication.
    - Many clinics are adopting a 'treat now' policy whereby the ARV regimen is started on the first encounter with the clinic. In such instances, resistance tests are obtained and the regimen(s) adjusted as indicated once the resistance test data return.

What Regimen to Start

- Design a regimen consisting of:

Dual nucleoside / nucleotide reverse transcriptase inhibitor **(NRTI component) PLUS** either a	• Non-nucleoside reverse transcriptase inhibitor **(NNRTI) OR** • Protease Inhibitor **(PI) OR** • Integrase strand-transfer inhibitor **(INSTI)**
Note: Prefer combination that includes Tenofovir-AF over original Tenofovir-DF (in selected patients, a combination of Dolutegravir + Lamivudine can be used)	

NRTI: e.g., Tenofovir (TAF or TDF), Abacavir (ABC), Emtricitabine (FTC), or Lamivudine (3TC)
NNRTI: e.g., Efavirenz (EFV), Rilpivirine (RPV), or Etravirine (ETV)
PI: e.g., Darunavir (DRV) or Atazanavir (ATV) [both boosted with either Ritonavir (/r) or Cobicistat (Cobi)]
INSTI: e.g., Bictegravir (BIC), Dolutegravir (DTG), Elvitegravir (ETG), or Raltegravir (RAL)

- Selection of components is influenced by many factors, including:
    - Results of viral resistance testing
    - **Pregnancy:** EFV is now permitted for use in pregnancy; DTG and TAF not recommended yet for pregnant women owing to higher drug levels in fetus and reports of higher than expected neural tube defects in newborn with dolutegravir *(DOI: 10.1056/NEJMc1807653, 2018)*
    - Potential drug interactions or adverse drug effects; special focus on tolerability (even low grade side effects can profoundly affect adherence)
    - Co-morbidities (e.g., lipid effects of PIs, liver or renal disease, cardiovascular disease risk, chemical dependency, psychiatric disease)
    - Convenience of dosing. Co-formulations increase convenience, but sometimes prescribing the two constituents individually is preferred, as when dose-adjustments are needed for renal disease
    - HLA-B5701 testing required prior to using ABC

TABLE 14C (2)

RECOMMENDED AND ALTERNATIVE TREATMENT REGIMENS FOR HIV INFECTED ADULTS				
	Frequency & Formulation	**Drug/Dose**	**Components**	**Comments**
Recommended	Once daily, single tablet	**Biktarvy** 1 tablet once daily	Bictegravir (BIC) + FTC + TAF	
		Triumeq 1 tablet once daily	ABC + 3TC + DTV	Only if HLA-B* 5701 neg (See Warnings)
	Once daily, separate tablets	**Descovy** + **Dolutegravir** 1 tablet each once daily	(FTC + TAF) + DTV	
Alternative	Once daily, single tablet combinations	**Atripla** 1 tablet once daily qhs	TDF + FTC + EFV	
		Complera/Eviplera 1 tablet once daily with food	FTC + TDF + RPV	Avoid when VL >100,000 cells/mL
		Delstrigo 1 tablet once daily	Doravirine (DOR) + 3TC + TDF	
		Dovato 1 tablet once daily	DTG +3TC	Avoid when M184V or M184I resistance mutation present or in patients with HBV co-infection
		Genvoya 1 tablet once daily	EVG + Cobi + FTC + TAF	
		Odefsey 1 tablet once daily	FTC + TAF + RPV	
		Stribild 1 tablet once daily	EVG + Cobi + FTC + TDF	
		Symtuza 1 tablet once daily	DRV + Cobi + FTC + TAF	
Alternative	NNRTI-based, multi-tablet	**Efavirenz** (EFV) 1 tablet once daily + (**Descovy** or **Truvada** or **Epzicom/Kivexa**) 1 tablet once daily	**Descovy**: FTC + TAF; **Truvada**: FTC + TDF; **Epzicom/Kivexa**: ABC + 3TC; **Evotaz**: ATV + Cobi; **/r**: Ritonavir boosted; **Prezcobix**: DRV + Cobi	Epzicom/Kivexa: take qhs. Avoid when VL >100,000 cells/mL. Use only if HLA-B* 5701 neg; see Warnings. Rilpivirine-based regimens should not be used in patients with VL > 100,000 c/mL (except if RPV is used with DTG)
		Rilpivirine (RPV) 1 tablet once daily + (**Descovy** or **Truvada** or **Epzicom/Kivexa**) 1 tablet once daily		
		Doravirine 1 tablet once daily + (**Descovy** or **Truvada** or **Epzicom/Kivexa**) 1 tablet once daily		
	PI-based (boosted), multi-tablet	**Evotaz** 1 tablet once daily + (**Descovy** or **Truvada** or **Epzicom/Kivexa**) 1 tablet once daily		
		Atazanavir/r 1 tablet once daily + (**Descovy** or **Truvada** or **Epzicom/Kivexa**) 1 tablet once daily		
		Prezcobix 1 tablet once daily + (**Descovy** or **Truvada** or **Epzicom/Kivexa**) 1 tablet once daily		
		Darunavir/r 1 tablet once daily + (**Descovy** or **Truvada** or **Epzicom/Kivexa**) 1 tablet once daily		
	INSTI-based, multi-tablet	**Descovy** 1 tablet once daily + **Raltegravir** (RAL) 600 mg 2 tablets once daily		
		Truvada 1 tablet once daily + **RAL** 600 mg 2 tablets once daily		
		Truvada + **Dolutegravir** (DTG) 1 tablet each once daily		
		Epzicom/Kivexa + **DTG** 1 tablet each once daily		
	Dual therapy	**DTG** + (**3TC** or **FTC**) 1 tablet each once daily		
		DTG + **RPV** 1 tablet each once daily		

TABLE 14C (3)

Legend, Warnings and Notes Regarding Regimens

- Legend
    - **NNRTI** = Non-nucleoside reverse transcriptase inhibitor
    - **PI** = Protease inhibitor
    - **INSTI** = Integrase strand-transfer inhibitor
- Warnings
    - Epzicom/Kivexa (ABC/3TC) containing regimens: Use only in patients who are HLA-B5701 negative.
    - Use ABC with caution in those with HIV RNA > 100,000 c/mL at baseline (this does not apply when DTG is the anchor drug of the regimen).
- Notes
    - Co-formulations increase convenience, but sometimes prescribing the components individually is preferred, e.g., when dose adjustments are needed for renal impairment.
    - Rilpivirine (RPV) with 2 nucleosides should be used only in patients with a baseline HIV RNA level < 100,000 c/mL. However, RPV can be used in combination with DTG in those with > 100,000 c/mL.
    - Higher rates of renal dysfunction occur when TDF is combined with boosted PIs; TAF is the preferred drug in this setting. Conversely, TDF does not have nearly as much renal toxicity when paired with non-boosted PI drugs.
    - RAL reformulated as 600 mg tablet. Preferred dose is 2 tablets (1200 mg) once daily.

Other drugs that may be used in selected populations (typically not used as initial therapy)

- FDC DTG/RPV can be used to simplify 3-drug regimen to 2-drugs when initial regimen successful (< 50 c/ml for > 6 months), no baseline pre-Rx resistance mutations, and no virologic failure.
- ETV and RPV are options for some patients who have NNRTI resistance mutations, e.g., K103N, at baseline. Expert consultation is recommended.
- Boosted PIs can be administered once or twice daily.
- Both Ritonavir and Cobicistat are available as PI-boosting agents.
- Non-boosted PIs are no longer recommended.

Pregnancy Considerations

- Timing of initiation of therapy and drug choice must be individualized.
- Viral resistance testing should be performed.
- Long-term effects of agents are unknown.
- Efavirenz is a permitted alternative in pregnancy.
- DTG, BIC, Cobi, and TAF based regimens should NOT be used in pregnancy until further data are available.
- If recommended drugs are not available, remember that certain drugs are contraindicated, e.g., Didanosine plus Stavudine.

Other Special Populations

- Primary (acute) HIV (INSTI preferred).
- Hepatitis B/C co-infection (See Table 14E & 14F) (Should always use a TDF or TAF-based regimen).
- Opportunistic infection (Treat early in course of Rx of OI; use DTG or BIC if possible owing to fewer drug-drug interactions).

TABLE 14C (4)

Selected Characteristics of Antiretroviral Drugs (*CPE = CSF penetration effectiveness: 1-4)

1. **Selected Characteristics of Nucleoside or Nucleotide Reverse Transcriptase Inhibitors (NRTIs)**

All agents have Black Box warning: Risk of lactic acidosis/hepatic steatosis. Also, risk of fat redistribution/accumulation. For combinations, *see warnings for component agents.*

* **CPE (CNS Penetration Effectiveness) value:** 1= Low Penetration; 2 - 3 = Intermediate Penetration; 4 = Highest Penetration into CNS *(AIDS 25:357, 2011)*

Generic/ Trade Name	Pharmaceutical Prep.	Usual Adult Dosage & Food Effect	% Absorbed, po	Serum $T\frac{1}{2}$, hrs	Intracellular $T\frac{1}{2}$, hrs	CPE*	Elimination	Major Adverse Events/Comments *(See Table 14D)*
Abacavir (ABC; Ziagen)	300 mg tabs or 20 mg/mL oral solution	300 mg po bid or 600 mg po q24h. Food OK	83	1.5	20	1	Liver metab., renal excretion of metabolites, 82%	**Hypersensitivity reaction:** fever, rash, N/V, malaise, diarrhea, abdominal pain, respiratory symptoms. (Severe reactions may be ↑ with 600 mg dose.) **Do not rechallenge!** Report to 800-270-0425. **Test HLA-B*5701 before use.** ***See Comment Table 14D.*** Studies raise concerns re ABC/3TC regimens in pts with VL ≥ 100,000 *(www.niaid.nih.gov/news/newsreleases/2008/actg5202bulletin.htm)*. Controversy re increased CV events with use of ABC. Large meta-analysis shows no increased risk *(JAIDS 61, 441, 2012)*
Abacavir (ABC)/lamivudine (Epzicom or Kivexa)	Film coated tabs ABC 600 mg + 3TC 300 mg	1 tab once daily (not recommended)	*(See individual components)*					*(See for individual components)* **Black Box warning**— limited data for VL >100,000 copies/mL. Not recommended as initial therapy because of inferior virologic efficacy.
Abacavir (ABC)/ lamivudine (3TC)/ dolutegravir (DTG) (Triumeq)	Film coated tabs: ABC 600 mg + 3TC 300 mg + DTG 50 mg	1 tab po once daily	*(See individual components)*					
Abacavir (ABC)/ lamivudine (3TC)/ zidovudine (AZT) (Trizivir)	Film-coated tabs: ABC 300 mg + 3TC 150 mg + ZDV 300 mg	1 tab po bid (not recommended for wt <40 kg or CrCl <50 mL/min or impaired hepatic function)	*(See individual components)*					
Didanosine (ddI; Videx or Videx EC)	125, 200, 250, 400 enteric-coated caps; 100, 167, 250 mg powder for oral solution;	≥60 kg Usually 400 mg enteric-coated po q24h 0.5 hr before or 2 hrs after meal. Do not crush. <60 kg: 250 mg EC po q24h. Food ↓ levels. *See Comment*	30–40	1.6	25–40	2	Renal excretion, 50%	**Pancreatitis,** peripheral neuropathy, lactic acidosis & hepatic steatosis (rare but life-threatening, esp. combined with stavudine in pregnancy). Retinal, optic nerve changes. **The combination ddI + TDF is generally avoided, but if used,** reduce dose of ddI-EC from 400 mg to 250 mg EC q24h (or from 250 mg EC to 200 mg EC for adults <60 kg). **Monitor for ↑ toxicity & possible ↓ in efficacy of this combination; may result in ↓ CD4.**
Dolutegravir (DTG)/ Rilpivirine (RPV) (Juluca)	Film-coated tabs: DTG 50 mg + RPV 25 mg	1 tab once daily with meal	*(See individual components)*					Contraindicated if prior hypersensitivity reaction to DTV or RPV; do not co-administer with dofetilide or with drugs that significantly decrease RPV plasma concentrations. Warnings: Severe skin and hypersensitivity reactions (rash) and sometimes liver injury reported with DTV and RPV. **Common AEs:** diarrhea and headache.

TABLE 14C (5)

Generic/ Trade Name	Pharmaceutical Prep.	Usual Adult Dosage & Food Effect	% Absorbed, po	Serum $T\frac{1}{2}$, hrs	Intracellular $T\frac{1}{2}$, hrs	CPE*	Elimination	Major Adverse Events/Comments *(See Table 14D)*
Selected Characteristics of Antiretroviral Drugs (*CPE = CSF penetration effectiveness: 1-4)								
1. **Selected Characteristics of Nucleoside or Nucleotide Reverse Transcriptase Inhibitors (NRTIs)** *(continued)*								
Dolutegravir (DTG)/ Lamivudine (3TC) (Dovato)	Film-coated tabs: DTG 50 mg + 3TC 300 mg	1 tab once daily with or without food	*(See individual components)*					Do not use if baseline M184V or I mutation is present. Contraindicated in those with HIV-HBV co-infection unless other HBV specific agent is also administered.
Emtricitabine (FTC, Emtriva)	200 mg caps; 10 mg per mL oral solution.	200 mg po q24h. Food OK	93 (caps), 75 (oral sol'n)	Approx. 10	39	3	Renal excretion 86%	Well tolerated; headache, nausea, vomiting & diarrhea occasionally, skin rash rarely. Skin hyperpigmentation. Differs only slightly in structure from lamivudine (5-fluoro substitution). **Exacerbation of Hep B reported in pts after stopping FTC.** Monitor at least several months after stopping FTC in Hep B pts; some may need anti-HBV therapy.
Emtricitabine/ tenofovir disoproxil fumarate (Truvada)	Film-coated tabs: FTC 200 mg + TDF 300 mg	1 tab po q24h for CrCl ≥50 mL/min. Food OK	92/25	10/17	—	*(See individual components)*	Primarily renal/renal	*See Comments for individual agents* **Black Box warning—Exacerbation of HepB after stopping FTC;** but preferred therapy for those with Hep B/HIV co-infection.
Emtricitabine/ Tenofovir/Efavirenz (Atripla)	Film-coated tabs: FTC 200 mg + TDF 300 mg + Efavirenz 600 mg	1 tab po q24h on an empty stomach, preferably at bedtime. Do not use if CrCl <50 mL/min	*(See individual components)*					Not recommended for pts <18 yrs. *(See warnings for individual components).* **Exacerbation of Hep B** reported in pts discontinuing component drugs; some need anti-HBV therapy (tenofovir preferred). **Pregnancy category D-** Efavirenz may cause fetal harm. Avoid in pregnancy or in women who may become pregnant.
Emtricitabine/ Tenofovir/ Rilpivirine (Complera/Eviplera)	Film-coated tabs: FTC 200 mg + TDF 300 mg + RPL 25 mg	1 tab po q24h with food	*(See individual components)*					*See individual components.* Preferred use in pts with HIV RNA level <100,000 c/mL. Should not be used with PPI agents.
Lamivudine (3TC; Epivir)	150, 300 mg tabs; 10 mg/mL oral solution	150 mg po bid or 300 mg po q24h. Food OK	86	5–7	18	2	Renal excretion, minimal metabolism	**Use HIV dose, not Hep B dose.** Usually well-tolerated. **Risk of exacerbation of Hep B after stopping 3TC.** Monitor at least several months after stopping 3TC in Hep B pts; some may need anti-HBV therapy.
Lamivudine/ abacavir (Epzicom)	Film-coated tabs: 3TC 300 mg + abacavir 600 mg	1 tab po q24h. Food OK Not recommended for CrCl <50 mL/min or impaired hepatic function	86/86	5–7/1.5	16/20	*(See individual components)*	Primarily renal/ metabolism	*See Comments for individual agents.* **Note abacavir hypersensitivity Black Box warnings** (severe reactions may be somewhat more frequent with 600 mg dose) and 3TC Hep B warnings. Test HLA-B*5701 before use.

TABLE 14C (6)

Generic/ Trade Name	Pharmaceutical Prep.	Usual Adult Dosage & Food Effect	% Absorbed, po	Serum $T_{1/2}$, hrs	Intracellular $T_{1/2}$, hrs	CPE*	Elimination	Major Adverse Events/Comments *(See Table 14D)*
Selected Characteristics of Antiretroviral Drugs (*CPE = CSF penetration effectiveness: 1-4)								
1. **Selected Characteristics of Nucleoside or Nucleotide Reverse Transcriptase Inhibitors (NRTIs)** *(continued)*								
Lamivudine/ zidovudine (Combivir)	Film-coated tabs: 3TC 150 mg + ZDV 300 mg	1 tab po bid. Not recommended for CrCl <50 mL/min or impaired hepatic function Food OK	86/64	5-7/0.5-3	—	*(See individual compo- nents)*	Primarily renal/ metabolism with renal excretion of glucuronide	*See Comments for individual agents* **Black Box warning**—exacerbation of Hep B in pts stopping 3TC
Stavudine (d4T; Zerit)	15, 20, 30, 40 mg capsules; 1 mg per mL oral solution	≥60 kg: 40 mg po bid <60 kg: 30 mg po bid Food OK	86	1.2–1.6	3.5	2	Renal excretion, 40%	Not recommended by DHHS as initial therapy because of adverse reactions. **Highest incidence of lipoatrophy, hyperlipidemia, & lactic acidosis of all NRTIs.** Pancreatitis. Peripheral neuropathy. *(See Didanosine comments.)*
Tenofovir disoproxil fumarate (TDF; Viread)—a nucleotide	300 mg tabs	CrCl ≥50 mL/min: 300 mg po q24h. Food OK; high-fat meal ↑ absorption	39 (with food) 25 (fasted)	17	>60	1	Renal excretion	Headache, N/V. **Cases of renal dysfunction reported:** check renal function before using (dose reductions necessary if CrCl <50 cc/min); avoid concomitant nephrotoxic agents. One study found ↑ renal function at 48-wks in pts receiving TDF with a PI (mostly lopinavir/ritonavir) than with a NNRTI *(JID 197:102, 2008)*. Avoid concomitant ddI. Atazanavir & lopinavir/ritonavir ↑ tenofovir concentrations: monitor for adverse effects. **Black Box warning—exacerbations of Hep B reported after stopping tenofovir.** Monitor liver enzymes if TDF stopped on HBV pts.
Tenofovir alafenamide (TAF)	25 mg (10 mg when used with Cobi or RTV)	CrCl >30 mL/min Food OK; high-fat meal ↑ absorption						
Zidovudine (ZDV, AZT; Retrovir)	100 mg caps, 300 mg tabs; 10 mg per mL IV solution; 10 mg/mL oral syrup	300 mg po q12h. Food OK	64	1.1	11	4	Metabolized to glucuronide & excreted in urine	Bone marrow suppression, GI intolerance, headache, insomnia, malaise, myopathy.
2. **Selected Characteristics of Non-Nucleoside Reverse Transcriptase Inhibitors (NNRTIs)**								
Delavirdine (Rescriptor)	100, 200 mg tabs	400 mg po three times daily. Food OK	85	5.8	3		Cytochrome P450 (3A inhibitor). 51% excreted in urine (<5% unchanged)	Rash severe enough to stop drug in 4.3%. ↑ AST/ALT, headaches. **Use of this agent is not recommended.**
Doravirine (Pifeltro)	100 mg tabs	100 mg po q24h. Food OK.	64	20	ND	ND	Metabolism; 6% excreted in urine unchanged	GI, dizziness, headache, fatigue, abnormal dreams. **Co-administration with strong CYP3A4 inducers is contraindicated.** No issues with acid-suppressing agents. Retains activity against viruses containing many common NNRTI resistance mutations. Also available in combination with TDF and 3TC as Delstrigo.

TABLE 14C (7)

Generic/ Trade Name	Pharmaceutical Prep.	Usual Adult Dosage & Food Effect	% Absorbed, po	Serum T½, hrs	Intracellular T½, hrs	CPE	Elimination	Major Adverse Events/Comments *(See Table 14D)*
Selected Characteristics of Antiretroviral Drugs (*CPE = CSF penetration effectiveness: 1-4)								
2. **Selected Characteristics of Non-Nucleoside Reverse Transcriptase Inhibitors (NNRTIs)** *(continued)*								
Efavirenz (Sustiva) New Guidelines indicate is OK to use in pregnant women (WHO Guidelines) or continue EFV in women identified as pregnant (HHS Guidelines).	50, 100, 200 mg capsules; 600 mg tablet	600 mg po q24h at bedtime, without food. Food may ↑ serum conc., which can lead to ↑ in risk of adverse events.	42	40–55 *See Comment*	3		Cytochrome P450 2B6 (3A mixed inducer/ inhibitor). 14-34% excreted in urine as glucuroni-dated metabolites, 16–61% in feces	Severe rash in 1.7%. High frequency of CNS AEs: somnolence, dreams, confusion, agitation. Serious psychiatric symptoms. Certain CYP2B6 poly-morphisms may predict exceptionally high plasma levels with standard doses *(CID 45:1230, 2007)*. False-pos. cannabinoid screen. Very long tissue T½. **If rx to be discontinued, stop Efavirenz 1–2 wks before stopping companion drugs.** Otherwise, risk of developing Efavirenz resistance, as after 1–2 days only Efavirenz in blood &/or tissue. Some bridge this gap by adding a PI to the NRTI backbone after Efavirenz is discontinued. *(CID 42:401, 2006)*
Etravirine (Intelence)	100 mg tabs 200 mg tabs	200 mg twice daily after a meal. May also be given as 400 mg once daily	Unknown (↓ systemic exposure if taken fasting)	41	2		Metabolized by CYP 3A4 (inducer) & 2C9, 2C19 (inhibitor). Fecal extraction.	For pts with HIV-1 resistant to NNRTIs & others. Active in vitro against most such isolates. Rash common, but rarely can be severe. Potential for multiple drug interactions. Generally, multiple mutations are required for high-level resistance. *See Table 14D, page 209 for specific mutations and effects.* Because of interactions, do not use with boosted atazanavir, boosted tipranavir, unboosted PIs, or other NNRTIs.
Nevirapine (Viramune) Viramune XR	200 mg tabs; 50 mg per 5 mL oral suspension; XR 400 mg tabs	200 mg po q24h x 14 days & then 200 mg po bid *(see comments & **Black Box warning**)* Food OK. **If using Viramune XR, Still need the lead in dosing of 200 mg q24h prior to using 400 mg/d**	>90	25–30	4		Cytochrome P450 (3A4, 2B6) inducer; 80% excreted in urine as glucuronidat-ed metaboli-tes, 10% in feces	**Black Box warning—fatal hepatotoxicity.** Women with CD4 >250 esp. vulnerable, inc. pregnant women. Avoid in this group unless benefits clearly > risks *(www.fda.gov/cderdrug/advisory/nevirapine.htm)*. Intensive monitoring for liver toxicity required. Men with CD4 >400 also at ↑ risk. Severe rash in 7%, **severe or life-threatening skin reactions** in 2%. Do not restart if any suspicion of such reactions. 2 wks dose escalation period may ↓ skin reactions. Because of long T½, consider continuing companion agents for several days if nevirapine is discontinued.

TABLE 14C (8)

Generic/ Trade Name	Pharmaceutical Prep.	Usual Adult Dosage & Food Effect	% Absorbed, po	Serum T½, hrs	Intracellular T½, hrs	CPE	Elimination	Major Adverse Events/Comments *(See Table 14D)*
Selected Characteristics of Antiretroviral Drugs (*CPE = CSF penetration effectiveness: 1-4)								
2. **Selected Characteristics of Non-Nucleoside Reverse Transcriptase Inhibitors (NNRTIs)** *(continued)*								
Rilpivirine (Edurant)	25 mg tabs	25 mg daily with food	absolute bioavailability unknown; 40% lower Cmax in fasted state	50	unknown		Metabolized by Cyp3A4 in liver; 25% excreted unchanged in feces.	QTc prolongation with doses higher than 50 mg per day. Common AEs: depression, insomnia, headache, and rash. Do not co-administer with carbamazepine, phenobarbitol, phenytoin, rifabutin, rifampin, rifapentine, proton pump inhibitors, or multiple doses of dexamethasone. A fixed dose combination of rilpivirine + TDF/FTC (Complera/Eviplera) is approved. **Needs stomach acid for absorption. Do not administer with PPI.**

3. **Selected Characteristics of Protease Inhibitors (PIs)**

All PIs: Glucose metabolism: new diabetes mellitus or deterioration of glucose control; fat redistribution; possible hemophilia bleeding; hypertriglyceridemia or hypercholesterolemia. Exercise caution re: potential drug interactions & contraindications. QTc prolongation has been reported in a few pts taking PIs; some PIs can block HERG channels in vitro *(Lancet 365:682, 2005)*.

Generic/ Trade Name	Pharmaceutical Prep.	Usual Adult Dosage & Food Effect	% Absorbed, po	Serum T½, hrs	CPE*	Elimination	Major Adverse Events/Comments *(See Table 14D)*
Atazanavir (Reyataz)	100, 150, 200, 300 mg capsules	400 mg po q24h with food. Ritonavir-boosted dose (atazanavir 300 mg po q24h + ritonavir 100 mg po q24h), with food, is recommended for ART-experienced pts. Use boosted dose when combined with either Efavirenz 600 mg po q24h or TDF 300 mg po q24h. If used with buffered ddI, take with food 2 hrs pre or 1 hr post ddI.	Good oral bioavailability; food enhances bioavailability & ↓ pharmacokinetic variability. Absorption ↓ by antacids, H_2-blockers, proton pump inhibitors. Avoid unboosted drug with PPIs/H2-blockers. Boosted drug can be used with or >10 hr after H2-blockers or >12 hr after a PPI, if limited doses of the acid agents are used.	Approx. 7	2	Cytochrome P450 (3A4, 1A2 & 2C9 inhibitor) & UGT1A1 inhibitor, 13% excreted in urine (7% unchanged), 79% excreted in feces (20% unchanged)	Lower potential for ↑ lipids. Asymptomatic unconjugated hyperbilirubinemia common; jaundice especially likely in Gilbert's syndrome *(JID 192:1381, 2005)*. Headache, rash, GI symptoms. Prolongation of PR interval (1st degree AV block) reported. Caution in pre-existing conduction system disease. Efavirenz & Tenofovir ↓ atazanavir exposure: use atazanavir/ritonavir regimen; also, atazanavir ↑ tenofovir concentrations—watch for adverse events. In rx-experienced pts taking TDF and needing H2 blockers, atazanavir 400 mg with ritonavir 100 mg can be given; do not use PPIs. Rare reports of renal stones.
Darunavir (Prezista)	400 mg, 600 mg, 800 mg tablets	[600 mg darunavir + 100 mg ritonavir] po bid, with food or **[800 mg darunavir (two 400 mg tabs or one 800 mg tab) + 100 mg ritonavir] po once daily with food (Preferred regimen in ART naïve pts)**	82% absorbed (taken with ritonavir). Food ↑ absorption.	Approx 15 hr (with ritonavir)	3	Metabolized by CYP3A and is a CYP3A inhibitor	Contains sulfa moiety. Rash, nausea, headaches seen. Coadmin of certain drugs cleared by CYP3A is contraindicated *(see label)*. Use with caution in pts with hepatic dysfunction. (FDA warning about occasional hepatic dysfunction early in the course of treatment). Monitor carefully, esp. first several months and with pre-existing liver disease. May cause hormonal contraception failure.

TABLE 14C (9)

Generic/ Trade Name	Pharmaceutical Prep.	Usual Adult Dosage & Food Effect	% Absorbed, po	Serum $T\frac{1}{2}$, hrs	CPE*	Elimination	Major Adverse Events/Comments *(See Table 14D)*
Selected Characteristics of Antiretroviral Drugs (*CPE = CSF penetration effectiveness: 1-4)							
3. **Selected Characteristics of Protease Inhibitors (PIs)** *(continued)*							
Fosamprenavir (Lexiva)	700 mg tablet, 50 mg/mL oral suspension	1400 mg (two 700 mg tabs) po bid **OR** with ritonavir: [1400 mg fosamprenavir (2 tabs) + ritonavir 100 mg or 200 mg] po q24h **OR** [700 mg fosamprenavir (1 tab) + ritonavir 100 mg] po bid	Bioavailability not established. Food OK	7.7 Amprenavir	3	Hydrolyzed to amprenavir, then acts as cytochrome P450 (3A4 substrate, inhibitor, inducer)	Amprenavir prodrug. Contains sulfa moiety. Potential for serious drug interactions *(see label)*. Rash, including Stevens-Johnson syndrome. Once daily regimens: (1) not recommended for PI-experienced pts, (2) additional ritonavir needed if given with Efavirenz *(see label)*. Boosted twice daily regimen is recommended for PI-experienced pts. Potential for PI cross-resistance with darunavir.
Indinavir (Crixivan)	100, 200, 400 mg capsules Store in original container with desiccant	Two 400 mg caps (800 mg) po q8h, without food or with light meal. Can take with enteric-coated Videx. *[If taken with ritonavir (e.g., 800 mg indinavir + 100 mg ritonavir po q12h), no food restrictions]*	65	1.2–2	4	Cytochrome P450 (3A4 inhibitor)	**Maintain hydration. Nephrolithiasis,** nausea, inconsequential ↑ of indirect bilirubin (jaundice in Gilbert syndrome), ↑ AST/ALT, headache, asthenia, blurred vision, metallic taste, hemolysis. ↑ urine WBC (>100/hpf) has been assoc. with nephritis/ medullary calcification, cortical atrophy.
Lopinavir + ritonavir (Kaletra)	(200 mg lopinavir + 50 mg ritonavir), and (100 mg lopinavir + 25 mg ritonavir) tablets. Tabs do not need refrigeration. Oral solution: (80 mg lopinavir + 20 mg ritonavir) per mL. Refrigerate, but can be kept at room temp. (≤77°F) x 2 mos.	(400 mg lopinavir + 100 mg ritonavir)—2 tabs po bid. Higher dose may be needed in non-rx-naïve pts when used with Efavirenz, nevirapine, or unboosted fosamprenavir. [Dose adjustment in concomitant drugs may be necessary*; see Table 22B.*	No food effect with tablets.	5–6	3	Cytochrome P450 (3A4 inhibitor)	Nausea/vomiting/diarrhea (worse when administered with zidovudine), ↑ AST/ ALT, pancreatitis. Oral solution 42% alcohol. Lopinavir + ritonavir can be taken as a single daily dose of 4 tabs (total 800 mg lopinavir + 200 mg ritonavir), except in treatment-experienced pts or those taking concomitant Efavirenz, nevirapine, amprenavir, or nelfinavir. Possible PR and QT prolongation. Use with caution in those with cardiac conduction abnormalities or when used with drugs with similar effects.
Nelfinavir (Viracept)	625, 250 mg tabs; 50 mg/gm oral powder	Two 625 mg tabs (1250 mg) po bid, with food	20–80 Food ↑ exposure & ↓ variability	3.5–5	1	Cytochrome P450 (3A4 inhibitor)	Diarrhea. Coadministration of drugs with life-threatening toxicities & which are cleared by CYP34A is contraindicated. Not recommended in initial regimens because of inferior efficacy; **prior concerns about EMS now resolved. Acceptable choice in pregnant women although it has inferior virologic efficacy than most other ARV anchor drugs**.

TABLE 14C (10)

Generic/ Trade Name	Pharmaceutical Prep.	Usual Adult Dosage & Food Effect	% Absorbed, po	Serum $T\frac{1}{2}$, hrs	CPE	Elimination	Major Adverse Events/Comments *(See Table 14D)*
Selected Characteristics of Antiretroviral Drugs (*CPE = CSF penetration effectiveness: 1-4)							
3. **Selected Characteristics of Protease Inhibitors (PIs).** *(continued)*							
Ritonavir (Norvir)	100 mg capsules; 600 mg per 7.5 mL solution. Refrigerate caps but not solution. Room temperature for 1 mo. is OK.	Full dose not recommended *(see comments)*. **With rare exceptions, used exclusively to enhance pharmacokinetics of other PIs, using lower ritonavir doses.**	Food ↑ absorption	3–5	1	Cytochrome P450. Potent 3A4 & 2 d6 inhibitor	Nausea/vomiting/diarrhea, extremity & circumoral paresthesias, hepatitis, pancreatitis, taste perversion, ↑ CPK & uric acid. **Black Box warning**—potentially fatal drug interactions. Many drug interactions— *see Table 22A–Table 22B.*
Saquinavir (Invirase—hard gel caps or tabs) **+ ritonavir**	Saquinavir 200 mg caps, 500 mg film-coated tabs; ritonavir 100 mg caps	[2 tabs saquinavir (1000 mg) + 1 cap ritonavir (100 mg)] po bid with food	Erratic, 4 (saquinavir alone). Much more reliably absorbed when boosted with ritonavir.	1–2	1	Cytochrome P450 (3A4 inhibitor)	Nausea, diarrhea, headache, ↑ AST/ALT. Avoid rifampin with saquinavir + ritonavir: ↑ hepatitis risk. **Black Box warning**—Invirase to be used only with ritonavir. Possible QT prolongation. Use with caution in those with cardiac conduction abnormalities or when used with drugs with similar effects.
Tipranavir (Aptivus)	250 mg caps. Refrigerate unopened bottles. Use opened bottles within 2 mo. 100 mg/mL solution	[500 mg (two 250 mg caps) + ritonavir 200 mg] po bid with food.	Absorption low, ↑ with high fat meal, ↓ with Al^{+++} & Mg^{++} antacids.	5.5-6	1	Cytochrome 3A4 but with ritonavir, most of drug is eliminated in feces.	Contains sulfa moiety. **Black Box warning—reports of fatal/nonfatal intracranial hemorrhage, hepatitis, fatal hepatic failure.** Use cautiously in liver disease, esp. hepB, hepC; contraindicated in Child-Pugh class B-C. Monitor LFTs. Coadministration of certain drugs contraindicated *(see label)*. **For highly ART-experienced pts or for multiple-PI resistant virus.** Do not use tipranavir and etravirine together owing to 76% reduction in etravirine levels.

4. **Selected Characteristics of Fusion Inhibitors**

Generic/ Trade Name	Pharmaceutical Prep.	Usual Adult Dosage	% Absorbed	Serum $T\frac{1}{2}$, hrs	CPE*	Elimination	Major Adverse Events/Comments *(See Table 14D)*
Enfuvirtide (T20, Fuzeon)	Single-use vials of 90 mg/mL when reconstituted. Vials should be stored at room temperature. Reconstituted vials can be refrigerated for 24 hrs only.	90 mg (1 mL) subcut. bid. Rotate injection sites, avoiding those currently inflamed.	84	3.8	1	Catabolism to its constituent amino acids with subsequent recycling of the amino acids in the body pool. Elimination pathway(s) have not been performed in humans. Does not alter the metabolism of CYP3A4, CYP2 d6, CYP1A2, CYP2C19 or CYP2E1 substrates.	Local reaction site reactions 98%, 4% discontinue; erythema/induration ~80–90%, nodules/cysts ~80%. **Hypersensitivity reactions reported** (fever, rash, chills, N/V, ↓ BP, &/or ↑ AST/ALT)—do not restart if occur. Including background regimens, peripheral neuropathy 8.9%, insomnia 11.3%, ↓ appetite 6.3%, myalgia 5%, lymphadenopathy 2.3%, eosinophilia ~10%. ↑ incidence of bacterial pneumonias.

TABLE 14C (11)

Generic/ Trade Name	Pharmaceutical Prep.	Usual Adult Dosage & Food Effect	% Absorbed	Serum T½, hrs	CPE	Elimination	Major Adverse Events/Comments *(See Table 14D)*
Selected Characteristics of Antiretroviral Drugs (*CPE = CSF penetration effectiveness: 1-4)							
5. **Selected Characteristics of CCR-5 Co-receptor Antagonists**							
Maraviroc (Selzentry)	150 mg, 300 mg film-coated tabs	Without regard to food: - 150 mg bid if concomitant meds include CYP3A inhibitors including PIs (except tipranavir/ritonavir) and delavirdine (with/ without CYP3A inducers) - 300 mg bid without significantly interacting meds including NRTIs, tipranavir/ritonavir, neverapine - 600 mg bid if concomitant meds include CYP3A inducers, including Efavirenz (without strong CYP3A inhibitors)	Est. 33% with 300 mg dosage	14-18	3	CYP3A and P-glycoprotein substrate. Metabolites (via CYP3A) excreted feces > urine	**Black Box Warning-Hepatotoxicity,** may be preceded by rash, ↑ eos or IgE. NB: no hepatoxicity was noted in MVC trials. Black box inserted owing to concern about potential CCR5 class effect. Data lacking in hepatic/renal insufficiency; ↑ concern with either could ↑ risk of ↓BP. Currently for treatment-experienced patients with multi-resistant strains. **Document CCR-5-tropic virus before use, as treatment failures assoc. with appearance of CXCR-4 or mixed-tropic virus.**
6. **Selected Characteristics of Integrase Strand Transfer Inhibitors (INSTI)**							
Raltegravir (Isentress)	600 mg film-coated tabs	600 mg po bid without regard to food	Unknown	~ 9	3	Glucuronidation via UGT1A1, with excretion into feces and urine. (Therefore does NOT require ritonavir boosting)	For naïve patients and treatment experienced pts with multiply-resistant virus. Well-tolerated. Nausea, diarrhea, headache, fever similar to placebo. CK↑ & rhabdomyolysis reported: unclear relationship. Increased depression in those with a history of depression. Low genetic barrier to resistance. Increase in CPK, myositis, rhabdomyolysis have been reported. Rare Stevens Johnson Syndrome. Better oral absorption if chewed *(CID 57:480, 2013)*.
Bictegravir (part of Biktarvy)	50 mg (per Biktarvy tab)	50 mg once daily with or without food	No data	17.3	No data	Mainly metabolized by CYP3A enzymes; also glucuronidated by UGT1A1.	Indicated (as Biktarvy) for treatment naive pts and as replacement for prior or existing therapy. Generally well tolerated. Expect increased serum creatinine by 0.1-0.15 mg/dL due to inhibition of proximal tubular secretion; does not reflect a reduced GFR. **Black box warning: possible acute exacerbation of hep B** in co-infected patients who discontinue Biktarvy.

TABLE 14C (12)

Generic/ Trade Name	Pharmaceutical Prep.	Usual Adult Dosage & Food Effect	% Absorbed	Serum $T^{1}/_{2}$, hrs	CPE	Elimination	Major Adverse Events/Comments *(See Table 14D)*
6. **Selected Characteristics of Strand Transfer Integrase Inhibitors** *(continued)*							
Elvitegravir/ cobicistat (Stribild)	150 mg - 150 mg	150 mg-150 mg once daily with or without food	<10%	12.9 (Cobi), 3.5 (ELV)	Un-known	The majority of **elvitegravir** metabolism is mediated by CYP3A enzymes. Elvitegravir also undergoes glucuronidation via UGT1A1/3 enzymes. **Cobicistat** is metabolized by CYP3A and to a minor extent by CYP2D6	For both treatment naïve patients and treatment experienced pts with multiply-resistant virus. Generally well-tolerated. Use of cobicistat increases serum creatinine by ~ 0.1 mg/dl via inhibition of proximal tubular enzyme; this does not result in reduction in true GFR but will result in erroneous apparent reduction in eGFR by MDRD or Cockcroft Gault calculations. Usual AEs are similar to those observed with ritonavir (cobi) and tenofovir/FTC.
Dolutegravir (Tivicay)	50 mg	50 mg po once daily 50 mg po bid (if INSTI resistance present or if co-admin with EFV, FOS, TIP, or RIF	Unknown	14	4	Glucuronidation via UGT1A1 (therefore does not require ritonavir or cobicistat boosting)	Hypersensitivity (rare); Most common: insomnia (3%) headache (2%), N/V (1%), rash (<1%). Watch for IRIS; Watch for elevated LFTs in those with HCV

Other Considerations in Selection of Therapy

Caution: Initiation of ART may result in immune reconstitution syndrome with significant clinical consequences. *See Table 11B, of Sanford Guide to HIV/AIDS Therapy (AIDS Reader 16:199, 2006).*

1. Resistance testing: Given current rates of resistance, resistance testing is recommended in all patients prior to initiation of therapy, including those with acute infection syndrome (may initiate therapy while waiting for test results and adjusting Rx once results return), at time of change of therapy owing to antiretroviral failure, when suboptimal virologic response is observed, and in pregnant women. **Resistance testing NOT recommended if pt is off ART for >4 weeks or if HIV RNA is <1000 c/mL.** *See Table 6F of Sanford Guide to HIV/AIDS Therapy.*
2. Drug-induced disturbances of glucose & lipid metabolism *(see Table 14D)*
3. Drug-induced lactic acidosis & other FDA "box warnings" *(see Table 14D)*
4. Drug-drug interactions *(see Table 22B)*
5. Risk in pregnancy *(see Table 8)*
6. Use in women & children *(see Table 14C)*
7. Dosing in patients with renal or hepatic dysfunction *(see Table 17A & Table 17B)*

* **CPE (CNS Penetration Effectiveness) value:** 1= Low Penetration; 2 - 3 = Intermediate Penetration; 4 = Highest Penetration into CNS *(AIDS 25:357, 2011)*

TABLE 14D - ANTIRETROVIRAL DRUGS & ADVERSE EFFECTS
(www.aidsinfo.nih.gov)

DRUG NAME(S): GENERIC (TRADE)	MOST COMMON ADVERSE EFFECTS	MOST SIGNIFICANT ADVERSE EFFECTS
Nucleoside Reverse Transcriptase Inhibitors (NRTI) Black Box warning for all nucleoside/nucleotide RTIs: lactic acidosis/hepatic steatosis, potentially fatal. Also carry Warnings that fat redistribution and immune reconstitution syndromes (including autoimmune syndromes with delayed onset) have been observed		
Abacavir (Ziagen)	Headache 7–13%, nausea 7–19%, diarrhea 7%, malaise 7-12%	**Black Box warning-Hypersensitivity reaction (HR)** in 8% with malaise, fever, GI upset, rash, lethargy & respiratory symptoms most commonly reported; myalgia, arthralgia, edema, paresthesia less common. **Discontinue immediately if HR suspected. Rechallenge contraindicated; may be life-threatening.** Severe HR may be more common with once-daily dosing. **HLA-B*5701 allele** predicts ↑ risk of HR in Caucasian pop.; excluding pts with B*5701 markedly ↓'d HR incidence *(NEJM 358:568, 2008; CID 46:1111-1118, 2008)*. DHHS guidelines recommend testing for B*5701 and use of abacavir-containing regimens only if HLA-B*5701 negative; Vigilance essential in all groups. Possible increased risk of MI with use of abacavir had been suggested *(JID 201:318, 2010)*. Other studies found no increased risk of MI *(CID 52: 929, 2011)*. A meta-analysis of randomized trials by FDA also did not show increased risk of MI *(www.fda.gov/drugs/drugsafety/ucm245164.htm)*. Nevertheless, care is advised to optimize potentially modifiable risk factors when abacavir is used.
Didanosine (ddI) (Videx)	Diarrhea 28%, nausea 6%, rash 9%, headache 7%, fever 12%, hyperuricemia 2%	**Pancreatitis 1–9%. Black Box warning—Cases of fatal & nonfatal pancreatitis** have occurred in pts receiving ddI, especially when used in combination with d4T or d4T + hydroxyurea. Fatal lactic acidosis in pregnancy with ddI + d4T. Peripheral neuropathy in 20%, 12% required dose reduction. ↑ toxicity if used with ribavirin. Use with TDF generally avoided (but would require dose reduction of ddI) because of ↑ toxicity and possible ↓ efficacy; may result in ↓ CD4. Rarely, retinal changes or optic neuropathy. Diabetes mellitus and rhabdomyolysis reported in post-marketing surveillance. Possible increased risk of MI under study *(www.fda.gov/CDER; JID 201:318, 2010)*. Non-cirrhotic portal hypertension with ascites, varices, splenomegaly reported in post-marketing surveillance. *See also Clin Infect Dis 49:626, 2009; Amer J Gastroenterol 104:1707, 2009.*
Emtricitabine (FTC) (Emtriva)	Well tolerated. Headache, diarrhea, nausea, rash, skin hyperpigmentation	Potential for lactic acidosis (as with other NRTIs). Also **in Black Box—severe exacerbation of hepatitis B on stopping drug reported—monitor clinical/labs for several months after stopping in pts with hepB.** Anti-HBV rx may be warranted if FTC stopped.
Lamivudine (3TC) (Epivir)	Well tolerated. Headache 35%, nausea 33%, diarrhea 18%, abdominal pain 9%, insomnia 11% (all in combination with ZDV). Pancreatitis more common in pediatrics.	**Black Box warning.** Make sure to use HIV dosage, not Hep B dosage. **Exacerbation of hepatitis B on stopping drug. Patients with hepB who stop lamivudine require close clinical/lab monitoring for several months.** Anti-HBV rx may be warranted if 3TC stopped.
Stavudine (d4T) (Zerit)	Diarrhea, nausea, vomiting, headache	**Peripheral neuropathy** 15–20%. Pancreatitis 1%. Appears to produce lactic acidosis, hepatic steatosis and lipoatrophy/lipodystrophy more commonly than other NRTIs. **Black Box warning—Fatal & nonfatal pancreatitis with d4T + ddI.** Use with TDF generally avoided (but would require dose reduction of ddI) because of ↑ toxicity and possible ↓ efficacy; may result in ↓ CD4. Rarely, retinal changes or optic neuropathy. Diabetes mellitus and rhabdomyolysis reported in post-marketing surveillance. **Fatal lactic acidosis/steatosis in pregnant women receiving d4T + ddI.** Fatal and non-fatal lactic acidosis and severe hepatic steatosis can occur in others receiving d4T. Use with particular caution in patients with risk factors for liver disease, but lactic acidosis can occur even in those without known risk factors. Possible ↑ toxicity if used with ribavirin. Motor weakness in the setting of lactic acidosis mimicking the clinical presentation of Guillain-Barré syndrome (including respiratory failure) (rare).
Zidovudine (ZDV, AZT) (Retrovir)	Nausea 50%, anorexia 20%, vomiting 17%, **headache 62%.** Also reported: asthenia, insomnia, myalgias, nail pigmentation. Macrocytosis expected with all dosage regimens.	**Black Box warning—hematologic toxicity, myopathy. Anemia** (<8 gm, 1%), granulocytopenia (<750, 1.8%). Anemia may respond to epoetin alfa if endogenous serum erythropoietin levels are ≤500 milliUnits/mL. Possible ↑ toxicity if used with ribavirin. Co-administration with Ribavirin not advised. Hepatic decompensation may occur in HIV/HCV co-infected patients receiving zidovudine with interferon alfa ± ribavirin.

TABLE 14D (2)

DRUG NAME(S): GENERIC (TRADE)	MOST COMMON ADVERSE EFFECTS	MOST SIGNIFICANT ADVERSE EFFECTS
Nucleotide Reverse Transcriptase Inhibitor (NtRTI) Black Box warning for all nucleoside/nucleotide RTIs: lactic acidosis/hepatic steatosis, potentially fatal. Also carry Warnings that fat redistribution and immune reconstitution syndromes (including autoimmune syndromes with delayed onset) have been observed *(continued)*		
Tenofovir disoproxil fumarate (TDF) (Viread) ; Tenofovir alafenamide (TAF)	Diarrhea 11%, nausea 8%, vomiting 5%, flatulence 4% (generally well tolerated)	**Black Box Warning—Severe exacerbations of hepatitis B reported in pts who stop tenofovir.** Monitor carefully if drug is stopped; anti-HBV rx may be warranted if TDF stopped. Reports of renal injury from TDF, including Fanconi syndrome *(CID 37:e174, 2003; J AIDS 35:269,204; CID 42:283, 2006)*. Fanconi syndrome and diabetes insipidus reported with TDF + ddI *(AIDS Reader 19:114, 2009)*. Modest decline in renal function appears greater with TDF than with NRTIs (CID 51:296, 2010) or TAF and may be greater in those receiving TDF with a PI instead of an NNRTI *(JID 197:102, 2008; AIDS 26:567, 2012)*. In a VA study that followed >10,000 HIV-infected individuals, TDF exposure was significantly associated with increased risk of proteinuria, a more rapid decline in renal function and chronic kidney disease *(AIDS 26:867, 2012)*. Monitor Ccr, serum phosphate and urinalysis, especially carefully in those with pre-existing renal dysfunction or nephrotoxic medications. TDF, but not TAF, also appears to be associated with increased risk of bone loss. In a substudy of an ACTG comparative treatment trial, those randomized to TDF-FTC experienced greater decreases in spine and hip bone mineral density (BMD) at 96 weeks compared with those treated with ABC-3TC *(JID 203:1791, 2011)*. Consider monitoring BMD in those with history of pathologic fractures, or who have risks for osteoporosis or bone loss.
Non-Nucleoside Reverse Transcriptase Inhibitors (NNRTI). Labels caution that fat redistribution and immune reconstitution can occur with ART.		
Doravirine (Pifeltro)	Nausea (5-7%), diarrhea (3-5%), abdominal pain (1-5%), headache (4-6%), fatigue (4-6%), rash (2%). Dizziness: 9% (37% with Atripla). Sleep disturbances: 12% (26% with Atripla). Better lipid profile than efavirenz- or PI-based regimens.	Co-administration with drugs that are strong CYP3A inducers will significantly decrease Doravirine plasma concentrations. Monitor for IRIS during initiation of therapy.
Efavirenz (Sustiva)	**CNS side effects 52%;** symptoms include dizziness, insomnia, somnolence, impaired concentration, psychiatric sx, & abnormal dreams; symptoms are worse after 1st or 2nd dose & improve over 2–4 weeks; discontinuation rate 2.6%. Rash 26% (vs. 17% in comparators); often improves with oral antihistamines; discontinuation rate 1.7%. Can cause false-positive urine test results for cannabinoid with CEDIA DAU multi-level THC assay. Metabolite can cause false-positive urine screening test for benzodiazepines *(CID 48:1787, 2009)*.	**Caution:** CNS effects may impair driving and other hazardous activities. Serious neuropsychiatric symptoms reported, including severe depression (2.4%) & suicidal ideation (0.7%). Elevation in liver enzymes. Fulminant hepatic failure has been reported *(see FDA label)*. **Teratogenicity reported in primates; pregnancy category D—may cause fetal harm, avoid in pregnant women or those who might become pregnant.** NOTE: No single method of contraception is 100% reliable. Barrier + 2nd method of contraception advised, continued 12 weeks after stopping Efavirenz. Contraindicated with certain drugs metabolized by CYP3A4. Slow metabolism in those homozygous for the CYP-2B6 G516T allele can result in exaggerated toxicity and intolerance. This allele much more common in blacks and women *(CID 42:408, 2006)*. Stevens-Jonson syndrome and erythema multiforme reported in post-marketing surveillance.
Etravirine (Intelence)	Rash 9%, generally mild to moderate and spontaneously resolving; 2% dc clinical trials for rash. More common in women. Nausea 5%.	Severe rash (erythema multiforme, toxic epidermal necrolysis, Stevens-Johnson syndrome) has been reported. Hypersensitivity reactions can occur with rash, constitutional symptoms and organ dysfunction, including hepatic failure *(see FDA label)*. Potential for CYP450-mediated drug interactions. Rhabdomyolysis has been reported in post-marketing surveillance.

TABLE 14D (3)

DRUG NAME(S): GENERIC (TRADE)	MOST COMMON ADVERSE EFFECTS	MOST SIGNIFICANT ADVERSE EFFECTS
Non-Nucleoside Reverse Transcriptase Inhibitors (NNRTI) *(continued)*		
Nevirapine (Viramune)	**Rash 37%:** usually occurs during 1st 6 wks of therapy. Follow recommendations for 14-day lead-in period to ↓ risk of rash *(see Table 14C)*. Women experience 7-fold ↑ in risk of severe rash *(CID 32:124, 2001)*. 50% resolve within 2 wks of dc drug & 80% by 1 month. 6.7% discontinuation rate.	**Black Box warning—Severe life-threatening skin reactions reported:** Stevens-Johnson syndrome, toxic epidermal necrolysis, & hypersensitivity reaction or drug rash with eosinophilia & systemic symptoms (DRESS) *(ArIM 161:2501, 2001)*. For severe rashes, dc drug immediately & do not restart. In a clinical trial, the use of prednisone ↑ the risk of rash. **Black Box warning—Life-threatening hepatotoxicity reported,** 2/3 during the first 12 wks of rx. Overall 1% develops hepatitis. Pts with pre-existing ↑ in ALT or AST &/or history of chronic Hep B or C ↑ susceptible *(Hepatol 35:182, 2002)*. Women with CD4 >250, including pregnant women, at ↑ risk. Avoid in this group unless no other option. Men with CD4 >400 also at ↑ risk. Monitor pts intensively (clinical & LFTs), esp. during the first 12 wks of rx. If clinical hepatotoxicity, severe skin or hypersensitivity reactions occur, dc drug & never rechallenge.
Rilpivirine (Edurant)	Headache (3%), rash (3%; led to discontinuation in 0.1%), insomnia (3%), depressive disorders (4%). Psychiatric disorders led to discontinuation in 1%. Increased liver enzymes observed.	Drugs that induce CYP3A or increase gastric pH may decrease plasma concentration of rilpivirine and co-administration with rilpivirine should be avoided. Among these are certain anticonvulsants, rifamycins, PPIs, dexamethasone and St. John's wort. At supra-therapeutic doses, rilpivirine can increase QTc interval; use with caution with other drugs known to increase QTc. May cause depressive disorder, including suicide attempts or suicidal ideation. Overall, appears to cause fewer neuropsychiatric side effects than Efavirenz *(JAIDS 60:33, 2012)*.
Protease inhibitors (PI)		
Diarrhea is common AE (**crofelemer** 125 mg bid may help, but expensive). Abnormalities in glucose metabolism, dyslipidemias, fat redistribution syndromes are potential problems. Pts taking PI may be at increased risk for developing osteopenia/osteoporosis. Spontaneous bleeding episodes have been reported in HIV+ pts with hemophilia being treated with PI. Rheumatoid complications have been reported *(An Rheum Dis 61:82, 2002)*. Potential for QTc prolongation *(Lancet 365:682, 2005)*. **Caution for all PIs**—Coadministration with drugs dependent on CYP3A or other enzymes for elimination & for which ↑ levels can cause serious toxicity may be contraindicated. ART may result in immune reconstitution syndromes, which may include early or late presentations of autoimmune syndromes. Increased premature births among women receiving ritonavir-boosted PIs as compared with those receiving other antiretroviral therapy, even after accounting for other potential risk factors *(CID 54: 1348, 2012)*.		
Atazanavir (Reyataz)	Asymptomatic unconjugated hyperbilirubinemia in up to 60% of pts, jaundice in 7–9% [especially with Gilbert syndrome *(JID 192: 1381, 2005)*]. Moderate to severe events: Diarrhea 1–3%, nausea 6–14%, abdominal pain 4%, headache 6%, rash 20%.	Prolongation of PR interval (1st degree AV block in 5-6%) reported; rarely 2° AV block. QTc increase and torsades reported *(CID 44:e67, 2007)*. Acute interstitial nephritis *(Am J Kid Dis 44:E81, 2004)* and urolithiasis (atazanavir stones) reported *(AIDS 20:2131, 2006; NEJM 355:2158, 2006)*. Potential ↑ transanimases in pts co-infected with HBV or HCV. Severe skin eruptions (Stevens-Johnson syndrome, erythema multiforme, and toxic eruptions, or DRESS syndrome) have been reported.
Darunavir (Prezista)	With background regimens, headache 15%, nausea 18%, diarrhea 20%, ↑ amylase 17%. Rash in 10% of treated; 0.5% discontinuation.	Hepatitis in 0.5%, some with fatal outcome. Use caution in pts with HBV or HCV co-infections or other hepatic dysfunction. Monitor for clinical symptoms and LFTs. Stevens-Johnson syndrome, toxic epidermal necrolysis, erythema multiforme. Contains sulfa moiety. Potential for major drug interactions. May cause failure of hormonal contraceptives.
Fosamprenavir (Lexiva)	Skin rash ~ 20% (moderate or worse in 3–8%), nausea, headache, diarrhea.	Rarely Stevens-Johnson syndrome, hemolytic anemia. Pro-drug of amprenavir. Contains sulfa moiety. Angioedema and nephrolithiasis reported in post-marketing experience. Potential increased risk of MI *(see FDA label)*. Angioedema, oral paresthesias, myocardial infarction and nephrolithiasis reported in post-marketing experience. Elevated LFTs seen with higher than recommended doses; increased risk in those with pre-existing liver abnormalities. Acute hemolytic anemia reported with amprenavir.
Indinavir (Crixivan)	↑ in indirect bilirubin 10–15% (≥2.5 mg/dl, with overt jaundice especially likely in those with Gilbert syndrome *(JID 192: 1381, 2005)*. Nausea 12%, vomiting 4%, diarrhea 5%. Metallic taste. Paronychia and ingrown toenails reported *(CID 32:140, 2001)*.	**Kidney stones.** Due to indinavir crystals in collecting system. Nephrolithiasis in 12% of adults, higher in pediatrics. Minimize risk with good hydration (at least 48 oz. water/day) *(AAC 42:332, 1998)*. Tubulointerstitial nephritis/renal cortical atrophy reported in association with asymptomatic ↑ urine WBC. Severe hepatitis reported in 3 cases *(Ln 349:924, 1997)*. Hemolytic anemia reported.

TABLE 14D (4)

DRUG NAME(S): GENERIC (TRADE)	MOST COMMON ADVERSE EFFECTS	MOST SIGNIFICANT ADVERSE EFFECTS
Protease inhibitors (PI) *(continued)*		
Lopinavir/Ritonavir (Kaletra)	GI: **diarrhea** 14–24%, nausea 2–16%. More diarrhea with q24h dosing.	Lipid abnormalities in up to 20–40%. Possible increased risk of MI with cumulative exposure *(JID 201:318, 2010)*. ↑ PR interval, 2º or 3º heart block described. Post-marketing reports of ↑ QTc and torsades: avoid use in congenital QTc prolongation or in other circumstances that prolong QTc or increase susceptibility to torsades. Hepatitis, with hepatic decompensation; caution especially in those with pre-existing liver disease. Pancreatitis. Inflammatory edema of legs *(AIDS 16:673, 2002)*. Stevens-Johnson syndrome & erythema multiforme reported. Note high drug concentration in oral solution. Toxic potential of oral solution (contains ethanol and propylene glycol) in neonates.
Nelfinavir (Viracept)	Mild to moderate **diarrhea** 20%. Oat bran tabs, calcium, or oral anti-diarrheal agents (e.g., loperamide, diphenoxylate/atropine sulfate) can be used to manage diarrhea.	Potential for drug interactions. Powder contains phenylalanine.
Ritonavir (Norvir) (Currently, primary use is to enhance levels of other anti-retrovirals, because of ↑ toxicity/ interactions with full-dose ritonavir)	GI: bitter aftertaste ↓ by taking with chocolate milk, Ensure, or Advera; nausea 23%, ↓ by initial dose esc (titration) regimen; vomiting 13%; diarrhea 15%. Circumoral paresthesias 5–6%. Dose >100 mg bid assoc. with ↑ GI side effects & ↑ in lipid abnormalities.	**Black Box** warning relates to many important drug-drug interactions—inhibits P450 CYP3A & CYP2 D6 system—may be life-threatening *(see Table 22A)*. Several cases of iatrogenic Cushing's syndrome reported with concomitant use of ritonavir and corticosteroids, including dosing of the latter by inhalation, epidural injection or a single IM injection. Rarely Stevens-Johnson syndrome, toxic epidermal necrolysis anaphylaxis. Primary A-V block (and higher) and pancreatitis have been reported. Hepatic reactions, including fatalities. Monitor LFTs carefully during therapy, especially in those with pre-existing liver disease, including HBV and HCV.
Saquinavir (Invirase: hard cap, tablet)	**Diarrhea,** abdominal discomfort, nausea, headache	**Warning—Use Invirase only with ritonavir.** Avoid garlic capsules (may reduce SQV levels) and use cautiously with proton-pump inhibitors (increased SQV levels significant. Use of saquinavir/ritonavir can prolong QTc interval or may rarely cause 2º or 3º heart block; torsades reported. Contraindicated in patients with prolonged QTc or those taking drugs or who have other conditions (e.g., low K+ or Mg++) that pose a risk with prolonged QTc *(http://www.fda.gov/drugs/DrugSafety/ucm230096.htm, accessed May 25, 2011)*. Contraindicated in patients with complete AV block, or those at risk, who do not have pacemaker. Hepatic toxicity encountered in patients with pre-existing liver disease or in individuals receiving concomitant rifampin. Rarely, Stevens Johnson syndrome.
Tipranavir (Aptivus)	Nausea & vomiting, diarrhea, abdominal pain. Rash in 8-14%, more common in women, & 33% in women taking ethinyl estradiol. Major lipid effects.	**Black Box Warning—associated with hepatitis & fatal hepatic failure.** Risk of hepatotoxicity increased in hepB or hepC co-infection. Possible photosensitivity skin reactions. Contraindicated in Child-Pugh Class B or C hepatic impairment. **Associated with fatal/nonfatal intracranial hemorrhage (can inhibit platelet aggregation).** Caution in those with bleeding risks. Potential for major drug interactions. Contains sulfa moiety and vitamin E.
Fusion Inhibitor		
Enfuvirtide (T20, Fuzeon)	Local injection site reactions (98% at least 1 local ISR, 4% dc because of ISR) (pain & discomfort, induration, erythema, nodules & cysts, pruritus, & ecchymosis). Diarrhea 32%, nausea 23%, fatigue 20%.	↑ Rate of bacterial pneumonia (3.2 pneumonia events/100 pt yrs), **hypersensitivity reactions** ≤1% (rash, fever, nausea & vomiting, chills, rigors, hypotension, & ↑ serum liver transaminases); can occur with reexposure. Cutaneous amyloid deposits containing enfuvirtide peptide reported in skin plaques persisting after discontinuation of drug *(J Cutan Pathol 39:220, 2012)*.
CCR5 Co-receptor Antagonists		
Maraviroc (Selzentry)	With ARV background: Cough 13%, fever 12%, rash 10%, abdominal pain 8%. Also, dizziness, myalgia, arthralgias. ↑ Risk of URI, HSV infection.	**Black box warning-Hepatotoxicity.** May be preceded by allergic features (rash, ↑eosinophils or ↑IgE levels). Use with caution in pt with HepB or C. Cardiac ischemia/infarction in 1.3%. May cause ↓BP, orthostatic syncope, especially in patients with renal dysfunction. Significant interactions with CYP3A inducers/inhibitors. Long-term risk of malignancy unknown. Stevens-Johnson syndrome reported post-marketing. Generally favorable safety profile during trial of ART-naïve individuals *(JID 201: 803, 2010)*.

TABLE 14D (5)

DRUG NAME(S): GENERIC (TRADE)	MOST COMMON ADVERSE EFFECTS	MOST SIGNIFICANT ADVERSE EFFECTS
Integrase Inhibitors		
Bictegravir (part of Biktarvy)	Reported in at least 5% of patients: nausea, diarrhea, headache. May increase serum creatinine 0.1-0.15 mg/dL due to inhibition of proximal tubular secretion of creatinine (does not reflect a decrease in GFR).	**Black Box Warning:** possible severe hepatitis B exacerbation in co-infected patients who discontinue therapy. Monitor for IRIS if treating an ARV-naive patient with a lower CD4 cell count (<150/microliter).
Dolutegravir (Tivicay)	Insomnia and headache (2-4%)	Rash, liver injury reported. Increased ALT/AST in 203%. Competition with creatinine for tubular secretion increased serum creatinine by a mean of 0.1 mg/dL with no change in GFR.
Elvitegravir+ Cobicistat (Stribild), Elvitegravir (Vitekta)	Nausea and diarrhea are the two most common AEs. Increased serum creatinine 0.1-0.15 mg/dL due to inhibition of prox. tubular enzymes by cobicistat with no decrease in GFR.	**Same Black Box warnings as ritonavir and tenofovir (TDF and TAF)**. Rare lactic acidosis syndrome. Owing to renal toxicity, should not initiate Rx when pre-Rx eGFR is <70 cc/min. Follow serial serum creatinine and urinary protein and glucose. Discontinue drug if serum Cr rises >0.4 mg/dl above baseline value.
Raltegravir (Isentress)	Diarrhea, headache, insomnia, nausea. LFT ↑ may be more common in pts co-infected with HBV or HCV.	Hypersensitivity reactions can occur. Rash, Stevens-Johnson syndrome, toxic epidermal necrolysis reported. Hepatic failure reported. ↑CK, myopathy and rhabdomyolysis reported *(AIDS 22:1382, 2008)*. ↑ of preexisting depression reported in 4 pts; all could continue raltegravir after adjustment of psych. meds *(AIDS 22:1890, 2008)*. Chewable tablets contain phenylalanine.

TABLE 14E – HEPATITIS A & HBV TREATMENT

For HBV Activity Spectra, *see Table 4C, page 87*

Hepatitis A Virus (HAV)

1. Outbreaks in homeless populations. Vaccination is primary defense *(https://emergency.cdc.gov/han/han00412.asp)*.
2. **Drug/Dosage:** No therapy recommended. If within 2 wks of exposure, prophylactic IVIG 0.02 mL per kg IM times 1 protective. Hep A vaccine equally effective as IVIG in randomized trial and is emerging as preferred Rx *(NEJM 357:1685, 2007)*.
3. **HAV Superinfection:** 40% of pts with chronic Hepatitis C virus (HCV) infection who developed superinfection with HAV developed fulminant hepatic failure *(NEJM 338:286, 1998)*. Similar data in pts with chronic Hepatitis B virus (HBV) infection that suffer acute HAV *(Ann Trop Med Parasitol 93:745, 1999)*. **Hence, need to vaccinate all HBV and HCV pts with HAV vaccine.**

Hepatitis B Virus (HBV): Treatment

	ALT	HBV DNA	HBe Ag	Recommendation
Immune-Tolerant Phase	Normal	>1x106 IU/mL	Positive	**Monitor:** ALT levels be tested at least every 6 months for adults with immune tolerant CHB to monitor for potential transition to immune-active or - inactive CHB. **NB: For those over 40 years of age + liver fibrosis, TREAT as Immune Active (below)**
HBeAg+ Immune Active Phase	Elevated	>20,000 IU/mL	Positive	**TREAT (Duration of therapy+):** Tenofovir (indefinitely; esp. if fibrosis) OR Entecavir (indefinitely; esp. if fibrosis) OR Peg-IFN++ (48 weeks of Rx)
Inactive CHB Phase	Normal	<2,000 IU/mL	Negative	**Monitor:** ALT levels at least once / year
HBeAg-neg Immune Reactivation Phase	Elevated	>2,000 IU/mL	Negative	**TREAT (Duration of therapy+):** Tenofovir (indefinitely; esp. if fibrosis) OR Entecavir (indefinitely; esp. if fibrosis) OR Peg-IFN++ (48 weeks of Rx)

+ Duration of therapy largely unknown; most experts favor indefinite Rx, esp. among those with moderate to advanced fibrosis or inflammation (liver biopsy). Ref: *JAMA 2018,319:1802*.
++ Peg-INF contraindicated in patients with decompensated cirrhosis, autoimmune disease, uncontrolled psychiatric disease, cytopenias, severe cardiac disease, and uncontrolled seizures

For details of therapy, especially in special populations (e.g., pregnant women, children) *see updated AASLD Guidelines (Hepatology, 2015 Nov 13. doi: 10.1002/hep.2)*

HBV Treatment Regimens. Single drug therapy is usually sufficient; combination therapy recommended for HIV co-infection.

	Drug/Dose	Comments
Preferred Regimens	**Pegylated-Interferon-alpha 2a** 180 µg sc once weekly OR **Entecavir** 0.5 mg po once daily OR **Tenofovir alafenamide (TAF/Vemlidy)** 25 mg po once daily	PEG-IFN: Treat for 48 weeks Entecavir: Do not use Entecavir if Lamivudine resistance present. Entecavir/Tenofovir: Treat for at least 24-48 weeks after seroconversion from HBeAg to anti-HBe (if no mod-adv fibrosis present). Indefinite chronic therapy for HBeAg negative patients. Renal impairment dose adjustments necessary.
Alternative Regimens	**Lamivudine** 100 mg po once daily OR **Telbivudine** 600 mg po once daily OR **Emtricitabine** 200 mg po once daily (investigational) OR **Adefovir** 10 mg po once daily OR **Tenofovir disoproxil (TDF)** 300 mg po once daily	These alternative agents are rarely used except in combination. When used, restrict to short term therapy owing to high rates of development of resistance. Not recommended as first-line therapy. Use of Adefovir has mostly been replaced by Tenofovir-based regimens.
Preferred Regimen for HIV-HBV Co-Infected Patient	**Truvada** (TDF + FTC) or **Descovy** (TAF + FTC) po once daily + another anti-HIV drug	ALL patients if possible as part of a fully suppressive anti-HIV/anti-HBV regimen. Continue therapy indefinitely.

TABLE 14F – HCV TREATMENT REGIMENS AND RESPONSE

For HCV Activity Spectra, *see Table 4C, page 87*

1. **Indications for Treatment.** Treatment is indicated for **all patients** with chronic HCV. Rx should be initiated urgently for those with more advanced fibrosis (F3 / F4) and those with underlying co-morbid conditions due to HCV. Type and duration of Rx is based on genotype and stage of fibrosis. Pegylated interferon (Peg-IFN) is no longer a recommended regimen; all DAA regimens with or without ribavirin are the preferred choice.
2. **Definitions of Response to Therapy.**

End of Treatment Response (ETR)	Undetectable at end of treatment.
Relapse	Undetectable at end of therapy (ETR) but rebound (detectable) virus within 24 weeks after therapy stopped.
Sustained Virologic Response (SVR)	CURE! Still undetectable at end of therapy and beyond 12-24 weeks after therapy is stopped.

3. **HCV Treatment Regimens**
   - Biopsy is a 'gold standard' for staging HCV infection and is helpful in some settings to determine the ideal timing of HCV treatment. When bx not obtained, "non-invasive" tests are often employed to assess the relative probability of advanced fibrosis or cirrhosis. Fibroscan (elastography) is now approved in the US and most of the world as a means of assessing liver fibrosis. Elastography values of >10 kPa (Kilopascals) correlates with significant fibrosis (F3 or F4 disease).
   - Resistance tests: Genotypic resistance assays are available that can determine polymorphisms associated with reduction in susceptibility to some DAAs (Direct Acting Agents, e.g., protease inhibitors). **However, resistance tests are recommended only for those who have failed treatment with a prior NS5A or protease inhibitor regimen.**
   - **Patients with decompensated cirrhosis should only be treated by hepatologists owing to the risk of rapid clinical deterioration while receiving treatment for HCV.**
   - **IMPORTANT NOTE REGARDING TREATMENT DECISION-MAKING:** Newer drugs are in development and options for Rx are changing rapidly (i.e., several times per year). Monitor updates at *webedition.sanfordguide.com or hcvguidelines.org.*
   - **Black Box Warning for ALL Direct Acting Agents (DAA):** Cases of HBV reactivation, occasionally fulminant, during or after DAA therapy have been reported in HBV/HCV coinfected patients who were not already on HBV suppressive therapy. *See U.S. FDA Drug Safety Announcement, Oct 4, 2016.* **For HCV/HBV coinfected patients who are HBsAg+ and are not already on HBV suppressive therapy, monitoring HBV DNA levels during and immediately after DAA therapy for HCV is recommended and antiviral treatment for HBV should be given if treatment criteria for HBV are met.** *See HBV treatment.*

CURRENT DRUGS FOR INITIAL TREATMENT FOR PATIENTS WITH CHRONIC HCV

- Drugs and regimens are evolving. For updates go to: webedition.sanfordguide.com and *www.hcvguidelines.org*

Agents/Abbreviation	Tradename	Formulation/Dosing Specifics
Daclatasvir (DCV)	Daklinza	60 mg tab po once daily. Note: decrease dose to 30 mg/d when co-administered with a strong CYP3A inhibitor, e.g., several ARV drugs; increase dose to 90 mg/d when co-administered with a mild-moderate CYP3A inducer. Contraindicated when co-administered with a strong CYP3A inducer.
Elbasvir + **Grazoprevir**	Zepatier	Fixed dose combination (Elbasvir 50 mg + Grazoprevir 100 mg) 1 tab po once daily
Glecaprevir + **Pibrentasvir**	Mavyret	Fixed dose combination (Glecaprevir 100 mg + Pibrentasvir 40 mg) 3 tabs once daily with food
Paritaprevir/ritonavir + **Ombitasvir** (PrO)	Technivie	Fixed dose combination (Paritaprevir 150 mg/ritonavir 100 mg + Ombitasvir 25 mg) 1 tab once daily
Paritaprevir/ritonavir + **Ombitasvir** + **Dasabuvir** (PrOD)	Viekira Pak	Fixed dose combination [(Paritaprevir 150 mg/ritonavir 100 mg + Ombitasvir 25 mg) 1 tab once daily + Dasabuvir 250 mg] 1 tab twice daily with food
	Viekira XR	Extended release fixed dose combination [(Dasabuvir 200 mg + Paritaprevir 50 mg/ritonavir 33.3 mg + Ombitasvir 8.33 mg) 3 tabs once daily with food
Simeprevir (SMV)	Olysio	150 mg tab po once daily with food
Sofosbuvir (SOF)	Sovaldi	400 mg tab po once daily
Sofosbuvir + **Ledipasvir**	Harvoni	Fixed dose combination (Sofosbuvir 400 mg + Ledipasvir 90 mg) 1 tab po once daily
Sofosbuvir + **Velpatasvir**	Epclusa	Fixed dose combination (Sofosbuvir 400 mg + Velpatasvir 100 mg): 1 tab po once daily
Sofosbuvir + **Velpatasvir** + **Voxilaprevir**	Vosevi	Fixed dose combination (Sofosbuvir 400 mg + Velpatasvir 100 mg + Voxilaprevir 100 mg): 1 tab po once daily with food
Ribavirin	Ribavirin, Copegus	Weight-based daily dosing: 1000 mg (Wt <75 kg) or 1200 mg (Wt >75 kg). Low dose: 600 mg/day. Taken with food
Pegylated interferon (alfa 2a)	Roferon, Intron-A, Peg-Intron, Pegasys	180 mcg sc per week (rarely used any more)

TABLE 14F (2)

HCV RECOMMENDED TREATMENT REGIMENS (P = Primary regimen, A = Alternative regimen, Regimens from prior page)

HCV Mono Infection					
Genotype	**P/A**	**Regimen**	**Cirrhosis**	**Duration**	**Comments**
1-6	P	**Epclusa** 1 tab po once daily	With or without	12 weeks	Pan-genotypic DAAs
	P	**Mavyret** 3 tabs po once daily	Without With	8 weeks 12 weeks	
1a	P	**Epclusa** 1 tab po once daily	With or without	12 weeks	
	P	**Harvoni** 1 tab po once daily	Without* With**	8 weeks 12 weeks	* If patient is non-black, HIV-uninfected, non-cirrhotic, and HCV RNA <6 million c/mL ** If patient is black, HIV-co-infected, compensated cirrhosis, or HCV RNA >6 million c/mL
	P	**Mavyret** 3 tabs po once daily	Without With	8 weeks 12 weeks	
	P	**Zepatier** 1 tab po once daily	With or without	12 weeks	If no baseline high-fold NS5A resistance associated mutations
	A	**Viekira Pak** (as directed) + **RBV**	Without only	12 weeks	RBV dosing is wt-based
	A	(**DCV + SOF**) po once daily	Without only	12 weeks	
	A	(**SOF + SMV ± RBV**) po divided twice daily	Without only	12 weeks	RBV dosing is wt-based
1b	P	**Epclusa** 1 tab po once daily	With or without	12 weeks	
	P	**Harvoni** 1 tab po once daily	Without* With**	8 weeks 12 weeks	* If patient is non-black, HIV-uninfected, non-cirrhotic, and HCV RNA <6 million c/mL ** If patient is black, HIV-co-infected, compensated cirrhosis, or HCV RNA >6 million c/mL
	P	**Mavyret** 3 tabs po once daily	Without With	8 weeks 12 weeks	
	P	**Zepatier** 1 tab po once daily	With or without	12 weeks	
	A	**Viekira Pak** (as directed)	With or without	12 weeks	
	A	(**DCV + SOF**) po once daily	Without only	12 weeks	
	A	(**SOF + SMV ± RBV**) po divided twice daily	Without only	12 weeks	RBV dosing is wt-based
2	P	**Epclusa** 1 tab po once daily	With or without	12 weeks	
	P	**Mavyret** 3 tabs po once daily	Without With	8 weeks 12 weeks	
	A	(**DCV + SOF**) po once daily	Without With	12 weeks 16-24 weeks	
3	P	**Epclusa** 1 tab po once daily	With or without	12 weeks	Do not use in cirrhosis if RAV Y93H is present
	P	**Mavyret** 3 tabs po once daily	Without With	8 weeks 12 weeks	
	A	**Vosevi** 1 tab po once daily	With	12 weeks	RAS Y93H is present
	A	(**DCV + SOF**) po once daily	Without With	12 weeks 16-24 weeks	

TABLE 14F (3)

Genotype	P/A	Regimen	Cirrhosis	Duration	Comments
HCV Mono Infection *(continued)*					
4	P	**Epclusa** 1 tab po once daily	With or without	12 weeks	
	P	**Harvoni** 1 tab po once daily	Without* With**	8 weeks 12 weeks	* If patient is non-black, HIV-uninfected, non-cirrhotic, and HCV RNA <6 million c/mL ** If patient is black, HIV-co-infected, compensated cirrhosis, or HCV RNA >6 million c/mL
	P	**Mavyret** 3 tabs po once daily	Without With	8 weeks 12 weeks	
	P	**Zepatier** 1 tab po once daily	With or without	12 weeks	
	A	**Technivie** once daily	Without	12 weeks	
	A	**Technivie** once daily + **RBV** twice daily	With	12 weeks	RBV dosing is wt-based
5 & 6	P	**Epclusa** 1 tab po once daily	With or without	12 weeks	
	P	**Harvoni** 1 tab po once daily	Without* With**	8 weeks 12 weeks	* If patient is non-black, HIV-uninfected, non-cirrhotic, and HCV RNA <6 million c/mL ** If patient is black, HIV-co-infected, compensated cirrhosis, or HCV RNA >6 million c/mL
	P	**Mavyret** 3 tabs po once daily	Without With	8 weeks 12 weeks	
HCV-HIV Co-infection					
1a & 1b	P/A	Same as for HCV Mono Infection		8-12 weeks*	Watch for drug-drug interactions. * 8 weeks ONLY in HCV Rx naive co-infected patients receiving **Mavyret**; otherwise, minimum 12 weeks with any other regimen
2	P/A	Same as for HCV Mono Infection		8- 12 weeks*	Watch for drug-drug interactions. * 8 weeks ONLY in HCV Rx naive co-infected patients receiving **Mavyret**; otherwise, minimum 12 weeks with any other regimen
3	P/A	Same as for HCV Mono Infection			Watch for drug-drug interactions.
4, 5, 6		Not enough experience; if treatment required, use same as for HCV Mono Infection			
Decompensated Cirrhosis					
1, 4, 5, 6	P	**Epclusa** 1 tab po once daily + **RBV**		12 weeks	RBV dosing is wt-based. If RBV-intolerant, treat without RBV for 24 weeks. If prior SOF or NS5A treatment experience, RBV alone for 24 weeks.
	P	**Harvoni** 1 tab po once daily + low dose **RBV**		12 weeks	If RBV-intolerant, treat without RBV for 24 weeks. If prior SOF or NS5A treatment experience, RBV alone for 24 weeks.
1, 4	P	(**DCV + SOF**) po once daily + low dose **RBV**		12 weeks	24 weeks if RBV intolerant
2, 3	P	**Epclusa** 1 tab po once daily + **RBV**		12 weeks	RBV dosing is wt-based. If RBV-intolerant, treat without RBV for 24 weeks. If prior SOF or NS5A treatment experience, RBV alone for 24 weeks.
	P	(**DCV + SOF**) po once daily + low dose **RBV**		12 weeks	24 weeks if RBV intolerant

TABLE 14F (4)

Post-Liver Transplant					
Genotype	P/A	Regimen	Cirrhosis	Duration	Comments
1, 4, 5, 6	P	**Mavyret** 3 tabs po once daily	Without	12 weeks	Alternative if compensated cirrhosis
	P	**Harvoni** 1 tab po once daily + **RBV**	With or without	12 weeks	RBV dosing is wt-based. Dose as tolerated.
	A	(**DCV + SOF**) po once daily + low dose **RBV**	Without	12 weeks	
1, 4	A	(**SOF + SMV ± RBV**) po divided twice daily	Without	12 weeks	RBV dosing is wt-based.
2, 3	P	**Mavyret** 3 tabs po once daily	Without	12 weeks	Alternative if compensated cirrhosis
	P	(**DCV + SOF**) po once daily + low dose **RBV**	With	12 weeks	Compensated or decompensated
	A	**Epclusa** 1 tab po once daily + **RBV**	With	12 weeks	Compensated or decompensated. RBV dosing is wt-based
	A	**SOF + RBV** po daily		24 weeks	RBV initial dose 600 mg/day, increased monthly by 200 mg/day as tolerated up to max wt-based dose

TABLE 15A – ANTIMICROBIAL PROPHYLAXIS FOR SELECTED BACTERIAL INFECTIONS*

CLASS OF ETIOLOGIC AGENT/DISEASE/CONDITION	PROPHYLAXIS AGENT/DOSE/ROUTE/DURATION	COMMENTS
Group B streptococcal disease (GBS), neonatal: Approaches to management (CDC Guidelines, *MMWR 59 (RR-10):1, 2010; CID 2017;65(S2):S143*)		
Pregnant women—intrapartum antimicrobial prophylaxis procedures: 1. Screen all pregnant women with vaginal & rectal swab for GBS at 35–37 wks gestation (unless other indications for prophylaxis exist: GBS bacteriuria during this pregnancy or previously delivered infant with invasive GBS disease; even then cultures may be useful for susceptibility testing). Use transport medium; GBS survive at room temp. up to 96 hrs. **Rx during labor if swab culture positive.** 2. Rx during labor if previously delivered infant with invasive GBS infection, or if any GBS bacteriuria during this pregnancy. 3. Rx if GBS status unknown but if any of the following are present: (a) delivery at <37 wks gestation [*see MMWR 59 (RR-10): 1, 2010* algorithms for preterm labor and preterm premature rupture of membranes]; or (b) duration of ruptured membranes ≥18 hrs; or (c) intrapartum temp. ≥100.4ºF (≥38.0ºC). If amnionitis suspected, broad-spectrum antibiotic coverage should include an agent active vs. group B streptococci. 4. Rx if positive intra-partum NAAT for GBS. 5. Unless other conditions exist, Rx not indicated if: negative vaginal/rectal cultures at 35-37 wks gestation or C-section performed before onset of labor with intact amniotic membranes (use standard surgical prophylaxis).		**Regimens for prophylaxis against early-onset group B streptococcal disease in neonate used during labor:** **Pen G** 5 million Units IV (initial dose) then 2.5 to 3 million Units IV q4h until delivery Alternative: **AMP** 2 gm IV (initial dose) then 1 gm IV q4h until delivery Penicillin-allergic patients: • Patient not at high risk for anaphylaxis: **Cefazolin** 2 gm IV (initial dose) then 1 gm IV q8h until delivery • Patient at high risk for anaphylaxis from β-lactams: ○ If organism is both clindamycin- and erythromycin-susceptible, **or** is erythromycin-resistant, but clindamycin-susceptible confirmed by D-zone test (or equivalent) showing lack of inducible resistance: **Clinda** 900 mg IV q8h until delivery ○ If susceptibility of organism unknown, lack of inducible resistance to clindamycin has not been excluded, or patient is allergic to clindamycin: **Vanco** 1 gm IV q12h until delivery
Neonate of mother given prophylaxis	*See detailed algorithm in MMWR 59 (RR-10):1, 2010.*	
Preterm, premature rupture of the membranes: Grp B strep-negative women Cochrane Database Rev *12:CD00:1058, 2013; Obstet Gyn 124:515:2014; Am J Ob-Gyn 207:475. 2012.*	(**AMP** 2 gm IV q6h + **Erythro** 250 mg IV q6h) x 48 hrs, then (**Amox** 250 mg po q8h + **Erythro base** 333 mg po q8h) x 5 days *(ACOG Practice Bulletin: Obstet Gynecol 127: e39, 2016).*	
Post-splenectomy bacteremia. Usually encapsulated bacteria: pneumococci, meningococci, H. flu type B; bacteremia: Enterobacter, S. aureus, Capnocytophaga, P. aeruginosa. Also at risk for fatal malaria, severe babesiosis. Asplenia review *(Chest 2016,150:1394)*	Protein conjugate and polysaccharide vaccines at age and timing appropriate intervals (Adults: *www.cdc.gov/vaccines/schedules/downloads/adult/adult-combined-schedule.pdf.* Children: *www.cdc.gov/vaccines/schedules/downloads/child/0-18yrs-child-combined-schedule.pdf).* Daily Prophylaxis in asplenic child (daily until age 5 yrs or minimum of 1 yr rx): **Amox** 125 mg po bid (age 2 mo-3 yr); **Amox** 250 mg po bid (age >3 yr-5 yr). If allergic, e.g. rash only: **Cephalexin** 250 mg po bid. If IgE-mediated reaction, no good choice. Fever in Children & Adults: **Amox-clav** 875/125 po bid (adult), 90 mg/kg po div bid (child); Alternative: (**Levo** 750 mg po or **Moxi** 400 mg po) once daily. Seek immediate medical care. Some recommend **Amox** 2 gm po before sinus or airway procedures.	

TABLE 15A (2)

CLASS OF ETIOLOGIC AGENT/DISEASE/CONDITION	PROPHYLAXIS AGENT/DOSE/ROUTE/DURATION	COMMENTS
Sexual Exposure		
Sexual assault survivor [likely agents and risks, *see CDC Guidelines at MMWR 64(RR-3):1, 2015*]. For review of overall care: *NEJM 365:834, 2011.*	[**Ceftriaxone** 250 mg IM + **Azithro** 1 gm po once + (**Metro** 2 gm po once or **Tinidazole** 2 gm po once)]. Can delay Metro/Tinidazole if alcohol was recently ingested.	• Obtain expert individualized advice re: forensic exam and specimens, pregnancy (incl. emergency contraception), physical trauma, psychological support • Test for chlamydia and gonococci at sites of penetration or attempted penetration by NAATs. Obtain molecular tests for trichomonas and check vaginal secretions for BV and candidiasis. • Serological evaluation for syphilis, HIV, HBV, HCV • Initiate post-exposure protocols for HBV vaccine, HIV post-exposure prophylaxis as appropriate • HPV vaccine recommended for females 9-26 or males 9-21, if not already immunized • Follow-up in 1 week to review results, repeat negative tests in 1-2 weeks to detect infections not detected previously, repeat syphilis testing 4-6 weeks and 3 months, repeat HIV testing 6 weeks and 3-6 months. • Check for anogenital warts at 1-2 months. Notes: If ceftriaxone not available, can use cefixime 400 mg po once in its place for prevention of gonorrhea, but the latter is less effective for pharyngeal infection and against strains with reduced susceptibility to cephalosporins. For non-pregnant individuals who cannot receive cephalosporins, treatment with (Gemifloxacin 320 mg po once + azithro 2 gm po once) or (Gentamicin 240 mg IM once + azithro 2 gm po once) can be substituted for ceftriaxone/azithro.
Contact with specific sexually transmitted diseases. *See comprehensive guidelines for specific pathogens in MMWR 64(RR-3):1, 2015.*		
Syphilis exposure		Presumptive rx for exposure within 3 mos., as tests may be negative. *See Table 1, page 26.* If exposure occurred >90 days prior, establish dx or treat empirically.
Sickle-cell disease. Likely agent: S. pneumoniae *(see post-splenectomy, above)* Ref.: *NEJM 376: 1561, 2017*	Children <5 yrs: **Pen V** 62.5 to 125 mg po bid ≥5 yrs: **Pen V** 250 mg po bid. (Alternative in children: **Amox** 20 mg/kg/day)	Start prophylaxis by 2 mos. *(Pediatrics 106:367, 2000);* continue until at least age 5. When to d/c must be individualized. Age-appropriate vaccines, including pneumococcal, Hib, influenza, meningococcal. Treating infections, consider possibility of penicillin non-susceptible pneumococci. May need malaria prophylaxis entire life.

TABLE 15B – ANTIBIOTIC PROPHYLAXIS TO PREVENT SURGICAL INFECTIONS IN ADULTS*

2013 Guidelines: Am J Health Syst Pharm 70:195, 2013; Med Lett 58:63, 2016

General Comments:

- To be optimally effective, antibiotics must be started within 60 minutes of the surgical incision. Vancomycin and FQs may require 1-2 hr infusion time, so start dose 2 hrs before the surgical incision.
- Most applications employ a single preoperative dose or continuation for less than 24 hrs.
- For procedures lasting >2 half-lives of prophylactic agent, intraoperative supplementary dose(s) may be required.
- Dose adjustments may be desirable in pts with BMI >30.
- Prophylaxis does carry risk: e.g., C. difficile colitis, allergic reactions
- Active S. aureus screening, decolonization & customized antimicrobial prophylaxis demonstrated efficacious in decreasing infections after hip, knee & cardiac surgery *(JAMA 313:2131 & 2162, 2015)*.
- See additional details for prevention of surgical site infections by CDC *(JAMA Surg 152: 784, 2017)* and Am Coll Surg/Surg Infect Soc *(J Am Coll Surg 224: 59, 2016)*. Both support no further antibiotics once surgical wound is closed, although latter includes possible exceptions: breast reconstruction, joint arthroplasty, and cardiac procedures.

Use of Vancomycin:

- For many common prophylaxis indications, vancomycin is considered an alternative to β-lactams in pts allergic to or intolerant of the latter.
- Vancomycin use may be justifiable in centers where rates of post-operative infection with methicillin-resistant staphylococci are high or in pts at high risk for these.
- Unlike β-lactams in common use, vancomycin has no activity against gram-negative organisms. **When gram-negative bacteria are a concern following specific procedures, it may be necessary or desirable to add a second agent with appropriate in vitro activity.** This can be done using cefazolin with vancomycin in the non-allergic pt, or in pts intolerant of β-lactams using vancomycin with another ram-negative agent (e.g., aminoglycoside, fluoroquinolone, possibly aztreonam, if pt not allergic; local resistance patterns and pt factors would influence choice).
- Infusion of vancomycin, especially too rapidly, may result in hypotension or other manifestations of histamine release (red person syndrome). Does not indicate an allergy to vancomycin.

TYPE OF SURGERY	PROPHYLAXIS	COMMENTS
Cardiovascular Surgery		
Antibiotic prophylaxis in cardiovascular surgery has been proven beneficial in the following procedures: • Reconstruction of abdominal aorta • Procedures on the leg that involve a groin incision • Any vascular procedure that inserts prosthesis/ foreign body • Lower extremity amputation for ischemia • Cardiac surgery • Permanent Pacemakers *(Circulation 121:458, 2010)* • Heart transplant • Implanted cardiac defibrillators	**Cefazolin** 1–2 gm (Wt <120 kg) or 3 gm (Wt >120 kg) IV as a single dose or q8h for 1–2 days or **Cefuroxime** 1.5 gm IV as a single dose or q12h for total of 6 gm or **Vanco** 1 gm IV as single dose or q12h for 1–2 days. For pts weighing >90 kg, use vanco 1.5 gm IV as a single dose or q12h for 1-2 days. Re-dose cefazolin q4h if CrCl>30 mL/min or q8h if CrCl ≤30 mL/min Consider **intranasal Mupirocin** evening before, day of surgery & bid for 5 days post-op in pts with pos. nasal culture for S. aureus. Mupirocin resistance has been encountered.	**Timing & duration:** Single infusion just before surgery as effective as multiple doses. No prophylaxis needed for cardiac catheterization. For prosthetic heart valves, customary to stop prophylaxis either after removal of retrosternal drainage catheters or just a 2nd dose after coming off bypass. **Vanco** may be preferable in hospitals with ↑ freq of MRSA, in high-risk pts, those colonized with MRSA or for Pen-allergic pts. Clindamycin 900 mg IV is another alternative for Pen-allergic or Vanco-allergic pt. Implanted devices ref: *JAC 70:325, 2015.* For insertion of ventricular assist devices, prophylaxis same as for cardiac surgery (e.g., cefazolin ± vancomycin) *(CID 64: 222, 2017)*.
Gastric, Biliary and Colonic Surgery		
Gastroduodenal/Biliary		
Gastroduodenal, includes percutaneous endoscopic gastrostomy (high risk only), pancreaticoduodenectomy (Whipple procedure)	**Cefazolin** (1-2 gm IV) or **Cefoxitin** (1-2 gm IV) or **Cefotetan** (1-2 gm IV) or **Ceftriaxone** (2 gm IV) as a single dose (some give additional doses q12h for 2–3 days). *See Comment*	Gastroduodenal (PEG placement): High-risk is marked obesity, obstruction, ↓ gastric acid or ↓ motility. Re-dose Cefazolin q4h and Cefoxitin q2h if CrCl >30 mL/min; q8h and q4h, respectively, if CrCl ≤30 mL/min
Biliary, includes laparoscopic cholecystectomy	Low risk, laparoscopic: No prophylaxis Open cholecystectomy: **Cefazolin, Cefoxitin, Cefotetan, Ampicillin-sulbactam**	Biliary high-risk or open procedure: age >70, acute cholecystitis, non-functioning gallbladder, obstructive jaundice or common duct stones. With cholangitis, treat as infection, not prophylaxis.
Endoscopic retrograde cholangiopancreatography	No rx without obstruction. If obstruction: **CIP** 500–750 mg po or 400 mg IV 2 hrs prior to procedure or **Pip-tazo** 4.5 gm IV 1 hr prior to procedure	Most studies show that **achieving adequate drainage** will prevent post-procedural cholangitis or sepsis and no further benefit from prophylactic antibiotics; greatest benefit likely when complete drainage cannot be achieved. *See Gastroint Endosc 81: 81, 2015 for American Society of Gastrointestinal Endoscopy recommendations for ERCP; Gut 58:868, 2009.*

TABLE 15B (2)

TYPE OF SURGERY	PROPHYLAXIS	COMMENTS
Gastric, Biliary and Colonic Surgery *(continued)*		
Colorectal, elective colectomies Recommend combination of: • Mechanical bowel prep • po antibiotic *(See Comment)* • IV antibiotic Ref: *Am J Health Sys Pharm 70:195, 2013*	**Parenteral regimens** (emergency or elective): [**Cefazolin** 1-2 gm IV + **Metro** 0.5 gm IV] *(see Comment)* or **Cefoxitin** or **Cefotetan** 1-2 gm IV (if available) or **Ceftriaxone** 2 gm IV + **Metro** 0.5 gm IV or **ERTA** 1 gm IV Beta-lactam allergy, *see Comment*	**Oral regimens: Neomycin** + **Erythro**. Pre-op day: (1) 10 am 4L polyethylene glycol electrolyte solution (Colyte, GoLYTELY) po over 2 hr. (2) Clear liquid diet only. (3) 1 pm, 2 pm & 11 pm, Neomycin 1 gm + Erythro base 1 gm po. (4) NPO after midnight. Alternative regimens have been less well studied; GoLYTELY 1-6 pm, then Neomycin 2 gm po + Metronidazole 2 gm po at 7 pm & 11 pm. **Beta lactam allergy: Clinda** 900 mg IV + (**Gent** 5 mg/kg or **Aztreonam** 2 gm IV or **CIP** 400 mg IV)
Ruptured viscus: *See Peritoneum/Peritonitis, Secondary, Table 1, page 50.*		
Head and Neck Surgery		
	Cefazolin 2 gm IV (Single dose) (some add **Metro** 500 mg IV) OR **Clinda** 600-900 mg IV (single dose) ± **Gent** 5 mg/kg IV (single dose) *(See Table 10C for weight-based dose calculation)*.	Antimicrobial prophylaxis in head & neck surg appears efficacious only for procedures involving oral/ pharyngeal mucosa (e.g., laryngeal or pharyngeal tumor) but even with prophylaxis, wound infection rate can be high. **Clean, uncontaminated head & neck surg does not require prophylaxis.** Re-dose cefazolin q4h if CrCl>30 mL/min or q8h if CrCl ≤30 mL/min
Neurosurgical Procedures		
Clean, non-implant; e.g., elective craniotomy	**Cefazolin** 1-2 gm IV once. Alternative: **Vanco** 1 gm IV once; for pts weighing >90 kg, use vanco 1.5 gm IV as single dose.	Clindamycin 900 mg IV is alternative for vanco-allergic or beta-lactam allergic pt. Re-dose cefazolin q4h if CrCl>30 mL/min or q8h if CrCl ≤30 mL/min
Clean, contaminated (cross sinuses, or naso/oropharynx)	**Clinda** 900 mg IV (single dose)	British recommend Amoxicillin-Clavulanate 1.2 gm IV[NUS] or (Cefuroxime 1.5 gm IV + Metronidazole 0.5 gm IV)
CSF shunt surgery, intrathecal pumps:	**Cefazolin** 1-2 gm (Wt <120 kg) or 3 gm (Wt >120 kg) IV once. Alternative: **Vanco** 1 gm IV once; for pts weighing >90 kg, use vanco 1.5 gm IV as single dose OR **Clinda** 900 mg IV.	Randomized study in a hospital with high prevalence of infection due to methicillin-resistant staphylococci showed Vancomycin was more effective than cefazolin in preventing CSF shunt infections *(J Hosp Infect 69:337, 2008)*. Re-dose cefazolin q4h if CrCl >30 mL/min or q8h if CrCl ≤30 mL/min
Obstetric/Gynecologic Surgery		
Vaginal or abdominal hysterectomy	**Cefazolin** 1–2 gm or **Cefoxitin** 1–2 gm or **Cefotetan** 1–2 gm or **Amp-sulb** 3 gm IV 30 min. before surgery.	Alternative: (**Clinda** 900 mg IV or **Vanco** 1 gm IV) + (**Gent** 5 mg/kg x 1 dose or **Aztreonam** 2 gm IV or **CIP** 400 mg IV) OR (**Metro** 500 mg IV + **CIP** 400 mg IV)
Cesarean section for premature rupture of membranes or active labor	**Cefazolin** 1-2 gm IV x 1 dose Alternative: **Clinda** 900 mg IV + (**Gent** 5 mg/kg IV or **Tobra** 5 mg/kg IV) x 1 dose. Increased risk of infection vs. cefazolin *(Obstet Gyn 2018;132:948)*.	Administering prophylaxis before the skin incision reduces surgical site infections. **In non-elective C-section,** addition of **Azithro** 500 mg IV in addition to standard antibiotics significantly decreased endometritis and wound infections *(NEJM 375: 1231, 2016)*. **In obesity**, give standard pre-op prophylaxis, then (Cephalexin 500 mg po q8h + Metro 500 mg po q8h) x 18 hrs *(JAMA 2017;318:1012 & 1026)*
Surgical Abortion (1st trimester)	1st trimester: **Doxy** 300 mg po: 100 mg 1 hr before procedure + 200 mg post-procedure.	Meta-analysis showed benefit of antibiotic prophylaxis in all risk groups.
Ophthalmic Surgery	(**Neomycin-Gent-Polymyxin B** or **Gati** or **Moxi**) eye drops, 1 drop q5-15 min x 5 doses	Some add **Cefazolin** 100 mg under conjunctiva at end of surgery.

TABLE 15B (3)

TYPE OF SURGERY	PROPHYLAXIS	COMMENTS
Orthopedic Surgery		
Hip arthroplasty, spinal fusion	Same as cardiac surgery	Customarily stopped after "Hemovac" removed. 2013 Guidelines recommend stopping prophylaxis within 24 hrs of surgery *(Am J Health Syst Pharm 70:195, 2013)*.
Total joint replacement (other than hip)	**Cefazolin** 1–2 gm IV pre-op (± 2nd dose) or **Vanco** 1 gm IV. For pts weighing >90 kg, use vanco 1.5 gm IV as single dose or **Clinda** 900 mg IV.	2013 Guidelines recommends stopping prophylaxis within 24 hrs of surgery *(Am J Health Syst Pharm 70:195, 2013)*. Usual to administer before tourniquet inflation. Intranasal mupirocin if colonized with S. aureus.
Open reduction of closed fracture with internal fixation	**Ceftriaxone** 2 gm IV once	3.6% (ceftriaxone) vs 8.3% (for placebo) infection found in Dutch trauma trial *(Ln 347:1133, 1996)*. Several alternative antimicrobials can ↓ risk of infection *(Cochrane Database Syst Rev 2010: CD 000244)*.
Prophylaxis to protect prosthetic joints from hematogenous infection related to distant procedures (patients with plates, pins and screws only are not considered to be at risk)	• A prospective, case-control study concluded that antibiotic prophylaxis for dental procedures did not decrease the risk of hip or knee prosthesis infection *(Clin Infect Dis 50:8, 2010)*. • An expert panel of the American Dental Association concluded that, in general, prophylactic antibiotics are not recommended prior to dental procedures to prevent prosthetic joint infection *(J Amer Dental Assoc 146: 11, 2015)*. • Individual circumstances should be considered; when there is planned manipulation of tissues thought to be actively infected, antimicrobial therapy for the infection is likely to be appropriate.	
Peritoneal Dialysis Catheter Placement	**Vanco** single 1 gm IV dose 12 hrs prior to procedure	Effectively reduced peritonitis during 14 days post-placement in 221 pts: Vanco 1%, Cefazolin 7%, placebo 12% (p=0.02) *(Am J Kidney Dis 36:1014, 2000)*.
Urologic Surgery/Procedures • See *Best Practice Policy Statement* of Amer. Urological Assoc. (AUA) *(J Urol 179:1379, 2008)* and 2013 Guidelines *(Am J Health Syst Pharm 70:195, 2013)*. • Selection of agents targeting urinary pathogens may require modification based on local resistance patterns; ↑ TMP-SMX and/or fluoroquinolone (FQ) resistance among enteric gram-negative bacteria is a concern.		
Cystoscopy	• Prophylaxis generally not necessary if urine is sterile (however, AUA recommends FQ or TMP-SMX for those with several potentially adverse host factors (e.g., advanced age, immunocompromised state, anatomic abnormalities, etc.) • Treat patients with UTI prior to procedure using an antimicrobial active against pathogen isolated	
Cystoscopy with manipulation	**CIP** 500 mg po (**TMP-SMX** 1 DS tablet po may be an alternative in populations with low rates of resistance)	Procedures mentioned include ureteroscopy, biopsy, fulguration, TURP, etc. Treat UTI with targeted therapy before procedure if possible.
Transrectal prostate biopsy	**CIP** 500 mg po 12 hrs prior to biopsy and repeated 12 hrs after 1st dose. *See Comment.*	Bacteremia 7% with **CIP** vs 37% with **Gent** *(JAC 39:115, 1997)*. **Levofloxacin** 500 mg 30-60 min before procedure was effective in low risk pts; additional doses were given for ↑ risk (J Urol 168:1021, 2002). Serious bacteremias due to FQ-resistant organisms have been encountered in patients receiving FQ prophylaxis. Screening stool cultures pre-procedure for colonization with FQ-resistant organisms is increasingly utilized to inform choice of prophylaxis (Clin Infect Dis 60: 979, 2015). One study showed non-significant decrease in risk of infection with culture-directed antimicrobial prophylaxis (Urology 146: 11, 2015). Pre-operative prophylaxis should be determined on an institutional basis based on susceptibility profiles of prevailing organisms. Although 2nd or 3rd generation Cephalosporins or addition of single-dose gentamicin has been suggested, infections due to ESBL-producing and gent-resistant organisms have been encountered *(Urol 74:332, 2009)*. Meta-analysis found fosfomycin trometamol more effective than FQ in preventing infection after transrectal prostate biopsy *(World J Urol: 36: 323, 2018)*.
Other		
Breast surgery, herniorrhaphy, thoracotomy	**Cefazolin** 1-2 gm IV x 1 dose or **Amp-sulb** 3 gm IV x 1 dose or **Clinda** 900 mg IV x 1 dose or **Vanco** 1 gm IV x 1 dose (1.5 gm if wt >90 kg)	*Am J Health Syst Pharm 70:195, 2013.*
Vascular surgery: aneurysm repair, revascularization	**Cefazolin** 2 gm IV x 1 dose	

TABLE 15C – ANTIMICROBIAL PROPHYLAXIS FOR THE PREVENTION OF BACTERIAL ENDOCARDITIS IN PATIENTS WITH UNDERLYING CARDIAC CONDITIONS*

In 2007, the American Heart Association guidelines for the prevention of bacterial endocarditis were updated. The resulting document *(Circulation 2007; 116:1736-1754 and http://circ.ahajournals.org/cgi/reprint/116/15/1736)*, which was also endorsed by the Infectious Diseases Society of America, represents a significant departure from earlier recommendations.

- Antibiotic prophylaxis for dental procedures is now directed at individuals who are likely to suffer the most devastating consequences should they develop endocarditis. Prophylaxis to prevent endocarditis is no longer specified for gastrointestinal or genitourinary procedures. The following is adapted from and reflects the new AHA recommendations. *See original publication for explanation and precise details.*

SELECTION OF PATIENTS FOR ENDOCARDITIS PROPHYLAXIS				
FOR PATIENTS WITH ANY OF THESE HIGH-RISK CARDIAC CONDITIONS ASSOCIATED WITH ENDOCARDITIS:	**WHO UNDERGO DENTAL PROCEDURES INVOLVING:**	**WHO UNDERGO INVASIVE RESPIRATORY PROCEDURES INVOLVING:**	**WHO UNDERGO INVASIVE PROCEDURES OF THE GI OR GU TRACTS:**	**WHO UNDERGO PROCEDURES INVOLVING INFECTED SKIN AND SOFT TISSUES:**
Prosthetic heart valves Previous infective endocarditis Congenital heart disease with any of the following: • Completely repaired cardiac defect using prosthetic material (Only for 1st 6 months) • Partially corrected but with residual defect near prosthetic material • Uncorrected cyanotic congenital heart disease • Surgically constructed shunts and conduits Valvulopathy following heart transplant [Benefit unclear in pt with ventricular assist device *(CID 64: 222, 2017)*.]	Any manipulation of gingival tissue, dental periapical regions, or perforating the oral mucosa. **PROPHYLAXIS RECOMMENDED‡** *(see Dental Procedures Regimens table below)* (Prophylaxis is *not* recommended for routine anesthetic injections (unless through infected area), dental x-rays, shedding of primary teeth, adjustment of orthodontic appliances or placement of orthodontic brackets or removable appliances.)	Incision of respiratory tract mucosa **CONSIDER PROPHYLAXIS** *(see Dental Procedures Regimens table)* OR For treatment of established infection **PROPHYLAXIS RECOMMENDED** *(see Dental Procedures Regimens table for oral flora,* but include anti-staphylococcal coverage when *S. aureus* is of concern)	PROPHYLAXIS is no longer recommended solely to prevent endocarditis, **but the following approach is reasonable:** For patients with enterococcal UTIs • treat before elective GU procedures • include enterococcal coverage in perioperative regimen for non-elective procedures† For patients with existing GU or GI infections or those who receive perioperative antibiotics to prevent surgical site infections or sepsis • it is reasonable to include agents with anti-enterococcal activity in perioperative coverage†	Include coverage against staphylococci and β-hemolytic streptococci in treatment regimens

† Agents with anti-enterococcal activity include penicillin, ampicillin, amoxicillin, vancomycin and others. Check susceptibility if available. *(See Table 5 for highly resistant organisms.)*
‡ 2008 AHA/ACC focused update of guidelines on valvular heart disease use term "is reasonable" to reflect level of evidence *(Circulation 118:887, 2008)*.

PROPHYLACTIC REGIMENS FOR DENTAL PROCEDURES		
SITUATION	**AGENT**	**REGIMEN[1]**
Usual oral prophylaxis	**Amox**	Adults 2 gm, children 50 mg per kg; orally, 1 hour before procedure
Unable to take oral medications	**AMP[2]**	Adults 2 gm, children 50 mg per kg; IV or IM, within 30 min before procedure.
Allergic to penicillins	**Cephalexin[3]** OR	Adults 2 gm, children 50 mg per kg; orally, 1 hour before procedure
	Clinda OR	Adults 600 mg, children 20 mg per kg; orally, 1 hour before procedure
	Azithro or **Clarithro**	Adults 500 mg, children 15 mg per kg; orally, 1 hour before procedure
Allergic to penicillins and unable to take oral medications	**Cefazolin[3]** OR	Adults 1 gm, children 50 mg per kg; IV or IM, within 30 min before procedure
	Clinda	Adults 600 mg, children 20 mg per kg; IV or IM, within 30 min before procedure

1 Children's dose should not exceed adult dose. AHA document lists all doses as 30-60 min before procedure.
2 AHA lists Cefazolin or Ceftriaxone (at appropriate doses) as alternatives here.
3 Cephalosporins should not be used in individuals with immediate-type hypersensitivity reaction (urticaria, angioedema, or anaphylaxis) to penicillins or other β-lactams. AHA proposes ceftriaxone as potential alternative to cefazolin; and other 1st or 2nd generation cephalosporin in equivalent doses as potential alternatives to cephalexin.

TABLE 15D – MANAGEMENT OF EXPOSURE TO HIV-1 AND HEPATITIS B AND C*

OCCUPATIONAL EXPOSURE TO BLOOD, PENILE/VAGINAL SECRETIONS OR OTHER POTENTIALLY INFECTIOUS BODY FLUIDS OR TISSUES WITH RISK OF TRANSMISSION OF HEPATITIS B/C AND/OR HIV-1 (E.G., NEEDLESTICK INJURY)

Free consultation for occupational exposures, call (PEPline) 1-888-448-4911. *[Information also available at www.aidsinfo.nih.gov]*

General steps in management:

1. Wash clean wounds/flush mucous membranes immediately (use of caustic agents or squeezing the wound is discouraged; data lacking regarding antiseptics).
2. Assess risk by doing the following: (a) Characterize exposure; (b) Determine/evaluate source of exposure by medical history, risk behavior, & testing for hepatitis B/C, HIV; (c) Evaluate and test exposed individual for hepatitis B/C & HIV.

Hepatitis B Occupational Exposure Prophylaxis *(MMWR 62(RR-10):1-19, 2013)*

Exposed Person Vaccine Status	Exposure Source		
	HBs Ag+	**HBs Ag–**	**Status Unknown or Unavailable for Testing**[†]
Unvaccinated	Give HBIG 0.06 mL per kg IM & initiate HB vaccine	Initiate HB vaccine	Initiate HB vaccine
Vaccinated (antibody status unknown)	Do anti-HBs on exposed person: If titer ≥10 milli-International units per mL, no rx If titer <10 milli-International units per mL, give HBIG + 1 dose HB vaccine**	No rx necessary	Do anti-HBs on exposed person: If titer ≥10 milli-International units per mL, no rx § If titer <10 milli-International units per mL, give 1 dose of HB vaccine**

§ Persons previously infected with HBV are immune to reinfection and do not require postexposure prophylaxis.

For known vaccine series responder (titer ≥10 milli-International units per mL), monitoring of levels or booster doses not currently recommended. Known non-responder (<10 milli-International units per mL) to 1º series HB vaccine & exposed to either HBsAg+ source or suspected high-risk source—rx with HBIG & re-initiate vaccine series **or** give 2 doses HBIG 1 month apart. For non-responders after a 2nd vaccine series, 2 doses HBIG 1 month apart is preferred approach to new exposure.

If known high risk source, treat as if source were HBsAG positive.

** Follow-up to assess vaccine response or address completion of vaccine series.

Hepatitis B Non-Occupational Exposure & Reactivation of Latent Hepatitis B

Non-Occupational Exposure *(MMWR 59(RR-10):1, 2010)*

- Exposure to blood or sexual secretion of HBsAg-positive person
  - Percutaneous (bite, needlestick)
  - Sexual assault
- Initiate immunoprophylaxis within 24 hrs or sexual exposure & no more than 7 days after parenteral exposure
- Use Guidelines for occupational exposure for use of HBIG and HBV vaccine

Reactivation of Latent HBV *(AnIM 164:30 & 64, 2016)*

- Patients requiring administration of anti-CD 20 monoclonal antibodies as part of treatment selected malignancies, rheumatoid arthritis and vasculitis are at risk for reactivation of latent HBV
- Use of two FDA-approved anti-CD 20 drugs: ofatumumab (Arzerra) & rituximab (Rituxan) put patients at risk
- Prior to starting anti-CD 20 drug, test for latent HBV with test for HBsAg and Anti IgG HB core antibody & perhaps HIV PCR. Positive HBsAg and/or Anti IgG HBc AB = occult Hepatitis B
- **If pt has latent (occult) HBV & anti-CD 20 treatment is necessary, treatment should include an effective anti-HBV drug**

Hepatitis C Exposure

Determine antibody to hepatitis C for both exposed person &, if possible, exposure source. If source + or unknown and exposed person negative, follow-up HCV testing for HCV RNA (detectable in blood in 1-3 weeks) and HCV antibody (90% who seroconvert will do so by 3 months) is advised. **No recommended prophylaxis;** immune serum globulin not effective. Monitor for early infection, as therapy may ↓ risk of progression to chronic hepatitis. Persons who remain viremic 8-12 weeks after exposure should be treated with a course of pegylated interferon *(Gastro 130:632, 2006 and Hpt 43:923, 2006). See Table 14F*. Case-control study suggested risk factors for occupational HCV transmission include percutaneous exposure to needle that had been in artery or vein, deep injury, male sex of HCW, & was more likely when source VL >6 log10 copies/mL.

TABLE 15D (2)

A. HIV OCCUPATIONAL EXPOSURE

The decision to initiate post-exposure prophylaxis (PEP) is a clinical judgment made in concert with the exposed individual and is based on three factors:

1. Type of exposure
   a. Potentially infectious substances include: blood, unfixed tissues, CSF; semen and vaginal secretions (these have not been implicated in occupational transmission of HIV); synovial, pleural, peritoneal, ascitic, and amniotic fluids; other visibly bloody fluids.
   b. Fluids of low or negligible risk for transmission, unless visibly bloody include: urine, sweat, vomitus, stool, saliva, nasal secretions, tears, and sputum. **PEP is not indicated.**
   c. If the exposure occurred to intact skin, regardless of whether the substance is potentially infectious or not, and regardless of the HIV status of the source patient, **PEP is not indicated.**
   d. If the exposure occurred to mucous membranes (e.g., blood splash to the eye) or non-intact skin (e.g., abraded skin, open wound, dermatitis) or occurred percutaneously as a consequence of a needle stick, scalpel, or other sharps injury or cut, then **PEP may be indicated.** Human bites resulting in a break in the skin could theoretically transmit HIV, particularly if oral blood is present, although these have not been implicated in occupational transmission of HIV.

2. Likelihood that the source patient is HIV infected
   a. If the exposure constitutes a risk of HIV transmission as described above and the source patient is **known positive for HIV**, then **PEP should be instituted** immediately, within hours of exposure (Animal studies show PEP less effective when started >72h post-exposure but interval after which PEP not beneficial is unknown; initiation of PEP after a longer interval may be considered if exposure risk of transmission is extremely high).
   b. If exposure constitutes a risk of HIV transmission, and the HIV status is **unknown**, but patient is **likely to be HIV infected** or there is a **reasonable suspicion** for infection based on HIV risk factors, then **PEP should be initiated pending confirmation of the source patient's HIV status.**
      i. If a rapid HIV test of the source patient can be performed, it is reasonable to withhold therapy pending results of this test and initiating PEP if the test is positive.
      ii. If rapid testing cannot be performed, PEP should be initiated pending results of source patient testing and discontinued if the test returns negative.
      iii. NOTE: Antibody testing is sufficient to rule out HIV infection, unless the source patient has suspected acute retroviral syndrome, in which case HIV viral load testing is recommended.
   c. If the **source is unknown** or the source is known but status and risk cannot be determined, the decision to initiate PEP should be made on a case-by-case basis in **consultation with an expert** (PEPline at *http://www.nccc.ucsf.edu/about_nccc/pepline/)* (1-888-448-4911), guided by the severity of the exposure and epidemiologic likelihood of HIV exposure.

3. Adverse effects and potential for drug interactions with the PEP regimen
   a. Newer agents are better tolerated and should allow a higher proportion of exposed healthcare providers to complete the prescribed four-week course of therapy. Doses of some agents may need to be adjusted based on renal function.
   b. Information about drug interactions is available in Tables 16A and 16B, in the package insert and on-line at *hivinsite.ucsf.edu*
   c. Breast feeding and pregnancy are not contraindications to PEP (efavirenz is contraindicated during pregnancy).

PEP Algorithm

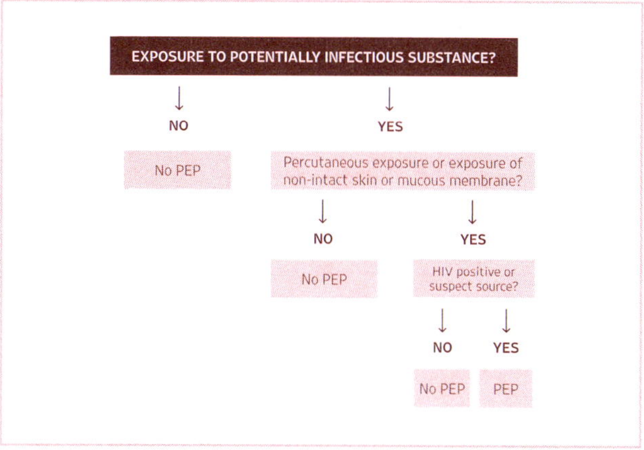

TABLE 15D (3)

REGIMENS FOR PEP: a 4-week course of 3 or more drugs now routinely recommended for all PEP

Preferred	• **Descovy** (FTC 200 mg + TAF)(but not recommended if CrCl <30 mL/min) po once daily + (**Raltegravir** 1200 mg (two 600 tabs) once daily or **Dolutegravir** 50 mg orally daily) or **Bictegravir** (FTC + TAF fixed dose formulation) one tab once daily • Creatinine clearance < 30 ml/min: [**Tenofovir disoproxil fumarate** (TDF) 300 mg q72-96h + **Emtricitabine** (FTC) 200 mg q72-96h + (**Dolutegravir** 50 mg po once daily OR **Raltegravir** 400 mg po twice daily]
Alternative	**Descovy** po once daily + ([DRV 800 mg po once daily + RTV 100 mg po once daily] or [**Prezcobix** (DRV 800 mg + Cobi 150 mg) one tab once daily])
	Descovy po once daily + **Lopinavir-Ritonavir** 800/200 mg po once daily
	Creatinine clearance < 30 ml/min: Renally adjusted doses of **Zidovudine** + **Lamivudine** + **Darunavir** 800 mg po once daily + **Ritonavir** 100 mg po once daily

1. Abacavir, efavirenz, enfuvirtide, maraviroc should be used only in consultation with an expert.
2. Didanosine, nelfinavir, tipranavir, stavudine (d4T) and nevirapine (contraindicated) are not recommended.
3. If transmission of drug resistant virus is suspected, the regimen should be appropriately modified in consultation with an expert to include agents to which it is likely to be susceptible.
4. **Descovy is the preferred substitute for Truvada** given lower potential for renal injury and osteomalacia for TAF vs. TDF. Note that Descovy is not recommended for CrCl <30 mL/min.
5. Do not use dolutegravir in pregnancy.

FOLLOW-UP

1. Complete blood count, renal and hepatic panels recommended at baseline and repeated at 2 weeks with further testing if results are abnormal.
2. HIV antibody testing to monitor seroconversion should be performed at baseline, 6 weeks, 12 weeks, and 6 months post-exposure.
3. If a 4th generation p24 antigen-HIV antibody test is used, testing may be terminated at 4 months.
4. Extended follow-up for 12 months is recommended if HCV conversion occurred upon exposure to an HIV-HCV co-infected patient.

B. HIV NON-OCCUPATIONAL EXPOSURE

- Risk of transmission of HIV via sexual contact or needle sharing may reach or exceed that of occupational needlestick exposure, thus HIV post-exposure prophylaxis (PEP) not later than 72 hours (and ideally within a few hours) of the exposure is recommended for HIV-negative persons non-occupationally exposed to blood or other potentially infected fluids from an HIV+ source.
- Substantial risk of HIV acquisition from HIV+ source
  - Exposure of vagina, rectum, eye, mouth, mucous membrane, non-intact skin, percutaneous contact
  - With blood semen, vaginal secretions, rectal secretions, breast milk, or anybody visibly contaminated with blood
- Negligible risk of HIV acquisition regardless of HIV status for any exposure to
  - Urine, nasal secretions, saliva, sweat, or tears if not visibly contaminated with blood
- PEP not effective and not recommended if ≥73 hours after an exposure.
- 4-week course of 3 ARV drugs is recommended for PEP.

Preferred Regimens

Age	Regimen
Age ≥13 years (not pregnant women; avoid TAF and dolutegravir with pregnancy. Use TDF 300 mg + FTC 200 mg instead of Descovy as part of regimen), CrCl ≥30 ml/min	**Descovy** (Emtricitabine [FTC] 200 mg + Tenofovir alafenamide fumerate [TAF]) + (**Dolutegravir** 50 mg po once daily OR **Raltegravir** 400 mg po twice daily) OR **Bictegravir** (FTC + TAF fixed dose formulation) one tab once daily (*See comments*; not recommended if CrCl is <30 ml/min).
Age ≥13 years (includes pregnant women), CrCl <30 ml/min	**Tenofovir disoproxil fumarate** (TDF) 300 mg q72-96h + **Emtricitabine** (FTC) 200 mg q72-96h + (**Dolutegravir** 50 mg po once daily OR **Raltegravir** 1200 po once daily)
Children aged 2-12 years	**TDF** + **FTC** + **Raltegravir**, each dose adjusted for age and weight
Children aged 4 weeks to <2 years	**Zidovudine** + **Lamivudine** + (**Raltegravir** OR **Lopinavir-Ritonavir**) each as an oral solution dose adjusted for age and weight
Children aged birth to 27 days	Consult a pediatric HIV specialist

Alternative Regimens

Age	Regimen
Age ≥13 years (in pregnancy use TDF 300 mg + FTC 200 mg instead of Descovy), CrCl ≥30 ml/min	**Descovy** (FTC 200 mg + Tenofovir alafenamide fumerate [TAF]) + **Darunavir** 800 mg po once daily + **Ritonavir** 100 mg po once daily (See comments; not recommended if creatinine clearance is <30 ml/min).
Age ≥13 years (includes pregnant women), CrCl <30 ml/min	Renally adjusted doses of **Zidovudine** + **Lamivudine** + **Darunavir** 800 mg po once daily + Ritonavir 100 mg po once daily
Children aged 2-12 years	**Zidovudine** + **Lamivudine** + (**Raltegravir** OR **Lopinavir-Ritonavir**) once daily each dose adjusted for age and weight OR **TDF** + **FTC** + (**Lopinavir-Ritonavir** OR [**Darunavir** + **Ritonavir**]) each dose adjusted for age and weight
Children aged 4 weeks to <2 years	**Zidovudine** + **FTC** + (**Raltegravir** OR [**Lopinavir-Ritonavir**]) each as an oral solution dose adjusted for age and weight

TABLE 15E – PREVENTION OF SELECTED OPPORTUNISTIC INFECTIONS IN HUMAN HEMATOPOIETIC CELL TRANSPLANTATION (HCT) OR SOLID ORGAN TRANSPLANTATION (SOT) IN ADULTS WITH NORMAL RENAL FUNCTION

General comments: Medical centers performing transplants will have detailed protocols for the prevention of opportunistic infections which are appropriate to the infections encountered, patients represented and resources available at those sites. Regimens continue to evolve and protocols adopted by an institution may differ from those at other centers. Care of transplant patients should be guided by physicians with expertise in this area.

References:
For HCT: Expert guidelines endorsed by the IDSA, updating earlier guidelines *(MMWR 49 (RR-10):1, 2000)* in: *Biol Blood Marrow Transpl 15:1143, 2009*. These guidelines provide recommendations for prevention of additional infections not discussed in this table and provide more detailed information on the infections included here.

For SOT: Recommendations of an expert panel of The Transplantation Society for management of CMV in solid organ transplant recipients in: *Transplantation 89:779, 2010*. Timeline of infections following SOT in: *Amer J Transpl 9 (Suppl 4):S3, 2009.*

OPPORTUNISTIC INFECTION	TYPE OF TRANSPLANT	PROPHYLACTIC REGIMENS
CMV (Recipient + **or** Donor +/Recipient –) Ganciclovir resistance: risk, detection, management *(CID 68:1420, 2019; Clin Transplant, 33: e13512, 2019)*	SOT	**Prophylaxis: Valganciclovir** 900 mg po q24h Alternatives include **Ganciclovir** 1000 mg po 3 x/day, **Ganciclovir** 5 mg/kg IV 1 x/day, **Valacyclovir** 2 gm po 4 x/day *(kidney only, see comment)*, CMV IVIG or IVIG. **Also consider preemptive therapy** (monitor weekly for CMV viremia by PCR (or antigenemia) for 3-6 months post transplant. If viremia detected, start Valganciclovir 900 mg po bid or Ganciclovir 5 mg/kg IV q12h until clearance of viremia, but for not less than 2 weeks followed by secondary prophylaxis or preemptive approach. Prophylaxis vs pre-emptive rx compared: *CID 58:785, 2014*. CMV hyper IVIG is as adjunct to prophylaxis in high-risk lung, heart/lung, heart, or pancreas organ transplant recipients. Dosing: 150 mg/kg within 72 hrs of transplant and at 2, 4, 6 and 8 weeks; then 100 mg/kg at weeks 12 and 16.
	HCT	**Preemptive Strategy:** Monitor weekly for CMV viremia by PCR (or antigenemia) for 3-6 months post transplant with consideration for more prolonged monitoring in patients at risk for late-onset CMV disease (chronic GVHD, requiring systemic treatment, patients receiving high-dose steroids, T-cell depleted or cord blood transplant recipients, and CD4 <100 cells/mL). Start treatment with identification of CMV viremia or antigenemia as above. Consider prophylaxis (beginning post-engraftment) with **Valganciclovir** 900 mg po q24h or **Letermovir** 480 mg po/IV once daily. *National Comprehensive Cancer Network Guidelines on Prevention and Treatment of Cancer-Related Infections, Version 1.2018.*
Hepatitis B	SOT	For anti-viral agents with activity against HBV, *see Table 14B, page 191*. For discussion of prevention of HBV re-infection after transplantation and prevention of donor-derived infection *see Am J Transplant 9: S116, 2013.*
	HCT	Patients who are anti-HBC positive and anti-HBs positive, but without evidence of active viral replication, can be monitored for ↑LFTs and presence of +HBV-DNA, and given pre-emptive therapy at that time. Alternatively, prophylactic anti-viral therapy can be given, commencing before transplant. (*See guidelines for other specific situations: Biol Blood Marrow Transpl 15:1143, 2009.*) These guidelines recommend Lamivudine 100 mg po q24h as an anti-viral.
Herpes simplex	SOT	**Acyclovir** 400 mg po bid, starting early post-transplant *(Clin Microbiol Rev 10:86, 1997)*.
	HCT	**Acyclovir** 250 mg/m² IV bid **or Acyclovir** 400 mg to 800 mg po bid, from conditioning to engraftment or resolution or mucositis. For those requiring prolonged suppression of HSV, the higher dose (Acyclovir 800 mg po bid) is recommended to minimize the risk of emerging resistance.

TABLE 15E (2)

OPPORTUNISTIC INFECTION	TYPE OF TRANSPLANT	PROPHYLACTIC REGIMENS
Aspergillus spp.	SOT	Lung and heart/lung transplant: Inhaled **Ampho B** and/or a mold active oral azole are commonly used, but optimal regimen not defined. Aerosolized **Ampho B** 6 mg q8h (or 25 mg/day) OR aerosolized **LAB** 25 mg/day OR **Vori** 200 mg po bid OR **Itra** 200 mg po bid. 59% centers employ universal prophylaxis for 6 months in lung transplant recipients with 97% targeting Aspergillus. Most use Voriconazole alone or in combination with inhaled Amphotericin B *(Am J Transplant 11:361, 2011).* Consider restarting prophylaxis during periods of intensified immune suppression. Liver transplant: Consider only in high-risk, re-transplant and/or those requiring renal-replacement therapy. Recommendations on aspergillus prophylaxis in SOT can be found at *(Clin Transplant, 33: e13544, 2019).*
	HCT/Heme malignancy	Indications for prophylaxis against aspergillus include AML and MDS with neutropenia and HCT with GVHD. Posaconazole 200 mg po tid approved this indication *(NEJM 356:335, 2007 and NEJM 356:348,2007).* Posaconazole ER tablets, also approved for prophylaxis (300 mg po BID x 1 day, then 300 daily). Retrospective analysis suggests that Voriconazole would have efficacy in steroid-treated patients with GVHD *(Bone Marrow Transpl 45:662, 2010),* but is not approved for this indication. Caspofungin is more effective than fluconazole in preventing invasive fungal infection *(JAMA 322;1673,2019).* Amphotericin B and echinocandins are alternatives as well.
Candida spp.	SOT	Consider in select, high risk patients (liver, small bowel, pancreas): Consider in select, high-risk patients (re-transplants, dialysis). **Flu** 400 mg daily for 4 weeks post-transplant *(Clin Transplant 33: e13623, 2019).*
	HCT	Recipient with positive serology, no active infection at time of transplant: **Flu** 400 mg once daily x 1 year; then 200 mg once daily indefinitely. Recipient of organ from donor with positive serology, no active infection: o Lung transplant recipients: **Flu** 400 mg once daily, indefinitely. o Other organ recipients: **Flu** 400 mg once daily x 1 year; then 200 mg once daily indefinitely. Recipient residing in an endemic area who underwent an organ transplant (primary prevention): **Flu** 200 mg once daily x 6-12 months post transplantation *(Clin Infect Dis 63:e112, 2016).*
Coccidioides immitis	Any	**Flu** 200-400 mg po q24h *(Transpl Inf Dis 5:3, 2003; Clin Transplant, 33:e13553, 2019)* for approach at one center in endemic area; e.g., for positive serology without evidence of active infection, Flu 400 mg q24h for first year post-transplant, then 200 mg q24h thereafter.
Pneumocystis jirovecii	SOT	**TMP-SMX:** 1 single-strength tab po q24h or 1 double-strength tab po once daily for 3 to 7 days per week. Duration: kidney: 6 mos to 1 year; heart, lung, liver: ≥ 1 year to life-long *(Clin Transplant 33: e13587, 2019).*
	HCT	**TMP-SMX:** 1 single-strength tab po q24h or 1 double-strength tab po once daily or once a day for 3 days per week, from engraftment to ≥ 6 mos post transplant.
Toxoplasma gondii	SOT	**TMP-SMX** (1 SS tab po q24h or 1 DS tab po once daily) x 3-7 days/wk for 6 mos post-transplant. *(See Clin Micro Infect 14:1089, 2008).*
	HCT	**TMP-SMX:** 1 single-strength tab po q24h or 1 double-strength tab po once daily or once a day for 3 days per week, from engraftment to ≥ 6 mos post transplant for seropositive allogeneic transplant recipients.
Trypanosoma cruzi	Heart	May be transmitted from organs or transfusions *(CID 48:1534, 2009).* Inspect peripheral blood of suspected cases for parasites *(MMWR 55:798, 2006).* Risk of reactivation during immunosuppression is variable *(JAMA 298:2171, 2007; JAMA 299:1134, 2008; J Cardiac Fail 15:249, 2009).* If known Chagas disease in donor or recipient, contact CDC for treatment options *(phone 770-488-7775 or in emergency 770-488-7100). Am J Transplant 11:672, 2011.*

TABLE 16 – PEDIATRIC DOSING (AGE >28 DAYS)

Editorial Note

There is limited data on when to switch adolescents to adult dosing. In general, pediatric weight based dosing is appropriate through mid puberty (Tanner 3) if no maximum dose is specified. Some change to adult dosing at 40 kg. If in doubt, when treating serious infections in peri-pubertal adolescents with drugs that have large margins of safety (e.g. Beta lactams and carbapenems) it may be safer to err on the side of higher doses.

DRUG	DOSE (AGE >28 DAYS) (Daily maximum dose shown, when applicable)
ANTIBACTERIALS	
Aminoglycosides	
Amikacin	15-20 mg/kg q24h; 5-7.5 mg/kg q8h
Gentamicin	5-7 mg/kg q24h; 2.5 mg/kg q8h
Tobramycin	5-7 mg/kg q24h; 2.5 mg/kg q8h.
Beta-Lactams	
Carbapenems	
Ertapenem	30 mg/kg/day (divided q12h). Max per day: 1 gm
Imipenem	Age ≥3 mon: 15-25 mg/kg q6h Age 4 wks to 3 mon, wt ≥1.5 kg: 25 mg/kg q6h Age 1 wk to 4 wks, wt ≥1.5 kg: 25 mg/kg q8h Age <1 wk, wt ≥1.5 kg: 25 mg/kg q12h Max 4 gm
Meropenem	60 mg/kg/day (divided q8h); Meningitis: 120 mg/kg/day (divided q8h).
Cephalosporins (po)	
Cefaclor	20-40 mg/kg/day (divided q8-12h). Max per day: 1 gm
Cefadroxil	30 mg/kg/day (divided q12h). Max per day: 2 gm
Cefdinir	14 mg/kg/day (divided q12-24h)
Cefixime	8 mg/kg/day (divided q12-24h)
Cefpodoxime	10 mg/kg/day (divided q12h). Max per day: 400 mg
Cefprozil	15-30 mg/kg/day (divided q12h) -- use 30 for AOM
Ceftibuten	9 mg/kg/day (divided q12-24h). Max per day: 1 gm
Cefuroxime axetil	20-30 mg/kg/day (divided q12h) -- use 30 for AOM. Max per day: 1 gm
Cephalexin	25-100 mg/kg/day (divided q6h). Max per day: 4 gm
Loracarbef	15-30 mg/kg/day (divided q12h). Max per day: 800 mg
Cephalosporins (IV)	
Cefazolin	50-150 mg/kg/day (divided q6-8h). Max per day: 6 gm
Cefepime (non-Pseudomonal)	100 mg/kg/day (divided q8h)
Cefepime (Pseudomonal)	150 mg/kg/day (divided q8h)
Cefotaxime	150-200 mg/kg/day (divided q6-8h). Meningitis: 300 mg/kg/day (divided q6h)
Cefotetan	60-100 mg/kg/day (divided q12h). Max per day: 6 gm
Cefoxitin	80-160 mg/kg/day (divided q6-8h)
Ceftaroline	Age 0 to <2 mon (skin only): 6 mg/kg q8h (GA ≥34 wk, postnatal ≥12 days) Age 2 mon to <2 yrs: 8 mg/kg q8h Age 2 yrs to <18 yrs, ≤33 kg: 12 mg/kg q8h Age ≥2 yrs to <18 yrs, >33 kg: 400 mg q8h or 600 mg q12h
Ceftazidime	150-200 mg/kg/day (divided q8h) CF: 300 mg/kg/day (divided q8h)
Ceftazidime-avibactam	Age 2 to <18 yrs: 62.5 (50/12.5) mg/kg q8h Age 6 mon to <2 yrs: 62.5 (50/12.5) mg/kg q8h Age 3 mon to <6 mon: 50 (40/10) mg/kg q8h / Max 2.5 gm
Ceftizoxime	150-200 mg/kg/day (divided q6-8h)
Ceftriaxone	50-100 mg/kg q24h; Meningitis: 50 mg/kg q12h
Cefuroxime	150 mg/kg/day (divided q8h); Meningitis: 80 mg/kg q8h
Penicillins	
Amoxicillin	25-50 mg/kg/day (divided q8h)
Amoxicillin (AOM, pneumonia)	80-100 mg/kg/day (divided q8-12h; q12h for AOM)
Amoxicillin-clavulanate 7:1 formulation	45 mg/kg/day (divided q12h)
Amoxicillin-clavulanate 14:1 (AOM)	90 mg/kg/day (divided q12h) for wt <40 kg
Ampicillin (IV)	200 mg/kg/day (divided q6h); Meningitis: 300-400 mg/kg/day (divided q6h)
Ampicillin-sulbactam	100-300 mg/kg/day (divided q6h)
Cloxacillin (po)	If <20 kg: 25-50 mg/kg/day (divided q6h); Otherwise dose as adult
Dicloxacillin (mild - moderate)	12.5-25 mg/kg/day (divided q6h)
Dicloxacillin (osteo articular infection)	100 mg/kg/day (divided q 6h)
Flucloxacillin	Age 2-10: 50% of adult dose; Age<2: 25% of adult dose
Nafcillin	150-200 mg/kg/day (divided q6h)
Oxacillin	150-200 mg/kg/day (divided q6h)
Penicillin G	150,000-300,000 units/kg/day (divided q4-6h). Max per day: 12-20 million units
Penicillin VK	25-75 mg/kg/day (divided q6-8h)

TABLE 16 (2)

DRUG	DOSE (AGE >28 DAYS) (Daily maximum dose shown, when applicable)
ANTIBACTERIALS *(continued)*	
Penicillins *(continued)*	
Piperacillin-tazobactam	300 mg/kg/day (divided q6h)
Temocillin	25 mg/kg q12h
Fluoroquinolones * Approved only for CF, anthrax, and complicated UTI	
Ciprofloxacin (po)	20-40 mg/kg/day (divided q12h) *. Max per day: 1.5 gm
Ciprofloxacin (IV)	20-30 mg/kg/day (divided q12h) *. Max per day: 1.2 gm
Levofloxacin (IV/po)	16-20 mg/kg/day (divided q12h) *. Max per day: 750 mg
Lincosamides	
Clindamycin (po)	30-40 mg/kg/day (divided q6-8h)
Clindamycin (IV)	20-40 mg/kg/day (divided q6-8h)
Lincomycin	10-20 mg/kg/day (divided q8-12h)
Lipopeptides	
Daptomycin, cSSSI (infusion only, up to 14 days)	Age 12-17: 5 mg/kg (over 30 min) q24h Age 7-11: 7 mg/kg (over 30 min) q24h Age 2-6: 9 mg/kg (over 60 min) q24h Age 1 to <2: 10 mg/kg (over 60 min) q24h
Daptomycin, S. aureus bacteremia (infusion only, up to 42 days)	Age 12-17: 7 mg/kg (over 30 min) q24h Age 7-11: 9 mg/kg (over 30 min) q24h Age 1-6: 12 mg/kg (over 60 min) q24h
Macrolides	
Azithromycin (po)	5-12 mg/kg/day (once daily)
Azithromycin (IV)	10 mg/kg/day (once daily)
Clarithromycin	15 mg/kg/day (divided q12h). Max per day: 1 gm
Erythromycin (po, IV)	40-50 mg/kg/day (divided q6h)
Monobactams	
Aztreonam	90-120 mg/kg/day (divided q8h). Max per day: 8 gm
Tetracyclines	
Doxycycline (po/IV)	2-4.4 mg/kg/day (divided q12h). Max per day: 200 mg. Max duration: 21 days
Minocycline (po, age >8)	4 mg/kg/day (divided q12h)
Sarecycline	Age >9 yrs, Wt 33-54 kg: 60 mg po q24h Age >9 yrs, Wt 55-84 kg: 100 mg po q24h Age >9 yrs, Wt 85-136 kg: 150 mg po q24h
Tetracycline	Age >8: 25-50 mg/kg/day (divided q6h). Max per day: 2 gm
Other	
Chloramphenicol (IV)	50-100 mg/kg/day (divided q6h). Max per day: 2-4 gm
Colistin	2.5-5 mg/kg/day (divided q6-12h) CF: 3-8 mg/kg/day (divided q8h)
Fosfomycin (po)	2 gm once
Fosfomycin (IV)(very limited data)	Premature (gest+postnatal age <40 wk): 100 mg/kg/day (divided q12h) Neonate (gest+postnatal age 40-44 wk): 200 mg/kg/day (divided q8h) Infant (age 1-12 mon, ≤10 kg): 200-300 mg/kg/day (divided q8h) Age 1-12 years, 10-40 kg: 200-400 mg/kg/day (divided q6-8h) Age ≥12 years: use adult recommendations
Fusidic acid (po)	Age 1-5: 250 mg q8h Age 6-12: 250-500 mg q8h
Linezolid	Age ≥12 yrs: use adult dosing Age 7 days to <12 yrs: 10 mg/kg (IV/po) q8h Age <7 days, GA <34 wks: 10 mg/kg (IV/po) q12h
Methenamine hippurate (age 6-12)	500-1000 mg q12h
Methenamine mandelate	Age >2 to 6: 50-75 mg/kg/day (divided q6-8h) Age 6-12: 500 mg q6h
Metronidazole (po)	30-40 mg/kg/day (divided q6h)
Metronidazole (IV)	22.5-40 mg/kg/day (divided q6h)
Nitrofurantoin (po Cystitis)	5-7 mg/kg/day (divided q 6h)
Nitrofurantoin (po UTI prophylaxis)	1-2 mg/kg/day (once daily)
Polymyxin B (age 2 and older)	2.5 mg/kg (load), then 1.5 mg/kg q12h
Rifampin (meningococcal prophylaxis)	10 mg/kg q12h x2 days
Tinidazole (age >3 for Giardia, amebiasis)	50 mg/kg q24h x1-5 days. Max per day: 2 gm
Sulfadiazine	120-150 mg/kg/day (divided q4-6h). Max per day: 6 gm
TMP-SMX (UTI and other)	8-12 mg TMP/kg/day (divided q12h)
TMP-SMX (PCP)	15-20 mg TMP/kg/day (divided q12h)
Trimethoprim	4 mg/kg/day (divided q12h)
Vancomycin (IV)	60 mg/kg/day (divided q6-8h) Ideally target AUC>400, but if not available, trough target is 10-15 μg/mL
Vancomycin (po for C. difficile)	40 mg/kg/day (divided q6h)

TABLE 16 (3)

DRUG	DOSE (AGE >28 DAYS) (Daily maximum dose shown, when applicable)
ANTIMYCOBACTERIALS	
Bedaquiline	Age ≥12, wt ≥30 kg: 400 mg qd x2 wks, then 200 mg thrice weekly x22 wks
Capreomycin	15-30 mg/kg/day (divided q12-24h). Max per day: 1 gm
Cycloserine	10-15 mg/kg/day (divided q12h). Max per day: 1 gm
Ethambutol	15-25 mg/kg/day (once daily). Max per day: 2.5 gm
Ethionamide	15-20 mg/kg/day (divided q12h). Max per day: 1 gm
Isoniazid (daily dosing)	10-15 mg/kg/day (once daily). Max per day: 300 mg
Isoniazid (2 x/week)	20-30 mg/kg twice weekly. Max per day: 900 mg
Kanamycin	15 -30 mg/kg/day (divided q12-24h). Max per day: 1 gm
Para-aminosalicylic acid	200-300 mg/kg/day (divided q6-12h)
Pyrazinamide (daily)	15-30 mg/kg/day (once daily). Max per day: 2 gm
Pyrazinamide (2 x/week)	50 mg/kg/day (2 days/week). Max per day: 2 gm
Rifabutin (MAC prophylaxis)	5 mg/kg/day (once daily). Max per day: 300 mg
Rifabutin (active TB)	10-20 mg/kg/day (once daily). Max per day: 300 mg
Rifampin	10-20 mg/kg/day (divided q12-24h). Max per day: 600 mg
Streptomycin (age 2 and older)	20-40 mg/kg/day (once daily). Max per day: 1 gm
ANTIFUNGALS	
Amphotericin B deoxycholate	0.5-1 mg/kg/day (once daily)
Amphotericin B lipid complex	5 mg/kg/day (once daily)
Anidulafungin	1.5-3 mg/kg loading dose then .75-1.5 mg/kg/day (once daily)
Caspofungin	70 mg/m2 loading dose then 50 mg/m2 (once daily)
Fluconazole	6 mg/kg/day for oral/esophageal Candida; 12 mg/kg/day for invasive disease
Griseofulvin	Tinea capitis: micro susp 20-25 mg/kg/day, ultra tab 10-15 mg/kg/day (duration ≥6 weeks, continue until clinically clear) Tinea corporis: micro susp 10-20 mg/kg/day x 2-4 weeks Tinea pedis: micro susp 10-20 mg/kg/day x 4-8 weeks
Isavuconazonium sulfate (prodrug of Isavuconazole)	Not known; adult dose 372 mg q8h x 3 doses loading dose then 744 mg/day (divided q12h)
Itraconazole	5-10 mg/kg/day (divided q12h)
Ketoconazole	3.3-6.6 mg/kg/day (once daily)
Micafungin	Age >4 mon: 2 mg/kg q24h (max 100 mg) for candidiasis; for EC use 3 mg/kg q24h if <30 kg, 2.5 mg/kg q24h (max 150 mg) if >30 kg
Nystatin	Adolescents, children: 500,000 units (5 mL) swish & swallow qid Infants: 200,000 units (2 mL) qid Premature infants: 100,000 units (1 mL) qid
Posaconazole	Not known; adult dose 300 mg bid loading dose then 300 mg/day (extended release)
Terbinafine	Tinea capitis: 4-6 mg/kg/day (tabs) Wt 10-20 kg: 62.5 mg q24h Wt 20-40 kg: 125 mg q24h Wt >40 kg: 250 mg q24h Duration: 2 wks for T. tonsurans, 4 wks for M. canis
Voriconazole	12-20 mg/kg/day (divided q12h) (Variable bioavailability and metabolism. Adjust to trough level 1-6 mcg/mL)
ANTIPARASITICS	
Fexinidazole	Age ≥6 yr, wt ≥20 kg: use adult dose
Triclabendazole	Age ≥6 years: 10 mg/kg po q12h x2 doses
ANTIRETROVIRALS	
Abacavir (ABC)	Oral soln, age <3 mon: not approved Oral soln, age ≥3 mon: 8 mg/kg q12h or 16 mg/kg q24h (start soln q12h) Tabs, wt-based: 14 to <20 kg: 150 mg q12h (300 mg q24h also ok) ≥20 to <25 kg: 150 mg qAM, 300 mg qPM (450 mg q24h also ok) ≥25 kg: 300 mg q12h (600 mg q24h also ok) Adolescent: 300 mg q12h or 600 mg q24h
Atazanavir (ATV)	Neonates: not recommended Age ≥3 mon, oral powder: 5 to <15 kg: ATV 200 mg + RTV 80 mg q24h (5 to <10 kg, can't tolerate ATV 200 mg, PI naive: ATV 150 mg + RTV 80 mg q24h with close monitoring of VL) 15 to <25 kg: ATV 250 mg + RTV 80 mg q24h ≥25 kg: ATV 300 mg + RTV 100 mg q24h Age >6 yrs, capsules: 15 to <35 kg: ATV 200 mg + RTV 100 mg q24h ≥35 kg: ATV 300 mg + RTV 100 mg q24h Adolescents: 400 mg q24h, or ATV 300 mg + RTV 100 mg q24h

TABLE 16 (4)

DRUG	DOSE (AGE >28 DAYS) (Daily maximum dose shown, when applicable)
ANTIRETROVIRALS *(continued)*	
Darunavir (DRV)	Neonate: not approved Age <3 or wt <10 kg: avoid use Age ≥3 yr, tx naive or exp ± one or more DRV mutations: 10 to <11 kg: 200 mg (+ RTV 32 mg) q12h 11 to <12 kg: 220 mg (+ RTV 32 mg) q12h 12 to <13 kg: 240 mg (+ RTV 40 mg) q12h 13 to <14 kg: 260 mg (+ RTV 40 mg) q12h 14 to <15 kg: 280 mg (+ RTV 48 mg) q12h 15 to <30 kg: 375 mg (+ RTV 48 mg) q12h 30 to <40 kg: 450 mg (+ RTV 100 mg) q12h ≥40 kg: 600 mg (+ RTV 100 mg) q12h Adolescent (age ≥12 yrs): ≥30 to <40 kg, tx naive/exp ± ≥1 DRV mut: 450 mg (+ RTV 100 mg) q12h ≥40 kg, tx naive/exp, no DRV mut: 800 mg (+ RTV 100 mg) q24h ≥40 kg, tx exp, ≥1 DRV mut: 600 mg (+ RTV 100 mg) q12h
Didanosine (ddI)	Age 2 wk to 3 mon: 50 mg/m2 q12h Age ≥3 mon to 8 mon: 100 mg/m2 q12h Age >8 mon: 120 mg/m2 q12h (240 mg/m2 q24h if age 3-21 yr and tx naive) EC caps (age 6-18 yr): 20 to <25 kg, 200 mg q24h 25 to <60 kg, 250 mg q24h ≥60 kg, 400 mg q24h
Dolutegravir (DTG)	Wt <25 kg: no recommendation made Wt 25 to <40 kg: 50 mg q24h (tx naive or tx exp/INSTI-naive, no inducers Wt ≥40 kg: 50 mg q24h ↑ to q12h if given w/EFV, FPV/r, TPV/r, CBZ, rifampin
Efavirenz (EFV)	Neonates: not approved for use Age ≥3 yr: 10 to <15 kg, 200 mg q24h 15 to <20 kg, 250 mg q24h 20 to <25 kg, 300 mg q24h 25 to <32.5 kg, 350 mg q24h 32.5 to <40 kg, 400 mg q24h ≥40 kg, 600 mg q24h Age 3 mon to <3 yr, wt ≥3.5 kg: not recommended (variable PK)
Elvitegravir (EVG)	As Vitekta, not for use in children age <18 yrs
Emtricitabine (FTC)	Oral soln: 0 to ≤3 mon, 3 mg/kg q24h 3 mon to 17 yr: 6 mg/kg (max 240 mg) q24h ≥18 yr, 240 mg q24h Caps, wt >33 kg: 200 mg q24h
Enfuvirtide (T-20)	Age <6 yrs: not approved for use Age 6-16 yr: 2 mg/kg (max 90 mg) sc q12h Age >16 yr: 90 mg sc q12h
Etravirine (ETR)	Age 2-18 yr: 10 to <20 kg, 100 mg q12h 20 to <25 kg, 125 mg q12h 25 to <30 kg, 150 mg q12h ≥30 kg, 200 mg q12h Age <2 yr: not recommended
Fosamprenavir (FPV)	Neonate: use not recommended Age 2-5 yrs (ARV naive): 30 mg/kg q12h (not recommended) Age 6 mon to 18 yrs (ARV naive or experienced): <11 kg: 45 mg/kg q12h (+ RTV 7 mg/kg q12h) 11 to <15 kg: 30 mg/kg q12h (+ RTV 3 mg/kg q12h) 15 to <20 kg: 23 mg/kg q12h (+ RTV 3 mg/kg q12h) ≥20 kg: 18 mg/kg q12h (+ RTV 3 mg/kg q12h) Adolescent, ARV naive: 700 mg q12h (+ RTV 100 mg q12h), or 1400 mg q24h (+ RTV 100-200 mg q24h) Adolescent, ARV exp: 700 mg q12h (+ RTV 100 mg q12h)
Indinavir (IDV)	Neonate/infant: not approved for use Children: not approved for use Adolescent: 800 mg q12h (+ RTV 100-200 mg q12h)
Lamivudine (3TC)	Oral solution: Age 0 to <4 wks: 2 mg/kg q12h Age ≥4 wks to <3 mon: 4 mg/kg q12h Age ≥3 mon to <3 yrs: 5 mg/kg (max 150 mg) q12h Age ≥3 yr: 5 mg/kg (max 150 mg) q12h, OR 10 mg/kg (max 300 mg) q24h Tabs: 14 to <20 kg: 75 mg q12h (or 150 mg q24h) ≥20 to <25 kg: 75 mg qam + 150 mg qpm (or 225 mg q24h) ≥25 kg: 150 mg q12h (or 300 mg q24h)

TABLE 16 (5)

DRUG	DOSE (AGE >28 DAYS) (Daily maximum dose shown, when applicable)
ANTIRETROVIRALS *(continued)*	
Maraviroc (MVC)	Age ≥2 yrs, w/3A4 inhibitor: 10 to <20 kg: 50 mg q12h (tab or soln) 20 to <30 kg: 80 mg soln q12h or 75 mg tab q12h 30 to <40 kg: 100 mg q12h (tab or soln) ≥40 kg, 150 mg q12h (tab or soln) Age ≥2 yrs, no interacting meds: <30 kg: not recommended ≥30 kg: 300 mg q12h (tab or soln) Age ≥2 yrs, w/3A4 inducer: not recommended
Nelfinavir (NFV)	Neonate (NICHD/HPTN 040/PACTG 1043): Wt 1.5 to 2 kg: 100 mg q12h Wt >2 to 3 kg: 150 mg q12h Wt >3 kg: 200 mg q12h Age 2-13 yrs: 45-55 mg/kg q12h (8th CROI 2001, #250) Adolescent: 1250 mg q12h
Nevirapine (NVP)	Neonate, 34-37 wk EGA: 4 mg/kg q12h (no lead-in); increase to 6 mg/kg q12h after one week Neonate, ≥37 wk EGA to <1 mon: 6 mg/kg q12h (no lead-in) Neo prophylaxis: 2 mg/kg at birth, 48 hr after dose 1, 96 hr after dose 2 1 mon to <8 yr: 7 mg/kg or 200 mg/m2 q12h ≥8 yr: 4 mg/kg or 120-150 mg/m2 q12h Adolescens: 200 mg q24h x14 days, then 200 mg q12h (or 400 mg XR q24h)
Raltegravir (RAL)	Film-coated tab: ≥40 kg, tx-naive or suppr on 400 mg q12h: 1200 mg q24h ≥25 kg: 400 mg q12h <25 kg: use chew tabs Chewable tab: 11 to <14 kg, 75 mg q12h 14 to <20 kg, 100 mg q12h 20 to <28 kg, 150 mg q12h 28 to <40 kg, 200 mg q12h ≥40 kg, 300 mg q12h Oral susp, age ≥4 weeks: 3 to <4 kg, 25 mg q12h 4 to <6 kg, 30 mg q12h 6 to <8 kg, 40 mg q12h 8 to <11 kg, 60 mg q12h 11 to <14 kg, 80 mg q12h 14 to <20 kg, 100 mg q12h Oral susp, neonate, full term, age 1-4 weeks: 2 to <3 kg: 8 mg q12h 3 to <4 kg: 10 mg q12h 4 to <5 kg: 15 mg q12h Oral susp, neonate, full term, age 0-1 week: 2 to <3 kg: 4 mg q24h 3 to <4 kg: 5 mg q24h 4 to <5 kg: 7 mg q24h Preterm or low birth weight: no data
Rilpivirine (RPV)	Adolescent ≥12 yrs, ≥35 kg: 25 mg q24h
Ritonavir (RTV)	Neonates: dose not established Peds dose: 350-400 mg/m2 q12h (not recommended) Used as pharmacologic enhancer
Saquinavir (SQV)	Neonate/infant: not approved for use Age <2 yrs: dose not determined Age ≥2 yrs: Wt 5 to <15 kg: 50 mg/kg q12h (+RTV 3 mg/kg q12h) Wt 15 to <40 kg: 50 mg/kg q12h (+RTV 2.5 mg/kg q12h) Wt ≥40 kg: 50 mg/kg q12h (+RTV 100 mg q12h) Adolescent (age ≥16 yrs): 1 gm q12h (+RTV 100 mg q12h)
Stavudine (d4T)	Age 0-13 days: 0.5 mg/kg q12h Age ≥14 days, <30 kg: 1 mg/kg q12h ≥30 kg: 30 mg q12h
Tenofovir alafenamide (TAF)	≥12 yrs, wt ≥35 kg: 10 mg q24h (part of Genvoya) 25 mg q24h (part of Descovy, Odefsey) Vemlidy not approved for patients <18 yrs of age
Tenofovir (TDF)	Age 2 to <12 yr: 8 mg/kg powder (max 300 mg) q24h [1 scoop=40 mg] Tablets, weight-based: 17 to <22 kg: 150 mg q24h 22 to <28 kg: 200 mg q24h 28 to <35 kg: 250 mg q24h ≥35 kg: 300 mg q24h

TABLE 16 (6)

DRUG	DOSE (AGE >28 DAYS) (Daily maximum dose shown, when applicable)
ANTIRETROVIRALS *(continued)*	
Tipranavir (TPV)	Age <2 yrs: use not approved Age ≥2 to 18 yrs: by BSA: 375 mg/m2 q12h (+RTV 150 mg/m2 q12h) by wt: 14 mg/kg q12h (+RTV 6 mg/kg q12h) (not recommended for tx naive pts) Adolescent: 500 mg q12h (+RTV 200 mg q12h) (not recommended for tx naive pts)
Zidovudine (ZDV)	Neonate, EGA <30 wks: age 0-4 weeks: 2 mg/kg po q12h or 1.5 mg/kg IV q12h (increase to 3 mg/kg po q12h at age 4 weeks) Neonate, EGA ≥30 to <35 wks: age 0-2 weeks: 2 mg/kg po q12h or 1.5 mg/kg IV q12h (increase to 3 mg/kg po q12h at age 2 weeks) EGA ≥35 wks, age 0-4 wks: 4 mg/kg q12h or 3 mg/kg IV q12h Infant/child (EGA ≥35 wks, age ≥4 wks): 4 to <9 kg: 12 mg/kg po q12h 9 to <30 kg: 9 mg/kg po q12h ≥30 kg: 300 mg q12h Dosing by BSA: 180-240 mg/m2 po q12h Adolescent: 300 mg po q12h
Antiretroviral combination products	
Atripla (EFV/FTC/TDF)	Age ≥12 yr, wt ≥40 kg: one tab q24h
Biktarvy (BIC/FTC/TAF)	Wt ≥25 kg: one tab q24h
Combivir (3TC/AZT)	Age ≥12 yr, wt ≥30 kg: one tab q12h
Complera (RPV/FTC/TDF)	Age ≥12 yr, wt ≥35 kg: one tab q24h
Descovy (FTC/TAF)	Age ≥12 yr, wt ≥35 kg: one tab q24h
Epzicom (ABC/3TC)	Wt ≥25 kg: one tab q24h
Evotaz (ATV/cobi)	Age <18: not recommended
Genvoya (EVG/cobi/FTC/TAF)	Age ≥12 yr, wt ≥35 kg: one tab q24h
Kaletra (LPV/RTV)	Age <14 days: avoid use. Age 14 days to 12 mon: 300 mg/75 mg per m2 q12h. Age >12 mon to 18 yrs: 300 mg/75 mg per m2 q12h (tx-experienced); 230 mg/57.5 mg per m2 q12h (tx-naive)
Odefsey (RPV/FTC/TAF)	Age ≥12 yr, wt ≥35 kg: one tab q24h
Prezcobix (DRV/cobi)	Age <18: not recommended
Symfi (EFV 600/3TC/TDF)	Wt ≥40 kg: one tab q24h Symfi Lo (EFV 400/3TC/TDF) Wt ≥35 kg: one tab q24h
Stribild (EVG/cobi/FTC/TDF)	Age ≥12 yr, wt ≥35 kg: one tab q24h
Symtuza (DRV/cobi/FTC/TAF)	Age <18: not approved
Triumeq (DTG/ABC/3TC)	Wt ≥25 kg: one tab q24h *(DHHS guidelines, May 2019)*
Trizivir (ABC/3TC/ZDV)	Wt ≥30 kg: one tab q12h
Truvada (FTC/TDF)	Wt 17 to <22 kg: 100 mg/150 mg q24h; Wt 22 to <28 kg: 133 mg/200 mg q24h; Wt 28 to <35 kg: 167 mg/250 mg q24h; Wt ≥35 kg: 200 mg/300 mg q24h
ANTIVIRALS	
Acyclovir (IV) neonatal herpes simplex	60 mg/kg/day (divided q8h)
Acyclovir (IV) HSV encephalitis >3 months	30-45 mg/kg/day (divided q8h)
Acyclovir (IV) varicella immunocompromised	<1 year: 30 mg/kg/day (divided q8h); >1 year: 30 mg/kg/day or 1500 mg/m2/day (divided q8h)
Acyclovir (IV) HSV immunocompromised	30 mg/kg/day (divided q8h)
Cidofovir	Induction 5 mg/kg once weekly. Suppressive therapy 3 mg/kg once weekly (all with hydration + probenecid)
Entecavir (treatment-naive)	Wt 10-11 kg, 0.15 mg q24h; >11 to 14 kg, 0.2 mg q24h; >14 to 17 kg, 0.25 mg q24h; >17 to 20 kg, 0.3 mg q24h; >20 to 23 kg, 0.35 mg q24h; >23 to 26 kg, 0.4 mg q24h; >26 to 30 kg, 0.45 mg q24h; >30 kg, 0.5 mg q24h
Entecavir (lamivudine-experienced)	Wt 10-11 kg, 0.3 mg q24h; >11 to 14 kg, 0.4 mg q24h; >14 to 17 kg, 0.5 mg q24h; >17 to 20 kg, 0.6 mg q24h; >20 to 23 kg, 0.7 mg q24h; >23 to 26 kg, 0.8 mg q24h; >26 to 30 kg, 0.9 mg q24h; >30 kg, 1 mg q24h
Foscarnet	120-180 mg/kg/day (divided q8-12h)
Ganciclovir	Symptomatic congenital CMV 12 mg/kg/day (divided q12h). CMV tx or first 2 weeks after SOT: 10 mg/kg/day (divided q12h). Suppressive tx or prophylaxis 5 mg/kg/day (divided q24h)
Glecaprevir/pibrentasvir (Mavyret)	Age ≥12 yrs, wt ≥45 kg: 3 tabs q24h
Laninamivir	Treatment or prophylaxis, age <10 yrs: 20 mg inhaled x1 Treatment or prophylaxis, age ≥10 yrs: 40 mg inhaled x1

TABLE 16 (7)

DRUG	DOSE (AGE >28 DAYS) (Daily maximum dose shown, when applicable)
ANTIVIRALS *(continued)*	
Ledipasvir/sofosbuvir (Harvoni)	Age ≥3 yrs, wt ≥35 kg: 90 mg/400 mg q24h Age ≥3 yrs, wt 17 kg to <35 kg: 45 mg/200 mg q24h Age ≥3 yrs, wt <17 kg: 33.75 mg/150 mg q24h Geno 1, tx-naive, no cirr or comp: 12 wks Geno 1, tx-exp, no cirr: 12 wks Geno 1, tx-exp with comp: 24 wks Geno 1, tx-naive/exp with decomp cirr:12 wks (+ribavirin) Geno 1/4, tx-naive/exp LT recipients, no cirr or comp: 12 wks (+ribavirin) Geno 4/5/6, tx-naive/exp, no cirr or comp: 12 wks
Oseltamivir <1 year old	6 mg/kg/day (divided q12h)
Oseltamivir ≥1 year old	<15 kg: 30 mg bid; >15 to 23 kg: 45 mg bid; >23 to 40 kg: 60 mg bid; >40 kg: 75 mg bid (adult dose)
Peramivir	Not studied
Ribavirin (with sofosbuvir, Harvoni)	Wt <47 kg: 15 mg/kg/day (divided q12h) 47-49 kg: 600 mg/day (200 mg in am, 400 mg in pm) 50-65 kg: 800 mg/day (400 mg q12h) 66-80 kg: 1000 mg/day (400 mg in am, 600 mg in pm) >80 kg: 1200 mg/day (divided q12h)
Sofosbuvir (age ≥3 years)	Wt ≥35 kg: 400 mg q24h Wt 17 to <35 kg: 200 mg q24h Wt <17 kg: 150 mg q24h Geno 2, tx-naive/exp, no cirr or comp=12 wks (with ribavirin) Geno 3, tx-naive/exp, no cirr or comp=24 wks (with ribavirin)
Tecovirimat	Wt 13 to <25 kg: 200 mg bid x 14 days Wt 25 to <40 kg: 400 mg bid x 14 days Wt ≥40 kg: 600 mg bid x 14 days
Valacyclovir (Varicella or Herpes Zoster)	60 mg/kg/day (divided q8h)
Valganciclovir	Symptomatic congenital CMV: 32 mg/kg/day (divided q12h); Prevention of CMV after SOT: 7 mg x BSA x CrCl; (once daily; use Schwartz formula for CrCl).
Zanamivir (age >7 years)	10 mg (two 5-mg inhalations) q12h

TABLE 17A – DOSAGE OF ANTIMICROBIAL DRUGS IN ADULT PATIENTS WITH RENAL IMPAIRMENT

- For listing of drugs with NO need for adjustment for renal failure, *see Table 17B.*
- Adjustments for renal failure are based on an estimate of creatinine clearance (CrCl) which reflects the glomerular filtration rate.
- **Different methods for calculating estimated CrCl are suggested for non-obese and obese patients.**
  - Calculations for ideal body weight (IBW) in kg:
    - *Men:* 50 kg plus 2.3 kg/inch over 60 inches height.
    - *Women:* 45 kg plus 2.3 kg/inch over 60 inches height.
  - Obese is defined as 20% over ideal body weight or body mass index (BMI) >30

- Calculations of estimated CrCl *(References, see (NEJM 354:2473, 2006 (non-obese), AJM 84:1053, 1988 (obese))*
  - **Non-obese patient**—
    - Calculate ideal body weight (IBW) in kg (as above)-
    - Use the following formula to determine estimated CrCl

$$\frac{\text{(140 minus age)(IBW in kg)}}{\text{72 x serum creatinine}} = \text{CrCl in mL/min for men. Multiply answer by 0.85 for women (estimated)}$$

  - **Obese patient**—
    - Weight ≥20% over IBW or BMI >30
    - Use the following formulas to determine estimated CrCl

$$\frac{\text{(137 minus age) x [(0.285 x wt in kg) + (12.1 x ht in meters}^2\text{)}}{\text{51 x serum creatinine}} = \text{CrCl (obese male}$$

$$\frac{\text{(146 minus age) x [(0.287 x wt in kg) + (9.74 x ht in meters}^2\text{)}}{\text{60 x serum creatinine}} = \text{CrCl (obese female)}$$

Estimated CrCl is the most common method used for FDA-approved dose adjustments for renal insufficiency. The bulk of the data in this table are based on calculated estimates of CrCl. **Emerging methods use calculations designed to estimate the glomerular filtration rate (eGFR).** Going forward the FDA may require that renal dosing adjustments be based on estimated CrCl and/or eGFR. See *Adv Chronic Kid Dis 2018,25:14.*

Sources for drug dose adjustment for renal impairment: 1) Drug Prescribing in Renal Failure, 5th ed., Aronoff, et al *(eds)(Am College Physicians, 2007)*; 2) package inserts; 3) *AAC 63:e00583, 2019.*

- If estimated CrCl ≥90 mL/min, *see Tables 10A and 10D for dosing.*
- What weight should be used to calculate dosage on a mg/kg basis?
  - If less than 20% over IBW, use the patient's actual weight for all drugs.
  - **For obese patients** (≥20% over IBW or BMI >30).
    - **Aminoglycosides:** (IBW plus 0.4(actual weight minus IBW) = adjusted weight.
    - **Vancomycin:** actual body weight whether non-obese or obese.
    - **All other drugs:** *see Table 17C.*

- For slow or sustained extended daily dialysis **(SLEDD)** over 6-12 hours, adjust doses as for CRRT. For details, *see CID 49:433, 2009; CCM 39:560, 2011.*
- **SLED**: Limited data on dose adjustment for sustained low efficiency dialysis (SLED)*(Can J Kidney Health Dis 2018;5:1).*
- General reference: Drug Prescribing in Renal Failure, 5th ed., Aronoff, et al. (eds) *(Amer College Physicians, 2007 and drug package inserts).*

TABLE 17A (2)

ANTIMICROBIAL	Half-life, hrs (renal function normal)	Half-life, hrs (ESRD)	Dose (renal function normal)	CrCl >50-90	CrCl 10-50	CrCl <10	Hemodialysis	CAPD	CRRT
ANTIBACTERIAL ANTIBIOTICS AMINOGLYCOSIDES, MDD									
Amikacin[1,2]	2-3	30-70	7.5 mg/kg IM/IV q12h (once-daily dosing below)	7.5 mg/kg q12h	7.5 mg/kg q24h	7.5 mg/kg q48h	7.5 mg/kg q48h (+ extra 3.75 mg/kg AD)	15-20 mg lost per L of dialysate/day	7.5 mg/kg q24h
Plazomicin	3.5	No data	15 mg/kg IV q24h	≥60:15 mg/kg q24h	≥30 to <60: 10 mg/kg q24h	≥15 to <30: 10 mg/kg q48h; CrCl <15: No data	No data	No data	No data
Gentamicin, Netilmicin[NUS], Tobramycin[1,2,3]	2-3	30-70	1.7-2.0 mg/kg IM/IV q8h	1.7-2.0 mg/kg q8h	1.7-2.0 mg/kg q12-24h	1.7-2.0 mg/kg q48h	1.7-2.0 mg/kg q48h (+ extra 0.85-1.0 mg/kg AD)	3-4 mg lost per L of dialysate/day	1.7-2.0 mg/kg q24h
AMINOGLYCOSIDES, ODD *(see Table 10C)*									
			Dose for CrCl >80 (mg/kg q24h)	**CrCl 60-80 (mg/kg q24h)**	**CrCl 40-60 (mg/kg q24h)**	**CrCl 30-40 (mg/kg q24h)**	**CrCl 20-30 (mg/kg q48h)**	**CrCl 10-20 (mg/kg q48h)**	**CrCl 0-10 (mg/kg q72h and AD)**
Gentamicin, Tobramycin	2-3	30-70	5.1	4	3.5	2.5	4	3	2
Amikacin, Kanamycin, Streptomycin	2-3	30-70	15	12	7.5	4	7.5	4	3
Isepamicin[NUS]	2-3	30-70	8	8	8	8 mg/kg q48h	8	8 mg/kg q72h	8 mg/kg q96h
Netilmicin[NUS]	2-3	30-70	6.5	5	4	2	3	2.5	2
BETA-LACTAMS									
Carbapenems									
Doripenem	1	18	500 mg IV q8h	500 mg q8h	30-50: 250 mg q8h; 10-30: 250 mg q12h	No data	No data	No data	500 mg q8h *(JAC 69:2508, 2014)*
Ertapenem	4	>4	1 gm IV q24h	1 gm q24h	<30: 0.5 gm q24h	0.5 gm q24h	500 mg IV 3x/week AD *(AAC, Sep 2019)*	0.5 gm q24h	0.5-1 gm q24h
Imipenem-cilastatin	1	4	500 mg IV q6h OR 1 gm IV q8h Intermed susc: 1 gm IV q6h	60 to <90: 400-500 mg q6h Intermed susc: 750 mg q8h	30 to <60: 300 mg q6h OR 500 mg q8h Intermed susc: 500 mg q6h	15 to <30: 200 mg q6h OR 500 mg q12h Intermed susc: 500 mg q12h	200 mg q6h or 500 mg q12h (dose AD) Intermed susc: 500 mg q12h (dose AD)	125-250 mg q12h	0.5-1 gm q12h
Imipenem-cilastatin-relebactam	1 (IMP)	4 (IMP)	1.25 gm IV q6h	60-89: 1 gm q6h	30-59: 0.75 gm q6h; 15-29: 0.5 gm q6h	No data	0.5 gm q6h (dose AD)	No data	No data
Meropenem	1	10	1 gm IV q8h	1 gm q8h	25-50: 1 gm q12h; 10-25: 0.5 gm q12h	0.5 gm q24h	0.5 gm q24h (give dialysis day dose AD)	0.5 gm q24h	1 gm q12h

TABLE 17A (3)

ANTIMICROBIAL	Half-life, hrs (renal function normal)	Half-life, hrs (ESRD)	Dose (renal function normal)	CrCl >50-90	CrCl 10-50	CrCl <10	Hemodialysis	CAPD	CRRT
Carbapenems *(continued)*									
Meropenem-vaborbactam	Mer 1.2 Vab 1.7	Mer 10 Vab ND	2 gm/2 gm IV q8h	**eGFR** ≥50: 2 gm/2 gm q8h	**eGFR** 30-49: 1 gm/1 gm q8h; 15-29: 1 gm/1 gm q12h	**eGFR** <15: 0.5 gm/0.5 gm q12h	0.5 gm/0.5 gm q12h (AD)	No data	No data
Cephalosporins, IV, 1st gen									
Cefazolin	1.9	40-70	1-2 gm IV q8h	1-2 gm q8h	1-2 g q12h	1-2 gm q24-48h	1-2 gm q24-48h (+ extra 0.5-1 gm AD)	0.5 gm IV q12h	1-2 gm q12h
Cephalosporins, IV, 2nd gen									
Cefotetan	4	13-25	1-2 gm IV q12h	1-2 gm q12h	1-2 gm q24h	1-2 gm q48h	1-2 gm q24h (+ extra 1 gm AD)	1 gm q24h	750 mg q12h
Cefoxitin[4]	0.8	13-23	2 gm IV q8h	2 gm q8h	2 gm q8-12h	2 gm q24-48h	2 gm q24-48h (+ extra 1 gm AD)	1 gm q24h	2 gm q8-12h
Cefuroxime	1.5	17	0.75-1.5 gm IV q8h	0.75-1.5 gm q8h	0.75-1.5 gm q8-12h	0.75-1.5 gm q24h	0.75-1.5 gm q24h (give dialysis day dose AD)	0.75-1.5 gm q24h	0.75-1.5 gm q8-12h
Cephalosporins, IV, 3rd gen, non-antipseudomonal									
Cefotaxime[5]	1.5	15-35	2 gm IV q8h	2 gm q8-12h	2 gm q12-24h	2 gm q24h	2 gm q24h (+ extra 1 gm AD)	0.5-1 gm q24h	2 gm q12-24h
Ceftizoxime	1.7	15-35	2 gm IV q8h	2 gm q8-12h	2 gm q12-24h	2 gm q24h	2 gm q24h (+ extra 1 gm AD)	0.5-1 gm q24h	2 gm q12-24h
Ceftriaxone[5]	8	Unchanged	1-2 gm IV q12-24h	1-2 gm q12-24h	1-2 gm q12-24h	1-2 gm q12-24h	1-2 gm q12-24h	1-2 gm q12-24h	1-2 gm q12-24h
Cephalosporins, IV, Advanced									
Cefepime	2	18	2 gm IV q8h	>60: 2 gm q8-12h	30-60: 2 gm q12h; 11-29: 2 gm q24h	1 gm q24h	1 gm q24h (+ extra 1 gm AD)	1-2 gm q48h	2 gm q12-24h
Cefiderocol	2-3	ND	2 gm IV q8h	≥120: 2 gm q6h; 60-119: 2 gm q8h	30-59: 1.5 gm q8h; 15-29: 1 gm q8h	<15: 0.75 gm q12h	0.75 gm q12h (dose AD)	No data	No data
Ceftazidime	1.9	13-25	2 gm IV q8h	2 gm q8-12h	2 gm q12-24h	2 gm q24-48h	2 gm q24-48h (+ extra 1 gm AD)	No data	1-2 gm q12-24h (depends on flow rate)
Ceftolozane/tazobactam	ceftolozane 3.1	ceftolozane 40	IAI/UTI: 1.5 gm IV q8h HAP: 3 gm IV q8h	IAI/UTI: 1.5 gm q8h HAP: 3 gm q8h	CrCl 30-50: IAI/UTI 750 mg q8h HAP 1.5 gm q8h CrCl 15-29: IAI/UTI 375 mg q8h HAP 750 mg q8h	<15: see HD	IAI/UTI: 750 mg load, 150 mg q8h (dose AD) HAP: 2.25 gm load, 450 mg q8h (dose AD)	No data	No data

TABLE 17A (4)

ANTIMICROBIAL	Half-life, hrs (renal function normal)	Half-life, hrs (ESRD)	Dose (renal function normal)	CrCl >50-90	CrCl 10-50	CrCl <10	Hemodialysis	CAPD	CRRT
Cephalosporins, IV, anti-carbapenemase producing GNB									
Ceftazidime-avibactam	Ceftaz 2.8 Avi 2.7	Ceftaz 13-25	2.5 gm q8h	>50: 2.5 gm q8h	31-50: 1.25 gm q8h; 16-30: 0.94 gm q24h	6-15: 0.94 gm q48h; ≤5: 0.94 gm q48h	0.94 gm q48h (dose AD on dialysis days)	No data	1.25 gm q8h
Cefiderocol	2-3	No data	2 gm q8h	>120: 2 gm q6h 60-119: 2 gm q8h	30-59: 1.5 gm q8h 15-29: 1 gm q8h	0-15: 0.75 gm q12h	0.75 gm q12h (dose AD)	No data	No data
Cephalosporins, IV, anti-MRSA									
Ceftaroline	2.7	No data	600 mg (over 5-60 min) IV q12h	600 mg q12h	30-50: 400 mg q12h; 15-30: 300 mg q12h	<15: 200 mg q12h	200 mg q12h	No data	No data
Ceftobiprole[NUS]	2.9-3.3	21	500 mg IV q8-12h	500 mg q8-12h	30-50: 500 mg q12h over 2 hr; 10-30: 250 mg q12h over 2 hr	No data	No data	No data	No data
Cephalosporins, oral, 1st gen									
Cefadroxil	1.5	20	1 gm po q12h	1 gm q12h	1 gm, then 500 mg q12-24h	1 gm, then 500 mg q36h	1 gm, then 1 gm AD	500 mg q24h	No data
Cephalexin	1	20	500 mg po q6h	500 mg q6h	500 mg q12h	250 mg q12h	250 mg q12h (give one of the dialysis day doses AD)	500 mg q12h	No data
Cephalosporins, oral, 2nd gen									
Cefaclor	0.8	3	500 mg po q8h	500 mg q8h	500 mg q8h	500 mg q12h	500 mg q12h (give one of the dialysis day doses AD)	500 mg q12h	No data
Cefprozil	1.5	5-6	500 mg po q12h	500 mg q12h	500 mg q24h	250 mg q12h	250 mg q12h (give one of the dialysis day doses AD)	250 mg q24h	No data
Cefuroxime axetil	1.5	17	500 mg po q8h	500 mg q8h	500 mg q12h	500 mg q24h	500 mg q24h (give extra 250 mg AD)	500 mg q24h	No data
Cephalosporins, oral, 3rd gen									
Cefdinir	1.7	16	300 mg po q12h	30-49: 300 mg q12h 11-29: 300 mg q24h	300 mg q12h	300 mg q24h	300 mg q24h (dose AD on dialysis days)	300 mg q24h	No data
Cefditoren pivoxil	1.6	5	400 mg po q12h	400 mg q12h	200 mg q12h	200 mg 24h	200 mg q24h (dose AD on dialysis days)	200 mg q24h	No data

TABLE 17A (5)

ANTIMICROBIAL	Half-life, hrs (renal function normal)	Half-life, hrs (ESRD)	Dose (renal function normal)	CrCl >50-90	CrCl 10-50	CrCl <10	Hemodialysis	CAPD	CRRT
Cephalosporins, oral, 3rd gen *(continued)*									
Cefixime	3	12	400 mg po q24h	400 mg q24h	300 mg q24h	200 mg q24h	200 mg q24h (dose AD on dialysis days)	200 mg q24h	No data
Cefpodoxime proxetil	2.3	10	200 mg po q12h	200 mg q12h	200 mg q12h	200 mg q24h	200 mg q24h (dose AD on dialysis days)	200 mg q24h	No data
Ceftibuten	2.5	13	400 mg po q24h	400 mg q24h	200 mg q24h	100 mg q24h	100 mg q24h (dose AD on dialysis days)	100 mg po q24h	No data
Monobactams									
Aztreonam	2	6-8	2 gm IV q8h	2 gm q8h	1-1.5 gm q8h	1-2 gm q24h *(AAC 62:e01066-18, 2018)*	1-2 gm q24h (dose AD on dialysis days)	500 mg q8h	1-1.5 gm q8h
Penicillins (natural)									
Penicillin G	0.5	6-20	0.5-4 million U IV q4h	0.5-4 million U q4h	0.5-4 million U q8h	0.5-4 million U q12h	0.5-4 million U q12h (give one of the dialysis day doses AD)	0.5-4 million U q12h	1-4 million U q6-8h
Penicillin V	0.5	4.1	250-500 mg po q6-8h	250-500 mg q6-8h	250-500 mg q6-8h	250-500 mg q6-8h	250-500 mg q6-8h (give one or more doses AD)	250-500 mg q6-8h	No data
Penicillins (amino)									
Amoxicillin	1.2	5-20	250-500 mg po q8h	250-500 mg q8h	250-500 mg q8-12h	250-500 mg q24h	250-500 mg q24h (give dialysis day dose AD)	250 mg q12h	250-500 mg q8-12h
Amoxicillin ER	1.2-1.5	?	775 mg po q24h	775 mg q24h	30: No data, avoid usage	No data, avoid usage	No data	No data	No data
Amoxicillin/ Clavulanate[6]	amox 1.4, clav 1	amox 5-20, clav 4	500/125 mg po q8h	500/125 mg q8h	250-500 mg (amox component) q12h	250-500 mg (amox) q24h	250-500 mg (amox) q24h (give an extra dose AD on dialysis days)	No data	No data
Ampicillin	1.2	7-20	1-2 gm IV q4-6h	1-2 gm q4-6h	30-50: 1-2 gm q6-8h; 10-30: 1-2 gm q8-12h	1-2 gm q12h	1-2 gm q12h (give one of the dialysis day doses AD)	500 mg - 1 gm q12h	1-2 gm q8-12h
Ampicillin/Sulbactam	amp 1.4, sulb 1.7	amp 7-20, sulb 10	3 gm IV q6h	>60: 3 gm q6h	30-60: 3 gm q8h 10<30: 3 gm q12h	3 gm q24h	3 gm q24h (give AD on dialysis day)	3 gm q24h	3 gm q12h
Penicillins (penicillinase-resistant)									
Dicloxacillin	0.7	No change	125-500 mg po q6h	125-500 mg q6h	125-500 mg q6h	125-500 mg q6h			
Temocillin	4	No data	1-2 gm IV q12h	1-2 gm q12h	1-2 gm q24h	1 gm q48h	1 gm q48h (give AD on dialysis days)	1 gm q48h	No data

TABLE 17A (6)

ANTIMICROBIAL	Half-life, hrs (renal function normal)	Half-life, hrs (ESRD)	Dose (renal function normal)	CrCl >50-90	CrCl 10-50	CrCl <10	Hemodialysis	CAPD	CRRT
Penicillins (antipseudomonal)									
Piperacillin/ Tazobactam (non-Pseudomonas dose)	pip 1, Tazo 1	pip 3-5, Tazo 2.8	3.375 gm IV q6h (over 30 min)	>40: 3.375 gm q6h	20-40: 2.25 gm q6h; <20: 2.25 gm q8h	2.25 gm q8h	2.25 gm q12h (+ extra 0.75 gm AD)	2.25 gm q12h	2.25 gm q6h
Piperacillin/ Tazobactam (Pseudomonas dose)	pip 1, Tazo 1	pip 3-5, Tazo 2.8	4.5 gm IV q6h (over 30 min)	>40: 4.5 gm q6h	20-40: 3.375 gm q6h; <20: 2.25 gm q6h	2.25 gm q6h	2.25 gm q8h (+ extra 0.75 gm AD)	2.25 gm q8h	MIC ≤16: 3.375 gm (over 30 min) q6h; MIC >16 to 64: 4.5 gm (over 4h) q8h *(Pharmacother 35:600, 2015)*
FLUOROQUINOLONES									
Ciprofloxacin po (not XR)	4	6-9	500-750 mg po q12h	500-750 mg q12h	250-500 mg q12h	500 mg q24h	500 mg q24h (dose AD on dialysis days)	500 mg q24h	250-500 mg q12h
Ciprofloxacin XR po	5-7	6-9	500-1000 mg po q24h	500-1000 mg q24h	30-50: 500-1000 mg q24h; 10-30: 500 mg q24h	500 mg q24h	500 mg q24h (dose AD on dialysis days)	500 mg q24h	No data
Ciprofloxacin IV	4	6-9	400 mg IV q12h	400 mg q12h	400 mg q24h	400 mg q24h	400 mg q24h (dose AD on dialysis days)	400 mg q24h	200-400 mg q12h
Delafloxacin IV	4.2-8.5	No data	300 mg IV q12h	300 mg q12h	**eGFR** 30-50: 300 mg q12h; 15-29: 200 mg q12h	**eGFR**<15: No data	No data	No data	No data
Delafloxacin po	4.2-8.5	No data	450 mg po q12h	450 mg q12h	**eGFR** 15-50: 450 mg q12h	**eGFR**<15: No data	No data	No data	No data
Gatifloxacin[NUS]	7-8	11-40	400 mg po/IV q24h	400 mg q24h	400 mg, then 200 mg q24h	400 mg, then 200 mg q24h	200 mg q24h (give dialysis day dose AD)	200 mg q24h	400 mg, then 200 mg q24h
Gemifloxacin	7	>7	320 mg po q24h	320 mg q24h	160 mg q24h	160 mg q24h	160 mg q24h (give dialysis day dose AD)	160 mg q24h	No data
Levofloxacin	7	76	750 mg po/IV q24h	750 mg q24h	20-49: 750 mg q48h	<20: 750 mg x1, then 500 mg q48h	750 mg x1, then 500 mg q48h	750 mg x1, then 500 mg q48h	750 mg x1, then 500 mg q48h
Norfloxacin	3-4	8	400 mg po q12h	400 mg q12h	30-49: 400 mg q12h; 10-30: 400 mg q24h	400 mg q24h	400 mg q24h	400 mg q24h	Not applicable
Ofloxacin	7	28-37	200-400 mg po q12h	200-400 mg q12h	200-400 mg q24h	200 mg q24h	200 mg q24h (give dialysis day dose AD)	200 mg q24h	200-400 mg q24h
Prulifloxacin[NUS]	10.6-12.1	No data	600 mg po q24h	No data	No data	No data	No data	No data	No data

TABLE 17A (7)

ANTIMICROBIAL	Half-life, hrs (renal function normal)	Half-life, hrs (ESRD)	Dose (renal function normal)	CrCl >50-90	CrCl 10-50	CrCl <10	Hemodialysis	CAPD	CRRT
GLYCOPEPTIDES, LIPOGLYCOPEPTIDES, LIPOPEPTIDES									
Dalbavancin	147-258 (terminal)	No data	1 gm IV x1, then 500 mg IV in 7 days	1 gm x1, then 500 mg in 7 days	30-49: 1 gm x1, then 500 mg in 7 days; <30, non-regular HD: 750 mg x1, then 375 mg in 7 days		Regularly scheduled HD: 1 gm x1, then 500 mg in 7 days	No data	No data
Daptomycin	8-9	30	4-6 mg/kg IV q24h	4-6 mg/kg q24h	30-49: 4-6 mg/kg q24h; <30: 6 mg/kg q48h		6 mg/kg q48h after dialysis; consider 7-9 mg/kg if intradialytic dapto used *(Clin J Am Soc Nephrol 4:1190, 2009)*. If next planned dialysis is 72 hrs away, give 9 mg/kg *(AAC 57:864, 2013; JAC 69:200, 2014)*	6 mg/kg q48h	6 mg/kg q48h
Oritavancin	245 (terminal)	No data	1200 mg IV x1	1200 mg x1	<30: No data	No data	Not removed by hemodialysis	No data	No data
Teicoplanin[NUS]	70-100	up to 230	6 mg/kg IV q12h x3 doses (load), then 6 mg/kg q24h	30-80: load, then 6 mg/kg q48h	<30: load, then 6 mg/kg q72h	Load, then 6 mg/kg q72h	Load, then 6 mg/kg q72h. Give AD on dialysis day.	6 mg/kg q72h; for peritonitis see *Table 19*	6 mg/kg q48h
Telavancin	8.1	17.9	10 mg/kg IV q24h	10 mg/kg q24h	30-50: 7.5 mg/kg q24h; 10-30: 10 mg/kg q48h	10 mg/kg q48h	No data	No data	No data
Vancomycin[7]	4-6	200-250	15-30 mg/kg IV q12h	15-30 mg/kg q12h	15 mg/kg q24-96h	7.5 mg/kg q2-3 days	For trough conc of 15-20, give 15 mg/kg if next dialysis in 1 day; give 25 mg/kg if next dialysis in 2 days; give 35 mg/kg if next dialysis in 3 days *(CID 53:124, 2011)*	7.5 mg/kg q2-3 days	CAVH/CVVH: 500 mg q24-48h
MACROLIDES, AZALIDES, LINCOSAMIDES, KETOLIDES									
Azithromycin	68	Unchanged	250-500 mg IV/po q24h	250-500 mg q24h	250-500 mg q24h	250-500 mg q24h	250-500 mg q24h	250-500 mg q24h	250-500 mg q24h
Clarithromycin (not ER)	5-7	22	500 mg po q12h	500 mg q12h	500 mg q12-24h	500 mg q24h	500 mg q24h (dose AD on dialysis days)	500 mg q24h	500 mg q12-24h
Telithromycin[5]	10	15	800 mg po q24h	800 mg q24h	30-50: 800 mg 10-30: 600 mg q24h	600 mg q24h	600 mg q24h (give AD on dialysis days)	No data	No data

TABLE 17A (8)

ANTIMICROBIAL	Half-life, hrs (renal function normal)	Half-life, hrs (ESRD)	Dose (renal function normal)	CrCl >50-90	CrCl 10-50	CrCl <10	Hemodialysis	CAPD	CRRT
MISCELLANEOUS ANTIBACTERIALS									
Chloramphenicol[5]	4.1	Unchanged	50-100 mg/kg/day po/IV (divided q6h)	50-100 mg/kg/day (divided q6h)	50-100 mg/kg/day (divided q6h)	50-100 mg/kg/day (divided q6h)	50-100 mg/kg/day (divided q6h)	50-100 mg/kg/day (divided q6h)	50-100 mg/kg/day (divided q6h)
Fosfomycin IV[NUS]	5,7	50	12-24 gm/day (divided q8-12h) - depends on indication	12-24 gm/day (divided q8-12h) - depends on indication	>40: 100% of norm 40: 70% of norm 30: 60% of norm 20: 40% of norm (all div q8-12h)	10: 20% of norm (div q8-12h)	2 gm q48h (give AD)	No data	No data
Fosfomycin po	5.7	50	3 gm po x1		Do not use (low urine concentrations)				
Fusidic acid[NUS,5]	8.9-11	8.9-11	250-750 mg po q8-12h	250-750 mg q8-12h	250-750 mg q8-12h	250-750 mg q8-12h	250-750 mg q8-12h	250-750 mg q8-12h	250-750 mg q8-12h
Metronidazole[5]	6-14	7-21	7.5 mg/kg IV/po q6h	7.5 mg/kg q6h	7.5 mg/kg q6h	7.5 mg/kg q12h	7.5 mg/kg q12h (give one of the dialysis day doses AD)	7.5 mg/kg q12h	7.5 mg/kg q6h
Nitrofurantoin	1	-	100 mg po q12h (Macrobid)	100 mg q12h (Macrobid)	Avoid use	Avoid use	Avoid use	Avoid use	Avoid use
Tinidazole[5]	13	No data	2 gm po q24h x 1-5 days	2 gm q24h x1-5 days	2 gm q24h x1-5 days	2 gm q24h x1-5 days	2 gm q24h x1-5 days (+ extra 1 gm AD)	No data	No data
Trimethoprim	8-15	20-49	100-200 mg po q12h	100-200 mg q12h	>30: 100-200 mg q12h; 10-30: 100-200 mg q18h	100-200 mg q24h	100-200 mg q24h (give dialysis day dose AD)	100-200 mg q24h	100-200 mg q18h
TMP/SMX (treatment)	TMP 8-15, SMX 10	TMP 20-49, SMX 20-50	5-20 mg/kg/day po/IV (div q6-12h) base on TMP	5-20 mg/kg/day (divided q6-12h)	30-50: 5-20 mg/kg/day (div q6-12h); 10-29: 5-10 mg/kg/day (div q12h)	Not recommended (but if used: 5-10 mg/kg q24h)	Not recommended (but if used: 5-10 mg/kg q24h, give dialysis day dose AD)	Not recommended (but if used: 5-10 mg/kg q24h)	5 mg/kg q8h
TMP/SMX (prophylaxis)	as above	as above	1 DS tab po q24h or 3x/week	1 DS tab q24h or 3x/week	1 DS tab q24h or 3x/week	1 DS tab q24h or 3x/week			

TABLE 17A (9)

ANTIMICROBIAL	Half-life, hrs (renal function normal)	Half-life, hrs (ESRD)	Dose (renal function normal)	CrCl >50-90	CrCl 10-50	CrCl <10	Hemodialysis	CAPD	CRRT
OXAZOLIDINONES									
Linezolid	5	6-8	600 mg po/IV q12h	600 mg q12h (or 300 mg q12h for eGFR <60. (*AAC 2019;63: e00605-19*)	600 mg q12h (see rec for CrCl >50-90)	600 mg q12h (see rec for CrCl >50-90)	600 mg q12h (give one of the dialysis day doses AD)	600 mg q12h	600 mg q12h
Tedizolid	12	Unchanged	200 mg po/IV q24h	200 mg q24h	200 mg q24h	200 mg q24h	200 mg q24h	200 mg q24h	200 mg q24h
POLYMYXINS									
Colistin (polymyxin E) *See Table 10A* All doses refer to colistin base in mg	6.3-12	≥48	Load: (4) x (pt wt in kg). Use lower of ideal or actual wt. Load may exceed 300 mg. Start maintenance 12 hrs later.	≥90, 180 q12h; 80-<90, 170 mg q12h; 70-<80, 150 mg q12h; 60-<70, 137.5 mg q12h; 50-<60, 122.5 mg q12h	40-<50, 110 mg q12h; 30-<40, 97.5 mg q12h; 20-<30, 87.5 mg q12h; 10-<20, 80 mg q12h	5-<10, 72.5 mg q12h; <5, 65 mg q12h	On non-HD days, give 65 mg IV q12h. On HD days, add 40-50 mg to the daily dose after a 3-4 hr session. Give this supplement with the next regular dose after the dialysis has ended.	No data	Add 13 mg per hour of CRRT (or SLED) to the baseline dose of 65 mg q12h.
TETRACYCLINES, GLYCYLCYCLINES									
Tetracycline	6-12	57-108	250-500 mg po q6h	250-500 mg q8-12h	250-500 mg q12-24h	250-500 mg q24h	250-500 mg q24h	250-500 mg q24h	250-500 mg q12-24h
ANTIMETABOLITES									
Flucytosine[8]	3-5	75-200	25 mg/kg po q6h	25 mg/kg q6h	25 mg/kg q12h	25 mg/kg q24h	25 mg/kg q24h (give dialysis day dose AD)	0.5-1 gm q24h	25 mg/kg q12h
ALLYLAMINES, AZOLES									
Fluconazole	20-50	100	100-400 mg po/IV q24h	100-400 mg q24h	50-200 mg q24h	50-200 mg q24h	100-400 mg q24h (give dialysis day dose AD)	50-200 mg q24h	200-400 mg q24h
Itraconazole (IV)[5]	35-40	Unchanged	200 mg IV q12h	200 mg q12h	Do not use IV itraconazole if CrCl<30 due to accumulation of cyclodextrin vehicle				
Itraconazole (oral solution)[5]	35-40	Unchanged	100-200 mg po q12h	100-200 mg q12h	100-200 mg q12h	50-100 mg q12h	100 mg q12-24h	100 mg q12-24h	100-200 mg q12h
Terbinafine	36	No data	250 mg po q24h	250 mg q24h	Avoid use	Avoid use	Avoid use	Avoid use	Avoid use
Voriconazole (IV)[5]	dose-dependent	dose-dependent	6 mg/kg IV q12h x2 doses, then 4 mg/kg IV q12h	6 mg/kg q12h x2 doses, then 4 mg/kg q12h	If CrCl<50, IV vehicle (cyclodextrin) accumulates. Use oral or discontinue.		Avoid use	Avoid use	Avoid use

TABLE 17A (10)

ANTIMICROBIAL	Half-life, hrs (renal function normal)	Half-life, hrs (ESRD)	Dose (renal function normal)	CrCl >50-90	CrCl 10-50	CrCl <10	Hemodialysis	CAPD	CRRT
ANTIMYCOBACTERIALS **First line, tuberculosis**									
Ethambutol[9]	4	7-15	15-25 mg/kg po q24h	15-25 mg/kg q24h	CrCl 30-50: 15-25 mg/kg q24-36h; CrCl 10-30: 15-25 mg/kg q36-48h	15 mg/kg q48h	15 mg/kg q48h (administer AD on dialysis days)	15 mg/kg q48h	15-25 mg/kg q24h
Isoniazid (INH)[5]	0.7-4	8-17	5 mg/kg po q24h	5 mg/kg q24h	5 mg/kg q24h	5 mg/kg q24h	5 mg/kg q24h (administer AD on dialysis days)	5 mg/kg q24h	5 mg/kg q24h
Pyrazinamide	10-16	26	25 mg/kg (max 2.5 gm) po q24h	25 mg/kg q24h	21-50: 25 mg/kg q24h; 10-20: 25 mg/kg q48h	25 mg/kg q48h	25 mg/kg q48h (administer AD on dialysis days)	25 mg/kg q24h	25 mg/kg q24h
Rifabutin[5]	32-67	Unchanged	300 mg po q24h	300 mg q24h	150 mg q24h	150 mg q24h	No data	No data	No data
Rifampin[5]	1.5-5	up to 11	600 mg po q24h	600 mg q24h	300-600 mg q24h	300-600 mg q24h	300-600 mg q24h	300-600 mg q24h	300-600 mg q24h
Rifapentine	13.2-14.1	Unchanged	600 mg po 1-2x/wk	600 mg 1-2x/wk	600 mg 1-2x/wk	600 mg 1-2x/wk	600 mg 1-2x/wk	600 mg 1-2x/wk	600 mg 1-2x/wk
Streptomycin[1,2]	2-3	30-70	15 mg/kg (max 1 gm) IM q24h	15 mg/kg q24h	15 mg/kg q24-72h	15 mg/kg q72-96h	15 mg/kg q72-96h (+ extra 7.5 mg/kg AD)	20-40 mg lost per L of dialysate/day	15 mg/kg q24-72h
Second line, tuberculosis									
Bedaquiline	24-30 (terminal 4-5 mo)	No data	400 mg po q24h x2 wks, then 200 mg po 3x/wk x22 wks	400 mg q24h x2 wk, then 200 mg 3x/wks x22 wks	400 mg q24h x2 wks, then 200 mg 3x/wks x22 wks	Use with caution	Use with caution	Use with caution	Use with caution
Capreomycin	2-5	No data	15 mg/kg IM/IV q24h	15 mg/kg q24h	15 mg/kg q24h	15 mg/kg 3x/wk	15 mg/kg 3x/wk (give AD on dialysis days)	No data	No data
Cycloserine[10]	10	No data	250-500 mg po q12h	250-500 mg q12h	250-500 mg q12h-24h (dosing interval poorly defined)	500 mg q48h (or 3x/wk)	500 mg 3x/wk (give AD on dialysis days)	No data	No data
Ethionamide	2	9	500 mg po q12h	500 mg q12h	500 mg q12h	250 mg q12h	250 mg q12h	250 mg q12h	500 mg q12h
Kanamycin[1,2]	2-3	30-70	7.5 mg/kg IM/IV q12h	7.5 mg/kg q12h	7.5 mg/kg q24h	7.5 mg/kg q48h	7.5 mg/kg q48h (+ extra 3.25 mg/kg AD)	15-20 mg lost per L of dialysate/day	7.5 mg/kg q24h
Para-aminosalicylic acid (PAS)	0.75-1.0	23	4 gm po q12h	4 gm q12h	2-3 gm q12h	2 gm q12h	2 gm q12h (dose AD on dialysis days)	No data	No data

TABLE 17A (11)

ANTIMICROBIAL	Half-life, hrs (renal function normal)	Half-life, hrs (ESRD)	Dose (renal function normal)	CrCl >50-90	CrCl 10-50	CrCl <10	Hemodialysis	CAPD	CRRT
ANTIPARASITICS, ANTIMALARIALS									
Artemether/ lumefantrine (20 mg/120 mg)	art, DHA 1.6-2.2, lum 101-119	No data	4 tabs x1, 4 tabs in 8 hr, then 4 tabs q12h x2 days	4 tabs x1, 4 tabs in 8 hr, then 4 tabs q12h x2 days	4 tabs x1, 4 tabs in 8 hr, then 4 tabs q12h x2 days	4 tabs x1, 4 tabs in 8 hr, then 4 tabs q12h x2 days	No data	No data	No data
Atovaquone	67	No data	750 mg po q12h	750 mg q12h	30-50: 750 mg q12h; 10-30: use with caution	Use with caution	No data	No data	No data
Atovaquone/ Proguanil (250 mg/100 mg)	atov 67, pro 12-21	No data	4 tabs po q24h x3 days	4 tabs q24h x3 days	<30: use with caution	Use with caution	No data	No data	No data
Chloroquine phosphate	45-55 days (terminal)	No data	2.5 gm po over 3 days	2.5 gm over 3 days	2.5 gm over 3 days	2.5 gm over 3 days (consider reducing dose 50%)	2.5 gm over 3 days (consider reducing dose 50%)	No data	No data
Mefloquine	13-24 days	No data	750 mg po, then 500 mg po in 6-8 hrs	750 mg, then 500 mg in 6-8 hrs	750 mg, then 500 mg in 6-8 hrs	750 mg, then 500 mg in 6-8 hrs	No data	No data	No data
Quinine	9.7-12.5	up to 16	648 mg po q8h	648 mg q8h	648 mg q8-12h	648 mg q24h	648 mg q24h (give dialysis day dose AD)	648 mg q24h	648 mg q8-12h
OTHER									
Albendazole	8-12	No data	400 mg po q12-24h	400 mg q12-24h	400 mg q12-24h	400 mg q12-24h	No data	No data	No data
Dapsone	10-50	No data	100 mg po q24h	No data	No data	No data	No data	No data	No data
Ivermectin	20	No data	200 µg/kg/day po x1-2 days	200 µg/kg/day x1-2 days	200 µg/kg/day x1-2 days	200 µg/kg/day x1-2 days	No data	No data	No data
Miltefosine	7-31 days	No data	50 mg po q8h	No data	No data	No data	No data	No data	No data
Nitazoxanide	tizoxanide 1.3-1.8	No data	500 mg po q12h	No data	No data	No data	No data	No data	No data
Pentamidine	3-12	73-118	4 mg/kg IM/IV q24h	4 mg/kg q24h	4 mg/kg q24h	4 mg/kg q24-36h	4 mg/kg q48h (give dialysis day dose AD)	4 mg/kg q24-36h	4 mg/kg q24h

TABLE 17A (12)

ANTIMICROBIAL	Half-life, hrs (renal function normal)	Half-life, hrs (ESRD)	Dose (renal function normal)	CrCl >50-90	CrCl 10-50	CrCl <10	Hemodialysis	CAPD	CRRT
ANTIVIRALS HEPATITIS B									
Adefovir	7.5	15	10 mg po q24h	10 mg q24h	10 mg q48-72h	10 mg q72h	10 mg weekly (dose AD on dialysis days)	No data	No data
Entecavir	128-149	?	0.5 mg po q24h	0.5 mg q24h	0.15-0.25 mg q24h	0.05 mg q24h	0.05 mg q24h (dose AD on dialysis days)	0.05 mg q24h	No data
Telbivudine	40-49	No data	600 mg po q24h	600 mg q24h	30-49: 600 mg q48h; 10-30: 600 mg q72h	600 mg q96h	600 mg q96h (dose AD on dialysis days)	No data	No data
Tenofovir alafenamide	0.51	No data	25 mg po q24h	25 mg q24h	≥15: 25 mg q24h	<15, no HD: not recommended	25 mg q24h (dose AD on dialysis days)	No data	No data
HEPATITIS C (SINGLE AGENTS)									
Daclatasvir	12-15	No data	60 mg po q24h	60 mg q24h	60 mg q24h	60 mg q24h	No data	No data	No data
Ribavirin	44	No data	Depends on indication	No dosage adjustment	Use with caution	Use with caution	No data	No data	No data
Simeprevir	41	Unchanged	150 mg po q24h	150 mg q24h	Use with caution (no data for use in patients with CrCl<30)		No data	No data	No data
Sofosbuvir	sofosbuvir 0.5-0.75	Unchanged	400 mg po q24h	400 mg q24h	Use with caution (no data for use in patients with CrCl<30)		No data	No data	No data
HEPATITIS C (FIXED-DOSE COMBINATIONS)									
Epclusa (Velpatasvir, Sofosbuvir	velpat 15, sofos 0.5	No data	1 tab po q24h	1 tab po q24h	Use with caution (no data for use in patients with CrCl<30)		No data	No data	No data
Harvoni (Ledipasvir, Sofosbuvir)	ledipasvir 47	No data	1 tab po q24h	1 tab q24h	Use with caution (no data for use in patients with CrCl<30)		No data	No data	No data
Technivie (Ombitasvir, Paritaprevir, RTV)	ombit 28-34, parita 5.8	No data	2 tabs po q24h	2 tabs q24h	2 tabs q24h	2 tabs q24h	No data	No data	No data
Viekira Pak (Dasabuvir, Ombitasvir, Paritaprevir, RTV)	dasabuvir 5-8	No data	2 Ombit/Parita/RTV tabs q24h, Dasa 250 mg q12h	2 Ombit/Parita/RTV tabs q24h, Dasa 250 mg q12h	2 Ombit/Parita/RTV tabs q24h, Dasa 250 mg q12h	2 Ombit/Parita/RTV tabs q24h, Dasa 250 mg q12h	No data	No data	No data
Zepatier (Ebasvir, Grazoprevir)	elba 24, grazo 31	No data	1 tab po q24h	1 tab po q24h	1 tab po q24h	1 tab po q24h	1 tab po q24h	No data	No data

TABLE 17A (13)

ANTIMICROBIAL	Half-life, hrs (renal function normal)	Half-life, hrs (ESRD)	Dose (renal function normal)	CrCl >50-90	CrCl 10-50	CrCl <10	Hemodialysis	CAPD	CRRT
HERPESVIRUS									
Acyclovir (IV)[11]	2.5-3.5	20	5-12.5 mg/kg IV q8h	5-12.5 mg/kg q8h	5-12.5 mg/kg q12-24h	2.5-6.25 mg/kg q24h	2.5-6.25 mg/kg q24h (dose AD on dialysis days)	2.5-6.25 mg/kg q24h	5-10 mg/kg q24h
Acyclovir (po)	2.5-3.5	20	800 mg po q4h (5x/day)	800 mg q4h (5x/day)	>25: 800 mg q4h (5x/day); 10-25: 800 mg q8h	800 mg q12h	800 mg q12h (give extra dose AD)	800 mg q12h	No data
Cidofovir (induction)	2.6	No data	5 mg/kg IV q-week x2 weeks	>55: 5 mg/kg q-week x2 weeks	Contraindicated in patients with CrCl of 55 mL/min or less		Contraindicated	Contraindicated	Contraindicated
Cidofovir (maintenance)	2.6	No data	5 mg/kg IV every 2 weeks	>55: 5 mg/kg every 2 weeks	Contraindicated in patients with CrCl of 55 mL/min or less		Contraindicated	Contraindicated	Contraindicated
Famciclovir	penciclovir 2-3	10-22	500 mg po q8h (VZV)	500 mg q8h	500 mg q12-24h	250 mg q24h	250 mg q24h (dose AD on dialysis days)	No data	No data
Ganciclovir (IV induction)	3.5	30	5 mg/kg IV q12h	70-90, 5 mg/kg q12h; 50-69, 2.5 mg/kg q12h	25-49, 2.5 mg/kg q24h; 10-24, 1.25 mg/kg q24h	1.25 mg/kg 3x/week	1.25 mg/kg 3x/week (dose AD on dialysis days)	1.25 mg/kg 3x/week	CVVHF: 2.5 mg/kg q24h *(AAC 58:94, 2014)*
Ganciclovir (IV maintenance)	3.5	30	5 mg/kg IV q24h	2.5-5 mg/kg q24h	0.625-1.25 mg/kg q24h	0.625 mg/kg 3x/week	0.625 mg/kg 3x/week (dose AD on dialysis days)	0.625 mg/kg 3x/week	No data
Ganciclovir (oral)	3.5	30	1 gm po q8h	0.5-1 gm q8h	0.5-1 gm q24h	0.5 gm 3x/week	0.5 gm 3x/week (dose AD on dialysis days)	No data	No data
Letermovir	12	ND	480 mg po/IV q24h	480 mg q24h	480 mg q24h	No data	No data	No data	No data
Valacyclovir	3	14	1 gm po q8h (VZV)	1 gm q8h	1 gm q12-24h	0.5 gm q24h	0.5 gm q24h (dose AD on dialysis days)	0.5 gm q24h	1 gm q12-24h
Valganciclovir	ganciclovir 4	ganciclovir 67	900 mg po q12h	900 mg q12h	450 mg q24-48h	Do not use	*See prescribing information*	No data	No data
			CrCl above 1.4 mL/min/kg (foscarnet only)	**CrCl >1 to 1.4 mL/min/kg (foscarnet only)**	**CrCl >0.8 to 1.0 mL/min/kg (foscarnet only)**	**CrCl >0.6 to 0.8 mL/min/kg (foscarnet only)**	**CrCl >0.5 to 0.6 mL/min/kg (foscarnet only)**	**CrCl 0.4 to 0.5 mL/min/kg (foscarnet only)**	**CrCl <0.4 mL/min/kg (foscarnet only)**
Foscarnet (induction) special dosing scale	3 (terminal 18-88)	Very long	60 mg/kg IV q8h	45 mg/kg q8h	50 mg/kg q12h	40 mg/kg q12h	60 mg/kg q24h	50 mg/kg q24h	Not recommended
Foscarnet (maintenance) special dosing scale	3 (terminal 18-88)	Very long	90-120 mg/kg IV q24h	70-90 mg/kg q24h	50-65 mg/kg q24h	80-105 mg/kg q48h	60-80 mg/kg q48h	50-65 mg/kg q48h	Not recommended

TABLE 17A (14)

ANTIMICROBIAL	Half-life, hrs (renal function normal)	Half-life, hrs (ESRD)	Dose (renal function normal)	CrCl >50-90	CrCl 10-50	CrCl <10	Hemodialysis	CAPD	CRRT
INFLUENZA									
Amantadine	14.8	500	100 mg po q12h	100 mg q12h	100 mg q24-48h	100 mg weekly	100 mg weekly (give AD on dialysis days)	100 mg weekly	100 mg q24-48h
Oseltamivir	carboxylate 6-10	carboxylate >20	75 mg po q12h	>60: 75 mg q12h	31-60: 30 mg q12h; 10-30: 30 mg q24h	No recommendation unless HD	30 mg after each dialysis, no drug on non-HD days *(see comments)*	30 mg after a dialysis exchange	No data
Peramivir	20	No data	600 mg IV q24h	600 mg q24h	31-49: 200 mg q24h; 10-30: 100 mg q24h	100 mg x1, then 15 mg q24h	100 mg x1, then 100 mg 2 hrs AD on dialysis days only	No data	No data
Rimantadine[5]	24-36	prolonged	100 mg po q12h	100 mg q12h	100 mg q12-24h	100 mg q24h	No data	No data	Use with caution
ANTIRETROVIRALS (NRTIs)									
Abacavir (ABC)[5]	1.5	No data	600 mg po q24h	600 mg q24h	600 mg q24h	600 mg q24h	No data	No data	No data
Didanosine enteric coated (ddI)	1.6	4.5	400 mg EC po q24h	400 mg EC q24h	125-200 mg EC q24h	Do not use	No data	No data	No data
Emtricitabine capsules (FTC)	10	>10	200 mg po q24h	200 mg q24h	30-49: 200 mg q48h; 15-29: 200 mg q72h	<15: 200 mg q96h	200 mg q96h	No data	No data
Emtricitabine oral solution (FTC)	10	>10	240 mg po q24h	240 mg q24h	30-49: 120 mg q24h; 15-29: 80 mg q24h	<15: 60 mg q24h	60 mg q24h	No data	No data
Lamivudine (3TC)	5-7	15-35	300 mg po q24h (HIV dose)	300 mg q24h (HIV)	50-150 mg q24h (HIV)	25-50 mg q24h (HIV)	25-50 mg q24h (dose AD on dialysis days) (HIV)	25-50 mg po q24h (HIV)	100 mg first day, then 50 mg q24h (HIV)
Stavudine (d4T)	1.2-1.6	5.5-8	30-40 mg po q12h	30-40 mg q12h	15-20 mg q12h	≥60 kg: 20 mg q24h; <60 kg: 15 mg q24h	≥60 kg: 20 mg q24h; <60 kg: 15 mg q24h (dose AD on dialysis days)	No data	30-40 mg q12h
Tenofovir (TDF)	17	Prolonged	300 mg po q24h	300 mg q24h	30-49: 300 mg q48h; 10-29: 300 mg q72-96h	No data	300 mg after every 3rd dialysis, or q7 days if no dialysis	No data	No data
Zidovudine (ZDV)	0.5-3	1.3-3	300 mg po q12h	300 mg q12h	300 mg q12h	100 mg q8h	100 mg q8h (dose AD on dialysis days)	No data	300 mg q12h

TABLE 17A (15)

ANTIMICROBIAL	Half-life, hrs (renal function normal)	Half-life, hrs (ESRD)	Dose (renal function normal)	CrCl >50-90	CrCl 10-50	CrCl <10	Hemodialysis	CAPD	CRRT
FUSION/ENTRY INHIBITORS									
Enfuvirtide (ENF, T20)[5]	3.8	Unchanged	90 mg sc q12h	90 mg q12h	Not studied in patients with CrCl<35; DO NOT USE		Avoid use	Avoid use	Avoid use
Maraviroc (MVC)	14-18	No data	300 mg po q12h	300 mg q12h	No data	No data	No data	No data	No data
FIXED-DOSE COMBINATIONS									
Atripla (EFV/FTC/TDF)	*See components*	*See components*	1 tab po q24h	1 tab q24h	Do not use	Do not use	Do not use	Do not use	Do not use
Biktarvy (BIC-FTC-TAF)	*See components*	*See components*	1 tab po q24h	1 tab q24h	30-49: 1 tab q24h; do not use if CrCl <30	Do not use	Do not use	Do not use	Do not use
Cimduo (3TC-TDF)	*See components*	*See components*	1 tab po q24h	1 tab q24h	Do not use	Do not use	Do not use	Do not use	Do not use
Combivir (3TC/ZDV)	*See components*	*See components*	1 tab po q12h	1 tab q12h	Do not use	Do not use	Do not use	Do not use	Do not use
Complera, Eviplera (RPV/FTC/TDF)	*See components*	*See components*	1 tab po q24h	1 tab q24h	Do not use	Do not use	Do not use	Do not use	Do not use
Descovy (FTC-TAF)	*See components*	*See components*	1 tab po q24h	1 tab q24h	30-49: 1 tab q24h; do not use if CrCl <30	Do not use	Do not use	Do not use	Do not use
Dutrebis (3TC/RAL)	*See components*	*See components*	1 tab po q12h	1 tab q12h	Do not use	Do not use	Do not use	Do not use	Do not use
Epzicom, Kivexa (ABC/3TC)	*See components*	*See components*	1 tab po q24h	1 tab q24h	Do not use	Do not use	Do not use	Do not use	Do not use
Evotaz (ATV/cobi)[12]	*See components*	*See components*	1 tab po q24h	1 tab q24h	1 tab q24h	1 tab q24h	Do not use	No data	No data
Genvoya (EVG/FTC/TAF/cobi)	*See components*	*See components*	1 tab po q24h	1 tab po q24h	30-49: 1 tab po q24h; do not use if CrCl <30	Do not use	Do not use	Do not use	Do not use
Juluca (DTG-RPV)	*See components*	*See components*	1 tab po q24h	1 tab q24h	1 tab q24h	1 tab q24h	No data	No data	No data
Odefsey (RPV-FTC-TAF)	*See components*	*See components*	1 tab po q24h	1 tab q24h	30-49: 1 tab q24h; do not use if CrCl <30	Do not use	Do not use	Do not use	Do not use
Prezcobix (DRV/cobi)[12]	*See components*	*See components*	1 tab po q24h	1 tab q24h	1 tab q24h	1 tab q24h	1 tab q24h	1 tab q24h	1 tab q24h

TABLE 17A (16)

ANTIMICROBIAL	Half-life, hrs (renal function normal)	Half-life, hrs (ESRD)	Dose (renal function normal)	CrCl >50-90	CrCl 10-50	CrCl <10	Hemodialysis	CAPD	CRRT
FIXED-DOSE COMBINATIONS *(continued)*									
Symfi, Symfi Lo (EFV-3TC-TDF)	*See components*	*See components*	1 tab po q24h	1 tab q24h	Do not use	Do not use	Do not use	Do not use	Do not use
Stribild (EVG/FTC/TDF/cobi)	*See components*	*See components*	1 tab po q24h	Do not use if CrCl <70	Do not use	Do not use	Do not use	Do not use	Do not use
Symtuza (DRV-cobi-FTC-TAF)	*See components*	*See components*	1 tab po q24h	1 tab q24h	30-49: 1 tab q24h; do not use if CrCl <30	Do not use	Do not use	Do not use	Do not use
Triumeq (DTG/ABC/3TC)	*See components*	*See components*	1 tab po q24h	1 tab q24h	Do not use	Do not use	Do not use	Do not use	Do not use
Trizivir (ABC/3TC/ZDV)	*See components*	*See components*	1 tab po q12h	1 tab q12h	Do not use	Do not use	Do not use	Do not use	Do not use
Truvada (FTC/TDF)	*See components*	*See components*	1 tab po q24h	1 tab q24h	30-49: 1 tab q48h; do not use if CrCl <30	Do not use	Do not use	Do not use	Do not use

[1] High flux HD membranes lead to unpredictable drug Cl; measure post-dialysis drug levels.
[2] Check levels with CAPD, PK highly variable. Usual method w/CAPD: 2L dialysis fluid replaced qid (Example amikacin: give 8L x 20 mg lost/L = 160 mg amikacin IV supplement daily).
[3] Gentamicin SLEDD dose: 6 mg/kg IV q48h beginning 30 min before start of SLEDD *(AAC 54:3635, 2010)*.
[4] May falsely increase Scr by interference with assay.
[5] Dosage adjustment may be required in hepatic disease.
[6] Clav cleared by liver; thus, as dose of combination is decreased, a clav deficiency may occur (JAMA 285:386, 2001). If CrCl≤30, do not use 875/125 or 1000/62.5.
[7] New hemodialysis membranes increase Vancomycin clearance; check levels.
[8] Goal peak serum concentration: 25-100 µg/mL.
[9] Monitor serum concentrations if possible in dialysis patients.
[10] Goal peak serum concentration: 20-35 µg/mL.
[11] Rapid infusion can increase SCr.
[12] Do not use with Tenofovir if CrCl <70.

TABLE 17B – NO DOSAGE ADJUSTMENT WITH RENAL INSUFFICIENCY BY CATEGORY

Antibacterials		Antifungals	Anti-TBc	Antivirals		Antiparasitics
Azithromycin	Minocycline	Amphotericin B	Bedaquiline	Abacavir	Mavyret	Albendazole
Ceftriaxone	Moxifloxacin	Anidulafungin	Ethionamide	Atazanavir	Nelfinavir	Artesunate
Chloramphenicol	Nafcillin	Caspofungin	Isoniazid	Daclatasvir	Nevirapine	Ivermectin
Clindamycin	Omadacycline	Isavuconazonium sulfate	Rifampin	Darunavir	Raltegravir	Mefloquine
Dicloxacillin	Oritavancin	Itraconazole oral solution	Rifabutin	Dolutegravir	Ribavirin	Praziquantel
Doxycycline	Polymyxin B	Ketoconazole	Rifapentine	Efavirenz	Rilpivirine	Primaquine
Eravacycline	Rifamycin SV	Micafungin		Elvitegravir	Ritonavir	Pyrimethamine
Fidaxomicin	Rifaximin	Posaconazole, **po only**		Enfuvirtide[1]	Saquinavir	
Fusidic acid	Secnidazole	Voriconazole, **po only**		Epclusa[2]	Simeprevir[2]	
Lefamulin	Tedizolid			Etravirine	Sofosbuvir[2]	
Linezolid[3]	Tigecycline			Fosamprenavir	Technivie	
Quinupristin-Dalfopristin				Harvoni[2]	Tecovirimat	
				Ibalizumab-uiyk	Tipranavir	
				Indinavir	Viekira Pak	
				Letermovir	Viekira XR	
				Lopinavir	Zepatier	

[1] Enfuvirtide: Not studied in patients with CrCl <35 mL/min. DO NOT USE.
[2] No data for CrCl <30 mL/min
[3] Increased risk of bone marrow toxicity

TABLE 17C – ANTIMICROBIAL DOSING IN OBESITY

The number of obese patients is increasing. Intuitively, the standard doses of some drugs may not achieve effective serum concentrations. Pertinent data on anti-infective dosing in the obese patient is gradually emerging. Though some of the data needs further validation, the following table reflects what is currently known. **Obesity is defined as ≥20% over Ideal Body Weight (Ideal BW) or Body Mass Index (BMI) >30. Dose =** suggested body weight (BW) for dose calculation in obese patient, or specific dose if applicable. In general, the absence of a drug in the table indicates a lack of pertinent information in the published literature.

Drug	Dose	Comments
Acyclovir	Use **Adjusted BW** *(see Comments)* Example: for HSV encephalitis, give 10 mg/kg of Adjusted BW q8h	Unpublished data from 7 obese volunteers *(Davis, et al., ICAAC abstract, 1991)* suggested ideal BW, but newer and more convincing PK data suggest that adjusted BW better approximates drug exposure in normals *(AAC 60:1830, 2016)*.
Aminoglycosides	Use **Adjusted BW** Example: Critically ill patient, Gent or Tobra (not Amikacin) 7 mg/kg of Adjusted BW IV q24h *(see Comments)*	Adjusted BW = Ideal BW + 0.4(Actual BW – Ideal BW). Ref: *Pharmacother 27:1081, 2007*. Follow levels so as to lower dose once hemodynamics stabilize.
Anidulafungin	Consider dose increase if wt > 140 kg	PK modeling suggests a 25% increase in load and maintenance dose in pts > 140 kg results in exposure similar to non-obese pts receiving usual dose *(AAC 62:e00063-18, 2018)*.
Cefazolin (surgical prophylaxis)	No dose adjustment may be required: 2 gm x 1 dose (repeat in 3 hours?) *(see Comments)*	Conflicting data; unclear whether dose should be repeated, or if an even higher dose is required. Patients with BMI 40-80 studied. PK: 2-4 gm given to obese pts before c-section yielded inadequate conc in myometrium and subcutaneous adipose tissue despite adequate plasma conc. Refs: *Surg 136:738, 2004; Eur J Clin Pharmacol 67:985, 2011; Surg Infect 13:33, 2012; Pharmacother 37:1415, 2017.*
Cefepime	Modest dose increase: 2 gm IV q8h instead of the usual q12h	Data from 10 patients (mean BMI 48) undergoing bariatric surgery; regimen yields free T > MIC of 60% for MIC of 8 μg/mL. Ref: *Obes Surg 22:465, 2012.*
Cefotetan	No dose adjustment may be required. *(see Comments)*	No difference in surg wound infection rates between 2 and 3 gm prophylaxis doses in patients ≥120 kg, median BMI 42 kg/m² *(Surg Infect 19:504, 2018)*.
Cefoxitin	Larger dose possibly required but data insufficient for a firm recommendation *(see Comments)*	Single 40 mg/kg pre-op dose in obese pts (based on actual BW; range 4-7.5 gm) resulted in suboptimal achievement of pharmacodynamic targets in serum and tissue, although performance was better than a simulated 2 gm dose *(AAC 60:5885, 2016)*.
Clindamycin	Possibly use **Actual BW** *(see Comments)*	Combined PK modeling data from three prospective trials in children suggests actual BW to be most appropriate; no clinical outcome data available *(AAC 61:e02014, 2016)*.
Daptomycin	Use **Actual BW** Example: 4-12 mg/kg of Actual BW IV q24h	Data from a single-dose PK study in 7 obese volunteers. Ref: *Antimicrob Ag Chemother 51:2741, 2007*. New data suggest similar outcomes with ideal BW and actual BW *(AAC 58:88, 2014)*. Fixed, non-weight-based dosing in morbid obesity also suggested by a recent PK study *(Pharmacother 2018 June 15 [Epub ahead of print])*.
Fluconazole	Larger dose possibly required but data insufficient for a firm recommendation *(see Comments)*	Case reports suggest larger dose required in critically ill obese pts. Recent paper suggests that wt-based dosing (12 mg/kg load then 6 mg/kg/day using total BW) reaches desired PK/PD targets more reliably than fixed dosing; clinical validation required *(Pharmacother 17:1023, 1997; AAC 60:6550, 2016)*.

TABLE 17C (2)

Drug	Dose	Comments
Flucytosine	Use **Ideal BW** Example: Crypto meningitis, give 25 mg/kg of Ideal BW po q6h	Date from one obese patient with cryptococcal disease. Ref: *Pharmacother 15:251, 1995.*
Fosfomycin IV	**Unclear if dose adjustment is required, but data are emerging** *(see Comments)*	Lower Cmax (468 vs 594 mcg/mL) and higher Vd (24.4 vs 19 L) in 13 obese surgical patients given 8 gm IV dose x1 compared to non-obese; AUC difference NS but drug exposure significantly lower in sc tissue in obese patients. Difficult to translate to a dosing recommendation *(JAC 2019;74:2335).*
Levofloxacin	**No dose adjustment may be required** Example: 750 mg po/IV q24h *(see Comments)*	Data from 13 obese patients; variability in study findings renders conclusion uncertain. Refs: *AAC 55:3240, 2011; JAC 66:1653, 2011.* A recent PK study (requiring clinical validation) in patients with BMI of 40 or more suggests that higher doses may be necessary to achieve adequate drug exposure *(Clin Pharmacokin 53:753, 2014).*
Linezolid	**No dose adjustment may be required but data are inconsistent** Example: 600 mg po/IV q12h *(see Comments)*	Small numbers of patients have been studied. Data from 20 obese volunteers up to 150 kg body weight suggest standard doses provide AUC values similar to nonobese subjects. In a recent case report, standard dosing in a 265 kg male with MRSA pneumonia seemed to have reduced clinical effectiveness. Refs: *AAC 57:1144, 2013; Ann Pharmacother 47: e25, 2013.* In a PK/PD modeling study in 15 obese patients with MRSA pneumonia (MIC 1-4 µg/ml), standing dosing leads to low probability of target attainment in patients <65 years; clinical meaning is, at present, uncertain *(JAC 2019;74:667).*
Micafungin	Higher dose may be required. *(see Comments)*	PK/PD study suggests 100 mg q24h inadequate; 150 mg q24h adequate for *C. albicans* in pts ≤115 kg, 200 mg q24h in pts >115 kg. 200 mg q24h adequate for *C. glabrata* in pts ≤115 kg *(Crit Care 2018;22:94).* A more recent PK/PD study found that the maintenance dose should be 200 mg q24h in patients >125 kg if the Candida MIC is 0.016 µg/mL, and 300 mg q24h if the MIC is 0.032 µg/mL. A loading dose of twice the maintenance dose is also suggested *(JAC 2019;74:978).*
Oseltamivir	**No dose adjustment may be required** Example: 75 mg po q12h *(see Comments)*	Data from 10 obese volunteers, unclear if applicable to patients >250 kg (OK to give 150 mg po q12h). Ref: *J Antimicrob Chemother 66:2083, 2011.* Newer data consistent *(AAC 58:1616, 2014).*
Piperacillin-tazobactam	6.75 gm IV over 4 hours and dosed every 8 hours. No data for pt with impaired renal function	Data need confirmation. Based on 14 obese patients with actual BW >130 kg and BMI >40 kg/m^2. Ref: *Int J Antimicrob Ag 41:52, 2013.* High dose required to ensure adequate conc of both pip and tazo for pathogens with MIC ≤16 mcg/mL, but enhanced bleeding risk is a concern particularly in renal dysfunction.
Telavancin	If weight is 30% or more over ideal BW, dose using adjusted BW as for aminoglycosides.	The correct dosing weight to use for Telavancin is unclear. Actual BW may overdose and increase nephrotoxicity, ideal BW may underdose *(JAC 67:723, 2012; JAC 67:1300, 2012).* Problematic because serum levels are not routinely available.
Vancomycin	Use **Actual BW** Example: in critically ill patient give 25-30 mg/kg of Actual BW IV load, then 15-20 mg/kg of Actual BW IV q8h-12h (infuse over 1.5-2 hr). No single dose over 2 gm. Check trough levels.	Data from 24 obese patients; Vancomycin half-life appears to decrease with little change in Vd. Ref: *Eur J Clin Pharmacol 54:621, 1998.*
Voriconazole po	**No dose adjustment** required (use **Ideal BW**) *See Comments* Example: 400 mg po q12h x2 doses then 200 mg po q12h. Check trough concentrations (underdosing common with Voriconazole).	Data from a 2-way crossover study of oral Voriconazole in 8 volunteers suggest no adjustment required, but other data support use of adjusted BW. Best for now to use ideal BW and check serum concentrations *(AAC 55:2601, 2011; CID 53:745, 2011; CID 63:286, 2016).*

TABLE 17D – NO DOSING ADJUSTMENT REQUIRED IN OBESITY

The pharmacokinetics of antibacterials in obese patients is emerging, but only selected drugs have been evaluated. Those drugs where data justifies a dose adjustment in the obese are summarized in *Table 17C*. Those drugs where data indicates **NO NEED** for dose adjustment are listed below.

Drug	Drug
Ceftaroline	Imipenem/cilastatin
Ceftazidime/avibactam	Meropenem
Ceftolozane/tazobactam	Moxifloxacin
Dalbavancin	Oritavancin
Doripenem	Tedizolid
Ertapenem	Tigecycline

Ref: *Pharmacotherapy 37:1415, 2017*

TABLE 18 – ANTIMICROBIALS AND HEPATIC DISEASE: DOSAGE ADJUSTMENT*

The following alphabetical list indicates antibacterials excreted/metabolized by the liver **wherein a dosage adjustment may be indicated** in the presence of hepatic disease. Space precludes details; consult the PDR or package inserts for details. List is **not** all-inclusive:

Antibacterials		Antifungals	Antiparasitics	Antivirals§	
Ceftriaxone	Nafcillin	Caspofungin	Antimony, pentavalent	Abacavir	Indinavir
Chloramphenicol	Rifabutin	Itraconazole	Benznidazole	Atazanavir	Lopinavir/Ritonavir
Clindamycin	Rifampin	Voriconazole	Nifurtimox	Darunavir	Nelfinavir
Eravacycline	Synercid**		Praziquantel	Efavirenz	Nevirapine
Fusidic acid	Telithromycin++			Enfuvirtide	Ritonavir
Isoniazid	Tigecycline			Fosamprenavir	
Lefamulin (IV)	Tinidazole				
Metronidazole					

§ Ref. on antiretrovirals: *CID 40:174, 2005* ** Quinupristin-Dalfopristin ++ Telithro: reduce dose in renal & hepatic failure

TABLE 19 – TREATMENT OF CAPD PERITONITIS IN ADULTS

(Adapted from Guidelines – Int'l Soc Peritoneal Dialysis, *Periton Dialysis Intl 2016, 36:481*)

Principles: Empiric antibiotic therapy

- Initiate antibiotics asap after collection of peritoneal fluid & blood for culture
- Empiric regimens must be guided by local susceptibilities
    - Possible gram-positive infection: suggest either Cefazolin or Vanco
    - Possible gram-negative infection: suggest either Cefepime or aminoglycoside, e.g. Gentamicin
- No need to adjust intraperitoneal (IP) dose for residual renal function
- Can treat by IP route or systemic IV therapy, but Guidelines favor IP therapy

Intraperitoneal (IP) therapy

- Can be either continuous (drugs in each exchange) or intermittent (once daily)
- If intermittent, need antibiotic-containing dialysis fluid to dwell for minimum 6 hrs
- Vanco, aminoglycosides, cephalosporins can be combined in same dialysis bag; penicillins and aminoglycosides **cannot** be combined

Specific recommendations

IP Antibiotic Dosing Recommendations for Treatment of Peritonitis

	Intermittent (1 exchange daily)	Continuous (all exchanges)
Aminoglycosides:		
Amikacin	2 mg/kg daily	LD 25 mg/L, MD 12 mg/L
Gentamicin	0.6 mg/kg daily	LD 8 mg/L, MD 4 mg/L
Tobramycin	0.6 mg/kg daily	LD 3 mg/kg, MD 0.3 mg/kg
Cephalosporins:		
Cefazolin	15-20 mg/kg daily	LD 500 mg/L, MD 125 mg/L
Cefepime	1000 mg daily	LD 250-500 mg/L, MD 100-125 mg/L
Ceftazidime	1000-1500 mg daily	LD 500 mg/L, MD 125 mg/L
Ceftriaxone	1000 mg daily	No data
Penicillins:		
Penicillin G	No data	LD 50,000 unit/L, MD 25,000 unit/L
Amoxicillin	No data	MD 150 mg/L
Ampicillin	No data	MD 125 mg/L
Amp/sulb	2 gm/1 gm q12h	LD 750-100 mg/L, MD 100 mg/L
Pip/tazo	No data	LD 4 gm/0.5 gm, MD 1 gm/0.125 gm
Others:		
Aztreonam	2 gm daily	LD 1000 mg/L, MD 250 mg/L
Ciprofloxacin	No data	MD 50 mg/L
Clindamycin	No data	MD 600 mg/bag
Daptomycin	No data	LD 100 mg/L, MD 20 mg/L
Imipenem	500 mg in alternate exch	LD 250 mg/L, MD 50 mg/L
Polymyxin B	No data	MD 300,000 unit (30 mg)/bag
Meropenem	1 gm daily	No data
Teicoplanin	15 mg/kg every 5 days	LD 400 mg/bag, MD 20 mg/bag
Vancomycin	15-30 mg/kg every 5-7 days	LD 30 mg/kg, MD 1.5 mg/kg/bag
Antifungals:		
Fluconazole	IP 200 mg q24-48 hrs	No data
Voriconazole	IP 2.5 mg/kg daily	No data

LD = loading dose in mg; MD = maintenance dose in mg; IP = intraperitoneal
Ref: *Periton Dialysis Intl 2016;36:481*

Systemic dosing recommendations for treatment of CAPD peritonitis

- In general, IP dosing leads to high IP drug levels and, hence, IP is preferable to IV antibiotic administration
- See individual systemic drugs for dose recommendations for patients with end stage renal disease (ESRD)
- Do not co-administer the same drug IP and systemically (either po or IV)

Indications for removal of CAPD catheter

- Relapse with same organism within one month
- No clinical response within 5 days (failure)
- Infection at catheter exit site and/or catheter subcutaneous tunnel
- Fungal peritonitis
- Fecal flora peritonitis; sign of bowel wall erosion & perforation

TABLE 20A – ANTI-TETANUS PROPHYLAXIS, WOUND CLASSIFICATION, IMMUNIZATION

WOUND CLASSIFICATION		
Clinical Features	**Tetanus Prone**	**Non-Tetanus Prone**
Age of wound	>6 hours	≤6 hours
Configuration	Stellate, avulsion	Linear
Depth	>1 cm	≤1 cm
Mechanism of injury	Missile, crush, burn, frostbite	Sharp surface (glass, knife)
Devitalized tissue	Present	Absent
Contaminants (dirt, saliva, etc.)	Present	Absent

IMMUNIZATION SCHEDULE				
History of Tetanus Immunization	**Dirty, Tetanus-Prone Wound**		**Clean, non-Tetanus-Prone Wound**	
	Td[1,2]	Tetanus Immune Globulin	Td[1,2]	Tetanus Immune Globulin
Unknown or <3 doses[3]	Yes	Yes	Yes	No
3 or more doses	No[4]	No	No[5]	No

Ref: *MMWR 60:13, 2011; MMWR 61:468, 2012; MMWR 62:131, 2013 (pregnancy)*

[1] Td = Tetanus & diphtheria toxoids, adsorbed (adult). For adult who has not received Tdap previously, substitute one dose of Tdap for Td when immunization is indicated *(MMWR 61:468, 2012)*.
[2] For children <7 years, use DTaP unless contraindicated; for persons ≥7 years, Td is preferred to tetanus toxoid alone, but single dose of Tdap can be used if required for catch-up series.
[3] Individuals who have not completed vaccine series should do so.
[4] Yes, if >5 years since last booster.
[5] Yes, if >10 years since last booster.

TABLE 20B – RABIES POSTEXPOSURE PROPHYLAXIS

All wounds should be cleaned immediately & thoroughly with soap & water. This has been shown to protect 90% of experimental animals![1]

Exposure to animal saliva or nervous system tissue through a bite, scratch, or contamination of open wounds or mucous membranes *(www.cdc.gov/rabies/exposure/type.html)* or when such exposure cannot be reliably excluded (e.g., bat found in room of sleeping person).

Animal Type	Evaluation & Disposition of Animal	Recommendations for Prophylaxis
Dogs, cats, ferrets	Healthy & available for 10-day observation	Don't start unless animal develops sx, then immediately begin HRIG + vaccine
	Rabid or suspected rabid	Immediate HRIG + vaccine
	Unknown (escaped)	Consult public health officials
Skunks, raccoons, *bats, foxes, coyotes, most carnivores	Regard as rabid	Immediate prophylaxis unless brain of animal tests negative for rabies virus
Livestock, horses, rodents, rabbits; includes hares, squirrels, hamsters, guinea pigs, gerbils, chipmunks, rats, mice, woodchucks	Consider case-by-case	Consult public health officials. Bites of squirrels, hamsters, guinea pigs, gerbils, chipmunks, rats, mice, other small rodents, rabbits, and hares **almost never** require rabies post-exposure prophylaxis.

* Most recent cases of human rabies in U.S. due to contact (not bites) with silver-haired bats or rarely big brown bats but risk of acquiring rabies from non-contact bat exposure is exceedingly low *(CID 48:1493, 2009)*. For more detail, *see CID 30:4, 2000; JAVMA 219:1687, 2001; CID 37:96, 2003 (travel medicine advisory); Ln 363:959, 2004; EID 11:1921, 2005; MMWR 55 (RR-5), 2006.*

Postexposure Rabies Immunization Schedule

IF NOT PREVIOUSLY VACCINATED

Treatment	Regimen[2]
Local wound cleaning	**All postexposure treatment should begin with immediate, thorough cleaning of all wounds with soap & water.** Then irrigate with a virucidal agent such as povidone-iodine solution if available.
Human rabies immune globulin (HRIG)	20 IU per kg body weight given once on day 0. If anatomically feasible, the full dose should be infiltrated around the wound(s), the rest should be administered IM in the gluteal area. If the calculated dose of HRIG is insufficient to inject all the wounds, it should be diluted with normal saline to allow infiltration around additional wound areas. HRIG should **not** be administered in the **same syringe, or** into the **same anatomical site** as vaccine, or more than 7 days after the initiation of vaccine. Because HRIG may partially suppress active production of antibody, no more than the recommended dose should be given.[3]
Vaccine	Human diploid cell vaccine (HDCV), rabies vaccine adsorbed (RVA), or purified chick embryo cell vaccine (PCECV) 1 mL **IM (deltoid area[4])**, one each days 0, 3, 7, 14[5].

IF PREVIOUSLY VACCINATED[6]

Treatment	Regimen[2]
Local wound cleaning	All postexposure treatment should begin with immediate, thorough cleaning of all wounds with soap & water. Then irrigate with a virucidal agent such as povidone-iodine solution if available.
HRIG	HRIG should **not** be administered
Vaccine	HDCV or PCEC, 1 mL **IM (deltoid area[4])**, one each on days 0 & 3

CORRECT VACCINE ADMINISTRATION SITES

Age Group	Administration Site
Children & adults	**DELTOID[4]** only (**NEVER** in gluteus)
Infants & young children	Outer aspect of thigh (anterolateral thigh) may be used (**NEVER** in gluteus)

1 From *MMWR 48:RR-1, 1999; CID 30:4, 2000*; B. T. Matyas, Mass. Dept. of Public Health. *MMWR 57:1, 2008*
2 These regimens are applicable for all age groups, including children.
3 In most reported post-exposure treatment failures, only identified deficiency was failure to infiltrate wound(s) with HRIG *(CID 22:228, 1996)*. However, several failures reported from SE Asia in patients in whom WHO protocol followed *(CID 28:143, 1999)*.
4 The **deltoid** area is the **only** acceptable site of vaccination for adults & older children. For infants & young children, outer aspect of the thigh (anterolateral thigh) may be used. Vaccine should **NEVER** be administered in gluteal area.
5 Note that this is a change from previous recommendation of 5 doses (days 0, 3, 7, 14 & 28) based on new data & recommendations from ACIP. Note that the number of doses for persons with altered immunocompetence remains unchanged (5 doses on days 0, 3, 7, 14 & 28) and recommendations for pre-exposure prophylaxis remain 3 doses administered on days 0, 7 and 21 or 28 *(MMWR 59 (RR-2), 2010)*.
6 Any person with a history of pre-exposure vaccination with HDCV, RVA, PCECV; prior post-exposure prophylaxis with HDCV, PCEC or rabies vaccine adsorbed (RVA); or previous vaccination with any other type of rabies vaccine & a documented history of antibody response to the prior vaccination.

TABLE 21 - SELECTED DIRECTORY OF RESOURCES

ORGANIZATION	PHONE/FAX	WEBSITE(S)
ANTIPARASITIC DRUGS & PARASITOLOGY INFORMATION		
CDC Drug Line	Weekdays: 404-639-3670 Evenings, weekends, holidays: 404-639-2888	http://www.cdc.gov/ncidod/srp/drugs/drug-service.html
DPDx: Lab ID of parasites		www.dpd.cdc.gov/dpdx/default.htm
Malaria	daytime: 770-488-7788 other: 770-488-7100 US toll free: 855-856-4713	www.cdc.gov/malaria
Expert Compound. Pharm.	800-247-9767/Fax: 818-787-7256	www.expertpharmacy.org
World Health Organization (WHO)		www.who.int
Parasites & Health		www.dpd.cdc.gov/dpdx/HTML/Para_Health.htm
BIOTERRORISM		
Centers for Disease Control & Prevention	770-488-7100	www.bt.cdc.gov
Infectious Diseases Society of America	703-299-0200	www.idsociety.org
Johns Hopkins Center Civilian Biodefense		www.jhsph.edu
Center for Biosecurity of the Univ. of Pittsburgh Med. Center		www.upmc-biosecurity.org
US Army Medical Research Institute of Inf. Dis.		www.usamriid.army.mil
HEPATITIS B		
Hepatitis B Foundation		www.hepb.org, www.natap.org
HEPATITIS C		
CDC		www.cdc.gov/ncidod/diseases/hepatitis/C
Individual		http://hepatitis-central.com www.natap.org
HCV Guidelines		www.hcvguidelines.org
HIV		
General		
HIV InSite		http://hivinsite.ucsf.edu www.natap.org
European AIDS Clinical Society (EACS) Guidelines		https://eacs.sanfordguide.com
Drug Interactions		
Liverpool HIV Pharm. Group		www.hiv-druginteractions.org
Other		http://AIDS.medscape.com
Prophylaxis/Treatment of Opportunistic Infections; HIV Treatment		www.aidsinfo.nih.gov
IMMUNIZATIONS		
CDC, Natl. Immunization Program	404-639-8200	www.cdc.gov/vaccines/
FDA, Vaccine Adverse Events	800-822-7967	www.fda.gov/cber/vaers/vaers.htm
National Network Immunization Info.	877-341-6644	www.immunizationinfo.org
Influenza vaccine, CDC	404-639-8200	www.cdc.gov/vaccines/
Institute for Vaccine Safety		www.vaccinesafety.edu
Immunization, "Ask the experts"		www.immunize.org/asktheexperts
OCCUPATIONAL EXPOSURE, BLOOD-BORNE PATHOGENS (HIV, HEPATITIS B & C)		
Clinicians Consultation Center	888-448-4911	www.ucsf.edu/hivcntr
PEPline (exposed clinicians)		
WARMline (clinicians of HIV pts)		
Perinatal HIV Hotline	888-448-8765	www.ucsf.edu/hivcntr
Q-T$_c$ INTERVAL PROLONGATION BY DRUGS		www.qtdrugs.org; www.crediblemeds.org
TRAVELERS' INFO: Immunizations, Malaria Prophylaxis, More		
Amer. Soc. Trop. Med. & Hyg.		www.astmh.org
CDC, general	877-394-8747	http://www.cdc.gov/travel/default.asp
CDC, Malaria:		www.cdc.gov/malaria
Prophylaxis		http://www.cdc.gov/travel/default.asp
Medical Considerations Before Int'l Travel		*Med Lett 61:153, 2019*
Pan American Health Organization		www.paho.org
World Health Organization (WHO)		www.who.int/home-page

TABLE 22A – ANTI-INFECTIVE DRUG-DRUG INTERACTIONS

For HIV drug-drug interactions, see: *https://www.hiv-druginteractions.org/*. For Hepatitis C drug-drug interactions, see *https://www.hep-druginteractions.org/checker*

Anti-Infective agent	Other Drug	Effect on concentration (or other effect)	Suggested management
Abacavir	Methadone	↓ methadone	Monitor, adjust dosage
Amantadine	Alcohol	↑ CNS effects	Monitor
	Anticholinergic agents	↑ anticholinergic effects	Monitor
	Digoxin	↑ digoxin	Monitor, adjust dosage
Aminoglycosides (parenteral)	Amphotericin B (deoxycholate, lipid forms)	↑ nephrotoxicity	Avoid co-administration
	Cisplatin	↑ nephrotoxicity, ototoxicity	Avoid co-administration
	Cyclosporine	↑ nephrotoxicity	Avoid co-administration
	Furosemide	↑ ototoxicity	Monitor
	Neuromuscular blocking agents	↑ apnea or respiratory paralysis	Monitor
	NSAIDs	↑ nephrotoxicity	Monitor
	Non-polarizing muscle relaxants	↑ apnea	Monitor
	Radiographic contrast	↑ nephrotoxicity	Monitor
	Vancomycin	↑ nephrotoxicity	Avoid co-administration
Aminoglycosides (oral)(kanamycin, neomycin)	Warfarin	↑ warfarin	Monitor INR, adjust dosage
Ampho B (deoxycholate, lipid forms)	Digoxin	↑ toxicity of digoxin if pt hypokalemic	Monitor
Amoxicillin, ampicillin	Allopurinol	↑ frequency of rash	Monitor

Antiretroviral Drug Combinations

Combivir	Dovato	Cimduo	Odefsey	Atripla	Juluca	Biktarvy	Descovy	Delstrigo	Genvoya	Symfi (Lo)	Triumeq	Stribild	Truvada	Evotaz	Prezcobix	Trizivir	Temixys	Other Drug	Effect on concentration (or other effect)	Suggested management
									x			x		x	x			Alfuzosin	↑ alfuzosin	Contraindicated
														x	x			Amiodarone	↑ amiodarone	Monitor, adjust dosage
						x			x			x						Antacids	↓ INSTI component	Separate administration by 4 hr
	x										x							Antacids	↓ dolutegravir	Give ARVs 2 h pre, 6 h post
			x		x													Antacids	↓ dolutegravir and/or ↓ rilpivirine	Separate administration by 4-6 hr
														x				Antacids	↓ atazanavir	Give Evotaz 2 hr pre or post
									x			x						Antiarrhythmic agents	↑ antiarrhythmic agent	Monitor, adjust dosage
														x	x			Apixaban	↑ apixaban	Avoid co-administration
				x						x								Artemether-lumefantrine	↓ artemether, ↓ DHA, ↓ lumefantrine	Avoid co-administration
															x			Artemether-lumefantrine	Effect uncertain	Monitor
		x		x									x				x	Atazanavir/ritonavir	↓ atazanavir, ↑ tenofovir	Monitor or avoid
									x					x				Atorvastatin	↑ atorvastatin	Monitor, adjust dosage
												x			x			Atorvastatin	↑ atorvastatin	Max atorvastatin 20 mg daily
				x						x								Atorvastatin	↓ atorvastatin	Monitor, adjust dosage
x																x		Atovaquone	↑ zidovudine	Monitor

TABLE 22A (2)

Antiretroviral Drug Combinations *(continued)*

Combivir	Dovato	Cimduo	Odefsey	Atripla	Juluca	Biktarvy	Descovy	Delstrigo	Genvoya	Symfi (Lo)	Triumeq	Stribild	Truvada	Evotaz	Prezcobix	Trizivir	Temixys	Other Drug	Effect on concentration (or other effect)	Suggested management
				x						x								Atovaquone-proguanil	↓ atovaquone, ↓ proguanil	Avoid co-administration
														x	x			Avanafil	↑ avanafil	Avoid co-administration
									x			x		x	x			Beta blockers	↑ beta blockers	Monitor, adjust dosage
									x			x						Bosentan	↑ bosentan	Monitor, adjust dosage
														x	x			Bosentan	↓ protease inhibitor, ↓ cobicistat, ↑ bosentan	Monitor, adjust dosage
									x			x						Buprenorphine	↑ buprenorphine	Monitor, adjust dosage
														x	x			Buprenorphine/naloxone	Effect uncertain	Monitor, adjust dosage
				x						x								Bupropion	↓ bupropion	Monitor, adjust dosage
									x			x		x	x			Buspirone	↑ buspirone	Monitor, adjust dosage
						x												Calcium/iron containing supplements	↓ bictegravir	Take drug + supps w/food
	x										x							Calcium/iron containing supplements	↓ dolutegravir	Give ARVs 2 h pre, 6 h post
									x			x						Calcium/iron containing supplements	↓ elvitegravir	Separate admin by 4 hr
									x			x		x	x			Calcium channel blockers	↑ calcium channel blocker	Monitor, adjust dosage
										x								Calcium channel blockers	↓ calcium channel blocker	Monitor, adjust dosage
									x			x						Carbamazepine	↓ INSTI, ↓ cobicistat (↓ TAF in Genvoya)	Contraindicated
						x	x											Carbamazepine	↓ bictegravir and/or ↓ TAF	Avoid co-administration
				x						x								Carbamazepine	↓ carbamazepine, ↓ efavirenz	Avoid co-administration
	x										x							Carbamazepine	↓ dolutegravir	Give extra 50 mg DTG daily
			x		x													Carbamazepine	↓ dolutegravir and/or ↓ rilpivirine	Contraindicated
														x	x			Carbamazepine	↓ protease inhibitor, ↓ cobicistat	Contraindicated
								x										Carbamazepine	↓ doravirine	Contraindicated
									x			x						Clarithromycin	↑ clarithromycin and/or ↑ cobicistat	Monitor, adjust dosage
				x						x								Clarithromycin	↓ clarithromycin, ↑ 14-OH metabolite	Avoid co-administration
			x		x													Clarithromycin	↑ rilpivirine	Avoid co-administration
														x	x			Clarithromycin	↑ protease inhibitor, ↑ cobicistat, ↑ clarithromycin	Avoid co-administration
												x		x	x			Clonazepam	↑ clonazepam	Monitor
												x						Clorazepate	↑ clorazepate	Monitor, adjust dosage
									x			x		x	x			Colchicine	↑ colchicine	Adjust dosage or avoid
									x									Corticosteroids (not dex)	↑ corticosteroid	Use non-3A4 substrate steroids
									x			x						Cyclosporine	↑ cyclosporine, ↑ EVG, ↑ cobicistat	Monitor, adjust dosage
				x														Cyclosporine	↓ cyclosporine	Monitor, adjust dosage
														x	x			Cyclosporine	↑ cyclosporine	Monitor, adjust dosage
														x	x			Dabigatran	↑ dabigatran	Avoid co-administration

TABLE 22A (3)

Antiretroviral Drug Combinations *(continued)*

Combivir	Dovato	Cimduo	Odefsey	Atripla	Juluca	Biktarvy	Descovy	Delstrigo	Genvoya	Symfi (Lo)	Triumeq	Stribild	Truvada	Evotaz	Prezcobix	Trizivir	Temixys	Other Drug	Effect on concentration (or other effect)	Suggested management
		x											x				x	Darunavir/ritonavir	↑ tenofovir	Monitor
														x	x			Dasatinib	↑ dasatinib	Monitor, adjust dosage
									x			x						Dexamethasone	↑ dexamethasone, ↓ EVG, ↓ cobicistat	Consider alternative steroid
			x		x													Dexamethasone	↓ rilpivirine	Contraindicated
														x	x			Dexamethasone	↓ protease inhibitor, ↓ cobicistat, ↑ dexamethasone	Avoid co-administration
									x			x		x	x			Diazepam	↑ diazepam	Monitor, adjust dosage
													x				x	Didanosine	↑ didanosine	Monitor, adjust dosage
														x	x			Didanosine EC	↓ protease inhibitor, ↓ didanosine	Separate administration by 2 hr
									x			x		x	x			Digoxin	↑ digoxin	Monitor, adjust dosage
				x														Diltiazem	↓ diltiazem, metabolites	Monitor, adjust dosage
														x	x			Disopyramide	↑ disopyramide	Monitor
	x				x	x												Dofetilide	↑ dofetilide	Contraindicated
x																x		Doxorubicin	Antagonistic with zidovudine in vitro	Avoid co-administration
														x	x			Dronedarone	↑ dronedarone	Contraindicated
									x									Drospirenone	↑ drospirenone	Monitor, adjust dosage
											x							Efavirenz	↓ dolutegravir	Give extra 50 mg DTG daily
														x	x			Efavirenz	↓ protease inhibitor, ↓ cobicistat	Avoid co-administration
														x	x			Elbasvir/grazoprevir	↑ grazoprevir	Contraindicated
								x										Enzalutamide	↓ doravirine	Contraindicated
									x			x		x	x			Ergot derivatives	↑ ergot derivatives	Contraindicated
			x		x													Erythromycin	↑ rilpivirine	Avoid co-administration
														x	x			Erythromycin	↑ protease inhibitor, ↑ cobicistat, ↑ erythromycin	Avoid co-administration
														x	x			Eslicarbazepine	↓ protease inhibitor, ↓ cobicistat	Monitor or avoid
												x			x			Estazolam	↑ estazolam	Monitor, adjust dosage
									x									Ethinyl estradiol	↓ ethinyl estradiol	Monitor, adjust dosage
									x			x						Ethosuximide	↑ ethosuximide, ↓ EVG, ↓ cobicistat (Gen: ↓ TAF)	Monitor, adjust dosage
														x	x			Etravirine	↓ protease inhibitor, ↓ cobicistat	Avoid co-administration
														x	x			Everolimus	↑ everolimus	Avoid co-administration
														x	x			Fentanyl	↑ fentanyl	Monitor, adjust dosage
														x	x			Flecainide	↑ flecainide	Monitor
			x															Fluconazole	↑ rilpivirine, ↑ TAF	Monitor
x																x		Fluconazole	↑ zidovudine	Monitor
												x						Flurazepam	↑ flurazepam	Monitor, adjust dosage

TABLE 22A (4)

Antiretroviral Drug Combinations *(continued)*

Combivir	Dovato	Cimduo	Odefsey	Atripla	Juluca	Biktarvy	Descovy	Delstrigo	Genvoya	Symfi (Lo)	Triumeq	Stribild	Truvada	Evotaz	Prezcobix	Trizivir	Temixys	Other Drug	Effect on concentration (or other effect)	Suggested management
														x	x			Fluvastatin	↑ fluvastatin	Monitor, adjust dosage
											x							Fosamprenavir/ritonavir	↓ dolutegravir	Give extra 50 mg DTG daily
			x		x													H2-antagonists	↓ rilpivirine	Give H2 12 hr pre or 4 hr post
														x				H2-antagonists	↓ atazanavir (because of ↑ pH)	Limit H2 dose (see PI)
									x			x			x			Hormonal contraceptives	↓ ethinyl estradiol, ↑ progestogen	Use non-hormonal method
				x														Hormonal contraceptives	↓ ethinyl estradiol and/or ↓ progestogen	Use non-hormonal method
														x				Hormonal contraceptives	Effect uncertain	Use non-hormonal method
														x				Indinavir	Hyperbilirubinemia	Contraindicated
x																x		Indomethacin	↑ zidovudine toxic metabolite	Monitor
														x	x			Inhaled/nasal steroids	↑ steroid (if a CYP3A4 substrate)	Avoid co-administration
	x				x													Iron (oral)	↓ dolutegravir	Separate administration by 4-6 hr
														x				Irinotecan	↑ irinotecan	Contraindicated
									x			x						Itraconazole	↑ itraconazole, ↑ EVG, ↑ cobicistat	Max itra dose 200 mg qd
				x						x								Itraconazole	↓ itraconazole, ↓ OH-itraconazole	Avoid co-administration
			x															Itraconazole	↑ rilpivirine, ↑ TAF	Monitor
														x	x			Itraconazole	↑ protease inhibitor, ↑ cobicistat, ↑ itraconazole	Avoid co-administration
									x			x						Ketoconazole	↑ ketoconazole, ↑ EVG, ↑ cobicistat	Max keto dose 200 mg qd
				x														Ketoconazole	↓ ketoconazole	Monitor, adjust dosage
			x															Ketoconazole	↑ rilpivirine, ↑ TAF, ↓ ketoconazole	Monitor
														x	x			Ketoconazole	↑ protease inhibitor, ↑ cobicistat, ↑ ketoconazole	Avoid co-administration
														x				Lamotrigine	Effect uncertain	Monitor
												x						Ledipasvir/sofosbuvir	↑ tenofovir	Avoid co-administration
		x		x				x					x				x	Ledipasvir/sofosbuvir	↑ tenofovir	Monitor or avoid
														x	x			Lidocaine	↑ lidocaine	Monitor, adjust dosage
				x														Lopinavir/ritonavir	↓ lopinavir, ↑ tenofovir	Monitor, adjust dosage
		x											x				x	Lopinavir/ritonavir	↑ tenofovir	Monitor
									x			x		x	x			Lovastatin	↑ lovastatin	Contraindicated
									x			x		x	x			Lurasidone	↑ lurasidone	Contraindicated
				x														Maraviroc	↓ maraviroc	See maraviroc PI for help
														x	x			Maraviroc	↑ maraviroc	Consider MVC 150 mg bid
	x				x	x					x							Metformin	↑ metformin	Monitor, adjust dosage
			x	x	x					x	x							Methadone	↓ methadone	Monitor, adjust dosage
x																		Methadone	↑ zidovudine	Monitor

TABLE 22A (5)

Anti-Infective agent																		Other Drug	Effect on concentration (or other effect)	Suggested management
Antiretroviral Drug Combinations *(continued)*																				
Combivir	Dovato	Cimduo	Odefsey	Atripla	Juluca	Biktarvy	Descovy	Delstrigo	Genvoya	Symfi (Lo)	Triumeq	Stribild	Truvada	Evotaz	Prezcobix	Trizivir	Temixys			
																x		Methadone	↑ zidovudine, ↓ methadone	Monitor, adjust methadone
														x	x			Methadone	Effect uncertain	Monitor, adjust dosage
														x	x			Mexiletine	↑ mexiletine	Monitor
									x			x		x	x			Midazolam (IV)	↑ midazolam	Monitor, adjust dosage
									x			x		x	x			Midazolam (po)	↑ midazolam	Contraindicated
								x										Mitotane	↓ doravirine	Contraindicated
									x									Naloxone	↓ naloxone	Monitor
x																x		Nelfinavir	↓ zidovudine	Monitor
											x							Nevirapine	↓ dolutegravir	Avoid co-administration
														x	x			Nevirapine	↑ nevirapine, ↓ protease inhibitor?	Contraindicated
														x	x			Nilotinib	↑ nilotinib	Monitor, adjust dosage
														x				Omeprazole	↓ atazanavir (because of ↑ pH)	Limit omeprazole dose or avoid
									x			x						Oxcarbazepine	↓ elvitegravir, ↓ cobicistat	Use different anticonvulsant
	x					x	x				x							Oxcarbazepine	↓ INSTI and/or ↓ TAF	Avoid co-administration
			x		x													Oxcarbazepine	↓ dolutegravir and/or↓ rilpivirine	Contraindicated
														x	x			Oxcarbazepine	↓ protease inhibitor?, ↓ cobicistat	Monitor or avoid
								x										Oxcarbazepine	↓ doravirine	Contraindicated
															x			Oxycodone	↑ oxycodone	Monitor, adjust dosage
									x			x		x	x			Perphenazine	↑ perphenazine	Monitor, adjust dosage
									x			x						Phenobarbital	↓ EVG, ↓ cobicistat (Gen: ↓ TAF)	Contraindicated
														x	x			Phenobarbital	↓ protease inhibitor, ↓ cobicistat?	Contraindicated
				x														Phenobarbital	↓ phenobarbital, ↓ efavirenz	Monitor, adjust dosage
	x					x	x				x							Phenobarbital	↓ INSTI and/or ↓ TAF	Avoid co-administration
			x		x			x										Phenobarbital	↓ dolutegravir and/or ↓ NNRTI	Contraindicated
									x			x						Phenytoin	↓ EVG, ↓ cobicistat (Gen: ↓ TAF)	Contraindicated
				x														Phenytoin	↓ phenytoin, ↓ efavirenz	Monitor, adjust dosage
	x					x	x				x							Phenytoin	↓ INSTI and/or ↓ TAF	Avoid co-administration
			x		x													Phenytoin	↓ dolutegravir and/or ↓ rilpivirine	Contraindicated
														x	x			Phenytoin	↓ protease inhibitor, ↓ cobicistat?	Contraindicated
								x										Phenytoin	↓ doravirine	Contraindicated
									x			x		x	x			Pimozide	↑ pimozide	Contraindicated
				x						x								Posaconazole	↓ posaconazole	Avoid co-administration
			x															Posaconazole	↑ rilpivirine, ↑ TAF	Monitor

TABLE 22A (6)

Antiretroviral Drug Combinations *(continued)*

Combivir	Dovato	Cimduo	Odefsey	Atripla	Juluca	Biktarvy	Descovy	Delstrigo	Genvoya	Symfi (Lo)	Triumeq	Stribild	Truvada	Evotaz	Prezcobix	Trizivir	Temixys	Other Drug	Effect on concentration (or other effect)	Suggested management
				x						x								Pravastatin	↓ pravastatin	Monitor, adjust dosage
														x	x			Pravastatin	↑ pravastatin	Monitor, adjust dosage
x																x		Probenecid	↑ zidovudine	Monitor
														x	x			Propafenone	↑ propafenone	Monitor
			x		x													Proton-pump inhibitors	↓ rilpivirine	Contraindicated
									x			x		x	x			Quetiapine	↑ quetiapine	Adjust dosage or avoid
														x	x			Quinidine	↑ quinidine	Monitor, adjust dosage
				x														Raltegravir	↓ raltegravir	Monitor
														x	x			Ranolazine	↑ ranolazine	Contraindicated
x																x		Ribavirin	↑ anemia	Avoid co-administration
						x	x		x			x						Rifabutin	↓ INSTI and/or ↓ cobi and/or ↓ TAF	Avoid co-administration
														x	x			Rifabutin	↑ rifabutin	Monitor, adjust dosage
				x						x								Rifabutin	↓ rifabutin	↑ rif dosage by 50-100%
					x													Rifabutin	↓ rilpivirine	Give extra 25 mg RPV daily
			x															Rifabutin	↓ rilpivirine, ↓ TAF	Avoid co-administration
								x										Rifabutin	↓ doravirine	Extra 100 mg DOR 12 hr post
			x		x	x		x	x			x						Rifampin	↓ INSTI and/or ↓ NNRTI and/or ↓ cobi and/or ↓ TAF	Contraindicated
							x											Rifampin	↓ TAF	Avoid co-administration
	x										x							Rifampin	↓ dolutegravir	Give extra 50 mg DTG daily
										x								Rifampin	↓ efavirenz	Avoid co-administration
				x														Rifampin	↓ efavirenz	Consider extra efavirenz
x																x		Rifampin	↓ zidovudine	Monitor
														x	x			Rifampin	↓ protease inhibitor, ↓ cobicistat?	Contraindicated
						x	x		x			x						Rifapentine	↓ INSTI and/or ↓ cobicistat and/or ↓ TAF	Avoid co-administration
			x		x			x										Rifapentine	↓ dolutegravir and/or ↓ NNRTI	Contraindicated
															x			Rifapentine	↓ darunavir	Avoid co-administration
									x			x		x	x			Risperidone	↑ risperidone	Monitor, adjust dosage
														x	x			Rivaroxaban	↑ rivaroxaban	Avoid co-administration
														x				Rosuvastatin	↑ rosuvastatin	Max rosuva 10 mg daily
															x			Rosuvastatin	↑ rosuvastatin	Max rosuva 20 mg daily
									x			x		x	x			Salmeterol	↑ salmeterol	Avoid co-administration
				x						x								Sertraline	↓ sertraline	Monitor, adjust dosage
									x			x		x	x			Sildenafil (for ED)	↑ sildenafil	Monitor, adjust dosage

TABLE 22A (7)

Antiretroviral Drug Combinations *(continued)*

Combivir	Dovato	Cimduo	Odefsey	Atripla	Juluca	Biktarvy	Descovy	Delstrigo	Genvoya	Symfi (Lo)	Triumeq	Stribild	Truvada	Evotaz	Prezcobix	Trizivir	Temixys	Other Drug	Effect on concentration (or other effect)	Suggested management
									x			x		x	x			Sildenafil (for PAH)	↑ sildenafil	Contraindicated
				x						x								Simeprevir	↓ simeprevir	Avoid co-administration
														x	x			Simeprevir	↑ simeprevir	Avoid co-administration
									x			x		x	x			Simvastatin	↑ simvastatin	Contraindicated
										x								Simvastatin	↓ simvastatin	Monitor, adjust dosage
									x			x		x	x			Sirolimus	↑ sirolimus	Monitor, adjust dosage
				x														Sirolimus	↓ sirolimus	Monitor, adjust dosage
		x						x				x	x				x	Sofosbuvir/velpatasvir	↑ tenofovir	Monitor or avoid
				x														Sofosbuvir/velpatasvir	↑ tenofovir, ↓ velpatasvir	Avoid co-administration
													x				x	Sofosbuvir/velpatasvir/voxilaprevir	↑ tenofovir	Monitor
	x							x										Sorbitol	↓ lamivudine	Avoid co-administration
									x			x						SSRIs (not sertraline)	↑ SSRI	Monitor, adjust dosage
														x	x			SSRIs	Effect uncertain	Monitor, adjust dosage
			x		x			x	x			x						St. John's wort	↓ INSTI and/or ↓ NNRTI and/or ↓ cobicistat and/or ↓ TAF	Contraindicated
	x					x	x				x							St. John's wort	↓ INSTI and/or ↓ TAF	Avoid co-administration
														x	x			St. John's wort	↓ protease inhibitor, ↓ cobicistat?	Contraindicated
	x										x							Sucralfate	↓ dolutegravir	Give ARVs 2 h pre, 6 h post
									x			x		x	x			Tacrolimus	↑ tacrolimus	Monitor, adjust dosage
				x														Tacrolimus	↓ tacrolimus	Monitor, adjust dosage
									x			x		x	x			Tadalafil (for PAH)	↑ tadalafil	Monitor, adjust dosage
												x		x	x			Tadalafil (for ED)	↑ tadalafil	Monitor, limit tadalafil dosage
			x															Telithromycin	↑ rilpivirine	Avoid co-administration
														x	x			Telithromycin	↑ protease inhibitor, ↑ cobicistat, ↑ telithromycin	Avoid co-administration
														x				Tenofovir	↓ atazanavir, ↑ tenofovir	Monitor
									x			x		x	x			Thioridazine	↑ thioridazine	Monitor, adjust dosage
															x			Ticagrelor	↑ ticagrelor	Avoid co-administration
							x											Tipranavir/ritonavir	↓ TAF	Avoid co-administration
											x							Tipranavir/ritonavir	↓ dolutegravir	Give extra 50 mg DTG daily
x																x		TMP-SMX	↑ zidovudine	Monitor
														x	x			Tramadol	↑ tramadol	Monitor, adjust dosage
									x			x		x	x			Trazodone	↑ trazodone	Monitor, adjust dosage
									x			x		x	x			Triazolam	↑ triazolam	Contraindicated
									x			x		x	x			Tricyclic antidepressants	↑ TCA	Monitor, adjust dosage

TABLE 22A (8)

Anti-Infective agent																		Other Drug	Effect on concentration (or other effect)	Suggested management
Antiretroviral Drug Combinations *(continued)*																				
Combivir	Dovato	Cimduo	Odefsey	Atripla	Juluca	Biktarvy	Descovy	Delstrigo	Genvoya	Symfi (Lo)	Triumeq	Stribild	Truvada	Evotaz	Prezcobix	Trizivir	Temixys			
																	x	Trimethoprim	↑ lamivudine	Monitor (no dose adjustment)
x																x		Valproic acid	↑ zidovudine	Monitor
									x			x		x	x			Vardenafil (for ED)	↑ vardenafil	Monitor, adjust dosage
														x	x			Vinblastine	↑ vinblastine	Monitor, avoid if necessary
														x	x			Vincristine	↑ vincristine	Monitor, avoid if necessary
									x			x						Voriconazole	↑ voriconazole, ↑ EVG, ↑ cobicistat	Avoid co-administration
				x														Voriconazole	↑ voriconazole, ↑ efavirenz	Contraindicated
														x				Voriconazole	↑ atazanavir, ↑ cobicistat, ↑↓ voriconazole	Avoid co-administration
															x			Voriconazole	Effect uncertain	Avoid co-administration
				x					x	x		x		x	x			Warfarin	Effect uncertain	Monitor INR, adjust dosage
									x			x		x	x			Zolpidem	↑ zolpidem	Monitor, adjust dosage
Artemether-lumefantrine																		Amitriptyline	↑ amitriptyline, ↑ QT interval	Avoid co-administration
																		Carbamazepine	↓ artemether, ↓ DHA, ↓ lumefantrine	Contraindicated
																		Clomipramine	↑ clomipramine, ↑ QT interval	Avoid co-administration
																		Drugs that ↑ QT interval	↑ QT interval	Avoid co-administration
																		Flecainide	↑ flecainide, ↑ QT interval	Avoid co-administration
																		Hormonal contraceptives	↓ effectiveness	Use alternative method
																		Imipramine	↑ imipramine, ↑ QT interval	Avoid co-administration
																		Ketoconazole	↑ artemether, ↑ DHA, ↑ lumefantrine	Monitor, avoid if possible
																		Mefloquine (prior use)	↓ lumefantrine	Monitor, encourage food
																		NNRTI (HIV)	↑↓ artemether, ↑↓ DHA, ↑↓ lumefantrine	Monitor, avoid if possible
																		Phenytoin	↓ artemether, ↓ DHA, ↓ lumefantrine	Contraindicated
																		Protease inhibitors (HIV)	↑↓ artemether, ↑↓ DHA, ↑↓ lumefantrine	Monitor, avoid if possible
																		Rifampin	↓ artemether, ↓ DHA, ↓ lumefantrine	Contraindicated
																		St. John's wort	↓ artemether, ↓ DHA, ↓ lumefantrine	Contraindicated
Atovaquone																		Metoclopramide	↓ atovaquone	Monitor, adjust dosage
																		Tetracycline	↓ atovaquone	Monitor, adjust dosage

TABLE 22A (9)

Anti-Infective agent						Other Drug	Effect on concentration (or other effect)	Suggested management
Azole antifungal agents								
Fluconazole	Isavuconazole	Itraconazole	Ketoconazole	Posaconazole	Voriconazole			
x		x				Amitriptyline	↑ amitriptyline	Monitor, adjust dosage
	x					Atorvastatin	↑ atorvastatin	Monitor, adjust dosage
	x					Bupropion	↓ bupropion	Monitor, adjust dosage
x		x	x		x	Calcium channel blockers	↑ calcium channel blocker	Monitor, adjust dosage
	x	x	x		x	Carbamazepine	↓ azole	Avoid co-administration
x	x	x	x	x	x	Cyclosporine	↑ cyclosporine	Monitor, adjust dosage
		x	x			Didanosine	↓ absorption of azole	Avoid co-administration
	x			x		Digoxin	↑ digoxin	Monitor, adjust dosage
		x				Efavirenz	↓ Itraconazole, ↑ Efavirenz	Avoid co-administration
			x			Efavirenz	↓ Ketoconazole, ↑ Efavirenz	Avoid co-administration
				x		Efavirenz	↓ Posaconazole, ↑ Efavirenz	Avoid co-administration
					x	Efavirenz	↓ Voriconazole, ↑ Efavirenz	Avoid co-administration
		x	x	x		H2 blockers, antacids, sucralfate	↓ absorption of azole	Avoid co-administration
x		x	x	x	x	Phenytoin	↑ phenytoin, ↓ azole	Monitor, adjust dosage
		x	x			Isoniazid	↓ azole	Monitor, adjust dosage
	x					Lopinavir/ritonavir	↑ azole, ↑ lopinavir/ritonavir	Avoid co-administration
		x	x	x	x	Lovastatin, simvastatin	↑ statin	Monitor, adjust dosage
		x	x			Maraviroc	↑ maraviroc	Avoid co-administration
					x	Methadone	↑ methadone	Monitor, adjust dosage
				x		Metoclopramide	↓ posaconazole (susp form only)	Monitor, adjust dosage
x	x	x	x	x	x	Midazolam, triazolam	↑ midazolam, triazolam	Monitor, adjust dosage
	x					Mycophenolate	↑ mycophenolate	Monitor, adjust dosage
x		x			x	Oral hypoglycemics	↑ oral hypoglycemic	Monitor, adjust dosage
				x	x	Pimozide	↑ pimozide	Avoid co-administration
		x	x		x	Protease inhibitors	↑ protease inhibitor	Avoid co-administration
		x	x	x		Proton pump inhibitors	↓ azole, ↑ PPI (posa: susp form only)	Avoid co-administration
x	x			x		Proton pump inhibitors	↑ PPI (posa: tab form only)	Monitor, adjust dosage
					x	Proton pump inhibitors	↑ voriconazole, ↑ PPI	Monitor, adjust dosage
		x				Rituximab	Inhibits action of rituximab	Avoid co-administration
	x			x	x	Sirolimus	↑ sirolimus	Avoid co-administration
x	x	x	x	x	x	Tacrolimus	↑ tacrolimus	Avoid co-administration
x			x			Theophylline	↑ theophylline	Monitor, adjust dosage

TABLE 22A (10)

Anti-Infective agent						Other Drug	Effect on concentration (or other effect)	Suggested management
Azole antifungal agents *(continued)*								
Fluconazole	Isavuconazole	Itraconazole	Ketoconazole	Posaconazole	Voriconazole			
			x			Trazodone	↑ trazodone	Monitor, adjust dosage
x		x			x	Warfarin	↑ warfarin	Monitor INR, adjust dosage
x						Zidovudine	↑ zidovudine	Avoid co-administration
Bedaquiline						Carbamazepine	↓ bedaquiline	Avoid co-administration
						Ciprofloxacin	↑ bedaquiline	Avoid co-administration
						Clarithromycin	↑ bedaquiline	Avoid co-administration
						Efavirenz	↓ bedaquiline	Avoid co-administration
						Erythromycin	↑ bedaquiline	Avoid co-administration
						Etravirine	↓ bedaquiline	Avoid co-administration
						Fluconazole	↑ bedaquiline	Avoid co-administration
						Ketoconazole	↑ bedaquiline	Avoid co-administration
						Phenytoin	↓ bedaquiline	Avoid co-administration
						Rifabutin	↓ bedaquiline	Avoid co-administration
						Rifampin	↓ bedaquiline	Avoid co-administration
						Rifapentine	↓ bedaquiline	Avoid co-administration
						Ritonavir	↑ bedaquiline	Avoid co-administration
						St John's wort	↓ bedaquiline	Avoid co-administration
Caspofungin						Cyclosporine	↑ caspofungin	Monitor
						Tacrolimus	↓ tacrolimus	Monitor, adjust dosage
						Other CYP inducers	↓ caspofungin	Consider ↑ caspo dosage
Cephalexin						Metformin	↑ metformin	Monitor, adjust dosage
Chloramphenicol						Phenytoin	↑ phenytoin	Monitor, adjust dosage
						Iron salts, Vitamin B12	↓ response to iron salts, vitamin B12	Monitor
						HIV Protease inhibitors	↑ chloramphenicol, protease inhibitors	Avoid co-administration
Clindamycin						Kaolin	↓ absorption of clindamycin	Avoid co-administration
						Atracurium	↑ neuromuscular blockade	Avoid co-administration
						St. John's wort	↓ clindamycin	Monitor, adjust dosage
Cycloserine						Ethanol	↑ neurotoxicity	Monitor
						INH, ethionamide	↑ neurotoxicity	Monitor

TABLE 22A (11)

Anti-Infective agent	Other Drug	Effect on concentration (or other effect)	Suggested management
Dapsone	Didanosine	↓ absorption of dapsone	Avoid co-administration
	Oral contraceptives	↓ effectiveness of oral contraceptives	Use alternative method
	Pyrimethamine	↑ marrow toxicity	Monitor
	Zidovudine	↑ marrow toxicity	Monitor
Daptomycin	HMG-CoA inhibitors (statins)	↑ muscle toxicity	Monitor or avoid
Dicloxacillin	Warfarin	↓ warfarin (↓ INR)	Monitor INR, adjust dosage
Didanosine (ddI)	Allopurinol	↑ didanosine	Avoid co-administration
	Ethanol	↑ risk of pancreatitis	Monitor
	Fluoroquinolones	↓ FQ absorption	Avoid co-administration
	Drugs needing low pH for absorption	↓ absorption	Avoid co-administration
	Methadone	↓ didanosine	Avoid co-administration
	Pentamidine	↑ risk of pancreatitis	Monitor
	Ribavirin	↑ mitochondrial toxicity	Avoid co-administration
	Tenofovir	↑ didanosine	Adjust didanosine dosage
Doripenem	Probenecid	↑ doripenem	Adjust dosage or avoid
	Valproic acid	↓ valproic acid	Avoid co-administration
Doxycycline	Aluminum, bismuth, iron, magnesium salts	↓ doxycycline absorption	Avoid co-administration
	Barbiturates	↓ doxycycline	Avoid co-administration
	Carbamazepine	↓ doxycycline	Avoid co-administration
	Digoxin	↑ digoxin	Monitor, adjust dosage
	Phenytoin	↓ doxycycline	Avoid co-administration
	Warfarin	↑ warfarin	Monitor INR, adjust dosage
Entecavir	Crizotinib	↑ crizotinib	Monitor, avoid if possible
Eravacycline	Strong CYP3A4 inducer	↓ eravacycline	↑ dose to 1.5 mg/kg q12h
	Warfarin	↑ INR	Monitor INR, adjust dosage
Ertapenem	Probenecid	↑ ertapenem	Monitor or avoid
	Valproic acid	↓ valproic acid	Avoid co-administration
Ethambutol	Aluminum salts	↓ absorption of ethambutol, aluminum salts	Avoid co-administration
Fexinidazole	Alcohol	Disulfiram-like reaction	Avoid co-administration
	Beta-blockers	↑ risk of arrhythmia	Contraindicated
	Calcium channel blockers	↑ risk of arrhythmia	Contraindicated
	Corticosteroids	↑ risk of arrhythmia	Contraindicated
	Disulfiram	↑ risk of psychosis	Avoid co-administration
	Drugs that ↑ QT interval	↑ QT interval	Contraindicated
	Furosemide	↑ risk of arrhythmia	Contraindicated
	Thiazide diuretics	↑ risk of arrhythmia	Contraindicated
Flucloxacillin	Warfarin	↓ warfarin	Monitor INR, adjust dosage
	Voriconazole	↓ voriconazole	Monitor, adjust dosage

TABLE 22A (12)

Anti-Infective agent									Other Drug	Effect on concentration (or other effect)	Suggested management
Fluoroquinolones											
Ciprofloxacin	Delafloxacin	Gatifloxacin	Gemifloxacin	Levofloxacin	Moxifloxacin	Norfloxacin	Ofloxacin	Prulifloxacin			
x	x								Antacids	↓ FQ	Give FQ 2 hr pre or 6 hr post
								x	Antacids	↓ prulifloxacin	Give pruli 2 hr pre or 4 hr post
			x	x		x	x		Antacids	↓ FQ	Stagger admin by 2-3 hr
		x							Antacids	↓ gatifloxacin	Stagger admin by 4 hr
					x				Antacids	↓ moxifloxacin	Give moxi 4 hr pre or 8 hr post
x		x		x	x	x	x		Antiarrhythmics (Class IA/III)	↑ QT interval	Avoid co-administration
x						x			Caffeine	↑ caffeine	Monitor, adjust dosage
x									Calcium supplements	↓ ciprofloxacin	Give cipro 2 hr pre or 6 hr post
			x	x		x	x		Calcium supplements	↓ FQ	Stagger admin by 2-3 hr
					x				Calcium supplements	↓ moxifloxacin	Give moxi 4 hr pre or 8 hr post
								x	Calcium supplements	↓ prulifloxacin	Give pruli 2 hr pre or 4 hr post
								x	Cimetidine	↓ prulifloxacin	Give pruli 2 hr pre or 4 hr post
x						x			Clozapine	↑ clozapine	Monitor, adjust dosage
x						x			Cyclosporine	↑ cyclosporine	Monitor, adjust dosage
x	x								Didanosine	↓ FQ	Give FQ 2 hr pre or 6 hr post
			x	x		x	x		Didanosine	↓ FQ	Stagger admin by 2-3 hr
					x				Didanosine	↓ moxifloxacin	Give moxi 4 hr pre or 8 hr post
								x	Didanosine	↓ prulifloxacin	Give pruli 2 hr pre or 4 hr post
x						x			Duloxetine	↑ duloxetine	Monitor or avoid
x		x		x	x	x	x	x	Insulin	↑↓ blood glucose	Monitor
x	x								Iron supplements	↓ FQ	Give FQ 2 hr pre or 6 hr post
			x	x		x	x		Iron supplements	↓ FQ	Stagger admin by 2-3 hr
		x							Iron supplements	↓ gatifloxacin	Stagger admin by 4 hr
					x				Iron supplements	↓ moxifloxacin	Give moxi 4 hr pre or 8 hr post
								x	Iron supplements	↓ prulifloxacin	Give pruli 2 hr pre or 4 hr post
x									Methotrexate	↑ methotrexate	Monitor or avoid
								x	Nicardipine	↑ risk of prulifloxacin phototoxicity	Monitor or avoid
x		x	x	x		x	x	x	NSAIDs	↑ risk of CNS stimulation/seizures	Monitor or avoid
x		x		x	x	x	x	x	Oral hypoglycemics	↑↓ blood glucose	Monitor
x									Phenytoin	↑↓ phenytoin	Monitor, adjust dosage
x		x	x			x			Probenecid	↑ FQ	Monitor or avoid
					x				Rifampin	↓ moxifloxacin *(CID 2007;45:1001)*	Monitor, adjust dosage

TABLE 22A (13)

Anti-Infective agent									Other Drug	Effect on concentration (or other effect)	Suggested management
Fluoroquinolones *(continued)*											
Ciprofloxacin	Delafloxacin	Gatifloxacin	Gemifloxacin	Levofloxacin	Moxifloxacin	Norfloxacin	Ofloxacin	Prulifloxacin			
x						x			Ropinirole	↑ ropinirole	Monitor, adjust dosage
x									Sildenafil	↑ sildenafil	Monitor
x	x								Sucralfate	↓ FQ	Give FQ 2 hr pre or 6 hr post
			x	x		x	x		Sucralfate	↓ FQ	Stagger admin by 2-3 hr
		x							Sucralfate	↓ gatifloxacin	Stagger admin by 4 hr
								x	Sucralfate	↓ prulifloxacin	Give pruli 2 hr pre or 4 hr post
x						x	x	x	Theophylline	↑ theophylline	Monitor or avoid
x						x			Tizanidine	↑ tizanidine	Contraindicated
x				x	x	x	x	x	Warfarin	↑ warfarin, ↑ INR	Monitor INR, adjust dosage
x	x								Zinc	↓ FQ	Give FQ 2 hr pre or 6 hr post
			x	x		x	x		Zinc	↓ FQ	Stagger admin by 2-3 hr
		x							Zinc	↓ gatifloxacin	Stagger admin by 4 hr
					x				Zinc	↓ moxifloxacin	Give moxi 4 hr pre or 8 hr post
								x	Zinc	↓ prulifloxacin	Give pruli 2 hr pre or 4 hr post
Fosfomycin									Metoclopramide (w/po fosfomycin only)	↓ urinary excretion of fosfomycin	Avoid co-administration
									Probenecid	↓ urinary excretion of fosfomycin	Avoid co-administration
Fusidic acid									Atorvastatin	↑ atorvastatin (↑ risk of rhabdomyolysis)	Avoid co-administration
									Rifampin	↑ rifampin, ↓ fusidic acid	Monitor or avoid
									Simvastatin	↑ simvastatin (↑ risk of rhabdomyolysis)	Avoid co-administration
Ganciclovir									Imipenem	↑ risk of seizures	Monitor
									Probenecid	↑ ganciclovir	Monitor, adjust dosage
									Zidovudine	↓ ganciclovir, ↑ zidovudine	Adjust dosage or avoid
Griseofulvin									Barbiturates	↓ griseofulvin	Adjust dosage or avoid
									Cyclosporine	↓ cyclosporine	Monitor, adjust dosage
									Ethinyl estradiol	↓ ethinyl estradiol	Avoid co-administration
									Salicylates	↓ salicylates	Monitor, adjust dosage
									Warfarin	↓ warfarin	Monitor INR, adjust dosage

TABLE 22A (14)

Anti-Infective agent										Other Drug	Effect on concentration (or other effect)	Suggested management
Hepatitis C antivirals												
Epclusa	Zepatier	Daclatasvir	Simeprevir	Sofosbuvir	Harvoni	Technivie	Viekira Pak	Mavyret	Vosevi			
						x	x			Alfuzosin	Risk of hypotension	Avoid co-administration
						x	x			Alprazolam	↑ alprazolam	Monitor, adjust dosage
x		x		x	x				x	Amiodarone	Bradycardia	Avoid co-administration
			x			x	x			Amlodipine	↑ amlodipine	Monitor, adjust dosage
					x					Antacids	↓ ledipasvir	Separate administration
x									x	Antacids	↓ velpatasvir	Separate administration
								x		Atazanavir	↑ glecaprevir, ↑ pibrentasvir	Contraindicated
									x	Atazanavir	↑ voxilaprevir	Avoid co-administration
		x	x							Atazanavir / ritonavir	↑ hep C drug	Avoid co-administration
						x	x			Atazanavir / ritonavir	↑ paritaprevir	Avoid co-administration
x	x	x	x						x	Atorvastatin	↑ atorvastatin	Monitor, adjust dosage
								x		Atorvastatin	↑ atorvastatin	Avoid co-administration
						x	x			Bepridil	↑ bepridil	Monitor, adjust dosage
	x	x								Bosentan	↓ hep C drug	Adjust dosage or avoid
						x	x			Buprenorphine	↑ buprenorphine	Monitor, adjust dosage
x	x	x	x	x	x	x	x	x	x	Carbamazepine	↓ hep C drug(s)	Avoid co-administration
		x								Ciprofloxacin	↑ daclatasvir	Avoid co-administration
		x	x							Clarithromycin	↑ daclatasvir	Avoid co-administration
			x							Cobicistat	↑ simeprevir	Avoid co-administration
			x							Cyclosporine	↑ simeprevir	Avoid co-administration
						x	x			Cyclosporine	↑ cyclosporine	Adjust dosage or avoid
	x									Cyclosporine	↑ grazoprevir	Avoid co-administration
									x	Cyclosporine	↑ voxilaprevir	Avoid co-administration
								x		Cyclosporine	↑ glecaprevir, ↑ pibrentasvir	Avoid if stable cyclo >100 mg/d
		x								Dabigatran	↑ dabigatran	Avoid co-administration
								x	x	Dabigatran	↑ dabigatran	Monitor, adjust dosage
								x		Darunavir	↑ glecaprevir	Avoid co-administration
		x	x							Darunavir/ritonavir	↑ hep C drug	Avoid co-administration
						x	x			Darunavir/ritonavir	↓ darunavir/ritonavir	Avoid co-administration
	x									Darunavir/ritonavir	↑ grazoprevir	Avoid co-administration
		x	x							Dexamethasone	↓ hep C drug	Avoid co-administration
x		x	x		x	x		x	x	Digoxin	↑ digoxin	Monitor, adjust dosage
		x								Diltiazem	↑ daclatasvir	Avoid co-administration

TABLE 22A (15)

Epclusa	Zepatier	Daclatasvir	Simeprevir	Sofosbuvir	Harvoni	Technivie	Viekira Pak	Mavyret	Vosevi	Other Drug	Effect on concentration (or other effect)	Suggested management
Hepatitis C antivirals *(continued)*												
			x							Diltiazem	↑ diltiazem	Monitor, adjust dosage
			x			x	x			Disopyramide	↑ disopyramide	Monitor, adjust dosage
x	x	x	x					x	x	Efavirenz	↓ hep C drug(s)	Avoid co-administration
						x	x			Efavirenz	Increased LFTs	Monitor
						x	x			Ergot derivatives	Ergot toxicity	Avoid co-administration
		x								Erythromycin	↑ daclatasvir	Avoid co-administration
			x							Erythromycin	↑ simeprevir, erythromycin	Avoid co-administration
						x	x			Ethinyl estradiol	ALT elevations	Monitor
								x		Ethinyl estradiol	Effect uncertain	Avoid co-administration
	x	x	x							Etravirine	↓ hep C drug	Avoid co-administration
					x					Famotidine	↓ ledipasvir	Max fam 40 mg q12h
x									x	Famotidine	↓ velpatasvir	Max fam 40 mg q12h
			x							Felodipine	↑ felodipine	Monitor, adjust dosage
			x			x	x			Flecainide	↑ flecainide	Monitor, adjust dosage
		x	x							Fluconazole	↑ hep C drug	Avoid co-administration
						x	x			Fluticasone nasal	↑ fluticasone	Monitor, adjust dosage
	x	x						x	x	Fluvastatin	↑ fluvastatin	Monitor, adjust dosage
						x	x			Furosemide	↑ furosemide	Monitor, adjust dosage
							x			Gemfibrozil	↑ dasabuvir	Avoid co-administration
									x	H2-antagonists	↓ velpatasvir	Max fam 40 mg q12h (or equiv)
		x	x							Itraconazole	↑ hep C drug	Avoid co-administration
	x	x	x							Ketoconazole	↑ hep C drug	Avoid co-administration
						x	x			Ketoconazole	↑ ketoconazole	Monitor, adjust dosage
						x	x			Lidocaine	↑ lidocaine	Monitor, adjust dosage
								x		Lopinavir/ritonavir	↑ pibrentasvir	Avoid co-administration
						x	x			Lopinavir/ritonavir	↑ paritaprevir	Avoid co-administration
	x									Lopinavir/ritonavir	↑ grazoprevir	Avoid co-administration
									x	Lopinavir/ritonavir	↑ voxilaprevir	Avoid co-administration
	x		x						x	Lovastatin	↑ lovastatin	Monitor, adjust dosage
						x	x	x		Lovastatin	↑ lovastatin	Avoid co-administration
			x			x	x			Mexiletine	↑ mexiletine	Monitor, adjust dosage
			x							Midazolam	↑ midazolam	Monitor, adjust dosage
	x									Modafinil	↓ Zepatier	Avoid co-administration

TABLE 22A (16)

Hepatitis C antivirals *(continued)*

Epclusa	Zepatier	Daclatasvir	Simeprevir	Sofosbuvir	Harvoni	Technivie	Viekira Pak	Mavyret	Vosevi	Other Drug	Effect on concentration (or other effect)	Suggested management
		x								Nafcillin	↓ daclatasvir	Avoid co-administration
	x									Nafcillin	↓ Zepatier	Avoid co-administration
			x							Nicardipine	↑ nicardipine	Monitor, adjust dosage
			x							Nifedipine	↑ nifedipine	Monitor, adjust dosage
			x							Nisoldipine	↑ nisoldipine	Monitor, adjust dosage
					x				x	Omeprazole	↓ ledipasvir or ↓ velpatasvir	Max omep 20 mg q24h
x										Omeprazole	↓ velpatasvir	Avoid co-administration
						x	x			Omeprazole	↓ omeprazole	Monitor, adjust dosage
x			x	x	x				x	Oxcarbazepine	↓ hep C drug(s)	Avoid co-administration
x	x	x	x	x	x	x	x		x	Phenytoin	↓ hep C drug(s)	Avoid co-administration
x			x	x	x	x	x		x	Phenobarbital	↓ hep C drug(s)	Avoid co-administration
						x	x			Pimozide	Cardiac arrhythmias	Monitor
		x	x					x		Pitavastatin	↑ pitavastatin	Monitor, adjust dosage
									x	Pitavastatin	↑ pitavastatin	Avoid co-administration
		x	x							Posaconazole	↑ hep C drug	Avoid co-administration
		x	x			x	x		x	Pravastatin	↑ pravastatin	Monitor, adjust dosage
								x		Pravastatin	↑ pravastatin	↓ pravastatin dose by 50%
			x			x	x			Propafenone	↑ propafenone	Monitor, adjust dosage
						x	x			Quetiapine	↑ quetiapine	Monitor, adjust dosage
			x			x	x			Quinidine	↑ quinidine	Monitor, adjust dosage
x	x	x	x	x	x	x	x			Rifampin	↓ hep C drug(s)	Avoid co-administration
								x	x	Rifampin	↓ hep C drug(s)	Contraindicated
x			x	x	x				x	Rifabutin	↓ hep C drug(s)	Avoid co-administration
x		x	x	x	x				x	Rifapentine	↓ hep C drug(s)	Avoid co-administration
						x	x			Rilpivirine	↑ rilpivirine	Avoid co-administration
x	x	x	x		x		x	x		Rosuvastatin	↑ rosuvastatin	Monitor, adjust dosage
									x	Rosuvastatin	↑ rosuvastatin	Avoid co-administration
						x	x			Salmeterol	↑ salmeterol	Avoid co-administration
	x									Saquinavir	↑ grazoprevir	Avoid co-administration
			x			x	x			Sildenafil	↑ sildenafil	Monitor, adjust dosage
	x	x	x			x	x		x	Simvastatin	↑ simvastatin	Monitor, adjust dosage
								x		Simvastatin	↑ simvastatin	Avoid co-administration

TABLE 22A (17)

Hepatitis C antivirals *(continued)*

Epclusa	Zepatier	Daclatasvir	Simeprevir	Sofosbuvir	Harvoni	Technivie	Viekira Pak	Mavyret	Vosevi	Other Drug	Effect on concentration (or other effect)	Suggested management
			x							Sirolimus	↑ or ↓ sirolimus	Monitor, adjust dosage
x	x	x	x	x	x	x	x	x	x	St. John's wort	↓ hep C drug(s)	Avoid co-administration
	x					x	x			Tacrolimus	↑ tacrolimus	Monitor, adjust dosage
			x							Tadalafil	↑ tadalafil	Monitor, adjust dosage
x					x				x	Tenofovir DF	↑ tenofovir DF	Avoid co-administration
		x	x		x					Tipranavir/ritonavir	↑ or ↓ hep C drug	Avoid co-administration
x				x					x	Tipranavir/ritonavir	↓ hep C drug(s)	Avoid co-administration
	x									Tipranavir/ritonavir	↑ grazoprevir	Avoid co-administration
x										Topotecan	↑ topotecan	Avoid co-administration
			x			x	x			Triazolam	↑ triazolam	Avoid co-administration
			x							Vardenafil	↑ vardenafil	Monitor, adjust dosage
		x								Verapamil	↑ daclatasvir	Avoid co-administration
			x							Verapamil	↑ verapamil	Monitor, adjust dosage
		x	x							Voriconazole	↑ hep C drug	Avoid co-administration
						x	x			Voriconazole	↓ voriconazole	Avoid co-administration
				x						Warfarin	INR fluctuations	Monitor INR

Anti-Infective agent	Other Drug	Effect on concentration (or other effect)	Suggested management
Imipenem-cilastatin	BCG	↓ effectiveness of BCG	Avoid co-administration
	Ganciclovir	↑ risk of seizures	Monitor
	Probenecid	↑ imipenem	Monitor, adjust dosage
	Valproic acid	↓ valproic acid	Monitor, adjust dosage
Imipenem-cilastatin-relebactam	Ganciclovir	↑ risk of seizures	Avoid co-administration
	Valproic acid	↓ valproic acid	Avoid co-administration

Integrase Strand Transfer Inhibitors (INSTI)

Dolutegravir	Raltegravir	Other Drug	Effect on concentration (or other effect)	Suggested management
x		Al, Mg-containing antacid	↓ dolutegravir	Give DTG 2h pre or 6h post
	x	Al, Mg-containing antacid	↓ raltegravir	Avoid co-admin (HD, non-HD)
x		Calcium antacid or supplement	↓ dolutegravir	Give DTG 2h pre or 6h post
	x	Calcium antacid or supplement	↓ raltegravir	Non-HD ok; HD avoid co-admin
x		Carbamazepine	↓ dolutegravir	↑ DTG to 50 bid (check PI)
x		Dofetilide	↑ dofetilide	Contraindicated
x		Efavirenz	↓ dolutegravir	↑ DTG to 50 bid (check PI)
x		Etravirine	↓ dolutegravir	Coadminister with boosted PI

TABLE 22A (18)

Anti-Infective agent		Other Drug	Effect on concentration (or other effect)	Suggested management
Integrase Strand Transfer Inhibitors (INSTI) *(continued)*				
Dolutegravir	Raltegravir			
	x	Etravirine	↓ raltegravir	Non-HD ok; HD avoid co-admin
x		Fosamprenavir/ritonavir	↓ dolutegravir	↑ DTG to 50 bid (check PI)
x		INH/rifapentine	↓ dolutegravir, ↑ INH	Avoid co-administration
x		Iron supplements	↓ dolutegravir	Give DTG 2h pre or 6h post
x		Metformin	↑ metformin	Monitor, adjust dosage
x		Nevirapine	↓ dolutegravir	Avoid co-administration
x		Oxcarbazepine	↓ dolutegravir	Avoid co-administration
x		Phenobarbital	↓ dolutegravir	Avoid co-administration
x		Phenytoin	↓ dolutegravir	Avoid co-administration
x		Rifampin	↓ dolutegravir	↑ DTG to 50 bid (check PI)
	x	Rifampin	↓ raltegravir	Use Ral 800 bid (avoid HD)
x		St. John's wort	↓ dolutegravir	Avoid co-administration
x		Sucralfate	↓ dolutegravir	Give DTG 2h pre or 6h post
x		Tipranavir/ritonavir	↓ dolutegravir	↑ DTG to 50 bid (check PI)
	x	Tipranavir/ritonavir	↓ raltegravir	Non-HD ok; HD avoid co-admin
Isoniazid		Acetaminophen	↑ risk of hepatic injury	Monitor
		Alcohol	↑ risk of hepatic injury	Monitor, avoid if possible
		Aluminum salts	↓ absorption of INH	Avoid co-administration
		Carbamazepine	↑ carbamazepine	Monitor, adjust dosage
		Ketoconazole	↓ ketoconazole	Monitor, adjust dosage
		Oral hypoglycemics	↑ oral hypoglycemic	Monitor, adjust dosage
		Phenytoin	↑ phenytoin	Monitor, adjust dosage
		Theophylline	↑ theophylline	Monitor, adjust dosage
		Valproate	↑ valproate	Monitor, adjust dosage

TABLE 22A (19)

Anti-Infective agent			Other Drug	Effect on concentration (or other effect)	Suggested management
Integrase Strand Transfer Inhibitors (INSTI) *(continued)*					
Lefamulin			Alprazolam	↑ alprazolam	Monitor, adjust dosage
			Amiodarone	↑ amiodarone, ↑ QT interval	Avoid co-administration
			Antipsychotics	↑ QT interval	Avoid co-administration
			Diltiazem	↑ diltiazem	Monitor, adjust dosage
			Fluoroquinolones	↑ QT interval	Avoid co-administration
			Ketoconazole	↑ lefamulin	Avoid co-administration
			Macrolides	↑ QT interval	Avoid co-administration
			Midazolam (po)	↑ midazolam	Avoid co-administration
			Pimozide	↑ pimozide, ↑ QT interval	Contraindicated
			Procainamide	↑ QT interval	Avoid co-administration
			Quinidine	↑ quinidine, ↑ QT interval	Avoid co-administration
			Rifampin	↓ lefamulin	Avoid co-administration
			Simvastatin	↑ simvastatin	Monitor, adjust dosage
			Sotalol	↑ QT interval	Avoid co-administration
			Tricyclic antidepressants	↑ QT interval	Avoid co-administration
			Vardenafil	↑ vardenafil	Monitor, adjust dosage
			Verapamil	↑ verapamil	Monitor, adjust dosage
Linezolid			Adrenergic agents	Risk of hypertension	Monitor
			Aged, fermented, pickled or smoked foods	Risk of hypertension	Monitor
			Meperidine	Risk of serotonin syndrome	Monitor
			Rasagiline	Risk of serotonin syndrome	Monitor
			Rifampin	↓ linezolid	Adjust dosage or avoid
			Serotonergic drugs (SSRIs)	Risk of serotonin syndrome	Monitor
Macrolides					
Erythromycin	Azithromycin	Clarithromycin			
x		x	Alfentanil	↑ alfentanil	Monitor or avoid
x		x	Alprazolam	↑ alprazolam	Monitor, adjust dosage
x		x	Amiodarone	↑ amiodarone	Monitor or avoid
	x		Amiodarone	↑ QT interval	Monitor or avoid
x		x	Amlodipine	↑ amlodipine	Monitor or avoid
	x		Apixaban	↑ apixaban	Monitor or avoid
		x	Atazanavir	↑ clarithromycin, ↑ atazanavir	Monitor or avoid
x		x	Atorvastatin	↑ atorvastatin	Adjust dosage or avoid
	x		Betrixaban	↑ betrixaban	Monitor or avoid
x		x	Bromocriptine	↑ bromocriptine	Monitor or avoid
x		x	Carbamazepine	↑ carbamazepine	Monitor, adjust dosage
x		x	Cilostazol	↑ cilostazol	Monitor or avoid

TABLE 22A (20)

Anti-Infective agent			Other Drug	Effect on concentration (or other effect)	Suggested management
Macrolides *(continued)*					
Erythromycin	Azithromycin	Clarithromycin			
x			Clozapine	↑ clozapine	Monitor, adjust dosage
x		x	Colchicine (in renal/hepatic failure)	↑ colchicine	Contraindicated
x		x	Colchicine	↑ colchicine	Monitor, adjust dosage, avoid
			Corticosteroids	↑ corticosteroids	Monitor, adjust dosage
x	x	x	Cyclosporine	↑ cyclosporine	Monitor or avoid
	x		Dabigatran	↑ dabigatran	Monitor or avoid
x	x	x	Digoxin	↑ digoxin	Monitor, adjust dosage
x		x	Diltiazem	↑ diltiazem	Monitor or avoid
x		x	Disopyramide	↑ disopyramide	Monitor or avoid
x		x	Dofetilide	↑ dofetilide	Monitor or avoid
	x		Dofetilide	↑ QT interval	Monitor or avoid
	x		Edoxaban	↑ edoxaban	Monitor or avoid
		x	Efavirenz	↓ clarithromycin, ↑ 14-OH clarithro	Avoid co-administration
x		x	Ergot alkaloids	↑ ergot alkaloids	Contraindicated
		x	Etravirine	↓ clarithromycin	Avoid co-administration
	x		Everolimus	↑ everolimus	Monitor or avoid
		x	Itraconazole	↑ clarithromycin, ↑ itraconazole	Monitor, adjust dosage
x		x	Lovastatin	↑ lovastatin	Contraindicated
		x	Maraviroc	↑ maraviroc	Monitor, adjust dosage
x		x	Methylprednisolone	↑ methylprednisolone	Monitor
x		x	Midazolam	↑ midazolam	Monitor, adjust dosage
		x	Nateglinide	↑ nateglinide	Monitor or avoid
	x		Nelfinavir	↑ azithromycin	Monitor
		x	Nevirapine	↓ clarithromycin, ↑ 14-OH clarithro	Avoid co-administration
		x	Nifedipine	↑ nifedipine	Monitor or avoid
		x	Phenobarbital	↓ clarithromycin	Monitor or avoid
x			Phenytoin	↑ phenytoin	Monitor, adjust dosage
		x	Pioglitazone	↑ pioglitazone	Monitor or avoid
x		x	Pimozide	↑ pimozide	Contraindicated
		x	Pravastatin	↑ pravastatin	Adjust dosage or avoid
x	x		Procainamide	↑ QT interval	Monitor or avoid
		x	Quetiapine	↑ quetiapine	Monitor, adjust dosage
x		x	Quinidine	↑ quinidine	Monitor or avoid
	x		Quinidine	↑ QT interval	Monitor or avoid
		x	Repaglinide	↑ repaglinide	Monitor or avoid
x		x	Rifabutin	↓ macrolide, ↑ rifabutin	Monitor, adjust dosage

TABLE 22A (21)

Anti-Infective agent			Other Drug	Effect on concentration (or other effect)	Suggested management
Macrolides *(continued)*					
Erythromycin	Azithromycin	Clarithromycin			
		x	Rifampin	↓ clarithromycin, ↑ 14-OH clarithro	Avoid co-administration
		x	Rifapentine	↓ clarithromycin, ↑ 14-OH clarithro	Avoid co-administration
	x		Rivaroxaban	↑ rivaroxaban	Monitor or avoid
		x	Rosiglitazone	↑ rosiglitazone	Monitor or avoid
x		x	Sildenafil	↑ sildenafil	Adjust dosage or avoid
x		x	Simvastatin	↑ simvastatin	Contraindicated
	x		Sirolimus	↑ sirolimus	Monitor or avoid
x	x		Sotalol	↑ QT interval	Monitor or avoid
		x	St. John's wort	↓ clarithromycin	Monitor or avoid
x	x	x	Tacrolimus	↑ tacrolimus	Monitor or avoid
		x	Tadalafil	↑ tadalafil	Adjust dosage or avoid
x		x	Theophylline	↑ theophylline	Monitor or avoid
		x	Tolterodine	↑ tolterodine (if CYP2D6 deficient)	Monitor, adjust dosage
x		x	Triazolam	↑ triazolam	Monitor, adjust dosage
		x	Vardenafil	↑ vardenafil	Adjust dosage or avoid
x			Valproic acid	↑ valproic acid	Monitor, adjust dosage
x		x	Verapamil	↑ verapamil	Monitor or avoid
x		x	Vinca alkaloids	↑ vinca alkaloid	Avoid co-administration
x		x	Warfarin	↑ warfarin	Monitor INR, adjust dosage
		x	Zidovudine	↓ zidovudine	Separate admin by 2 hours
		x	Zolpidem	↑ zolpidem	Monitor, adjust dosage
Maraviroc			Carbamazepine	↓ maraviroc	↑ maraviroc dose
			Clarithromycin	↑ maraviroc	↓ maraviroc dose
			Itraconazole	↑ maraviroc	↓ maraviroc dose
			Ketoconazole	↑ maraviroc	↓ maraviroc dose
			Nefazodone	↑ maraviroc	↓ maraviroc dose
			Phenobarbital	↓ maraviroc	↑ maraviroc dose
			Phenytoin	↓ maraviroc	↑ maraviroc dose
			Rifabutin	↓ maraviroc	Monitor, adjust dosage
			Rifampin	↓ maraviroc	↑ maraviroc dose
Mefloquine			Beta blockers	↑ arrhythmias	Avoid co-administration
			Calcium channel blockers	↑ arrhythmias	Avoid co-administration
			Halofantrine	QT prolongation	Avoid co-administration
			Protease inhibitors	↓ mefloquine	Avoid co-administration
			Quinidine, quinine	↑ arrhythmias	Avoid co-administration
			Valproic acid	↓ valproic acid	Monitor, adjust dosage

TABLE 22A (22)

Anti-Infective agent					Other Drug	Effect on concentration (or other effect)	Suggested management
Meropenem					BCG	↓ effectiveness of BCG	Avoid co-administration
					Ganciclovir	↑ risk of seizures	Monitor
					Probenecid	↑ meropenem	Monitor, adjust dosage
					Valproic acid	↓ valproic acid	Avoid co-administration
Methenamine mand/hipp					Drugs that ↑ urine pH	↓ antibacterial effect	Acidify urine
Metronidazole					Alcohol	Disulfiram-like reaction	Avoid co-administration
					Busulfan	↑ busulfan	Avoid co-administration
					Chlorpropamide	↑ risk of hypoglycemia	Monitor, avoid if possible
					Disulfiram	Acute toxic psychosis	Monitor, avoid if possible
					Glimepiride	↑ risk of hypoglycemia	Monitor, avoid if possible
					Glipizide	↑ risk of hypoglycemia	Monitor, avoid if possible
					Glyburide	↑ risk of hypoglycemia	Monitor, avoid if possible
					Lithium	↑ lithium	Monitor, adjust dosage
					Nateglinide	↑ risk of hypoglycemia	Monitor, avoid if possible
					Phenobarbital	↑ phenobarbital	Monitor, adjust dosage
					Phenytoin	↑ phenytoin	Monitor, adjust dosage
					Rosiglitazone	↑ risk of hypoglycemia	Monitor, avoid if possible
					Tolbutamide	↑ risk of hypoglycemia	Monitor, avoid if possible
					Warfarin	↑ INR	Monitor INR, adjust dosage
Micafungin					Itraconazole	↑ itraconazole	Monitor, adjust dosage
					Nifedipine	↑ nifedipine	Monitor, adjust dosage
					Sirolimus	↑ sirolimus	Monitor, adjust dosage
Nafcillin					Warfarin	↓ warfarin (↓ INR)	Monitor INR, adjust dosage
Nitrofurantoin					Antacids	↓ nitrofurantoin	Monitor, adjust dosage
Non-Nucleoside RTIs							
Doravirine	Efavirenz	Etravirine	Nevirapine	Rilpivirine			
	x				Alprazolam	↑ or ↓ alprazolam	Monitor or avoid
	x		x		Amiodarone	↑ NNRTI, ↑ or ↓ amiodarone	Avoid co-administration
		x			Amiodarone	↓ amiodarone	Monitor, adjust dosage
				x	Amiodarone	↑ QT interval	Monitor or avoid
	x				Amlodipine	↑ or ↓ amlodipine	Monitor, adjust dosage
				x	Antacids (Al, Mg, Ca)	↓ rilpivirine	Separate admin by 4 hr
		x			Artemether-lumefantrine	↓ artemether, ↓ DHA, ↓ lumefantrine	Avoid co-administration
	x	x			Atorvastatin	↑ or ↓ atorvastatin	Monitor, adjust dosage
		x			Bepridil	↓ bepridil	Monitor, adjust dosage
		x			Buprenorphine	↓ buprenorphine	Monitor, adjust dosage
	x	x			Carbamazepine	↓ NNRTI, ↑ or ↓ carbamazepine	Avoid co-administration
			x		Carbamazepine	↓ nevirapine, ↓ carbamazepine	Monitor, adjust dosage

TABLE 22A (23)

Non-Nucleoside RTIs *(continued)*

Anti-Infective agent					Other Drug	Effect on concentration (or other effect)	Suggested management
Doravirine	Efavirenz	Etravirine	Nevirapine	Rilpivirine			
x				x	Carbamazepine	↓ NNRTI	Contraindicated
	x				Clarithromycin	↑ or ↓ clari metabolite, ↑ NNRTI	Monitor, adjust dosage
			x		Clarithromycin	↓ clarithromycin, ↑ 14-OH metabolite	Avoid co-administration
		x			Clarithromycin	↓ clarithro, ↑ 14-OH clarithro, ↑ etravirine	Avoid co-administration
				x	Clarithromycin	↑ rilpivirine	Avoid co-administration
			x		Clonazepam	↓ clonazepam	Monitor, adjust dosage
		x			Clopidogrel	↓ clopidogrel metabolite	Avoid co-administration
			x		Cyclophosphamide	↓ cyclophosphamide	Avoid co-administration
	x				Cyclosporine	↑ or ↓ cyclosporine	Avoid co-administration
			x		Cyclosporine	↓ cyclosporine, ↑ nevirapine	Avoid co-administration
		x			Cyclosporine	↓ cyclosporine	Monitor, adjust dosage
		x			Daclatasvir	↓ daclatasvir	Adjust daclatasvir dosage
	x				Dexamethasone	↓ NNRTI, ↑ or ↓ dexamethasone	Avoid co-administration
		x			Dexamethasone	↓ etravirine	Avoid co-administration
				x	Dexamethasone	↓ rilpivirine	Contraindicated
		x			Diazepam	↑ diazepam	Monitor, adjust dosage
		x			Digoxin	↑ digoxin	Monitor, adjust dosage
			x		Diltiazem	↓ diltiazem, ↑ nevirapine	Avoid co-administration
			x		Disopyramide	↓ disopyramide	Avoid co-administration
		x			Disopyramide	↓ disopyramide	Monitor, adjust dosage
		x			Dolutegravir	↓ dolutegravir	Co-administer a boosted PI
x					Efavirenz	↓ doravirine	Avoid co-administration
		x			Elbasvir-grazoprevir	↓ elbasvir, ↓ grazoprevir	Avoid co-administration
x					Enzalutamide	↓ doravirine	Contraindicated
	x		x		Ergotamine	↑ or ↓ ergotamine	Avoid co-administration
				x	Erythromycin	↑ rilpivirine	Avoid co-administration
			x		Ethinyl estradiol	↓ ethinyl estradiol, ↑ nevirapine	Monitor or avoid
			x		Ethosuximide	↓ ethosuximide	Monitor, adjust dosage
x					Etravirine	↓ doravirine	Avoid co-administration
			x		Fentanyl	↓ fentanyl	Avoid co-administration
	x				Fentanyl	↑ or ↓ fentanyl	Monitor
		x			Flecainide	↓ flecainide	Monitor, adjust dosage
		x	x	x	Fluconazole	↑ NNRTI	Monitor or avoid
		x			Fluvastatin	↑ fluvastatin	Monitor, adjust dosage
				x	H2 receptor antagonists	↓ rilpivirine	Give H2RA 12 hr pre/4 hr post
	x		x		Itraconazole	↓ itraconazole, ↑ NNRTI	Avoid co-administration

TABLE 22A (24)

Anti-Infective agent					Other Drug	Effect on concentration (or other effect)	Suggested management
Non-Nucleoside RTIs *(continued)*							
Doravirine	Efavirenz	Etravirine	Nevirapine	Rilpivirine			
		x			Itraconazole	↓ itraconazole, ↑ etravirine	Monitor, adjust dosage
				x	Itraconazole	↑ rilpivirine	Monitor
	x		x		Ketoconazole	↓ ketoconazole, ↑ NNRTI	Avoid co-administration
		x			Ketoconazole	↓ ketoconazole, ↑ etravirine	Monitor, adjust dosage
				x	Ketoconazole	↑ rilpivirine	Monitor
	x		x		Lidocaine	↑ or ↓ lidocaine	Avoid co-administration
		x			Lidocaine	↓ lidocaine	Monitor, adjust dosage
	x	x			Lovastatin	↑ or ↓ lovastatin	Monitor
	x				Mefloquine	↑ or ↓ mefloquine	Avoid co-administration
			x	x	Methadone	↓ methadone	Monitor, adjust dosage
	x				Methadone	↑ or ↓ methadone	Monitor
		x			Mexiletine	↓ mexiletine	Monitor, adjust dosage
	x				Midazolam	↑ or ↓ midazolam	Monitor or avoid
x					Mitotane	↓ doravirine	Contraindicated
x					Nevirapine	↓ doravirine	Avoid co-administration
			x		Nifedipine	↓ nifedipine	Avoid co-administration
	x				Oral contraceptives	↑ or ↓ oral contraceptive	Use alternative method
x				x	Oxcarbazepine	↓ NNRTI	Contraindicated
	x				PDE5 inhibitors	↑ or ↓ PDE5 inhibitor	Monitor, adjust dosage
	x				Phenobarbital	↓ NNRTI, ↑ or ↓ phenobarbital	Avoid co-administration
x				x	Phenobarbital	↓ NNRTI	Contraindicated
		x			Phenobarbital	↓ etravirine	Avoid co-administration
	x				Phenytoin	↓ NNRTI, ↑ or ↓ phenytoin	Avoid co-administration
x				x	Phenytoin	↓ NNRTI	Contraindicated
		x			Phenytoin	↓ etravirine	Avoid co-administration
	x				Pimozide	↑ or ↓ pimozide	Avoid co-administration
		x			Pitavastatin	↑ pitavastatin	Monitor, adjust dosage
	x				Posaconazole	↓ posaconazole, ↑ NNRTI	Avoid co-administration
		x		x	Posaconazole	↑ NNRTI	Monitor, adjust dosage
		x			Propafenone	↓ propafenone	Monitor, adjust dosage
		x			Protease inhibitors (HIV)	See Table 22B	See Table 22B
				x	Proton pump inhibitors	↓ rilpivirine	Contraindicated
		x			Quinidine	↓ quinidine	Monitor, adjust dosage
			x		Rifabutin	↑ rifabutin	Monitor or avoid
	x	x			Rifabutin	↑ or ↓ rifabutin, ↓ NNRTI	Avoid co-administration
x					Rifabutin	↓ doravirine	↑ DOR to 100 mg q12h

TABLE 22A (25)

Anti-Infective agent					Other Drug	Effect on concentration (or other effect)	Suggested management
Non-Nucleoside RTIs *(continued)*							
Doravirine	Efavirenz	Etravirine	Nevirapine	Rilpivirine			
				x	Rifabutin	↓ rilpivirine	↑ RPV to 50 mg q24h
		x	x		Rifampin	↓ NNRTI	Avoid co-administration
	x				Rifampin	↓ efavirenz	↑ EFV to 800 mg q24h
x				x	Rifampin	↓ NNRTI	Contraindicated
x				x	Rifapentine	↓ NNRTI	Contraindicated
		x			Rifapentine	↓ etravirine	Avoid co-administration
		x			Sildenafil	↓ sildenafil, ↓ N-desmethylsildenafil	Monitor, adjust dosage
		x			Simeprevir	↓ simeprevir	Avoid co-administration
	x		x		Sirolimus	↑ or ↓ sirolimus	Avoid co-administration
		x			Sirolimus	↓ sirolimus	Monitor, adjust dosage
	x				Simvastatin	↑ or ↓ simvastatin	Monitor
		x			Simvastatin	↓ simvastatin	Monitor, adjust dosage
	x	x	x		St. John's wort	↓ NNRTI	Avoid co-administration
x				x	St. John's wort	↓ NNRTI	Contraindicated
	x		x		Tacrolimus	↑ or ↓ tacrolimus	Avoid co-administration
		x			Tacrolimus	↓ tacrolimus	Monitor, adjust dosage
				x	Telithromycin	↑ rilpivirine	Avoid co-administration
	x				Triazolam	↑ or ↓ triazolam	Monitor or avoid
	x		x		Verapamil	↑ or ↓ verapamil, ↑ NNRTI	Avoid co-administration
	x				Voriconazole	↓ voriconazole, ↑ efavirenz	↑ vori, ↓ EFV to 300 mg q24h
				x	Voriconazole	↑ rilpivirine	Monitor
		x			Voriconazole	↑ voriconazole, ↑ etravirine	Monitor or avoid
	x	x	x		Warfarin	↑ or ↓ warfarin	Monitor INR, adjust dosage
Omadacycline					Antacids (Al, Mg, Ca, bismuth subsalicylate	↓ omadacycline	Separate administration by 4 hr
					Iron-containing preparations	↓ omadacycline	Separate administration by 4 hr
					Verapamil	↓ omadacycline	Monitor
					Warfarin	↑ INR	Monitor INR, adjust dosage
Oritavancin					Warfarin	↑ warfarin	Monitor INR, adjust dosage
Pentamidine (IV)					Amphotericin B	↑ risk of nephrotoxicity	Monitor
Piperacillin-Tazobactam					Methotrexate	↑ methotrexate	Monitor or avoid
Pivmecillinam					Probenecid	↑ mecillinam	Monitor, adjust dosage
					Valproic acid	Enhanced carnitine depletion	Avoid co-administration
Polymyxin B					Curare paralytics	Neuromuscular blockade	Avoid co-administration
					Aminoglycosides, amphotericin B, vancomycin	↑ nephrotoxicity risk	Avoid co-administration
Polymyxin E (colistin)					Curare paralytics	Neuromuscular blockade	Avoid co-administration
					Aminoglycosides, amphotericin B, vancomycin	↑ nephrotoxicity risk	Avoid co-administration

TABLE 22A (26)

Anti-Infective agent								Other Drug	Effect on concentration (or other effect)	Suggested management
Pretomanid								Efavirenz	↓ pretomanid	Avoid co-administration
								Methotrexate	↑ methotrexate	Monitor, adjust dosage
								Rifampin	↓ pretomanid	Avoid co-administration
Primaquine								Drugs causing hemolysis in G6PD-deficiency	↑ risk of hemolysis	Monitor
Pristinamycin								Cyclosporine	↑ cyclosporine	Monitor, adjust dosage
								Tacrolimus	↑ tacrolimus	Monitor, adjust dosage
Protease inhibitors										
Atazanavir/r	Darunavir/r	Fosamprenavir/r	Indinavir/r	Lopinavir/r	Nelfinavir	Saquinavir/r	Tipranavir/r			
	x	x	x	x	x	x	x	Alfuzosin	↑ alfuzosin	Contraindicated
		x				x		Alprazolam	↑ alprazolam	Monitor, adjust dosage
			x					Alprazolam	↑ alprazolam	Contraindicated
x	x	x		x				Amiodarone	↑ amiodarone	Monitor, adjust dosage, or avoid
			x		x	x	x	Amiodarone	↑ amiodarone	Contraindicated
	x	x				x		Amlodipine	↑ amlodipine	Monitor, adjust dosage
x								Antacids	↓ atazanavir	Give ATV 2 hr bef or 1 hr after
	x							Apixaban	↑ apixaban	Monitor, adjust dosage
	x							Artemether/lumefantrine	↑ artemether, ↓ DHA, ↑ lumefantrine	Monitor for QT prolongation
x	x	x	x	x	x	x		Atorvastatin	↑ atorvastatin	Monitor, adjust dosage
							x	Atorvastatin	↑ atorvastatin	Avoid co-administration
				x				Atovaquone	↓ atovaquone	Monitor, adjust dosage
	x			x				Avanafil	↑ avanafil	Avoid co-administration
				x				Bedaquiline	↑ bedaquiline	Avoid co-administration
x	x		x	x				Bepridil	↑ bepridil	Monitor, adjust dosage, or avoid
						x	x	Bepridil	↑ bepridil	Contraindicated
	x					x		Betamethasone	↑ betamethasone	Avoid co-administration
	x	x	x	x	x	x	x	Bosentan	↑ bosentan	Monitor, adjust dosage
x								Bosentan	↑ bosentan, ↓ atazanavir	Monitor, adjust dosage
	x							Budesonide	↑ budesonide	Avoid co-administration
x								Buprenorphine	↑ buprenorphine, ↑ norbuprenorphine	Monitor, adjust dosage
	x							Buprenorphine/naloxone	↑ norbuprenorphine	Monitor, adjust dosage
							x	Buprenorphine/naloxone	↓ tipranavir	Avoid co-administration
				x				Bupropion	↓ bupropion, ↓ metabolite	Monitor, adjust dosage
	x							Buspirone	↑ buspirone	Monitor, adjust dosage

TABLE 22A (27)

Anti-Infective agent								Other Drug	Effect on concentration (or other effect)	Suggested management
Protease inhibitors *(continued)*										
Atazanavir/r	Darunavir/r	Fosamprenavir/r	Indinavir/r	Lopinavir/r	Nelfinavir	Saquinavir/r	Tipranavir/r			
	x							Carbamazepine	↑ carbamazepine	Monitor, adjust dosage
x								Carbamazepine	↑ carbamazepine, ↓ atazanavir	Adjust dosage or avoid
		x	x	x	x	x	x	Carbamazepine	↓ protease inhibitor	Avoid co-administration
	x							Carvedilol	↑ carvedilol	Monitor, adjust dosage
						x		Chlorpromazine	↑ chlorpromazine	Contraindicated
	x			x				Clarithromycin	↑ clarithromycin (in renal impairment)	Monitor, adjust dosage
x			x				x	Clarithromycin	↑ clarithro, ↓ 14-OH clarithro, ↑ PI	Monitor, adjust dosage, or avoid
						x		Clarithromycin	↑ clarithromycin	Contraindicated
	x							Clonazepam	↑ clonazepam	Monitor
		x				x		Clorazepate	↑ clorazepate	Monitor, adjust dosage
						x		Clozapine	↑ clozapine	Contraindicated
x	x	x	x	x	x	x	x	Colchicine (in renal/hepatic failure)	↑ colchicine	Contraindicated
x	x	x	x	x	x	x	x	Colchicine	↑ colchicine	Monitor, adjust dosage, or avoid
x	x	x	x	x		x	x	Cyclosporine	↑ cyclosporine	Monitor, adjust dosage
					x			Cyclosporine	↑ cyclosporine, ↑ nelfinavir	Monitor, adjust dosage
	x			x				Dasatinib	↑ dasatinib	Monitor, adjust dosage
						x		Dasatinib	↑ dasatinib	Contraindicated
	x			x		x		Dexamethasone	↓ PI, ↑ dexamethasone	Avoid co-administration
		x						Dexamethasone	↓ amprenavir	Avoid co-administration
	x	x				x		Diazepam	↑ diazepam	Monitor, adjust dosage
	x					x		Digoxin	↑ digoxin	Monitor, adjust dosage
x	x	x				x	x	Diltiazem	↑ diltiazem	Monitor, adjust dosage
	x							Disopyramide	↑ disopyramide	Monitor, adjust dosage
						x		Disopyramide	↑ disopyramide	Contraindicated
				x				Disulfiram (w/Kaletra solution)	disulfiram-like reaction	Avoid co-administration
						x		Dofetilide	↑ dofetilide	Contraindicated
	x			x				Dronedarone	↑ dronedarone	Contraindicated
	x			x				Elbasvir/grazoprevir	↑ elbasvir, ↑ grazoprevir	Contraindicated
	x	x	x	x	x	x	x	Ergot alkaloids	↑ ergot alkaloid	Contraindicated
						x		Erythromycin	↑ erythromycin	Contraindicated
	x							Estazolam	↑ estazolam	Monitor, adjust dosage

TABLE 22A (28)

Protease inhibitors *(continued)*

Atazanavir/r	Darunavir/r	Fosamprenavir/r	Indinavir/r	Lopinavir/r	Nelfinavir	Saquinavir/r	Tipranavir/r	Other Drug	Effect on concentration (or other effect)	Suggested management
x	x			x	x	x	x	Ethinyl estradiol	↓ ethinyl estradiol	Use alternative method
		x						Ethinyl estradiol	↓ ethinyl estradiol, ↓ amprenavir	Use alternative method
	x							Everolimus	↑ everolimus	Avoid co-administration
x	x	x	x	x		x	x	Felodipine	↑ felodipine	Monitor, adjust dosage
	x			x				Fentanyl	↑ fentanyl	Monitor, adjust dosage
	x							Fesoterodine	↑ fesoterodine	Max feso dose 4 mg qd
	x							Flecainide	↑ flecainide	Monitor, adjust dosage
		x				x	x	Flecainide (with boosted PI)	↑ flecainide	Contraindicated
							x	Fluconazole	↑ tipranavir	Max flucon dose 200 mg qd
							x	Fluoxetine	↑ fluoxetine	Monitor, adjust dosage
		x				x		Flurazepam	↑ flurazepam	Monitor, adjust dosage
x	x	x	x		x	x	x	Fluticasone	↑ fluticasone	Avoid co-administration
						x		Fusidic acid	↑ saquinavir, ↑ ritonavir, ↑ fusidic acid	Avoid co-administration
	x							Glecaprevir/pibrentasvir	↑ glecaprevir, ↑ pibrentasvir	Avoid co-administration
						x		Halofantrine	↑ halofantrine	Contraindicated
						x		Haloperidol	↑ haloperidol	Contraindicated
x								H2 blockers	↓ atazanavir	Stagger admin, see PI
		x						H2 blockers	↓ amprenavir	Avoid co-administration
	x							Irinotecan	↑ irinotecan	Avoid co-administration
	x							Isavuconazole	↑ isavuconazole, ↑ darunavir	Monitor, adjust dosage
				x				Isavuconazole	↑ isavuconazole	Avoid co-administration
	x					x		Itraconazole	↑ protease inhibitor, ↑ itraconazole	Monitor, adjust dosage
x		x		x				Itraconazole	↑ itraconazole	Monitor, adjust dosage, or avoid
			x					Itraconazole	↑ indinavir	Monitor, adjust dosage, or avoid
	x							Ivabradine	↑ ivabradine	Contraindicated
	x							Ketoconazole	↑ ketoconazole, ↑ darunavir	Monitor, adjust dosage
x		x		x		x		Ketoconazole	↑ ketoconazole	Monitor, adjust dosage, or avoid
			x					Ketoconazole	↑ indinavir	Monitor, adjust dosage, or avoid
x				x				Lamotrigine	↓ lamotrigine	Monitor, adjust dosage, or avoid
x	x	x	x	x				Lidocaine	↑ lidocaine	Monitor, adjust dosage, or avoid
						x		Lidocaine	↑ lidocaine	Contraindicated

TABLE 22A (29)

Protease inhibitors *(continued)*

Atazanavir/r	Darunavir/r	Fosamprenavir/r	Indinavir/r	Lopinavir/r	Nelfinavir	Saquinavir/r	Tipranavir/r	Other Drug	Effect on concentration (or other effect)	Suggested management
	x							Lomitapide	↑ lomitapide	Contraindicated
	x	x	x	x	x	x	x	Lovastatin	↑ lovastatin	Contraindicated
x	x	x	x	x		x		Lurasidone	↑ lurasidone	Contraindicated
						x		Maraviroc	↑ maraviroc	Monitor, adjust dosage
							x	Meperidine	↓ meperidine, ↑ normeperidine	Avoid co-administration
	x	x		x	x	x	x	Methadone	↓ methadone	Monitor, adjust dosage, or avoid
	x					x		Methylprednisolone	↑ methylprednisolone	Avoid co-administration
	x							Metoprolol	↑ metoprolol	Monitor, adjust dosage
				x				Metronidazole (w/Kaletra soln)	Disulfiram-like reaction	Avoid co-administration
							x	Metronidazole	Disulfiram-like reaction	Monitor
	x							Mexiletine	↑ mexiletine	Monitor, adjust dosage
x	x	x	x	x		x	x	Midazolam (IV)	↑ midazolam	Monitor, adjust dosage
x	x	x	x	x	x	x	x	Midazolam (po)	↑ midazolam	Contraindicated
	x							Mometasone	↑ mometasone	Avoid co-administration
	x							Naloxegol	↑ naloxegol	Contraindicated
x	x	x	x	x		x	x	Nicardipine	↑ nicardipine	Monitor, adjust dosage
x	x	x	x	x		x		Nifedipine	↑ nifedipine	Monitor, adjust dosage
	x			x				Nilotinib	↑ nilotinib	Monitor, adjust dosage
		x				x	x	Nisoldipine	↓↑ nisoldipine	Monitor, adjust dosage
x	x	x	x	x	x	x	x	NNRTIs	See Table 22B	See Table 22B
	x				x			Norethindrone	↓ norethindrone	Use alternative method
x								Norethindrone	↑ norethindrone	Use alternative method
x								Norgestimate	↑ norgestimate	Use alternative method
x								Omeprazole	↓ atazanavir	Stagger admin, see PI
						x		Omeprazole	↑ saquinavir	Monitor, adjust dosage
	x						x	Omeprazole	↓ omeprazole	Monitor, adjust dosage
					x			Omeprazole	↓ omeprazole	Avoid co-administration
	x							Oxycodone	↑ oxycodone	Monitor, adjust dosage
	x	x						Paroxetine	↓ paroxetine	Monitor, adjust dosage
							x	Paroxetine	↑ paroxetine	Monitor, adjust dosage
	x							Perphenazine	↑ perphenazine	Monitor, adjust dosage

TABLE 22A (30)

Anti-Infective agent								Other Drug	Effect on concentration (or other effect)	Suggested management
Protease inhibitors *(continued)*										
Atazanavir/r	Darunavir/r	Fosamprenavir/r	Indinavir/r	Lopinavir/r	Nelfinavir	Saquinavir/r	Tipranavir/r			
	x							Phenobarbital	↓ phenobarbital	Monitor, adjust dosage
		x	x	x	x	x	x	Phenobarbital	↓ protease inhibitor	Avoid co-administration
x								Phenobarbital	↓ phenobarbital, ↓ atazanavir	Adjust dosage or avoid
	x							Phenytoin	↓ phenytoin	Monitor, adjust dosage
			x			x		Phenytoin	↓ protease inhibitor	Avoid co-administration
		x						Phenytoin (w/unboosted FPV)	↓ phenytoin	Avoid co-administration
x				x	x			Phenytoin	↓ phenytoin, ↓ protease inhibitor	Avoid co-administration
		x						Phenytoin (w/boosted FPV)	↑ amprenavir, ↓ phenytoin	Monitor, adjust dosage
							x	Phenytoin	↓ tipranavir	Avoid co-administration
	x	x	x	x	x	x	x	Pimozide	↑ pimozide	Contraindicated
	x							Pravastatin	↑ pravastatin	Monitor, adjust dosage
	x					x		Prednisone	↑ prednisone	Avoid co-administration
	x							Propafenone	↑ propafenone	Monitor, adjust dosage
		x				x	x	Propafenone (w/boosted PI)	↑ propafenone	Contraindicated
x	x	x	x	x		x	x	Quetiapine	↑ quetiapine	Monitor, adjust dosage, or avoid
x	x	x	x	x				Quinidine	↑ quinidine	Monitor, adjust dosage, or avoid
					x	x	x	Quinidine	↑ quinidine	Contraindicated
						x		Quinine	↑ quinine	Contraindicated
	x			x				Ranolazine	↑ ranolazine	Contraindicated
	x							Rifabutin	↑ rifabutin (+ metabolite), ↑ darunavir	Monitor, adjust dosage
x		x		x		x	x	Rifabutin	↑ rifabutin	Monitor, adjust dosage
			x		x			Rifabutin	↑ rifabutin, ↓ protease inhibitor	Monitor, adjust dosage, or avoid
	x	x	x		x		x	Rifampin	↓ protease inhibitor	Contraindicated
				x				Rifampin	↓ lopinavir, ↓ ritonavir, ↑ rifampin	Contraindicated
						x		Rifampin	↑ rifampin	Contraindicated
	x							Rifapentine	↓ darunavir	Avoid co-administration
	x							Risperidone	↑ risperidone	Monitor, adjust dosage
	x			x				Rivaroxaban	↑ rivaroxaban	Avoid co-administration
x	x		x	x	x			Rosuvastatin	↑ rosuvastatin	Monitor, adjust dosage
							x	Rosuvastatin	↑ rosuvastatin	Avoid co-administration
x	x	x	x	x	x	x	x	Salmeterol	↑ salmeterol	Avoid co-administration

TABLE 22A (31)

Protease inhibitors *(continued)*

Atazanavir/r	Darunavir/r	Fosamprenavir/r	Indinavir/r	Lopinavir/r	Nelfinavir	Saquinavir/r	Tipranavir/r	Other Drug	Effect on concentration (or other effect)	Suggested management
	x							Sertraline	↓ sertraline	Monitor, adjust dosage
x	x	x	x	x	x	x	x	Sildenafil (for ED)	↑ sildenafil	Monitor, adjust dosage
x	x	x	x	x	x	x	x	Sildenafil (for PAH)	↑ sildenafil	Contraindicated
	x							Simeprevir	↑ simeprevir, ↑ darunavir	Avoid co-administration
		x		x				Simeprevir	↑ simeprevir	Avoid co-administration
	x	x	x	x	x	x	x	Simvastatin	↑ simvastatin	Contraindicated
x	x		x	x			x	Sirolimus	↑ sirolimus	Monitor, adjust dosage
					x			Sirolimus	↑ sirolimus, ↑ nelfinavir	Monitor, adjust dosage
x								Sofosbuvir/velpatasvir/voxilaprevir	↑ voxilaprevir	Avoid co-administration
	x							Solifenacin	↑ solifenacin	Max solifenacin 5 mg qd
	x	x	x	x	x	x	x	St. John's wort	↓ protease inhibitor	Contraindicated
						x		Sunitinib	↑ sunitinib	Contraindicated
						x		Tacrolimus	↑ tacrolimus	Contraindicated
x	x	x	x	x			x	Tacrolimus	↑ tacrolimus	Monitor, adjust dosage
					x			Tacrolimus	↑ tacrolimus, ↑ nelfinavir	Monitor, adjust dosage
x	x	x	x	x	x	x	x	Tadalafil (for ED, PAH)	↑ tadalafil	Monitor, adjust dosage
	x							Timolol	↑ timolol	Monitor, adjust dosage
	x							Thioridazine	↑ thioridazine	Monitor, adjust dosage
						x		Thioridazine	↑ thioridazine	Contraindicated
	x							Ticagrelor	↑ ticagrelor	Avoid co-administration
	x							Tramadol	↑ tramadol	Monitor, adjust dosage
x	x	x	x	x	x		x	Trazodone	↑ trazodone	Monitor, adjust dosage
						x		Trazodone	↑ trazodone	Contraindicated
	x					x		Triamcinolone	↑ triamcinolone	Avoid co-administration
	x	x	x	x	x	x	x	Triazolam	↑ triazolam	Contraindicated
x	x	x				x	x	Tricyclic antidepressants	↑ TCA	Monitor, adjust dosage, or avoid
				x			x	Valproic acid	↓ valproic acid	Monitor, adjust dosage, or avoid
x	x	x	x	x	x	x	x	Vardenafil	↑ vardenafil	Monitor, adjust dosage
				x				Venetoclax	↑ venetoclax	Monitor, check venetoclax PI
			x					Venlafaxine	↓ indinavir	Monitor, adjust dosage, or avoid
x	x	x				x	x	Verapamil	↑ verapamil	Monitor, adjust dosage

TABLE 22A (32)

Anti-Infective agent								Other Drug	Effect on concentration (or other effect)	Suggested management
Protease inhibitors *(continued)*										
Atazanavir/r	Darunavir/r	Fosamprenavir/r	Indinavir/r	Lopinavir/r	Nelfinavir	Saquinavir/r	Tipranavir/r			
				x				Viekira (Pak, XR)	↑ ombitasvir, ↑ paritaprevir, ↑ ritonavir	Avoid co-administration
		x						Viekira Pak (w/boosted FPV)	↑ amprenavir, ↑ paritaprevir	Avoid co-administration
	x			x				Vinblastine	↑ vinblastine	Avoid co-administration
						x		Vincamine	↑ vincamine	Monitor, adjust dosage
	x			x				Vincristine	↑ vincristine	Avoid co-administration
	x			x				Voriconazole	↓ voriconazole	Avoid co-administration
x								Voriconazole	↓ atazanavir, ↓↑ voriconazole	Avoid co-administration
x	x	x		x	x	x	x	Warfarin	↓↑ warfarin	Monitor INR, adjust dosage
						x		Ziprasidone	↑ ziprasidone	Contraindicated
	x							Zolpidem	↑ zolpidem	Monitor, adjust dosage
Pyrimethamine								Lorazepam	↑ risk of hepatotoxicity	Monitor
								TMP-SMX	↑ risk of marrow suppression	Monitor
								Zidovudine	↑ risk of marrow suppression	Monitor
Quinine								Digoxin	↑ digoxin	Monitor, adjust dosage
								Mefloquine	↑ arrhythmias	Monitor
								Warfarin	↑ warfarin	Monitor INR, adjust dosage
Quinupristin-Dalfopristin								Calcium channel blockers	↑ calcium channel blocker	Monitor, adjust dosage
								Carbamazepine	↑ carbamazepine	Monitor, adjust dosage
								Cyclosporine	↑ cyclosporine	Monitor, adjust dosage
								Diazepam	↑ diazepam	Monitor, adjust dosage
								Docetaxel	↑ docetaxel	Avoid co-administration
								Lidocaine	↑ lidocaine	Monitor, adjust dosage
								Methylprednisolone	↑ methylprednisolone	Monitor, adjust dosage
								Midazolam	↑ midazolam	Monitor, adjust dosage
								Paclitaxel	↑ paclitaxel	Avoid co-administration
								Statins metabolized by CYP3A4	↑ statin	Monitor, adjust dosage
								Tacrolimus	↑ tacrolimus	Monitor, adjust dosage
								Vincristine	↑ vincristine	Avoid co-administration
Ribavirin								Didanosine	↑ didanosine	Avoid co-administration
								Stavudine	↓ stavudine	Avoid co-administration
								Zidovudine	↓ zidovudine	Avoid co-administration

TABLE 22A (33)

Anti-Infective agent			Other Drug	Effect on concentration (or other effect)	Suggested management
Rifamycins					
Rifabutin	Rifampin	Rifapentine			
	x		Amiodarone	↓ amiodarone	Monitor, adjust dosage
x	x	x	Amitriptyline	↓ amitriptyline	Adjust dosage or avoid
	x		Antacids	↓ rifampin	Adjust dosage or avoid
x	x		Atovaquone	↑ rifamycin, ↓ atovaquone	Adjust dosage or avoid
x	x	x	Caspofungin	↓ caspofungin	Adjust dosage or avoid
	x		Chlorpropamide	↓ chlorpropamide	Adjust dosage or avoid
		x	Clarithromycin	↓ clarithromycin	Adjust dosage or avoid
x	x		Clarithromycin	↑ rifamycin, ↓ clarithromycin	Adjust dosage or avoid
		x	Cyclosporine	↓ cyclosporine	Adjust dosage or avoid
x	x		Cyclosporine	↑ rifamycin, ↓ cyclosporine	Adjust dosage or avoid
x	x	x	Dapsone	↓ dapsone	Adjust dosage or avoid
	x		Desipramine	↓ desipramine	Adjust dosage or avoid
		x	Dexamethasone	↓ dexamethasone	Adjust dosage or avoid
x	x		Dexamethasone	↓ rifamycin, ↓ dexamethasone	Adjust dosage or avoid
x	x	x	Diazepam	↓ diazepam	Adjust dosage or avoid
	x		Digoxin	↓ digoxin	Adjust dosage or avoid
		x	Diltiazem	↓ diltiazem	Adjust dosage or avoid
x	x		Diltiazem	↑ rifamycin, ↓ diltiazem	Adjust dosage or avoid
x	x	x	Disopyramide	↓ disopyramide	Adjust dosage or avoid
x			Ethinyl estradiol	↑ rifabutin, ↓ ethinyl estradiol	Avoid co-administration
	x	x	Ethinyl estradiol	↓ ethinyl estradiol	Avoid co-administration
x			Fluconazole	↑ rifabutin, ↓ fluconazole	Adjust dosage or avoid
	x	x	Fluconazole	↓ fluconazole	Adjust dosage or avoid
	x		Fluvastatin	↓ fluvastatin	Adjust dosage or avoid
	x		Fusidic acid	↑ rifampin, ↓ fusidic acid	Monitor or avoid
x	x	x	Haloperidol	↓ haloperidol	Adjust dosage or avoid
x	x	x	Imipramine	↓ imipramine	Adjust dosage or avoid
	x		Isavuconazole	↓ isavuconazole	Avoid co-administration
x	x	x	Itraconazole	↓ itraconazole, ↑ rifabutin	Avoid co-administration
	x		Linezolid	↓ linezolid	Adjust dosage or avoid
	x		Lorlatinib	↓ lorlatinib, hepatotoxicity	Contraindicated
x	x	x	Methadone	↓ methadone	Adjust dosage or avoid
	x		Metoprolol	↓ metoprolol	Adjust dosage or avoid
	x		Moxifloxacin	↓ moxifloxacin	Monitor, adjust dosage
x	x	x	Nifedipine	↓ nifedipine	Monitor, adjust dosage
x	x	x	Nortriptyline	↓ nortriptyline	Monitor, adjust dosage

TABLE 22A (34)

Anti-Infective agent			Other Drug	Effect on concentration (or other effect)	Suggested management
Rifamycins *(continued)*					
Rifabutin	Rifampin	Rifapentine			
	x	x	Phenytoin	↓ phenytoin	Monitor, adjust dosage
x			Phenytoin	↓ rifabutin	Monitor, adjust dosage
x			Posaconazole	↑ rifabutin	Adjust dosage or avoid
x	x	x	Prednisone	↓ prednisone	Monitor, adjust dosage
	x		Propranolol	↓ propranolol	Monitor, adjust dosage
x		x	Quinidine	↓ quinidine	Monitor, adjust dosage
	x		Quinidine	↑ rifampin, ↓ quinidine	Monitor, adjust dosage
	x		Raltegravir	↓ raltegravir	Use RAL 800 mg bid; RAL HD not recommended
x		x	Tacrolimus	↓ tacrolimus	Monitor, adjust dosage
	x		Tacrolimus	↑ rifampin, ↓ tacrolimus	Monitor, adjust dosage
	x		Telithromycin	↓ telithromycin	Adjust dosage or avoid
	x		Terbinafine	↓ terbinafine	Adjust dosage or avoid
x	x	x	Theophylline	↓ theophylline	Monitor, adjust dosage
	x		Tinidazole	↓ tinidazole	Adjust dosage or avoid
x	x	x	Triazolam	↓ triazolam	Monitor, adjust dosage
	x		Trimethoprim-Sulfamethoxazole	↑ rifampin? ↓ TMP-SMX (likely)	Adjust dosage or avoid
x	x		Voriconazole	↑ rifamycin, ↓ voriconazole	Avoid co-administration
x	x	x	Warfarin	↓ warfarin	Avoid co-administration
	x		Zidovudine	↓ zidovudine	Avoid co-administration
Sarecycline			Antacids (Al, Ca, Mg)	↓ sarecycline	Separate dosing
			Bismuth subsalicylate	↓ sarecycline	Separate dosing
			Digoxin	↑ digoxin	Monitor, adjust dosage
			Iron-containing preparations	↓ sarecycline	Separate dosing
			Penicillin	↓ penicillin bactericidal activity	Avoid co-administration
			Retinoids	↑ intracranial pressure	Avoid co-administration
			Warfarin	↑ INR	Monitor INR, adjust dosage
Tafenoquine			Dofetilide	↑ dofetilide	Monitor, adjust dosage
			Metformin	↑ metformin	Monitor, adjust dosage
Tecovirimat			Midazolam	↓ midazolam	Monitor, adjust dosage
			Repaglinide	↑ repaglinide	Monitor blood glucose

TABLE 22A (35)

Anti-Infective agent	Other Drug	Effect on concentration (or other effect)	Suggested management
Telithromycin	Carbamazepine	↓ telithromycin	Adjust dosage or avoid
	Digoxin	↑ digoxin	Monitor, adjust dosage
	Ergot alkaloids	↑ ergot alkaloids	Avoid co-administration
	Itraconazole, ketoconazole	↑ telithromycin	Adjust dosage or avoid
	Metoprolol	↑ metoprolol	Monitor, adjust dosage
	Midazolam	↑ midazolam	Monitor, adjust dosage
	Warfarin	↑ warfarin	Monitor INR, adjust dosage
	Phenobarbital, phenytoin	↓ telithromycin	Adjust dosage or avoid
	Pimozide	↑ pimozide	Adjust dosage or avoid
	Simvastatin	↑ simvastatin	Monitor, adjust dosage
	Sotalol	↓ sotalol	Monitor, adjust dosage
	Theophylline	↑ theophylline	Monitor, adjust dosage
Tenofovir alafenamide (TAF)	Carbamazepine	↓ TAF	↑ TAF to 50 mg qd (for HBV)
	Oxcarbazepine	↓ TAF	Avoid co-administration
	Phenobarbital	↓ TAF	Avoid co-administration
	Phenytoin	↓ TAF	Avoid co-administration
	Rifabutin	↓ TAF	Avoid co-administration
	Rifampin	↓ TAF	Avoid co-administration
	Rifapentine	↓ TAF	Avoid co-administration
	St. John's wort	↓ TAF	Avoid co-administration
Terbinafine	Cimetidine	↑ terbinafine	Adjust dosage or avoid
	Phenobarbital	↓ terbinafine	Adjust dosage or avoid
Tetracyclines	Atovaquone	↓ atovaquone	Adjust dosage or avoid
	Digoxin	↑ digoxin	Monitor, adjust dosage
	Methoxyflurane	↑ methoxyflurane	Monitor, adjust dosage
	Sucralfate	↓ tetracycline absorption	Separate by ≥2 hrs
Tigecycline	Digoxin	↓ digoxin	Monitor, adjust dosage
	Oral contraceptives	↓ oral contraceptives	Use alternative method
	Warfarin	↑ warfarin	Monitor INR, adjust dosage
Tinidazole	Alcohol	Disulfiram-like reaction	Monitor
	Azole antifungals	↑ tinidazole	Monitor, adjust dosage

TABLE 22A (36)

Anti-Infective agent	Other Drug	Effect on concentration (or other effect)	Suggested management
Trimethoprim	ACE inhibitors	↑ serum K+	Avoid co-administration
	Amantadine	↑ amantadine	Monitor, adjust dosage
	Dapsone	↑ trimethoprim, ↑ dapsone	Monitor, adjust dosage
	Lamivudine	↑ lamivudine	Monitor (no adjustment)
	Methotrexate	↑ methotrexate	Monitor, adjust dosage
	Phenytoin	↑ phenytoin	Monitor, adjust dosage
	Potassium-sparing diuretics	↑ serum K+	Monitor
	Procainamide	↑ procainamide, ↑ NAPA	Monitor, adjust dosage
	Repaglinide	↑ repaglinide	Monitor blood glucose
Trimethoprim-Sulfamethoxazole	6-mercaptopurine	↓ 6-mercaptopurine	Monitor, adjust dosage
	ACE inhibitors	↑ serum K+	Monitor
	Amantadine	↑ amantadine	Monitor, adjust dosage
	Cyclosporine	↓ cyclosporine	Monitor, adjust dosage
	Loperamide	↑ loperamide	Monitor, adjust dosage
	Methotrexate	↑ methotrexate	Monitor, adjust dosage
	Oral contraceptives	↓ oral contraceptives	Use alternative method
	Phenytoin	↑ phenytoin	Monitor, adjust dosage
	Pimozide	↓ pimozide	Monitor, adjust dosage
	Spironolactone	↑ serum K+	Monitor
	Sulfonylureas	↑ sulfonylureas	Monitor blood glucose
	Warfarin	↑ warfarin	Monitor INR, adjust dosage
Zidovudine (ZDV, AZT)	Atovaquone	↑ zidovudine	Monitor
	Doxorubicin	Antagonistic in vitro	Avoid co-administration
	Fluconazole	↑ zidovudine	Monitor
	Indomethacin	↑ zidovudine toxic metabolite	Monitor
	Methadone	↑ zidovudine	Monitor
	Nelfinavir	↓ zidovudine	Monitor
	Probenecid	↑ zidovudine	Monitor
	Ribavirin	↑ anemia	Avoid co-administration
	Rifampin	↓ zidovudine	Monitor
	TMP-SMX	↑ zidovudine	Monitor
	Valproic acid	↑ zidovudine	Monitor

TABLE 22B – DRUG-DRUG INTERACTIONS BETWEEN NON-NUCLEOSIDE REVERSE TRANSCRIPTASE INHIBITORS (NNRTIS) AND PROTEASE INHIBITORS

(Adapted from Guidelines for the Use of Antiretroviral Agents in HIV-Infected Adults & Adolescents; *see www.aidsinfo.nih.gov*)

NAME (Abbreviation, Trade Name)	Atazanavir (ATV, Reyataz)	Darunavir (DRV, Prezista)	Fosamprenavir (FOS-APV, Lexiva)	Indinavir (IDV, Crixivan)	Lopinavir/Ritonavir (LP/R, Kaletra)	Nelfinavir (NFV, Viracept)	Saquinavir (SQV, Invirase)	Tipranavir (TPV)
Efavirenz (EFZ, Sustiva)	ATV AUC ↓ 74%. Dose: EFZ standard; ATA/RTV 300/100 mg q24h with food	Standard doses of both drugs	FOS-APV levels ↓ . Dose: EFZ standard; FOS-APV 1400 mg + RTV 300 mg q24h or 700 mg FOS-APV + 100 mg RTV q12h	Levels: IDV ↓ 31%. Dose: IDV 1000 mg q8h. EFZ standard	Level of LP ↓ 40%. Dose: LP/R 533/133 mg q12h, EFZ standard	Standard doses	Level: SQV ↓ 62%. Dose: SQV 400 mg + RTV 400 mg q12h	No dose change necessary
Etravirine (ETR, Intelence)	↑ ATV & ↑ ETR levels.	Standard doses of both drugs	↑ levels of FOS-APV.	↓ level of IDV.	↑ levels of ETR, **↓ levels of LP/R.**	↑ levels of NFV.	↓ ETR levels 33%; SQV/R no change. Standard dose of both drugs.	↓ levels of ETR, ↑ levels of TPV & RTV. **Avoid combination.**
Nevirapine (NVP, Viramune)	Avoid combination. ATZ increases NVP concentrations >25%; NVP decreases ATZ AUC by 42%	Standard doses of both drugs	Use with caution. NVP AUC increased 14% (700/100 Fos/rit; NVP AUC inc 29% (Fos 1400 mg bid).	IDV levels ↓ 28%. Dose: IDV 1000 mg q8h or combine with RTV; NVP standard	LP levels ↓ 53%. Dose: LP/R 533/133 mg q12h; NVP standard	Standard doses	Dose: SQV + RTV 400/400 mg, both q12h	**Standard doses**

TABLE 23 – LIST OF GENERIC AND TRADE NAMES

GENERIC NAME: TRADE NAMES

Abacavir: Ziagen
Abacavir + Lamivudine: Epzicom
Abacavir + Lamivudine + Dolutegravir: Triumeq
Abacavir + Lamivudine + Zidovudine: Trizivir
Acyclovir: Zovirax
Adefovir: Hepsera
Albendazole: Albenza
Amantadine: Symmetrel
Amikacin: Amikin
Amikacin liposomal: Arikayce
Amoxicillin: Amoxil, Polymox
Amoxicillin extended release: Moxatag
Amox./clav.: Augmentin, Augmentin ES-600; Augmentin XR
Amphotericin B: Fungizone
Ampho B-liposomal: AmBisome
Ampho B-lipid complex: Abelcet
Ampicillin: Omnipen, Polycillin
Ampicillin + Sulbactam: Unasyn
Artemether + Lumefantrine: Coartem
Atazanavir: Reyataz
Atovaquone: Mepron
Atovaquone + Proguanil: Malarone
Azithromycin: Zithromax
Azithromycin ER: Zmax
Aztreonam: Azactam, Cayston
Baloxavir marboxil: Xofluza
Bedaquiline: Sirturo
Benznidazole: Exeltis, Abarax
Bezlotoxumab: Zinplava
Bictegravir + FTC + TAF: Biktarvy
Caspofungin: Cancidas
Cefaclor: Ceclor, Ceclor CD
Cefadroxil: Duricef
Cefazolin: Ancef, Kefzol
Cefdinir: Omnicef
Cefditoren pivoxil: Spectracef
Cefepime: Maxipime
Cefiderocol: Fetroja
Cefixime[NUS]: Suprax
Cefoperazone + Sulbactam: Sulperazon[NUS]
Cefotaxime: Claforan
Cefotetan: Cefotan
Cefoxitin: Mefoxin
Cefpodoxime proxetil: Vantin
Cefprozil: Cefzil
Ceftaroline: Teflaro
Ceftazidime: Fortaz, Tazicef, Tazidime
Ceftazidime + Avibactam: Avycaz
Ceftibuten: Cedax
Ceftizoxime: Cefizox
Ceftobiprole: Zeftera
Ceftolozane + Tazobactam: Zerbaxa
Ceftriaxone: Rocephin
Cefuroxime: Zinacef, Ceftin
Cephalexin: Keflex
Cephradine: Anspor, Velosef
Chloroquine: Aralen
Cidofovir: Vistide
Ciprofloxacin: Cipro, Cipro XR
Clarithromycin: Biaxin, Biaxin XL
Clindamycin: Cleocin
Clofazimine: Lamprene
Clotrimazole: Lotrimin, Mycelex
Cloxacillin: Tegopen
Colistimethate: Coly-Mycin M
Cycloserine: Seromycin
Daclatasvir: Daklinza
Daptomycin: Cubicin
Dalbavancin: Dalvance
Darunavir: Prezista
Darunavir + Cobi + FTC + TAF: Symtuza
Delafloxacin: Baxdela
Dicloxacillin: Dynapen
Didanosine: Videx
Diethylcarbamazine: Hetrazan
Diloxanide furoate: Furamide
Dolutegravir: Tivicay
Dolutegravir + Emtricitabine: Dovato
Dolutegravir + Rilpivirine: Juluca
Doravirine + 3TC + TDF: Delstrigo
Doripenem: Doribax
Doxycycline: Vibramycin
Efavirenz: Sustiva
Efavirenz + Emtricitabine + Tenofovir: Atripla
Elbasvir + Grazoprevir: Zepatier
Elvitegravir + Cobicistat + Emtricitabine + Tenofovir: Stribild
Elvitegravir + Cobicistat + Emtricitabine + Tenofovir AF: Genvoya
Emtricitabine: Emtriva
Emtricitabine + Tenofovir: Truvada
Emtricitabine + Tenofovir + Rilpivirine: Complera
Enfuvirtide (T-20): Fuzeon
Entecavir: Baraclude
Eravacycline: Xerava
Ertapenem: Invanz
Erythromycin(s): Ilotycin
Ethyl succinate: Pediamycin
Glucoheptonate: Erythrocin
Estolate: Ilosone
Erythro + Sulfisoxazole: Pediazole
Ethambutol: Myambutol
Ethionamide: Trecator
Etravirine: Intelence
Famciclovir: Famvir
Fidaxomicin: Dificid
Fluconazole: Diflucan
Flucytosine: Ancobon
Fosamprenavir: Lexiva
Foscarnet: Foscavir
Fosfomycin: Monurol
Fusidic acid: Taksta
Ganciclovir: Cytovene
Gatifloxacin: Tequin
Gemifloxacin: Factive
Gentamicin: Garamycin
Grazoprevir + Elbasvir: Zepatier
Griseofulvin: Fulvicin
Halofantrine: Halfan
Ibalizumab-uiyk: Trogarzo
Idoxuridine: Dendrid, Stoxil
Imipenem + Cilastatin: Primaxin, Tienam
Imiquimod: Aldara
Imipenem + cilastatin + relebactam: Recarbrio
INH + RIF: Rifamate
INH + RIF + PZA: Rifater
Interferon alfa: Intron A
Interferon, pegylated: PEG-Intron, Pegasys
Interferon + Ribavirin: Rebetron
Indinavir: Crixivan
Isavuconazonium sulfate: Cresemba
Itraconazole: Sporanox
Iodoquinol: Yodoxin
Ivermectin: Stromectol, Sklice
Ketoconazole: Nizoral
Lamivudine: Epivir, Epivir-HBV
Lamivudine + Abacavir: Epzicom
Ledipasvir + Sofosbuvir: Harvoni
Lefamulin: Xenleta
Letermovir: Prevymis
Levofloxacin: Levaquin
Linezolid: Zyvox
Lopinavir + Ritonavir: Kaletra
Loracarbef: Lorabid
Mafenide: Sulfamylon
Maraviroc: Selzentry
Mebendazole: Vermox
Mefloquine: Lariam
Meropenem: Merrem
Meropenem + vaborbactam: Vabomere
Mesalamine: Asacol, Pentasa
Methenamine: Hiprex, Mandelamine
Metronidazole: Flagyl
Micafungin: Mycamine
Minocycline: Minocin
Moxifloxacin: Avelox
Mupirocin: Bactroban
Nafcillin: Unipen
Nelfinavir: Viracept
Nevirapine: Viramune
Nitazoxanide: Alinia
Nitrofurantoin: Macrobid, Macrodantin
Nystatin: Mycostatin
Ofloxacin: Floxin
Olysio: Simeprevir
Omadacycline: Nuzyra
Oritavancin: Orbactiv
Oseltamivir: Tamiflu
Oxacillin: Prostaphlin
Palivizumab: Synagis
Paritaprevir + Ritonavir + Ombitasvir: Technivie
Paritaprevir + Ritonavir + Ombitasvir + Dasabuvir: Viekira Pak
Paromomycin: Humatin
Pentamidine: NebuPent, Pentam 300
Peramivir: Rapivab
Piperacillin + Tazobactam: Zosyn, Tazocin
Piperazine: Antepar
Plazomicin: Zemdri
Podophyllotoxin: Condylox
Polymyxin B: Poly-Rx
Posaconazole: Noxafil
Praziquantel: Biltricide
Primaquine: Primachine
Proguanil: Paludrine
Prulifloxacin: Sword
Pyrantel pamoate: Antiminth
Pyrimethamine: Daraprim
Pyrimethamine + Sulfadoxine: Fansidar
Quinupristin + Dalfopristin: Synercid
Raltegravir: Isentress
Retapamulin: Altabax
Ribavirin: Virazole, Rebetol
Rifabutin: Mycobutin
Rifampin: Rifadin, Rimactane
Rifamycin: Aemcolo
Rifapentine: Priftin
Rifaximin: Xifaxan
Rilpivirine: Edurant
Rimantadine: Flumadine
Ritonavir: Norvir
Saquinavir: Invirase
Sarecycline: Seysara
Secnidazole: Solosec
Spectinomycin: Trobicin
Stavudine: Zerit
Stibogluconate: Pentostam
Silver sulfadiazine: Silvadene
Simeprevir: Olysio
Sofosbuvir: Sovaldi
Sulfamethoxazole: Gantanol
Sulfasalazine: Azulfidine
Sulfisoxazole: Gantrisin
Tafenoquine: Krintafel, Arakoda
Tecovirimat: Tpoxx
Tedizolid: Sivextro
Telaprevir: Incivek
Telavancin: Vibativ
Telbivudine: Tyzeka
Telithromycin: Ketek
Temocillin: Negaban, Temopen
Tenofovir AF-FTC: Descovy
Tenofovir alafenamide: Vemlidy
Tenofovir DF: Viread
Terbinafine: Lamisil
Thalidomide: Thalomid
Thiabendazole: Mintezol
Tigecycline: Tygacil
Tinidazole: Tindamax
Tipranavir: Aptivus
Tobramycin: Nebcin
Tretinoin: Retin A
Trifluridine: Viroptic
Trimethoprim: Primsol
Trimethoprim + Sulfamethoxazole: Bactrim, Septra
Valacyclovir: Valtrex
Valganciclovir: Valcyte
Vancomycin: Vancocin
Velpatasvir + Sofosbuvir: Epclusa
Voriconazole: Vfend
Zanamivir: Relenza
Zidovudine (ZDV): Retrovir
Zidovudine + 3TC: Combivir
Zidovudine + 3TC + Abacavir: Trizivir

TABLE 23 (2)
LIST OF TRADE AND GENERIC NAMES

TRADE NAMES: GENERIC NAME

Abelcet: Ampho B-lipid complex
Albenza: Albendazole
Aldara: Imiquimod
Alinia: Nitazoxanide
Altabax: Retapamulin
AmBisome: Ampho B-liposomal
Amikin: Amikacin
Amoxil: Amoxicillin
Ancef: Cefazolin
Ancobon: Flucytosine
Anspor: Cephradine
Antepar: Piperazine
Antiminth: Pyrantel pamoate
Aptivus: Tipranavir
Aralen: Chloroquine
Arakoda: Tafenoquine
Arikayce: Amikacin liposomal
Asacol: Mesalamine
Atripla: Efavirenz + Emtricitabine + Tenofovir
Augmentin, Augmentin ES-600 Augmentin XR: Amox./clav.
Avelox: Moxifloxacin
Avycaz: Ceftazidime + AvibactamAzactam: Aztreonam
Azulfidine: Sulfasalazine
Bactroban: Mupirocin
Bactrim: Trimethoprim + SMX
Baraclude: Entecavir
Baxdela: Delafloxacin
Biaxin, Biaxin XL: Clarithromycin
Biktarvy: Bictegravir + FTC + TAF
Biltricide: Praziquantel
Cancidas: Caspofungin
Cayston: Aztreonam (inhaled)
Ceclor, Ceclor CD: Cefaclor
Cedax: Ceftibuten
Cefizox: Ceftizoxime
Cefotan: Cefotetan
Ceftin: Cefuroxime axetil
Cefzil: Cefprozil
Cipro, Cipro XR: Ciprofloxacin & extended release
Claforan: Cefotaxime
Coartem: Artemether + Lumefantrine
Coly-Mycin M: Colistimethate
Combivir: Zidovudine + 3TC
Complera: Emtricitabine + Tenofovir + Rilpivirine
Cresemba: Isavuconazonium sulfate
Crixivan: Indinavir
Cubicin: Daptomycin
Cytovene: Ganciclovir
Daklinza: Daclatasvir
Dalvance: Dalbavancin
Daraprim: Pyrimethamine
Descovy: Tenofovir AF-FTC
Delstrigo: Doravirine + 3TC + TDF
Dificid: Fidaxomicin
Diflucan: Fluconazole
Doribax: Doripenem
Dovato: Dolutegravir + Emtricitabine
Duricef: Cefadroxil
Dynapen: Dicloxacillin
Edurant: Rilpivirine
Emtriva: Emtricitabine
Epclusa: Velpatasvir + Sofosbuvir
Epivir, Epivir-HBV: Lamivudine
Epzicom: Lamivudine + Abacavir
Exeltis: Benznidazole
Factive: Gemifloxacin
Famvir: Famciclovir
Fansidar: Pyrimethamine + Sulfadoxine
Fetroja: Cefiderocol
Flagyl: Metronidazole
Floxin: Ofloxacin
Flumadine: Rimantadine
Foscavir: Foscarnet
Fortaz: Ceftazidime
Fulvicin: Griseofulvin
Fungizone: Amphotericin B
Furadantin: Nitrofurantoin
Fuzeon: Enfuvirtide (T-20)
Gantanol: Sulfamethoxazole
Gantrisin: Sulfisoxazole
Garamycin: Gentamicin
Genvoya: Elvitegravir + Cobicistat + Emtricitabine + Tenofovir AF
Halfan: Halofantrine
Harvoni: Ledipasvir + Sofosbuvir
Hepsera: Adefovir
Herplex: Idoxuridine
Hiprex: Methenamine hippurate
Humatin: Paromomycin
Ilosone: Erythromycin estolate
Ilotycin: Erythromycin
Incivek: Telaprevir
Intelence: Etravirine
Intron A: Interferon alfa
Invanz: Ertapenem
Invirase: Saquinavir
Isentress: Raltegravir
Juluca: Dolutegravir + Rilpivirine
Kantrex: Kanamycin
Kaletra: Lopinavir + Ritonavir
Keflex: Cephalexin
Ketek: Telithromycin
Krintafel: Tafenoquine
Lamisil: Terbinafine
Lamprene: Clofazimine
Lariam: Mefloquine
Levaquin: Levofloxacin
Lexiva: Fosamprenavir
Lorabid: Loracarbef
Macrodantin, Macrobid: Nitrofurantoin
Malarone: Atovaquone + Proguanil
Mandelamine: Methenamine mandelate
Maxipime: Cefepime
Mefoxin: Cefoxitin
Mepron: Atovaquone
Merrem: Meropenem
Minocin: Minocycline
Mintezol: Thiabendazole
Monurol: Fosfomycin
Moxatag: Amoxicillin extended release
Myambutol: Ethambutol
Mycamine: Micafungin
Mycobutin: Rifabutin
Mycostatin: Nystatin
Nafcil: Nafcillin
Nebcin: Tobramycin
NebuPent: Pentamidine
Nizoral: Ketoconazole
Norvir: Ritonavir
Noxafil: Posaconazole
Nuzyra: Omadacycline
Olysio: Simeprevir
Omnicef: Cefdinir
Omnipen: Ampicillin
Orbactiv: Oritavancin
Pediamycin: Erythro. ethyl succinate
Pediazole: Erythro. ethyl succinate + sulfisoxazole
Pegasys, PEG-Intron: Interferon, pegylated
Pentam 300: Pentamidine
Pentasa: Mesalamine
Polycillin: Ampicillin
Polymox: Amoxicillin
Poly-Rx: Polymyxin B
Prevymis: Letermovir
Prezista: Darunavir
Priftin: Rifapentine
Primaxin: Imipenem + Cilastatin
Primsol: Trimethoprim
Prostaphlin: Oxacillin
Rapivab: Peramivir
Rebetol: Ribavirin
Rebetron: Interferon + Ribavirin
Recarbrio: Imipenem + cilastatin + relebactam
Relenza: Zanamivir
Retin A: Tretinoin
Retrovir: Zidovudine (ZDV)
Reyataz: Atazanavir
Rifadin: Rifampin
Rifamate: INH + RIF
Rifater: INH + RIF + PZA
Rimactane: Rifampin
Rocephin: Ceftriaxone
Selzentry: Maraviroc
Septra: Trimethoprim + Sulfamethoxazole
Seromycin: Cycloserine
Silvadene: Silver sulfadiazine
Sirturo: Bedaquiline
Sivextro: Tedizolid
Sklice: Ivermectin lotion
Solosec: Secnidazole
Sovaldi: Sofosbuvir
Spectracef: Cefditoren pivoxil
Sporanox: Itraconazole
Stoxil: Idoxuridine
Stribild: Elvitegravir + Cobicistat + Emtricitabine + Tenofovir
Stromectol: Ivermectin
Sulfamylon: Mafenide
Sulperazon[NUS]: Cefoperazone + Sulbactam
Suprax: Cefixime[NUS]
Sustiva: Efavirenz
Symmetrel: Amantadine
Symtuza: Darunavir + Cobi + TAF
Synagis: Palivizumab
Synercid: Quinupristin + Dalfopristin
Taksta: Fusidic acid
Talicia: Amoxicillin + Rifampin + Omeprazole
Tamiflu: Oseltamivir
Tazicef: Ceftazidime
Technivie: Paritaprevir + Ritonavir + Ombitasvir
Teflaro: Ceftaroline
Tegopen: Cloxacillin
Tequin: Gatifloxacin
Thalomid: Thalidomide
Tienam: Imipenem
Tinactin: Tolnaftate
Tindamax: Tinidazole
Tivicay: Dolutegravir
Tpoxx: Tecovirimat
Trogarzo: Ibalizumab-uiyk
Trecator SC: Ethionamide
Triumeq: Abacavir + Lamivudine + Dolutegravir
Trizivir: Zidovudine + 3TC + Abacavir
Trobicin: Spectinomycin
Truvada: Emtricitabine + Tenofovir
Tygacil: Tigecycline
Tyzeka: Telbivudine
Unasyn: Ampicillin/sulbactam
Unipen: Nafcillin
Vabomere: Meropenem + vaborbactam
Valcyte: Valganciclovir
Valtrex: Valacyclovir
Vancocin: Vancomycin
Vantin: Cefpodoxime proxetil
Velosef: Cephradine
Vemlidy: Tenofovir alafenamide
Vermox: Mebendazole
Vfend: Voriconazole
Vibativ: Telavancin
Vibramycin: Doxycycline
Videx: Didanosine
Viekira Pak: Paritaprevir + Ritonavir + Ombitasvir + Dasabuvir
Viracept: Nelfinavir
Viramune: Nevirapine
Virazole: Ribavirin
Viread: Tenofovir
Vistide: Cidofovir
Xenleta: Lefamulin
Xerava: Eravacycline
Xifaxan: Rifaximin
Xofluza: Baloxavir marboxil
Yodoxin: Iodoquinol
Zemdri: Plazomicin
Zerit: Stavudine
Zeftera: Ceftobiprole
Zepatier: Elbasvir + Grazoprevir
Zerbaxa: Ceftolozane + Tazobactam
Ziagen: Abacavir
Zinacef: Cefuroxime
Zinplava: Bezlotoxumab
Zithromax: Azithromycin
Zmax: Azithromycin ER
Zovirax: Acyclovir
Zosyn: Piperacillin + Tazobactam
Zyvox: Linezolid

INDEX

A

B